Lecture Notes of the In for Computer Sciences, and Telecommunications Engineering

MW01230423

431

More information about this series at https://link.springer.com/bookseries/8197

Hadas Lewy · Refael Barkan (Eds.)

Pervasive Computing Technologies for Healthcare

15th EAI International Conference, Pervasive Health 2021
Virtual Event, December 6–8, 2021
Proceedings

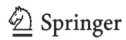 Springer

Editors
Hadas Lewy
Holon Institute of Technology
Holon, Israel

Refael Barkan
Holon Institute of Technology
Holon, Israel

ISSN 1867-8211 ISSN 1867-822X (electronic)
Lecture Notes of the Institute for Computer Sciences, Social Informatics
and Telecommunications Engineering
ISBN 978-3-030-99193-7 ISBN 978-3-030-99194-4 (eBook)
https://doi.org/10.1007/978-3-030-99194-4

This Springer imprint is published by the registered company Springer Nature Switzerland AG
The registered company address is: Gewerbestrasse 11, 6330 Cham, Switzerland

Preface

We are proud to introduce the proceedings of the 15th European Alliance for Innovation (EAI) International Conference on Pervasive Computing Technologies for Healthcare (Pervasive Health 2021).

This year was challenging in all dimensions of pervasive health due to the COVID-19 pandemic. Traditional ways of monitoring, diagnosing, treating, and communicating as well as relationships between healthcare providers and patients changed dramatically, at once, and challenged the healthcare sector, industry, and decision makers. The challenges were clinical, technological, legal, and social. However, the pandemic brought some opportunities and the new technologies that were developed and adapted for care as well as new care models are here to stay. Looking ahead we need to understand which care models and technologies should be implemented in future care and how can we implement the technologies and combine them with the "human factor" to yield the best results for future healthcare.

The Pervasive Health 2021 conference focused on "lessons learned from the first year of the COVID-19 pandemic" - new technologies and care models that were designed and developed to face the challenges. The conference also concentrated on ways healthcare systems should be re-designed in collaboration with the industry, academia, and decision makers to promote better care and at the same time to educate the next generation of healthcare professionals (especially physicians) to integrate new technologies into their clinical and administrative work in light of the new challenges they are facing. Therefore, we designed the conference program to consist of three main tracks: Hospital and Community Care, Homecare, and (Medical) Education. Each track included a keynote lecture, original research papers, and panel discussions with researchers, industry, and healthcare opinion leaders.

The program of Pervasive Health 2021 consisted of 37 peer-reviewed papers, which are presented in these proceedings, and 10 abstract-based presentations approved by the conference review committees. In addition, the conference program included 14 invited speakers and four panel discussions, with opinion leaders from academia, the healthcare sector, and the industry, focusing on Industry and Homecare Technologies, Privacy and Security in Homecare Technologies, Homecare and Technologies for the Elderly, and Education of the Next Generation of Healthcare Professionals in the Digital Era.

Aside from the high-quality paper presentations, the program included three invited keynote speakers: Eyal Zimlichman, Deputy Director, Chief Medical Officer, and Chief Innovation Officer at Sheba Medical Center (as well as the founder and director of Sheba's ARC Innovation Center), addressed Hospital and Community Care Challenges and the Role of Innovation in Future Healthcare. Abraham Seidmann from the Institute for Health System Innovation and Policy at Boston University, USA, discussed trends in Homecare and Future Healthcare, and Shmuel Reis, head of the Center for Medical Education at the Faculty of Medicine, Hebrew University, Israel (as well as a professor at the Department of Digital Medical Technologies, HIT, Israel) discussed the Education of the Next Generation of Healthcare Professionals, covering the use of technologies and re-design of healthcare services.

As part of the lessons learned regarding the need for healthcare systems to be re-designed, a workshop aimed at addressing the methodologies, approaches, and design of research and development for ageing population needs was led by Benjamin Salem from the School of Engineering at the University of Liverpool, UK.

We would like to thank all the researchers, practitioners, and technology developers from around the world—Israel, the USA, Canada, Bangladesh, the Philippines, Singapore, China, Nigeria, Brazil, and nine European countries—for the quality of research presented and for the stimulating discussions, as indicated by the contributions presented in this volume.

We thank also our partners—the European Alliance for Innovation (EAI)—for their collaboration and contribution to the success of this conference.

We strongly believe that the Pervasive Health 2021 conference provided an excellent forum for all interested parties to discuss all aspects (scientific, technological, and clinical) relevant to future healthcare design and the successful creation of a comprehensive ecosystem, involving healthcare organizations, academia, and the industry, shaping the future of healthcare.

Hadas Lewy
Refael Barkan
Gabriella Casalino
Yair Lempel
Boaz Tadmor
Tomas Karpati
Mordechay Shani

Organization

Steering Committee

Imrich Chlamtac	University of Trento, Italy
Mary Czerwinski	Microsoft Research, USA

Organizing Committee

General Chair

Hadas Lewy	Holon Institute of Technology, Israel

General Co-chair

Refael Barkan	HIT- Holon Institute of Technology, Israel

Technical Program Committee Chairs

Gabriella Casalino	Università degli Studi di Bari Aldo Moro, Italy
Hadas Lewy	HIT- Holon Institute of Technology, Israel
Refael Barkan	HIT- Holon Institute of Technology, Israel
Yair Lempel	HIT- Holon Institute of Technology, Israel
Boaz Tadmor	HIT- Holon Institute of Technology, Israel
Tomas Karpati	HIT- Holon Institute of Technology, Israel
Mordechay Shani	HIT- Holon Institute of Technology, Israel

Local Chair

Tony Levy	HIT- Holon Institute of Technology, Israel

Workshops Chairs

Hadas Lewy	HIT- Holon Institute of Technology, Israel
Refael Barkan	HIT- Holon Institute of Technology, Israel
Benjamin Salem	University of Liverpool, UK
Charlotte Magnusson	Lund University, Sweden
Vivian Motti	George Mason University, USA

Publications Chairs

Yair Lempel	HIT- Holon Institute of Technology, Israel
Nissim Harel	HIT- Holon Institute of Technology, Israel

Web Chair

Yair Lempel	HIT- Holon Institute of Technology, Israel

Panels Chair

Boaz Tadmor	HIT- Holon Institute of Technology, Israel

Technical Program Committee

Advait Balaji	Rice University, USA
Alar Kuusik	Tallinn University, Estonia
Alessio Vecchio	University of Pisa, Italy
Alvaro Uribe Quevedo	Ontario Tech University, Canada
Andreas Schrader	University of Lübeck, Germany
Andreas Triantafyllidis Aristotle	University of Thessaloniki, Greece
Angelica Ortiz de Gortari	University of Liège, Belgium
Ankur Bist	KIET Ghaziabad, India
Charlotte Tang	University of Michigan-Flint, USA
Dadmehr Rahbari	University of Qom, Iran
Daniel T. H. Lai	Victoria University, Australia
Daniel Tetteroo	Eindhoven University of Technology, The Netherlands
Faisal Hussain Al-Khawarizmi	University of Engineering and Technology, Lahore, Pakistan
Filipe Moutinho	UNINOVA-CTS, Portugal
Filipe Portela	University of Minho, Portugal
Francesco Ferrise	Politecnico di Milano, Italy
Geng Yang	Zhejiang University, China
Gennaro Vessio	University of Bari Aldo Moro, Italy
Helena Tendedez	Cera Care, UK
Jagmohan Chauhan	University of Southampton, UK
Jessica Pater	Parkview Research Center, USA
José Manuel Molina	UC3M, Spain
Manuel Santos	Universidade do Minho, Portugal
Marcin Grzegorzek	Universität zu Lübeck, Germany
Mounim A. El Yacoubi	Telecom SudParis, France
Nadja de Carolis	University of Bari Aldo Moro, Italy
Oluwafemi Sarumi	Federal University of Technology, Akure, Nigeria

Paolo Napoletano	University of Milano-Bicocca, Italy
Rogério Costa	Polytechnic Institute of Leiria, Portugal
Rosa Arriaga	Georgia Institute of Technology, USA
Rui Madeira	Nova University of Lisbon, Portugal
Salvatore Tedesco	University College Cork, Ireland
Stephen Schueller	University of California, Irvine, USA
Silvia Imbesi	University of Ferrara, Italy
Tomas Karpati	Holon Institute of Technology, Israel
Thomas Lux	Hochschule Niederrhein, Germany
Ugochukwu O. Matthew	Hussaini Adamu Federal Polytechnic, Nigeria
Vítor Carvalho	Polytechnic Institute of Cávado e Ave, Portugal

Contents

Technologies and Health Behavior

Design Contributions to Pervasive Health and Care Services

AI for COVID-19 Treatment
in Hospitals and Community Care

Clinical Decision Making and Outcome Prediction for COVID-19 Patients Using Machine Learning

Adamopoulou Maria[1,3]($\boxtimes$), Velissaris Dimitrios[2,3], Michou Ioanna[1,3], Matzaroglou Charalampos[1], Messaris Gerasimos[1,3], and Koutsojannis Constantinos[1]

[1] Department of Health Physics and Computational Intelligence, School of Health Rehabilitation Sciences, University of Patras, 251 00 Aigion, Greece
madamo@upatras.gr
[2] Department of Pathology, University of Patras, 265 04 Patras, Greece
[3] University Hospital of Patras, 265 04 Patras, Greece

Abstract. In this paper, we present the application of a Machine Learning (ML) approach that generates predictions to support healthcare professionals to identify the outcome of patients through optimization of treatment strategies. Based on Decision Tree algorithms, our approach has been trained and tested by analyzing the severity and the outcomes of 346 COVID-19 patients, treated through the first two pandemics "waves" in a tertiary center in Western Greece. Its' performance was achieved, analyzing entry features, as demographic characteristics, comorbidity details, imaging analysis, blood values, and essential hospitalization details, like patient transfers to Intensive Care Unit (ICU), medications, and manifestation responses at each treatment stage. Furthermore, it has provided a total high prediction performance (97%) and translated the ML analysis to clinical managing decisions and suggestions for healthcare institution performance and other epidemiological or postmortem approaches. Consequently, healthcare decisions could be more accurately figured and predicted, towards better management of the fast-growing patient subpopulations, giving more time for the effective pharmaceutical or vaccine armamentarium that the medical, scientific community will produce.

Keywords: COVID-19 · Clinical decision making · Machine learning · Patient management

1 Introduction

Several Artificial Intelligence (A.I.) applications on databases of Health Records (H.R.s) in hospitals have already been successfully established [1, 2]. COVID-19 pandemic has revealed A.I. approximations as first-line approaches for early infection detection and appropriate treatment [3–9]. Predictive analytics utilizes approaches to analyze medical information from H.R.s to predict future patient outcomes reducing costs [2, 3, 10, 11].

© ICST Institute for Computer Sciences, Social Informatics and Telecommunications Engineering 2022
Published by Springer Nature Switzerland AG 2022. All Rights Reserved
H. Lewy and R. Barkan (Eds.): PH 2021, LNICST 431, pp. 3–14, 2022.
https://doi.org/10.1007/978-3-030-99194-4_1

When each patient in the critical clinical condition is recognized adequately during hospital admission, they can immediately receive the appropriate treatment without [1, 3, 8, 12]. Early identification with higher accuracy than statistical approaches could further guide clinicians toward immediate intervention [13, 14]. According to several approaches, researchers managed to handle public health surveillance using AI and Big Data which appear to have enormous potential for the management of COVID-19 and other emergencies, and their role is anticipated to increase in the future. These approaches can now be used to track the spread of the virus in real-time, and plan and lift public health interventions accordingly, monitor their effectiveness, repurpose old compounds and discover new drugs, as well as identify potential vaccine candidates and enhance the response of communities and territories to the ongoing pandemic [9, 15, 16]. Based on Decision Tree algorithms, that more clear and easy to be used by the clinicians, our approach has been trained and tested by analyzing the severity and the outcomes of COVID-19 patients, treated through the first two pandemics "waves" in a tertiary center in Western Greece. Data were obtained using a software tool that was running parallel with Hospital Information System. Its' performance was achieved, analyzing entry features, as demographic characteristics, comorbidity details, imaging analysis, blood values, and essential hospitalization details, like patient transfers to Intensive Care Unit (ICU), medications, and manifestation responses at each treatment stage, of the COVID-19 patients finally collected.

Currently, A.I. systems, evaluating images to track the progression of COVID-19 patients, are already helping to identify urgent needs for ICU support [17]. Other approaches estimate individual patient's mortality probability by the use of an ML application on data of three biomarkers, showing more than 90% accuracy [18]. Another application was used to analyze images and then evaluate the infection with high accuracy performance classification [19]. Another ML-based model applying the Decision Tree (D.T.) algorithm used to recognize COVID-19 patients with severe illnesses after hospital admission providing 80% accuracy [20]. According to the patient clinical description at hospital admission, a Deep Learning (DL) approach, which can recognize COVID-19 patients at risk, tested providing accuracy at the level of 90%, respectively [21]. Additionally, according to an interesting approach, a human-machine collaborative design strategy is leveraged to create a human-driven principled network design for the detection of COVID-19 cases only from X-ray images [22]. According to another successful DL approach, recognizing areas with pathological artifacts on Ultrasound images was developed to identify the COVID-19 infection [23]. Other approaches have been discovered to analyze medical images, acquiring a prediction of 95.4% [24]. According to most published approaches, prediction models utilizing A.I. would improve with successive data for diagnosis to treatment, aiming to supplement decision-making by clinicians [8, 9, 13]. Specific patient populations can vary across countries, different institutions, and the ability of a predictive model to "learn" from its local patients provides more benefits than static modeling [3, 12]. Additionally, "best practices" could also be summarized, generalized, and introduced into published guidelines on use. In clinical decision-making, A.I. algorithms already successfully support medical staff, including entrance urgency classification decisions for the optimal use of institutional resources and analyzing the severity of the infection and patient progress [9].

An ML approach could be summarized in 4 general steps including, 1) data validation through preprocessing, 2) mining through output forecasting, 3) pattern/knowledge extraction through post-processing, and 4) final statistical evaluation and clinical Interpretation, usually in collaboration, with healthcare staff. This procedure is fulfilled for unsupervised or supervised learning approaches, dealing only with random data training and test sets targeting the highest possible accuracy levels (Fig. 1). After data analysis and interaction with medical experts, successful generalizations could be compared to published guidelines that usually do not consider workforce and appropriate resources for organizational modifications. ML approaches are well recognized for constructing risk models, selecting the predictors automatically from numerous features, minimizing random or systematic errors, and resulting generalizations [9, 11, 18, 19].

In the present paper, we describe an A.I. system incorporating ML in medical history and data that correlates, investigates, clarifies, evaluates, and saves clinical decisions, to D.T. structures [9]. Our approach first aims to reveal features for fast Triage-Classification based on minimum possible available tests, shortening life-threatening waiting times at emergency departments or Emergency Departments, which will be later enriched with other findings, as physical examination and laboratory results also be evaluated [24].

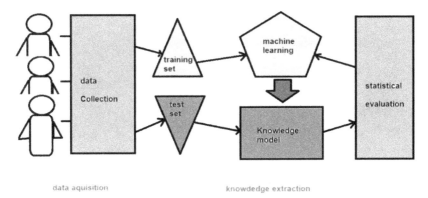

Fig. 1. Knowledge discovery from data collectors to new guidelines for new patients specifically during new or not well defined diseases

After severity estimation, secondly aims to achieve a patient-specific diagnosis, possible transfer to ICU, and evidence-based treatment planning, the use of the history and clinical examination information is expected to reach the acceptable accuracy in terms of risk assessment for the severity classification and subsequent first line life support to be followed with proper hospitalization. Based on laboratory tests, the possibility of achieving the diagnosis and appropriate treatment or other decisions as for secondary transfer to ICU according to patient response, the systems provide a probability for outcome prediction. The system finally aims, by improving class correlation of the parameters and mining process in ongoing clinical and laboratory data, the successful patient management according to available resources. The treatment response of each patient and relevant data consists of a new set of parameters at each specific step of the hospitalization period and characterize the current pathology of the patient accompanied with

predictions. The clinicians just enter the patient's medical information in terms of electronic forms as well as examination and treatment data at each stage. It is designed to
be globalized, through natural text analysis, along with the data mining process, as it
will be implemented with Natural Language Processing applications (Fig. 2). In the next
sections, the pilot's successful implementations are presented.

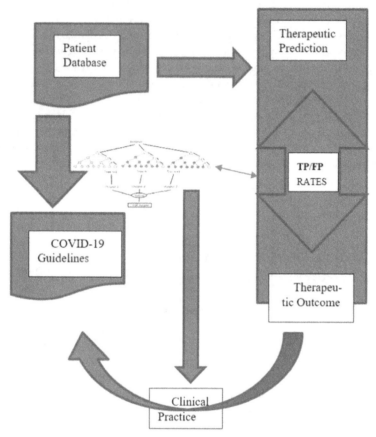

Fig. 2. Global system description and working flow for machine learning using decision trees
classifiers for COVID-19 patients' management

2   Materials and Methods

Existing data mining tools provide the implementation of different mining algorithms.
Most of them are free, open-source, easy to use software platforms. For our pilot implementation was used WEKA has been written in Java and is running on almost any operating system. WEKA collects A.I. algorithms and data preprocessing tools for ML and
supports evaluating, visualizing, and preparing the input data [25–27]. It also supports

different learning algorithms such as classification, clustering, and regression. D.T.s are classification algorithms functioning to predict an output based on decisions extracted from the input data mapped in tree structures [9, 22–25]. System's performance was achieved, analyzing several entry features, as demographic characteristics, comorbidity details, imaging analysis, blood values, and essential hospitalization details, like ICU transfers, medications, and manifestation responses at each treatment stage according to the patient database. Data was obtained with the use of specific software tool developed to access patient records from COVID clinics of during the pandemic "waves" in a tertiary center in Western Greece (University Hospital Patras University). A script was running parallel with Hospital Information System and every time that a new patient was characterized as COVID-patient a new record was developed in a parallel database including all appropriate useful information for our approach and finally the outcome of the hospitalization. Patient records were accessed after Hospital's Scientific Bioethics Committee Approval.

The proposed approach, that was based on D.T.s, and has been trained and tested by analyzing the severity and the outcomes of the 346 COVID-19 patients hospitalized through the first two pandemics "waves" Western Greece, as was described from the European Mortality Monitoring Activity database, supported by the European Centre for Disease Prevention and Control (ECDC) and the World Health Organization (WHO), in Patras University Hospital [28]. D.T.s additionally selected as the most acceptable form of knowledge representation for our clinicians. Urgency classification, ICU transfer risk, and final treatment outcome were the outputs at this stage of implementation (Table 1). First step was the preprocessing of patient data as there were detected no missing values. Data records were randomly partitioned to train (66%) and test (34%) sets. The division process was repeated for a number of times in order to avoid over-fitting. For the classification were used different classifiers but the best performance was obtained with *J48* (with Reduced Error Pruning enabled), as well as *Random Forest* (ensemble) classifiers, according to their total accuracy performance.

Treatment response as part of a set of parameters at each specific step of the hospitalization period accompanied with predictions that could be relevant in the management and targeted treatment of patients, with the potential to modify improving outcomes additionally to postmortem findings [29–31].

Statistical ranking to the output parameters was considered for the system's inputs to be at minimum performing the highest possible accuracy (Table 2). For our implementation, only several (up to 15) parameters were used for each patient, from the total (nearly 25) features and text records stored in H.R.s of Patras University Hospital. Features as patient sex, age, comorbid, grading of illness severity, blood test results, fever, oxygen saturation, heart rate, radiographic examination results, type of medication, days in each department or clinic, and treatment output are only a part of medical parameters that usually are recorded during hospitalization and stored in H.R.s.

According to our team physicians' advice, we did not take into account patient deaths after ICU transfer, but only before, because of a high frequency of nosocomial infections, equipment malfunction incidents, as well as the low learning curve of medical and nursing staff that was enrolled in emergency and ICU units in Greece, last year. Available

Table 1. Hospital patient data collected from digital health record database

Men	196		
Women	*150*		
Age yr.	*61.85 (16 – 97)*		
Comorbid	*206*		
Days in Hospital	*Mean 10.4 (0-90)*		
Severity classification	*60 low severity*	*243 medium severity*	*43 high severity*
ICU transfer	*5 patients treated*		
Treatment Outcome	*15 patients from 1ˢᵗ wave died*	*38 patients from 1ˢᵗ wave treated after hospitalization*	*17 patients from 1ˢᵗ wave immediately exited*
	49 patients from both waves died*	*118 patients from both waves treated after hospitalization*	*174 patients from both waves immediately exited*

*Before or after ICU transfer

Table 2. Part of the database's parameters after preprocessing with their values for patient management.

- *Sex with values {male, female}*
- *Age with numeric values*
- *Days In Hospital with numeric values*
- *Comorbid {yes, no} as well as*
- *Comorbid type with the corresponding values*
- *Blood_test results add to the percent of abnormal values*
- *Radiographic_Examination results with {free, spotted, diffused} values*
- *Medication type of specific medicines or combinations used*
- *Grading at emergency Unit with {low, mild, severe, urgent}*
- *Result {exit, hospitalization in COVID Clinic, transfer to ICU, death}*

data, including the "*third wave*" of COVID-19, is under consideration to calculate other parameters as patient risk per unit and total departmental or institutional performance.

3   Results

3.1   Experiments

Several available algorithms were used to succeed the higher possible accuracy of the system predictive model. Improved settings were used for optimization for improved results (Table 3). First, the system used for the 1st "wave" of patients performing data mining approach (75 patients). Finally, with the use of the same input parameters second "wave" data were analyzed using a mining approach (346 patients).

Table 3. Classification results for patient management prediction with the use of random forest ensemble classifier

Average evaluation	True positive rate	Fault positive rate	Precision	Recall	F measure	Correctly classified percent on test set data
Severity classification	0,92	0,18	0,93	0,92	0,92	**92%**
ICU transfer	1	0	1	1	1	**100%**
Days in hospital	1	0	1	1	1	**100%**
Treatment outcome	0,97	0,018	0,97	0,97	0,97	**97%**

The present ML was performed for patient outcome prediction for both pandemic waves. Initially, the system chooses the most appropriate features to be used for prediction according to their statistical ranking. The initial evaluation dealt with patient severity grading for proper Triage-Classification at emergency units. The most important parameters are usually on the top (root) of each D.T. For example, for urgency classification, only Radiographic evaluation (with free, spotted, diffused values), secondary supported with age and sex of the patient. The second evaluation dealt with patient transfer to ICU immediately from hospital emergency unit and hospitalization duration.

3.2 Results

Consequently, for ICU transfer decisions, essential features are urgency (from previous evaluation), comorbid and secondary age, and sex of the patient. Only for days of hospitalization prediction type of medication strategy was revealed as an important parameter, with secondary blood test results at each stage. Finally, for treatment outcome, the critical features are urgency (from previous evaluation), and only secondary blood test results, sex, and age features. The final results are very encouraging for our approximation, and the D.T.s are readily accepted by medical staff. The system proved 92% for triage classification, 100% for identifying patients that will need ICU transfer, 100% for total days of hospitalization, and 97% accuracy for the outcome, predictions. Consequently, if emergency units would like to identify the severity of the disease, physicians could safely evaluate all the X-ray imaging of each patient and later during hospitalization, only a part of available information to decide for further manifestations, transfer to ICU, etc. Furthermore, knowledge extraction revealed D.T.s were trained for future use of new patients by the medical staff (Figs. 3, 4 and 5).

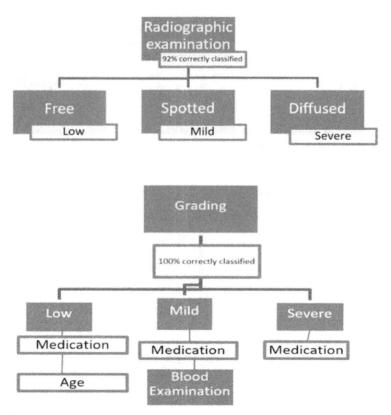

Fig. 3. Classification tree for Urgency evaluation at the emergency unit with the use of J48 classifier.

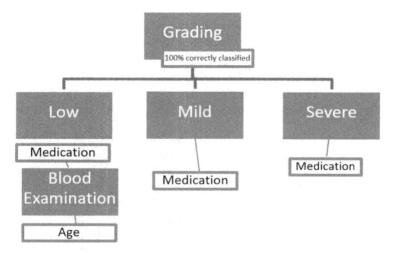

Fig. 4. Classification/decision tree for ICU transfer decision (part) with the use of J48 classifier.

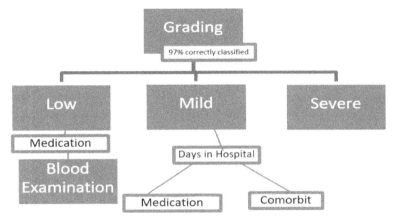

Fig. 5. Classification/decision tree for patient outcome (part) with the use of J48 classifier.

4 Discussion

Currently, pandemic waves push medical staff and infrastructures to their limits worldwide. Consequently, healthcare decisions can be more accurately figured and predicted, towards better management of the fast-growing patient subpopulations, giving more time for the effective pharmaceutical or vaccine armamentarium that the medical, scientific community will produce. According to our results, healthcare decisions could be accurately figured and predicted, towards better management of the fast-growing patient subpopulations, giving more time for the effective pharmaceutical or vaccine armamentarium produced by the medical, scientific community [9, 11]. Most published ML applications are used for detection/monitoring, prevention/treatment, and pathogenesis analysis of this virus [31]. More efforts have been focused on drug repurposing, analysis of dissemination patterns, and clinical radiographs. As all experts in biostatistics know, statistical approaches are affected not only by the selection of actual data that has been collected but also by "a priori" assumptions or guidelines of the researchers behind the experimental protocols [10]. Thinks are more difficult when an unknown disease with a fast-growing population appears. Similarities with past or early observations of an unknown fast-growing patient population usually cause delays or even incorrect treatment strategies targeting, for example, mostly to older men with comorbid, far from reality. This clinically "foggy" period can be easily understood, considering that our sample of the initial 75 patients hospitalized during the first pandemic wave was used a wide spectrum of available medications. This situation that lasted some months additionally overlapped medical or organizational errors revealed later during the second wave and at the beginning of the third wave, causing additional cost to our heavily threatened health system [18, 20]. ML methods can provide solutions for patient management support, which are not possible by the conventional statistical approaches [9]. Giving models of the dissemination pattern of the pandemic spread and its transmission processes, SVR, LSTM, and optimization problems, among other models, have been frequently used to investigate the COVID-19. Other models have been already effectively used to identify COVID-19 patients with the potential to develop more severe illnesses based on evaluating clinical information.

The proposed system will support clinicians for better services, improving patient outcomes, revealing faster diagnosis, reduce delays or mortality and give time for alternative medication. In addition, some algorithms can be employed to identify the patient possibility of severe illness by viruses [13]. Finally, for future work, our system could include an additional system for automatic detection of the disease according to automatic medical imaging analysis [32, 33].

5   Conclusions

New directions through managing the COVID-19 pandemic could include scoring the performance of the health care system and staff and adaptation to published protocols formulated after clinical research. An A.I. system could also be adopted using ML to estimate individuals' performance in working with patients that have been hired to work in the high-risk working areas as in ICUs. Currently, the system aims to support facing the third pandemic wave and is intended to face other types of respiratory pandemics in the future. Its' early-stage performance supports the importance of unsupervised ML in medical or other early-stage information databases to unknown infections. A.I. systems can be developed to provide managing decisions in such pandemics providing new directions for clinical research [31].

References

1. Chen, J., See, K.C.: Artificial intelligence for COVID-19: rapid review. J. Med. Internet Res. **22**(10), e21476 (2020)
2. Vaishya, R., Javaid, M., Khan, I.H., Haleem, A.: Artificial Intelligence (AI) applications for COVID-19 pandemic. Diab. Metab. Syndr. **14**(4), 337–339 (2020)
3. Mottaki, M.S., Mohammadipanah, F., Sajedi, H.: Contribution of machine learning approaches in response to COVID-19 infection. Inform. Med. Unlocked. **23**, 100526 (2021)
4. Wang, B., et al.: AI-assisted CT imaging analysis for COVID-19 screening: building and deploying a medical AI system. Appl. Soft Comput. **98**, 106897 (2021)
5. Mohanty, S., Rashid, M.H.A., Mridul, M., Mohanty, C., Swayamsiddha, S.: Application of artificial intelligence in COVID-19 drug repurposing. Diab. Metab. Syndr. **14**(5), 1027–1031 (2020)
6. Naseem, M., Akhund, R., Arshad, H., Ibrahim, M.T.: Exploring the potential of artificial intelligence and machine learning to combat COVID-19 and existing opportunities for LMIC: a scoping review. J. Prim. Care Community Health **11** (2020). https://doi.org/10.1177/215013 2720963634
7. Khemasuwan, D., Sorensen, J.S., Colt, H.G.: Artificial intelligence in pulmonary medicine: computer vision, predictive model and COVID-19. Eur. Respir. Rev. **29**(157), 200181 (2020)
8. Marchevsky, A.M., Patel, S., Wiley, K.J., et al.: Artificial neural networks and logistic regression as tools for the prediction of survival in patients with stages I and II non-small cell lung cancer. Model Pathol. **11**, 618–625 (1998)

9. Zampakis, P., et al.: Development of an intelligent system for the determination of rupture-related characteristics in intracranial aneurysms detected by Computed Tomography Angiography. Hellenic J. Radiol. **5**(4), 8–17 (2020)
10. Burke, H.B., Goodman, P.H., Rosen, D.B., Henson, D.E., Weinstein, J.N., Harrell, F.E., Jr., et al.: Artificial neural networks improve the accuracy of cancer survival prediction. Cancer **79**, 857–862 (1997)
11. Baxt, W.G.: Application of artificial neural networks to clinical medicine. Lancet **346**, 1135–1138 (1995)
12. Revuelta, I., et al.: A hybrid data envelopment analysis-artificial neural network prediction model for COVID-19 severity in transplant recipients. Artif. Intell. Rev. **23**, 1–32 (2021). https://doi.org/10.1007/s10462-021-10008-0
13. Bai, H.X., et al.: Performance of radiologists in differentiating COVID-19 from viral pneumonia on chest CT. Radiology **296**, E46–E54 (2020)
14. Jiang, X., Coffee, M., Bari, A.: Towards an artificial intelligence framework for data-driven prediction of coronavirus clinical severity. Comput. Mater. Continua **63**(1), 537–551 (2020)
15. Orsi, M.A., Oliva, G., Toluian, T., Pitino, C.V., Panzeri, M., Cellina, M.: Feasibility, reproducibility, and clinical validity of a quantitative chest X-ray assessment for COVID-19. Am. J. Trop. Med. Hyg. **103**, 822–827 (2020)
16. Bragazzi, N.L., Dai, H., Damiani, G., Behzadifar, M., Martini, M., Wu, J.: How big data and artificial intelligence can help better manage the COVID-19 pandemic. Int. J. Environ. Res. Public Health **17**, 3176 (2020)
17. Hurt, B., Kligerman, S., Hsiao, A.: Deep learning localization of pneumonia: 2019 coronavirus (COVID-19) outbreak. J. Thorac. Imaging **35**(3), W87–W89 (2020)
18. Yan, L., et al.: An interpretable mortality prediction model for COVID-19 patients. Nat. Mach. Intell. **2**(5), 283–288 (2020)
19. Carrer, L., et al.: Automatic pleural line extraction and COVID-19 scoring from lung ultrasound data. IEEE Trans. Ultrason. Ferroelectr. Freq. Control **67**, 2207–2217 (2020)
20. Hassanien, A., Elghamrawy, S.: Diagnosis and prediction model for COVID19 patients response to treatment based on convolutional neural networks and Whale optimization algorithm using CT images, medRxiv2020.04.16.20063990 (2020)
21. Liang, W., et al.: Early triage of critically ill COVID-19 patients using deep learning. Nat. Commun. **11**(1), 3543 (2020)
22. Wang, L., Lin, Z.Q., Wong, A.: Covid-net: a tailored deep convolutional neural network design for detection of covid-19 cases from chest x-ray images. Sci. Rep. **10**, 1–2 (2020)
23. Bai, X., Fang, C., Zhou, Y., Bai, S., Liu, Z., Chen, Q.: Predicting COVID-19 malignant progression with AI techniques. medRxiv (2020)
24. Roy, S., et al.: Deep learning for classification and localization of COVID-19 markers in point-of-care lung ultrasound. IEEE Trans. Med. Imaging **39**(8), 2676–2687 (2020)
25. Siegenthaler, W.: Differential diagnosis in internal medicine: from symptom to diagnosis, p. 1140 (2007)
26. Witten, I.H., Frank, E., Hall, M.A., Pal, C.J.: Data Mining: Practical Machine Learning tools and Techniques, 3rd edn. Morgan Kaufmann, Burlington (2011)
27. WEKA. Application of artificial neural networks to clinical medicine. Lancet q346, 1135–1138 (1995)
28. WEKA Machine Learning Group at the University of Waikato. http://www.cs.waikato.ac.nz/ml/index
29. https://www.euromomo.eu/graphs-and-maps#z-scores-by-country Accessed 02 Sep 2021
30. Sarica, A., Cerasa, A., Quattrone, A.: Random forest algorithm for the classification of neuroimaging data in Alzheimer's disease: a systematic review. Front. Aging Neurosci. **9**, 329 (2017)

31. Pfahringer, B.: Random model trees: an effective and scalable regression method. University of Waikato, New Zealand. http://www.cs.waikato.ac.nz/~bernhard
32. Sekhawat, V., Green, A., Mahadeva, U.: COVID-19 autopsies: conclusions from international studies. Diagn. Histopathol. **27**(3), 103–107 (2021)
33. Wong, H.Y.F., et al.: Frequency and distribution of chest radiographic findings in COVID-19 positive patients. Radiology **296**, E72–E78 (2020)

Building a Tool that Draws from the Collective Wisdom of the Internet to Help Users Respond Effectively to Anxiety-Related Questions

Benjamin T. Kaveladze[1]([✉]) [iD], George I. Kaveladze[2] [iD], Elad Yom-Tov[3,4] [iD], and Stephen M. Schueller[1,5] [iD]

[1] Department of Psychological Science, University of California, Irvine, Irvine, CA, USA
bkavelad@uci.edu
[2] The MITRE Corporation, Bedford, MA, USA
[3] Faculty of Industrial Engineering and Management, Technion - Israel Institute of Technology, Haifa, Israel
[4] Microsoft Research, Herzliya, Israel
[5] Department of Informatics, University of California, Irvine, Irvine, CA, USA

Abstract. Online anxiety support communities offer a valuable and accessible source of informational and emotional support for people around the world. However, effectively responding to posters' anxiety-related questions can be challenging for many users. We present our work in developing a web-based tool that draws from previous question-response interactions and trusted online informational resources to help users rapidly produce high-quality responses to anxiety-related questions. We describe our efforts in four parts: 1) Creating a machine learning classifier to predict response quality, 2) developing and evaluating a computational question-answering system that learns from previous questions and responses on support forums, 3) developing and evaluating a system to suggest online resources for anxiety-related questions, and 4) interviewing support community moderators to inform further system design. We discuss how this tool might be integrated into online anxiety support communities and consider challenges with the tool's functionality and implementation. We also provide the dataset we used to train the system to provide opportunities for other researchers to build on this work.

Keywords: Online mental health communities · Question answering · Big data · Online support provision · Anxiety

1 Introduction

1.1 Questions and Answers on Online Mental Health Communities

Mental health struggles are extremely common globally, but many people lack reliable access to professional mental healthcare or sensitive social networks from which they can draw support (Kohn et al. 2004). Online mental health support communities offer accessible opportunities for people to exchange advice and validation with others

H. Lewy and R. Barkan (Eds.): PH 2021, LNICST 431, pp. 15–27, 2022.
https://doi.org/10.1007/978-3-030-99194-4_2

who understand or share their struggles. These spaces take advantage of availability, anonymity, and ease of use to bypass common barriers to receiving mental health support, such as stigma, shyness, and physical isolation (Bargh 2002). As such, they can be especially crucial resources for young people or members of marginalized groups who might be concerned about the social consequences of seeking help from their in-person networks (O'Leary et al. 2017, Rains and Tsetsi 2017).

Subreddits are free, user-led online discussion forums hosted by Reddit.com. There are many subreddits related to mental health, each with its own subculture and unique forms of support (Sharma and De Choudhury 2018), but in the present work we focus on anxiety-related subreddits. While the norm of using Reddit anonymously precludes obtaining representative demographic information on subreddit users, most respondents to a survey of mental health subreddit users conducted in December 2019 (n > 300) were young (50% under 24), white (79%), female (56%), and American (59%, though respondents came from 44 countries in total); further, most rated their mental health as terrible or poor (82%) and had received professional mental healthcare in the past (87%) (Kaveladze and Schueller 2020).

Mental health subreddit users share a range of content, including uplifting messages, emotional "vents", and tips. However, many interactions across online mental health communities involve a user posting to ask for help with a personal problem (Kaveladze and Schueller 2020). After a question is submitted, other members comment on that submission to offer advice or support, typically within a few minutes to a few days later (De Choudhury and De 2014). Knowing how to respond effectively to a stranger's question about a private mental health issue can be challenging. As a result, many questions and support requests on these spaces go unanswered or receive unhelpful answers, and negativity and misinformation in responses are common issues (Kaveladze and Schueller 2020).

While every question is unique, we observe that many anxiety-related questions are similar to other questions that received effective responses in the past. We further observe that many of these responses are accessible via the internet, either in publicly-archived question-response interactions from online support communities or in online informational resources. Indeed, over 15,000 such question-response interactions occur annually on one popular anxiety subreddit. Thus, the internet provides a corpus of collective wisdom on responding to anxiety-related struggles that is unprecedented in its size and the diversity of its contributors. We aim to build an automated tool that leverages this corpus to help users respond to new anxiety-related questions. Specifically, the tool aims to help users craft high-quality and well-informed supportive responses quicker than they would otherwise.

1.2   Accessing Collective Wisdom from Mental Health Subreddits

Subreddits are particularly amenable to computational analyses because all posts are publicly available and because the Reddit API and interconnected data download tools like Pushshift enable large-scale downloads of post data (Baumgartner et al. 2020). Several studies have used computational approaches to study support interactions in online mental health communities. The majority of this research has examined help-seeking posts, identifying factors such as linguistic accommodation that predict posts' tendencies to receive responses expressing emotional and informational support (De Choudhury and De 2014; Sharma and De Choudhury 2018; Gkotsis et al. 2016). However, some research has explored the characteristics of helpful responses to posts on online mental health communities. Peng et al. (2021) found that mental health subreddit posters responded more positively to responses to their help-seeking posts that matched the kind of support they requested (informational vs. emotional). Also, Kavuluru et al. (2016) developed a computational model to predict responses' helpfulness from a suicide prevention perspective. Their model showed promising results, but it only included a few predictors from the response text and left out post metadata such as time to respond. We build on Kavuluru et al.'s approach, including a wider range of linguistic and metadata predictors aiming to create a more comprehensive model of response quality.

1.3   Project Summary

We describe the process of developing the helper tool in four parts, each with an overview, methods, and results section. Part 1 describes a machine learning classifier we built to label responses to anxiety-related questions as high- or low-quality. Part 2 describes a question-answering system we designed to take in anxiety-related questions and suggest responses pulled from a corpus of question-response interactions. Part 3 describes a system that matches questions to relevant online informational resources. Part 4 describes our current progress in designing the helper tool, including interviewing stakeholders and identifying challenges to the tool's effectiveness and implementation. This work's contribution is to inform efforts to improve supports for online mental health community members. In addition, we provide the dataset used to train our system for other researchers to learn from and improve on our method.

2   Creating the Helper Tool

2.1   Part 1: Creating a Machine Learning Classifier to Predict Response Quality

Overview. We drew from a corpus of 12,325 responses to 7,646 questions and associated metadata from two online support forums. Next, we gathered a subset of those responses and manually labeled the quality and type of support they offered. We then built a random forest classifier model (cross-validated AUC = 0.82) that labeled responses to anxiety-related questions as high- or low-quality.

Methods

Dataset. We examined two Anxiety-related subreddits that had been popular for several years (at the time of data collection, we observed that one subreddit often had over 1,000 subscribers logged into Reddit at any given time and the other often had over 250). Both of these subreddits required posters to tag their submissions with one of several flairs (subreddit-specific tags) describing their submission. We gathered submissions with the "Help" flair from one subreddit and with the "Advice needed" flair from the other subreddit as these flairs identified submissions asking questions. We also gathered comments associated with each of those posts. Next, we limited our dataset to comments responding to the submission, rather than those responding to other comments, and to posts, both submissions and comments, with fewer than 250 words and more than 5 words. We chose this word range as posts with 5 words or fewer may have been too vague to interpret and posts with more than 250 words may have taken too long for human raters to read. With these inclusion criteria, we used Python to query the Pushshift API and the Reddit API, yielding a dataset of 12,325 question-response pairs and their associated metadata posted between July of 2017 and February of 2021 on these two subreddits (Rossum and Drake 2009).

In addition to question and response text, we obtained post-level metadata on the date and time of posting and post score. A post's score is the sum of upvotes [+1] and downvotes [−1] that it receives – users with Reddit accounts can add one upvote or downvote to each post. The dataset also contained user-level metadata on karma (the sum of upvotes minus downvotes received across all of a user's Reddit posts) and account formation date/time. Finally, we created several textual variables for each post, including sentiment, readability, and the proportion of words matching several Linguistic Inquiry and Word Count (LIWC) dictionaries (negative, positive, feeling, anxiety, health, affiliative drive, body, anger, and sadness-related words) (Tausczik and Pennebaker 2010). We calculated average sentiment at the post level using the AFINN sentiment measure (Nielsen 2011), which provides values from −5 (negative sentiment) to 5 (positive sentiment) for emotionally-valenced words.

Data Privacy. All post data we analyzed in this work were publicly accessible and thus exempt from IRB review at the University of California, Irvine. However, most subreddit users likely do not expect that their posts will be used for research, making data privacy especially important. To help protect user privacy, we do not mention any potentially identifiable information and we removed the post authors' usernames and post text from the dataset we share.

Rating Response Quality. We selected a random sample of 790 question-response interactions from our dataset and recruited 365 crowdsourced workers from Amazon Mechanical Turk (Turkers) who self-identified as fluent English speakers to rate responses to 10 randomly chosen questions from the sample. Turkers were presented the question and response and asked to rate how well each response answered the question (not at all well [0] – very well [3]), whether the response provided emotional support (yes/no), and whether the response provided instrumental support (yes/no). Raters were told to imagine that they asked the question and received the response anonymously (Mazuz and Yom-Tov 2020). An example of a high-quality response to a mental health question is shown in Fig. 1.

To monitor the quality of the Turker ratings, we dropped rating data from Turkers who did at least one of the following: failed the attention check during the task, self-reported at the end that they just skipped through the task without reading, or gave the same rating to all 10 of the interactions they rated. Based on these exclusion criteria, we dropped ratings from 270/365 Turkers, leaving plausibly legitimate ratings from only 95 Turkers. To supplement the Turker ratings, we trained three research assistants to rate all 790 question-response interactions in the same way that the Turkers did. The research assistants provided reasonably consistent ratings (Krippendorff's alphas: subjective response quality = 0.68, emotional support = 0.69, informational support = 0.75). However, research assistants' and Turkers' ratings were less consistent (Krippendorff's alphas: subjective response quality = 0.54, emotional support = 0.36, informational support = 0.43). We transformed these ratings into a binary response quality variable, defining high-quality responses as those with ratings (averaged across all raters) above all three scale midpoints (1.5 for the subjective response quality scale, and 0.5 for the emotional support and informational support scales). Using this binary response quality variable, 399 responses were labeled as high-quality and 391 as low-quality.

Classification Model. We trained a random forest classification model (scikit-learn library, Pedregosa et al. 2011) on the human-rated dataset to predict if answers were of high quality. We used a random forest model because they are known to be the best overall models for structured data, together with SVMs and neural networks (see Fernández-Delgado et al. 2014 and the criticism thereof: Wainberg et al. 2016). The independent attributes of the model were syllable count, character count, word count, sentence count, readability (Flesch 1948), sentiment valence (Nielsen 2011), post score, percentage of words matching the LIWC "negative emotion", "positive emotion", "feeling", "anxiety", "health", "affiliative drive", "body", "anger", and "sadness" dictionaries (Nielsen 2011), posting date, and time of day of posting, all for both questions and responses. We also included question-asker and respondent account formation date and account karma as attributes. We used 10-fold cross-validation to assess the accuracy of the model.

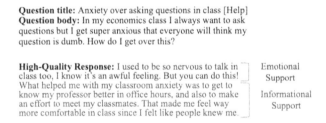

Fig. 1. An example of a high-quality response to an anxiety-related question, including emotional and informational support.

Results. In analyses, we used ordinary least squares regressions to detect linear relationships, Welch's t-tests to compare group means while accounting for unequal variance across groups, and Spearman's rank-order correlations (ρ) to track associations between non-normally distributed variables. All analyses were performed in the R statistical computing language using the "stats" package (R Core Team 2013). Data manipulation and figure creation used the "Tidyverse" family of packages in R (Wickham 2019).

Classification Model. Our cross-validated response quality classification model achieved a mean AUC of 0.82 and mean accuracy of 0.72. Each model feature's importance in the model is shown in Fig. 2. We applied this model to classify the 11,535 responses that had not been rated by humans.

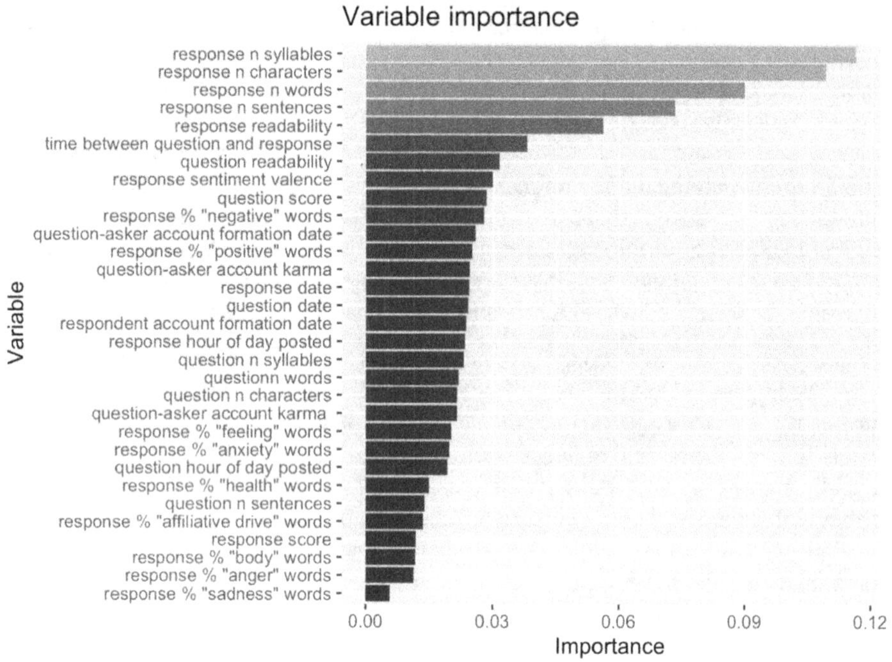

Variable importance

Fig. 2. Each feature's importance in the random forest model predicting response quality. Lighter blue signifies higher importance. Importance (GINI importance) was computed as the (normalized) total reduction of the criterion brought by that feature. "n syllables" refers to the number of syllables in the question or response text. "readability" refers to the Flesch reading ease score calculated on the response text (Flesch 1948). Time between question and response is the length of time between when the question was posted and the response was posted. Sentiment valence refers to the sentiment score using the AFINN sentiment measure (Nielsen 2011). Score refers to the sum of "upvotes" (+1) and "downvotes" (−1) on a post. % "negative words" refers to the percentage of words in a post that matched words from the "negative emotion" Linguistic Inquiry and Word Count (LIWC) dictionary (Tausczik and Pennebaker 2010). Account formation date refers to the date and time that a user's Reddit account was made. Account karma refers to the sum, across all a users' posts in their account history, of their posts' scores.

2.2 Part 2: Developing and Testing a Question-Answering System

Overview. We built on the predictive model from Part 1 to develop a question-answering (QA) system. Drawing from previous question-response interactions, the system aimed to match new anxiety-related questions to high-quality responses from previous interactions based on linguistic similarity. We then evaluated this tool's effectiveness with help from crowdworkers and found that it outperformed chance but did not provide acceptable responses for a majority of new questions.

Methods. Building on the original dataset of 12,365 question-response pairs, we gathered another 4,272 question-response pairs from the two subreddits posted between

May of 2020 and May of 2021, including their associated metadata. Using this dataset of 16,637 pairs, we developed a question-answering system to identify previous high-quality responses that might be relevant to a novel question.

Identifying Useful Responses. To identify potentially useful responses, we filtered the question-response pairs using the response quality classifier we developed in part 1, keeping only responses that the classifier labeled as high-quality.

Finding Similar Responses. Working under the assumption that similar questions could receive similar answers, we attempted to identify useful answers to new questions by finding the most similar past question that had a response classified as high-quality. However, questions are often lengthy and contain information that is sometimes irrelevant to the answer. Therefore, instead of finding the textual similarity between questions, we first applied abstractive summarization to all questions and then found the similarity among summarized questions.

Specifically, questions were summarized to a predefined length of 50 words using the Hugging Face summarization pipeline [huggingface.co]. In our work we used a maximal summary length of 50 words. We evaluated other lengths between 35 and 75 words but did not observe significant differences in performance. We estimated the similarity between questions using cosine similarity to the TF-IDF normalized word and bigram representation of the summarized questions.

Evaluation. Next, we recruited 106 crowdsourced workers from Prolific to test the QA system's effectiveness. Each participant viewed a series of responses to questions from the anxiety subreddits. Each of these responses was either 1) the original response to the question posted on Reddit, 2) a response to a question in our dataset that the QA system deemed was the closest, or 3) a randomly selected response to another question from our dataset. For each interaction, workers answered the following questions: "Does the response address the issues that the questions asked about? (y/n)" and "If you asked the question above, would you have been satisfied with the answer? (y/n)". Due to duplicate responses, there were 69 original question-response interactions but only 67 randomly selected responses and 60 QA system-selected "closest high-quality" responses. We conducted one-way ANOVAs to compare the means between types of responses, averaged across all raters (y = 1, n = 0), and ran planned Tukey's HSD tests to compare group means.

Results

Response Relevance and Satisfaction. The crowdsourced workers recruited from Prolific provided consistent ratings of response quality (Krippendorff's alphas = 0.73 for both response relevance and satisfaction). Average response relevance ratings were lowest for randomly selected responses (M = 0.18, SD = 0.38, n = 67), higher for closest high-quality responses (M = 0.26, SD = 0.44, n = 60), and highest for original responses (M = 0.52, SD = 0.50, n = 69), F = 55.88, p < 0.001, and a Tukey's HSD test found that all group means were significantly different (p's < 0.001). Response satisfaction ratings were lowest for randomly selected responses (M = 0.24, SD = 0.43, n = 67), higher for closest high-quality responses (M = 0.38, SD = 0.49, n = 60), and highest for original responses (M = 0.74, SD = 0.44, n = 69) (F = 116.20, p < 0.001), and a Tukey's HSD test found that all group means were significantly different (p's < 0.05).

2.3 Part 3: Developing a System to Suggest Online Resources for Anxiety-Related Question

Overview. To supplement the responses provided by the QA system, we developed a system to suggest relevant online resources for anxiety-related questions, The system recommended an appropriate resource 51% of the time, compared to 37% for a random choice.

Methods. We assembled a corpus of links to 80 online resources, 72 of which were from mhanational.org, a website providing free and accessible expert information about various mental health issues. The remaining 8 came from other informational websites. These resources provided information or other support for anxiety-related issues, such as advice on how to overcome social anxiety at parties or how to calm one's mind (corpus available online). A graduate student and undergraduate research assistant matched 250 questions from the dataset to an online resource from the corpus that they felt might be most helpful to the question-asker.

We developed a multiclass learning model to predict the appropriate online resources for particular questions. Our model ignored resources with fewer than 5 matched questions, leaving 26 online resources. The model was a Random Forest classifier with 10 trees and it used the TF-IDF representation of the words and bigrams of the questions to predict which of the information pages should be added to the answer. The model's performance was evaluated using 10-fold cross-validation.

Results. The online resource prediction model achieved 51% mean accuracy, compared to 37% mean accuracy for a model that did not use multiclass learning, and instead simply selected a resource for each question based only on the frequency with which that resource was chosen in the 250 training questions.

2.4 Part 4: Designing and Implementing the Helper Tool

Overview. We conducted interviews with moderators from mental health subreddits to gain stakeholder perspectives on how a tool using this QA system might be best designed and implemented. Some moderators expressed enthusiasm for the tool's potential to improve the quality and rapidity of responses, while other moderators were concerned that it could lead to less meaningful interactions in the community.

Methods. We reached out to nine moderators of mental health subreddits to invite them to participate in a semi-structured 30-min interview over video chat with one of the researchers on our team. During the interview, we walked moderators through a mockup of the tool (shown in Fig. 3) and asked them several questions regarding how helpful they felt it could be for moderators and users, how it could be improved to be more useful for subreddit users, and how comfortable they would be with the tool being used on mental health subreddits.

Results

Qualitative Interviews. Two mental health subreddits moderators agreed to participate in a video interview. These moderators were comfortable with the idea of the tool as we presented it and were not concerned about data privacy issues. The moderators felt that such a tool would help both moderators and non-moderators – many of whom struggle with how to formulate effective responses to mental health questions – to more rapidly and easily provide high-quality responses to mental health questions. One moderator noted that if the tool was available to all users, it would enable users to screen their own questions before posting, helping to deal with the common problem of similar questions being posted repeatedly on a subreddit by different users. One moderator also noted that the Reddit search tool did not function well at finding past responses that were relevant to a new question, so the tool could fill that role. Both moderators suggested it would be useful to make the tool integrate directly with the Reddit API so that it could be easily used while browsing the site. Both moderators also stressed that our research team should stay in communication with the mental health communities to get their input on the tool throughout the development process.

Two other mental health subreddit moderators responded to our invitations but turned down a full interview. One of these moderators stated over direct messages that they felt the tool idea was potentially dangerous for users' well-being because it would create a barrier to connection between support requesters and providers. The other moderator wrote that the tool sounded like it would not improve on the process of using the Reddit search function to find relevant past responses or using a web browser to find online informational resources.

2.5 Data Availability

The dataset we used to train the response quality classifier and the question-answering system, with usernames and post content removed, is available at https://github.com/benji700/qa_project/blob/main/anxiety_subreddit_data_complete.csv. In addition, the corpus of 80 online resources is available at https://github.com/benji700/qa_project/blob/main/MHA%20resources.xlsx.

3 Discussion

In the present work we described our progress in developing a tool to help users rapidly produce high-quality and well-informed responses to anxiety-related questions. Although automated tools exist to help Reddit moderators identify potentially problematic content, to our knowledge, no tools exist to improve response quality to mental health-related questions. Our work demonstrated both opportunities and challenges to designing such a tool.

The resultant tool takes in a text-based question and its associated post metadata from a subreddit and suggests 1) a previous response to a similar question and 2) a relevant online informational resource. We chose to include an online resource due to difficulty in identifying relevant responses to new questions and because many questions expressed recurring themes, so that a relatively small set of online informational resources might be useful to help answer many of those questions. Yet, our results show that both informational and emotional support can be valuable. Online informational resources might be able to provide better informational support, especially when those resources come from high-quality and authoritative sources. Emotional support, however, might need to come from humans who can understand and empathize with one's problems. Users may prefer human-generated responses when seeking empathic support online (Morris et al. 2018), and so efforts to remove a human component from mental health-related QA systems might face limitations.

Moderator perspectives on the tool were mixed. Those with positive impressions of the tool felt it could provide practical support for both moderators and subreddit members interested in rapidly helping posters, helping to offer timely support to more people. Even though they were positive about the tool, these moderators also stressed that if the tool were to be made publicly available for subreddit users, working closely with mental health communities would be essential. Moderators with less favorable impressions of the tool argued that making such a tool available to users would weaken the human connection between support requesters and support providers. They also predicted that the tool would be redundant with web browsers that could be used to look up the relevant information to write a high-quality response. These are useful considerations for other tools seeking to provide support for users on online mental health forums and it would be useful to consider the incremental or differential benefit of such a tool compared to tools like web browsers.

Our QA system and online resource suggestion system outperformed chance, but they did not produce useful suggestions reliably enough to be used without a human in the loop. Despite their inconsistent response quality, these systems might still help human response-providers to suggest higher-quality answers quicker. Even when imperfect, the tool's suggestions may provide useful starting points from which users can then build their own contoured responses. It is worth noting that in our initial hand-coding of responses to anxiety-related questions, about half of the responses were coded as low-quality, so even human-generated responses may not always be useful. Finally, if the tool's ability to produce relevant responses and online resources were to become much more reliable, it could be re-designed to be used by support-seekers themselves to find responses relevant to their own problems.

Next Steps and Future Directions. To improve the QA and online resource suggestion systems, we are designing the tool to produce more accurate recommendations over time based on feedback on response quality from its users. To begin gathering this user feedback, we will release the tool to a group of Reddit moderators and users who will use the tool and rate the quality of its suggestions. Even among this group, careful attention will be necessary to ensure that the tool's recommendations are safe and that users understand its limitations.

In addition to this iterative feedback from users, the suggestion systems could also be improved with a larger corpus of question-response interactions and a more elaborate model. Simplifying the data inputted into the system could also be relevant. For example, it is possible that the questions and responses from anxiety subreddits were too long for the QA system to parse the most relevant part of the question; Morris et al. (2018) designed a similar system using much shorter questions and responses and achieved more reliable response quality.

While the tool has demonstrated some potential, future work will be necessary to know if it can be a valuable contribution to online support communities. Open questions include if the tool produces responses that question-askers find useful, as well as whether people are willing to use the tool. These questions can be answered through experiments, case studies, or by making the tool publicly available and measuring user activity. Further, the tool will need to be refined through user experience research and with input from stakeholders in online mental health communities.

Limitations. First, although we were able to achieve reasonable inter-rater reliability in response quality ratings, our measure of response quality was not a precise estimate of our variable of interest: how much help seekers felt that a given response to their question was useful, informational, and empathic. An alternative strategy would have been to follow Peng et al. (2021) in evaluating help seekers' expressed satisfaction with responses (measured via linguistic analysis of their responses to other users' responses to their posts), although such an approach is also not ideal because many who asked a question do not react to responses they received. Second, our metrics of linguistic features such as sentiment and health-related words were imprecise because they were derived from a simple word-counting computational method and did not account for conversation norms on the subreddits we examined. These metrics would have been more valid with human coding, although such a strategy would have been too labor-intensive to perform on the full dataset and could also introduce bias from raters.

Conclusion. Our tool holds potential for improving the availability of effective support on online anxiety support communities by helping users to quickly produce high-quality responses to anxiety-related questions. As it continues, this project could also provide insights about the utility of crowdsourcing collective wisdom from the internet towards solving challenging personal problems. However, empirical research on our tool's effectiveness is necessary.

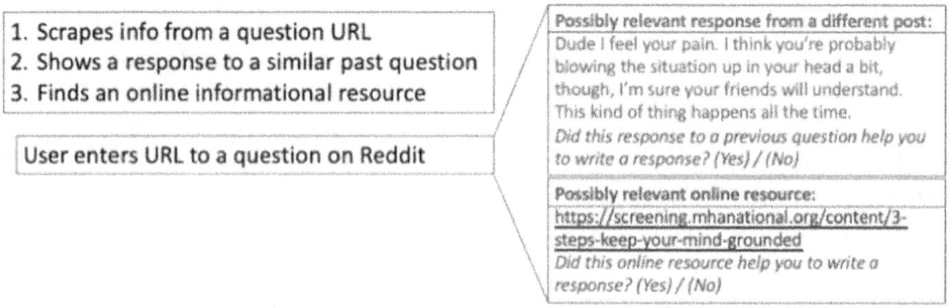

1. Scrapes info from a question URL 2. Shows a response to a similar past question 3. Finds an online informational resource

User enters URL to a question on Reddit

Possibly relevant response from a different post:
Dude I feel your pain. I think you're probably blowing the situation up in your head a bit, though, I'm sure your friends will understand. This kind of thing happens all the time.
Did this response to a previous question help you to write a response? (Yes) / (No)

Possibly relevant online resource:
https://screening.mhanational.org/content/3-steps-keep-your-mind-grounded
Did this online resource help you to write a response? (Yes) / (No)

Fig. 3. Design mockup for the response helper tool. Based on moderator feedback, input may instead be automatically scraped from Reddit as the tool user is browsing.

References

Bargh, J.A., McKenna, K.Y.A., Fitzsimons, G.M.: Can you see the real me? Activation and expression of the "true self" on the Internet. J. Soc. Issues **58**(1), 33–48 (2002). https://doi.org/10.1111/1540-4560.00247

Baumgartner, J., Zannettou, S., Keegan, B., Squire, M., Blackburn, J.: The pushshift reddit dataset. In: Proceedings of the International AAAI Conference on Web and Social Media, vol. 14, pp. 830–839 (2020)

De Choudhury, M., De, S.: Mental health discourse on reddit: self-disclosure, social support, and anonymity. In: Proceedings of the International AAAI Conference on Web and Social Media, vol. 8, no. 1 (2014)

Fernández-Delgado, M., Cernadas, E., Barro, S., Amorim, D.: Do we need hundreds of classifiers to solve real world classification problems? J. Mach. Learn. Res. **15**(1), 3133–3181 (2014)

Flesch, R.: A new readability yardstick. J. Appl. Psychol. **32**(3), 221 (1948)

Gkotsis, G., et al.: The language of mental health problems in social media. *CLPsych@HLT-NAACL* (2016). https://doi.org/10.18653/v1/W16-0307

Kaveladze, B., Schueller, S.: Mental health subreddits offer users valuable and unique support. Poster Session Presented at the 2020 Association for Psychological Science Virtual Poster Showcase (2020). https://imgur.com/a/RO1wHJd

Kavuluru, R., Williams, A.G., Ramos-Morales, M., Haye, L., Holaday, T., Cerel, J.: Classification of helpful comments on online suicide watch forums. In: ACM Conference on Bioinformatics, Computational Biology and Biomedicine, pp. 32–40 (2016). https://doi.org/10.1145/2975167.2975170

Kohn, R., Saxena, S., Levav, I., Saraceno, B.: The treatment gap in mental health care. Bull. World Health Organ. **82**, 858–866 (2004)

Mazuz, K., Yom-Tov, E.: Analyzing trends of loneliness through large-scale analysis of social media postings: observational study. JMIR Ment. Health **7**(4), e17188 (2020). https://doi.org/10.2196/17188

Morris, R.R., Kouddous, K., Kshirsagar, R., Schueller, S.M.: Towards an artificially empathic conversational agent for mental health applications: system design and user perceptions. J. Med. Internet Res. **20**(6), e1014 (2018)

Nielsen, F.Å.: A new ANEW: evaluation of a word list for sentiment analysis in microblogs. arXiv preprint arXiv:1103.2903 (2011)

O'Leary, K., Bhattacharya, A., Munson, S.A., Wobbrock, J.O., Pratt, W.: Design opportunities for mental health peer support technologies. In: Proceedings of the 2017 ACM Conference on Computer Supported Cooperative Work and Social Computing, pp. 1470–1484 (2017)

Pedregosa, F., et al.: Scikit-learn: machine learning in Python. J. Mach. Learn. Res. **12**, 2825–2830 (2011)

Peng, Z., Ma, X., Yang, D., Tsang, K.W., Guo, Q.: Effects of support-seekers' community knowledge on their expressed satisfaction with the received comments in mental health communities. In: Proceedings of the 2021 CHI Conference on Human Factors in Computing Systems, pp. 1–12 (2021)

R Core Team. R: A language and environment for statistical computing. R Foundation for Statistical Computing, Vienna, Austria (2019). https://www.R-project.org/

Rains, S.A., Tsetsi, E.: Social support and digital inequality: does internet use magnify or mitigate traditional inequities in support availability? Commun. Monogr. **84**(1), 54–74 (2017)

Sharma, E., De Choudhury, M.: Mental health support and its relationship to linguistic accommodation in online communities. In: Proceedings of the 2018 CHI Conference on Human Factors in Computing Systems, pp. 641:1–641:13 (2018). https://doi.org/10.1145/3173574.3174215

Tausczik, Y.R., Pennebaker, J.W.: The psychological meaning of words: LIWC and computerized text analysis methods. J. Lang. Soc. Psychol. **29**(1), 24–54 (2010)

Van Rossum, G., Drake, F.L.: Python 3 Reference Manual. CreateSpace, Scotts Valley (2009)

Wainberg, M., Alipanahi, B., Frey, B.J.: Are random forests truly the best classifiers? J. Mach. Learn. Res. **17**(1), 3837–3841 (2016)

Wickham, H., et al.: Welcome to the tidyverse. J. Open Source Softw. **4**(43), 1686 (2019). https://doi.org/10.21105/joss.01686

Technologies Implementation, Acceptance and Evaluation During the Pandemic

Aspects of Pervasive Health and Technology Use in Care Organizations During the Pandemic: Report from a Municipality Covid-19 Study

Erik Grönvall[1]([✉]) [iD] and Stefan Lundberg[2] [iD]

[1] IT University of Copenhagen, Rued Langgaards Vej 7, 2300 Copenhagen, Denmark
erig@itu.dk
[2] LCO Prime AB, Krokvägen 6, 12262 Enskede, Sweden
stefanl@lco.se

Abstract. The Covid-19 pandemic struck the world in spring 2019 and affected most people in the world. One group that suffered the most was older adults and others 'weak' citizens. In Sweden where the reported-on study was situated, especially people living in nursing homes and other care facilities suffered immensely, especially in the early stages of the pandemic. In this paper we report on perspectives and lessons learned from a survey compiled by 13 care managers in eleven Swedish municipalities followed by a workshop with ten of these municipality health managers. Our study showcase how technology has been a valuable tool for these organizations during the pandemic. While Internet-cameras in some instances has been used in private homes to facilitate 'remote monitoring', many of our findings points to aspects of managing care – a less studied aspect within the Pervasive health community.

Keywords: Municipality · Technology · Covid-19 · Lessons learned · Pandemic

1 Introduction

The ongoing Covid-19 pandemic has affected the whole world and challenged the care sector to the extreme. High mortality rates, especially among the older and institutionalized population were reported on in many countries at an early stage of the pandemic [1–3]. Sweden was one country that during the first year of the pandemic experienced high mortality numbers among care-receiving older adults, especially unmarried older adults [4]. In Sweden it is mostly the municipalities that have the responsibility to organize care-facilities, social care, and homecare. Consequently, many care- and organizational changes had to be made in the municipality care organizations as the pandemic spread and mortality increased, including the organization of elderly care facilities [5].

As part of an ongoing innovation project related to municipality care and social care a survey on the organizational effects of the pandemic was distributed to, and compiled by, care managers in 13 Swedish municipalities. The survey was followed-up by an online workshop. Our work did not have an outspoken technical agenda, but many of

H. Lewy and R. Barkan (Eds.): PH 2021, LNICST 431, pp. 31–39, 2022.
https://doi.org/10.1007/978-3-030-99194-4_3

the findings dealt with technology, or highlighted aspects of municipality care during a pandemic where technology can be part of a solution. The survey answers were analyzed and resulted in four broad themes, A) Information and information dissemination, B) Digital tools, C) Before and after a crisis, and D) Each crisis is different. These four themes were brought as input to the workshop and there further elaborated upon. The survey and workshop took place autumn 2020, what we then thought would be 'at the end' of the Covid-19 pandemic. While numerous large studies on the pandemic have been conducted [2, 6–8], the idea with our study was not to make a broad data-collection survey. Instead, the ambition was that the workshop would enable a discussion and collaborative reflection across the participants – using the survey data as a point of departure rather than the result. Combined, our survey data and workshop documentation provide insights into how the involved (small to midsize municipalities) experienced the pandemic and how they used (and not used) technology and pervasive healthcare technology as tools in managing the pandemic situation. Also, our data provides insights into challenges, for example organizational, where technology can be the solution, or part thereof.

2 Background and Case

Two representatives from a network of 13 Swedish municipalities and the authors of this paper collaboratively designed the study, in which all 13 municipalities agreed to participate. A study goal was for the municipalities to become better prepared for future pandemics and unforeseen crises situations based on shared experiences and lessons learned from working, and providing care, during Covid-19. The ambition was to have three workshops and using provocative design to stir reflection and discussion among the study participants. A motivation for the study was indeed not only to generate local data to complement national or large-scale studies but also to create a forum to discuss and reflect on the pandemic, its organizational and care-providing impact, and what lessons learned could be made to inform future crisis situations. Due to a new, second wave of Covid-19, the work was put on hold after the first workshop as the daily operation of managing the provision of care had to be prioritized.

3 Method

At the end, 13 people answered the survey, representing eleven out of the 13 municipalities. Eleven of the participants identified themselves as being Head of the social service office or having an equal position (titles and organizational structures may vary between municipalities, for example between a small and larger municipality). Additionally, one identified themselves as a dedicated Covid-19 pandemic coordinator and one as a Medical responsible nurse (i.e. a nurse with specific responsibilities in the Swedish municipal healthcare system). All municipality-participants in the herein reported-on study had through their work experienced the pandemic first-hand.

The survey was composed by three parts. The first part concerned background information about the respondent like what municipality they worked in and their formal role and position within the municipality. The second part was a set of Likert-scale questions related to the effects of the pandemic within the care organization. For example how the different social care areas (i.e. Elderly Care, Subsidies and services to certain disabled persons, Individual and Family care, Community Psychiatry, and Financial Assistance) had been affected by the pandemic and to what degree the municipality had manage to adapt the above areas in respect to the pandemic. The third part was composed by 14 open-ended free-text questions. These questions covered aspects of the initial situation, for example if there was a crisis management organization ready and how the pandemic had changed care work in the municipality. The survey asked the participants to also give examples of implemented changes that had worked and not worked during the pandemic. There were also questions directly related to equipment and technology, including what technologies worked and didn't work as planned during the pandemic. Some questions also asked the respondents to reflect on what experiences from the pandemic they found valuable to bring with them into the future, including a question where the respondents should mention three lessons learned from the Covid-19 pandemic that they deem important to handle a crisis five years from now. Finally, the survey had some concluding questions, including what part of the municipality care work, aspect, or routine they found most important to work with and develop based on the Covid-19 experience. The survey was distributed and compiled online. To prepare for the workshop, the survey results were first analyzed by the two authors independently and then together. The purpose with this first analysis was to get an overview of the main results and to extract themes for the workshop based on the survey answers.

The workshop was held online with ten of the original 13 participants, using Zoom [9] and the web-based tool Mural [10]. The main part of the 3-h long workshop used Mural to conduct a so-called Future Workshop. The participants were divided into two groups with one facilitator (i.e. one of the authors) per group. Each group then had to select one of the above outlined themes (derived from analyzing the survey results). The task was then to first identify all problematic aspects related to the selected theme, group these and translate the 'problems' into their positive counterpart. These positive statements were then used to envision possible futures where the current challenges did no longer exist. The participants had to envision opportunities to move from 'today' to 'the future'. Each group then selected three such 'transformations' and presented these in plenum.

4   Related Work

Since the start of the Covid-19 pandemic, a range of existing technologies (e.g. Zoom video calls) have pervade and new technologies have been developed to answer to healthcare challenges and needs raised by the pandemic and its effect on society. These studies include for example how to support individual's health [11], designing for mHealth support [12], and Covid-19 diagnostics using AI [13]. However, few studies have investigated needs and experiences of pervasive health technologies from the perspective of care providing organizations. A Google Scholar searching CSCW (Computer-Supported Collaborative Work) and Covid-19 also reveals publications that again cover other aspects of the pandemic, for example the use of Social Media [14, 15], remote working from home [16], distance learning [17], or organizational aspects from a SME perspective

[18], rather than a care organizations perspective on pervasive technology during the pandemic.

5   Empirical Data: Survey

The background survey was intended as a starting point for the envisioned three workshop. While limited in scope and number of answers, the survey by itself provides some interesting insights. The survey shows that among the main care areas of the municipalities, and from a pandemic perspective especially elderly care was rated as challenging (4,5/5 average) followed by subsidies and services to certain disabled persons (3,3/5 average). The survey also shows that these two areas are where the municipalities best have managed to adapt their work routines: Elderly care (4,7/5) and Subsidies and services to certain disabled persons (4,0/5). Across the care organization, the main challenges reported on relate to Leadership, Routines and organizations, Ways of working, and Manning. Least reported on challenges were related to Recruitment and competence support, Digital aids, Workspaces and its layouts, and Worries among clients.

According to the survey, most municipalities got 'up to speed' with handling the pandemic situation within a few weeks and about 50% of them could adapt existing emergency plans related to pandemics in general. The municipalities to a large degree used their existing communication channels, especially their Intranet in the early stage. One municipality mentions an early implementation of web-based courses and training for all relevant staff-members about hygiene, protective gears and clothes when caring for someone in a Covid-19 context.

An important observation made by the participants was that the crisis plans that were in place did not handle long-term and extensive crises as the one created by the pandemic. The crisis plans in the municipalities were created based on scenarios with a limited crisis, such as a large fire with harmful smoke development, or a train or car accident with many injured people to take care of. There were no plans to restructure the whole society, isolate certain groups due to risk of infection and still be able to provide the weakest and most vulnerable citizens with various necessities such as food, medicine, and nursing. Various authorities gave conflicting advice and guidelines, which created concerns and ambiguity at all levels within the municipal organization and its activities. The dissemination of information was rapid and sometimes inaccurate or based on rumours. The municipalities could sometimes feel that they were required to act in a certain way, but not because of instructions from the authorities but because of media and pressure from social media posts.

When asked about changes in the different organizations that worked well, 5 out of the 11 municipalities mentioned technology or technology-related aspects, like 'digital visits in homecare', information-flow and the use of Skype for meetings. That said, two municipalities also pointed to challenges with unclear flow of information and the 'communications area' in general. When directly asked about existing or new equipment and technology that worked very well during the pandemic, 12 out of 13 respondents mentioned different IT solutions (see Table 1). The one remaining respondent simply answered that there was nothing to mention.

While the municipalities have had overall positive experiences with implementing technology solutions, we can also see challenges. For example do the respondents answer

Table 1. Equipment and technology that worked well during the pandemic.

11	Digital meetings (Skype, Zoom, Teams)
3	Digital 'visits' in homecare, cameras for remote monitoring
2	I-pads for older adults and care facilities
1	Digital activities like web-based courses for staff
1	Online shopping in homecare

that they wanted more digital alternatives to visits in persons home (home care) and that they have experienced 'technology incompatibilities' that have slowed down the rollout of these solutions. A challenge is also when for example relatives (to a person referred with homecare) do not have sufficient technology skills while expected to operate these devices. Furthermore, while they have identified the Intranet as a communication channel and hub, they also report that much information ends up as email attachments. That in turn makes it difficult to sort and navigate the information. Working with technology, using for example Skype to talk with their clients' relatives, have reportedly strengthen the municipality care workers and their overall technical competences. A reported-on and partly technology-related downside has been the difficulty at times to manage information flows, including cases of disinformation.

6   Empirical Data: Workshop

As described in the Method section, an online Future workshop was conducted using Mural based on a first analysis of the survey results. Based on the survey data, four themes were developed and brought into the workshop. The four themes were: 1) Information and the spread of information, 2) Digital tools, 3) Before and after a crisis, and 4) Each crise is different.

The ten participants were divided into two groups and each group were appointed a facilitator (i.e. the authors) to guide the participants through the workshop. The two groups decided to work with the themes 1) Information and the spread of information and 3) Before and after a crisis. Based on the experiences from inside the municipalities during the pandemic, the workshop participants collaboratively generated 69 challenges or something that didn't work well related to these two themes. Each of the 69 challenges was then rewritten so rather than representing a challenge, or negative aspect, it became its positive counterpart. The challenge "Regions and municipalities manage important issues like personal protective gear differently" was for example rewritten as "Regions and municipalities manage important issues like personal protective gear in the same way". Each identified existing challenge thereby became an opportunity or goal to design for. Using Mural, these 'opportunities' were written down on digital post-its' and then organized into clusters. The two groups developed the following seven clusters: Readymade plans, Coordination and collaboration, Roles and responsibilities, Competence and knowledge, Structure and planning, Collaboration, and Communication. These seven clusters, while in need of further analysis and a deeper understanding of what they represent, were found at the workshop to cover important areas to consider for achieving an improved future pandemic- and crises response.

Working with the identified clusters, the two groups defined three summary statements each representing what they considered being the most important take-away messages: 1) **Clear division of responsibility and roles** is a condition for participation from politicians and the organization. 2) Create a more creative process regarding risk analysis together with **clearer roles** enables structures for new ways of working. 3) **Preventive information, clear definition of roles and responsibilities and good collaboration** leads to improved safety in an unsecure world. 4) A crisis can improve collaboration and development. We use **digital channels and tools** and contribute in creating **a more digital matureness-level** that in turn leads to new possibilities, the paradox of a crisis. 5) With established **communication-plans, clear messages and repetitions** will we create conditions to create calm and less stress for both co-workers and citizens. 6) The Pandemic plan is prepared and **contains clear division of responsibility**. The plan is **available digitally** and is implemented at a management level.

In the above six statements, some words are highlighted in bold font. These words are linked with opportunities for technology in aiding municipality care service delivery. These keywords highlight the importance of clear and defined roles, division of labor, and aspects of digitalization, including the need to use digital tools and increase an overall digital matureness-level. While being the result of a single, few-hours long online workshop, the clusters and the summary statements provide insights into current and potential future roles of technology in care management.

7   Discussion

The results of our study show that several technologies and services should be in place to better meet future crises. The municipality would benefit from a clear information strategy for a crisis that include both technology and services. Regular testing of the strategy (e.g. every second year) could help to both verify that important information reaches all staff, and to discover if new equipment has been added that is not managed by the crisis plan.

Technology, especially existing technology, have been an important tool for the municipalities in providing safe and qualitative care during the pandemic. They mention especially communication-software like Zoom and Skype, but also online cameras that can be used for 'online visits' and 'night check-ups'. Another important technology is the e-commerce which has shown to be an important tool during the pandemic to provide necessities such as food, medicine and clothing to people who have been isolated. It is our understanding that these technologies also have been used prior to the pandemic, but that they have got an increased spread and use in the care organizations due to the pandemic. This is a development much like other parts of society where we for example have witnessed an increased use of Zoom during the pandemic for professional meetings, remote teaching, but also to stay in contact with families and friends. While it is too early to uncover long-term effects, it is not unlikely that for example Zoom or similar platforms will be used also after the pandemic.

Mainly, the use of these systems has not been in direct care-situations but in care planning and care preparation – for example to train staff in upgraded hygiene routines.

As a result, the change in technology use and the introduction of new technology have mainly empowered the care organizations and individual caregivers. Our work points to mainly organizational gains by using for example Zoom. That said, iPads and other tablets have been used to support communication between care receivers and their families.

Similar to the Related work, our study also points to the need and use of online teaching and learning. Zoom can be one option, but the participants also mentioned specific online and web-based courses to train staff in for example new hygiene routines. An advantage with web-based courses is that they do not require course participants to meet at a specific place at a specific time, they can study when and where it suits them. New modules and materials can also be uploaded as recommendations change over time. It would also be useful with dedicated education and training for all staff in handling new digital equipment for communication and information. Such a training program could include both computer skills and practice in finding trustworthy and official information.

The participants have also understood that they must be able to take control of the information-flow in a crisis: To ensure that the information is correct and reaches everyone. There should for example be some routine to handle contradictory information from different authorities as both the municipality organizations, their employees and clients received information from many sources and through different channels. During the Covid-19 pandemic, information also came from both official and unofficial sources, and it can be difficult to understand what information is correct. During our work, it was noted that all these information sources require the municipalities to find new ways of working with information and information technology. While no solution was found during our work, the challenge of controlling information and the need to verify correctness of information was identified.

What stands out is that much of the technology that has been implemented and used by the municipality care organizations during the pandemic, represents relatively stand-alone solutions (e.g. Zoom and online shopping platforms) that can be used in parallel with existing platforms, systems and routines. Integration takes time and resources, and municipalities – like many other larger organizations – already have numerous systems they use. There has not been any evident 'integration work', where new technology has been integrated into existing systems. There is no doubt that pervasive healthcare systems and technologies can support care in both normal and crisis situations, but these systems should be built with integration in mind.

It is not unlikely that if we would have done the same survey and workshop with some of the nurses and care assistants actually visiting people's homes rather than responsible managers from the care providing organizations, we would have seen very different topics and results. Taking a top-down perspective we have however started to uncover organizational perspectives that influence how larger care organizations value and take up (for them) new care and care-related technology.

8   Conclusion

The reported-on work is based on limited data, namely a survey and one workshop. However, the participants all had key roles and responsibilities in their respective municipality to act on, and manage, the Covid-19 pandemic. The work differentiate itself from other

Related work as it focuses on the care providing organization and municipality perspective. The results should not be seen as definite, but rather as relevant points to consider for further work – being research on building future and resilient municipality-provided care scenarios or work within municipality organizations to define plans for managing future care crises. The survey indicates how the municipalities have used both existing and new technology as a resource during the pandemic, but they have also experienced challenges implementing and using, even mundane, technology solutions to provide and manage care. It is also important that all staff, clients, and family members have access to trusted information and hence that the care organization have a system and routines in place to handle that. It is also important to understand that it is the services, enabled through different technologies, that are more important to the municipality management than the service-enabling technology. Indeed, pervasive health goes beyond specific devices and technical solutions. This paper present aspects to consider when designing pervasive healthcare solutions for a care providing organizational context. Based on the presented work, the authors also like to invite the Pervasive Health community to consider the reality of care providing municipalities and organizations and the systems currently used by these organizations, and how to build pervasive healthcare applications and technologies to integrate with these systems. There is an opportunity for the field of pervasive health to, at a higher degree then today, design for social care organizations and their specific needs – both internally and towards their patients and other customers.

Acknowledgments. We like to extend our deepest gratitude to the municipality care managers that participated in our study. We also like to thank all people involved in setting up the study.

References

1. Liu, K., Chen, Y., Lin, R., Han, K.: Clinical features of COVID-19 in elderly patients: a comparison with young and middle-aged patients. J. Infect. **80**(6), e14–e18 (2020). https://doi.org/10.1016/j.jinf.2020.03.005
2. Kremer, H.-J., Thurner, W.: Age dependence in COVID-19 mortality in Germany. Dtsch Arztebl Int **117**(25), 432–433 (2020). https://doi.org/10.3238/arztebl.2020.0432
3. Yanez, N.D., Weiss, N.S., Romand, J.-A., Treggiari, M.M.: COVID-19 mortality risk for older men and women. BMC Public Health **20**(1), 1742 (2020). https://doi.org/10.1186/s12889-020-09826-8
4. Drefahl, S., et al.: A population-based cohort study of socio-demographic risk factors for COVID-19 deaths in Sweden. Nat. Commun. **11**(1), 5097 (2020). https://doi.org/10.1038/s41467-020-18926-3
5. Szebehely, M.: Internationella Erfarenheter av Covid-19 i Äldreboenden. Underlagsrapport till SOU 2020: 80 Äldreomsorgen under pandemin, Stockholm. Hentet fra (2020). https://www.regeringen.se/4af363/contentassets
6. Requia, W.J., Kondo, E.K., Adams, M.D., Gold, D.R., Struchiner, C.J.: Risk of the Brazilian health care system over 5572 municipalities to exceed health care capacity due to the 2019 novel coronavirus (COVID-19). Sci. Total Envirn. **730**, 139144 (2020)
7. Généreux, M., et al.: One virus, four continents, eight countries: an interdisciplinary and international study on the psychosocial impacts of the COVID-19 pandemic among adults. Int. J. Environ. Res. Public Health **17**(22), 8390 (2020)

8. Gloster, A.T., et al.: Impact of COVID-19 pandemic on mental health: an international study. PloS ONE **15**(12), e0244809 (2020)
9. Zoom (2021). https://zoom.us/. Accessed 8 Oct 2021
10. Mural webspace (2021). https://www.mural.co/. Accessed 8 Oct 2021
11. Ren, X., et al.: Weaving healthy behaviors into new technology routines: designing in (and for) the COVID-19 work-from-home period. In: Paper presented at the Companion Publication of the 2020 ACM Designing Interactive Systems Conference, Eindhoven, Netherlands (2020). https://doi.org/10.1145/3393914.3395911
12. Sharma, M.: m-health services for COVID-19 afflicted and infected victims. EAI Endorsed Trans. Pervasive Health Technol. **7**(27), e1 (2021)
13. Ko, H., et al.: COVID-19 pneumonia diagnosis using a simple 2D deep learning framework with a single chest CT image: model development and validation. J. Med. Internet Res. **22**(6), e19569 (2020)
14. Drouin, M., McDaniel, B.T., Pater, J., Toscos, T.: How parents and their children used social media and technology at the beginning of the COVID-19 pandemic and associations with anxiety. Cyberpsychol. Behav. Soc. Netw. **23**(11), 727–736 (2020)
15. Gleason, C., et al.: Disability and the COVID-19 pandemic: using Twitter to understand accessibility during rapid societal transition. In: The 22nd International ACM SIGACCESS Conference on Computers and Accessibility, pp 1–14 (2020)
16. Rudnicka, A., Newbold, J.W., Cook, D., Cecchinato, M.E., Gould, S., Cox, A.: Ework-life: developing effective strategies for remote working during the COVID-19 pandemic. In: Eworklife: Developing Effective Strategies for Remote Working During the COVID-19 Pandemic. The New Future of Work Online Symposium (2020)
17. Henriksen, D., Creely, E., Henderson, M.: Folk pedagogies for teacher transitions: approaches to synchronous online learning in the wake of COVID-19. J. Technol. Teach. Educ. **28**(2), 201–209 (2020)
18. Syed, H.A., et al.: Infrastructuring for organizational resilience: experiences and perspectives for business continuity. In: Proceedings of 19th European Conference on Computer-Supported Cooperative Work. European Society for Socially Embedded Technologies (EUSSET) (2021)

Acceptance Evaluation of a COVID-19 Home Health Service Delivery Relational Agent

Ashraful Islam[(✉)] and Beenish Moalla Chaudhry

School of Computing and Informatics, University of Louisiana at Lafayette,
Lafayette 70504, USA
{ashraful.islam1,beenish.chaudhry}@louisiana.edu

Abstract. Relational Agents (RAs) may be helpful in supporting the
social distancing mandate during the COVID-19 pandemic by providing
essential health services to patients at home and eliminating the need
for in-person hospital visits. We conceptualized and developed a prototypical RA to visualize how this can be done in four major COVID-19
related health scenarios. In this paper, we present acceptance evaluation of the proposed RA using a survey based approach. A total of 105
participants were asked to interact with and analyze the prototype. Participants then indicated perceived usefulness and willingness to accept
and use the proposed RA on Likert scales. The findings show that overall
80.77% of participants found the suggested RA useful. 59.67% of participants accepted it as an alternative to healthcare professionals as long
as the scenario is not life-threatening. Furthermore, 78.29% of the participants indicated that they would be willing to use the proposed RA,
if needed. Further research is needed to understand what factors can
improve the uptake of the proposed RA among individuals ≤ 30 years
and with no COVID-19 infection history.

Keywords: COVID-19 · Relational agent · Health service · mHealth ·
Healthcare professional · User-centered design

1 Introduction

A relational agent (RA) is a computational artifact (virtual agent (VA)) that is
able to maintain a long-term virtual socio-emotional relationship with its user.
An RA may be able to replace a healthcare professional (HCP) [12] and provide an alternative to telehealth services [19] by digitally delivering the required
healthcare services to patients remotely. RAs and their cousins, conversational
agents (CAs), have been previously used for providing health behavior education
and counseling to patients [2,12,14,18] in various settings. For example, Tielman
et al. [21,22] used RAs for delivering post-therapy stress management solutions
at home and for delivering motivational messages for treatment of post-traumatic

© ICST Institute for Computer Sciences, Social Informatics and Telecommunications Engineering 2022
Published by Springer Nature Switzerland AG 2022. All Rights Reserved
H. Lewy and R. Barkan (Eds.): PH 2021, LNICST 431, pp. 40–52, 2022.
https://doi.org/10.1007/978-3-030-99194-4_4

stress disorder (PTSD). It has also been demonstrated that RA-enabled health interventions can successfully improve healthcare access in remote areas [6,24].

During the COVID-19 pandemic, the need for social distancing prompted many researchers to explore alternate ways to deliver essential health services outside the healthcare settings. A variety of CA-based interventions were developed [7,15,16], wherein VAs helped patients check their symptoms and find answers to specific questions about COVID-19. Other solutions attempted to explore whether VAs can act as emotional support companions. Ouerhani et al. [17] proposed a cloud-based mobile CA that helped people cope with various emotions during COVID-19 quarantine period by increasing their consciousness about the real dangers of psychological disturbances, e.g., unintended and sudden fear, stress, anxiety, and depression, even the tendency of committing suicide. Ishii et al. [9] developed ERICA, an empathy-driven mobile VA that employs both verbal and non-verbal methods to help persons in self-quarantine feel less isolated. A user study with 19 participants showed that gestures and facial expressions of ERICA can be effective in showing empathy and attention.

While the existing research shows that the VA-based solutions have the potential to provide a variety of COVID-19 related services to people in the comfort of their own homes, there are three important limitations of these works. First, the existing VAs are mainly targeted towards healthy individuals. Second, it remains unknown whether general public is willing to accept a VA-based COVID-19 intervention. Third, it is unknown what socio-demographic factors might influence people's willingness to use and accept a such interventions in COVID-19 pandemic. To address these gaps, we designed an RA-based prototypical intervention [11], which targets four scenarios that a COVID-19 patient is likely to encounter during their journey through the disease. In this paper, we present a study wherein we investigated these questions.

2 Proposed System

2.1 Design Process

We followed the user-centered design (UCD) methodology to develop our RA-enabled intervention. The detailed design process of proposed RA is reported in forthcoming publications. In a nutshell, the design process is divided into four stages:

- **User Persona Creation:** Three user personas were identified in a prior study [10]. We conducted background research on the CDC's COVID-19 prevention guidelines [4] and analyzed published interviews with HCPs ($n = 19$). This led to the identification of three user personas (Table 1) at different stages of COVID-19. *Oli Smith*, an individual with no existing co-morbidity, was selected to play the roles of all these personas to emphasize the relationship building aspect of the RA.
- **Interaction Scenario Development:** At this point, another interview study was conducted with persons ($n = 12$) who had been infected with

COVID-19 and therefore had firsthand experience with each persona. The study's goal was to determine which tasks an RA should be able to perform for each persona. Based on the identified tasks, four potential RA-user inter-action scenarios were established. More details about the developed scenarios can be found in [11].

- **Interaction Dialogue Development:** Four sets of dialogues were formed for RA-user interaction for each scenario. These conversations were then validated and refined based on the input from another group of HCPs (n = 43) in a separate study.
- **Prototype Design:** A web-based conversational interface design tool named *BotSociety* [1] was used to build an interactive prototype for the proposed RA. Section 2.2 contains the details of the designed prototype.

Table 1. User personas identified in context of different COVID-19 scenarios.

Suspecting infection	Quarantining at home	Recovering after infection
Oli has been suffering from fever, cough, and headache many days. They are worried that they have caught the COVID-19 virus but they do not want to go for a test unless they are sure it is necessary. Moreover, they do not know where to go for testing and what precautions to take	Oli is experiencing mild COVID-19 symptoms. They do not require hospitalization at this time. However, they have been advised to self-isolate at home until symptoms subside. They want to know what they can do to accelerate recovery and prevent emergencies	Oli has recently recovered from severe COVID-19 symptoms that required hospitalization and a week in the intensive care unit (ICU). They are back at home and wish to recover as soon as possible. But they are experiencing PTSD and need both emotional and material assistance

2.2 Interactive Prototype

The RA interfaces were multi-modal consisting of verbal (voice recognition) and non-verbal (touch, prompts, visuals) interaction modes. Figure 1 illustrates the user interface of proposed RA. The voice prompts were also appeared as text on the interface to encourage user attention and engagement with the interface. The RA was designed to build a user model by tracking their input data (e.g., symptoms and interactions). The prototype interfaces enabled users to perform the following tasks (scenarios):

- **Testing Guidance:** The RA provides testing guidance to Oli who suspects getting infected by periodically engaging in a dialog to obtain up-to-date symptom status and health metrics (Fig. 2a). Also, the RA navigates Oli to the nearest COVID-19 testing center (Fig. 2b).
- **Support During Self-isolation:** The RA provides wellness tips and companionship to Oli during self-isolation at home. The RA also monitors their symptoms to avert and prevent emergencies (Fig. 2c).

- **Handling Emergency Situations**: The RA takes appropriate steps to detect critical situations and connects Oli to emergency services, if needed (Fig. 2d).
- **Post-infection Care**: The RA provides companionship and mental health counseling to help Oli recover from the stress of the infection during the recovery phase (Fig. 2e).

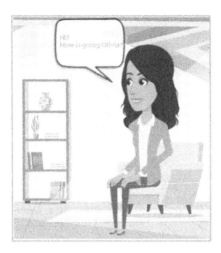

Fig. 1. The RA is available as an avatar as well as a chat interface, allowing Oli to choose between voice and text/touch modalities.

3   Preliminary Evaluation

The goal of the study was to assess whether people would find the proposed RA intervention beneficial and whether they would be willing to use and accept it. In addition, the following hypotheses were tested:

- perceived usefulness of the proposed system is dependent on history/status of infection, participants' demographics, and/or previous experience with mHealth apps,
- acceptance of the proposed system is dependent on history/status of infection, participants' demographics, and/or previous experience with mHealth apps,
- willingness to use the proposed system is dependent on history/status of infection, participants' demographics, and/or previous experience with mHealth apps.

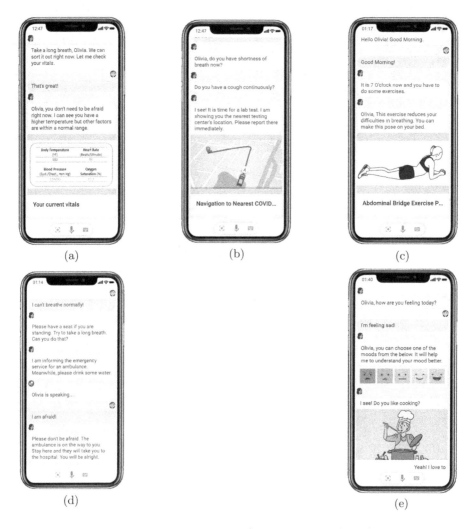

Fig. 2. Snippets from the prototype interface (smartphone view). The prototype can be simulated as a smartphone, tablet, and virtual assistant app, depending on the user's preference. (a) RA checks and displays Oli's physiological vitals; (b) RA navigates Oli to the nearest testing center; (c) RA helps Oli maintain healthy habits on a daily basis; (d) RA's interaction with Oli during an emergency situation; and (e) RA attempts to engage Oli in daily activities to reduce their PTSD symptoms.

3.1 Study Design

The research was approved by the ethical review board of our home institution. The survey started with a brief overview of the study followed by the informed consent process. After that, participants were requested to submit the basic demographic information (e.g., gender, age-range, education level, occupation, etc.). They also stated their COVID-19 infection status i.e., non-infected, currently infected, and already recovered. Then, participants were requested to interact with the RA and experience each interaction scenario (described earlier in Sect. 2.2) independently. Participants' interaction with each scenario lasted for 3–5 min. After reviewing the scenario, participants could re-review it, if they were interested.

After exploring each scenario (task) of the prototype, participants were asked to answer a series of questions aimed at assessing the quality of the interaction and helpfulness of the RA in each scenario. (The analysis of these data has been presented in a separate publication [11]). After completing their overall interaction with the prototype, participants were asked to assess the usefulness of the entire system on a Likert Scale. Participants then indicated their willingness to use the proposed RA on another Likert Scale. Finally, they indicated whether they were willing to accept the proposed system as an alternative to HCPs in non life-threatening situations.

3.2 Participants

We shared the survey link on different social media sites and email lists to obtain a diverse group of participants for the study. The following criteria were required for participation: (a) being at least 18 years old, (b) having a basic understanding of English, (c) having familiarity with a smartphone, and (d) having a basic understanding of how to operate a computer to explore the prototype. Participation was entirely voluntary, and no personally identifiable information, such as name, email address, or other contact information, was recorded. The average survey completion time was 45 min, and no incentives were given for completing the survey.

Our recruitment resulted in 105 (male = 74) responses from individuals between 18 and 64 years with a mean of 31.30 years and SD of 10.88 (18–30 years = 67, 31–40 years = 15, 41–50 years = 13, and 51–60 years = 10 individuals). Out of 52 infected participants, 26 participants were infected at the time of the survey, and 26 had already recovered. Table 2 contains detailed information on the participants' basic demographics and mHealth app experience. According to the survey responses, all participants held at least a high school diploma.

3.3 Measures and Data Analysis

Table 3 shows the metrics and questions that were used for evaluation. The survey responses were obtained in different ways, such as 5-point Likert scales (e.g., 1 stands for extremely disagree, 3 for neutral, and 5 for extremely agree), multiple-choice questions (yes, no, and neutral). Microsoft Excel, which provides various filters and functionalities, was used to conduct quantitative analysis, including descriptive and inferential analysis. The descriptive analysis consisted of calculating means, SD, percentages, and frequency distributions where necessary.

Table 2. Basic demographic and mHealth experience data of study participants.

Attribute		n
Infection Status		
	Non-Infected	53
	Infected	52
Gender		
	Male	74
	Female	31
mHealth App Experience		
	Yes	50
	No	47
	Not Sure	8
COVID-19 mHealth App Experience		
	Yes	24
	No	79
	Not Sure	2

We used two-sided Wilcoxon-Rank Sum test with continuity correction for determining statistical significance of the differences in medians of compared independent groups. This test was used because it is non-parametric and does not assume any underlying distribution for data being analyzed. Due to the small sample size, this test was assumed to be appropriate. The level of statistical significance was set at $p \leq 0.05$ for all measures.

3.4   Findings

Perceived Usefulness: Overall, 80.77% of participants thought that the modeled RA would be either very useful or useful to patients. However, 17.31% of participants were neutral about the model's usefulness, and 1.92% of participants did not think the model would benefit patients.

According to the Wilcoxon-Rank Sum test, there difference between the *perceived usefulness* scores of females versus males, and COVID-19 mHealth app experience versus no COVID-19 mHealth app experience were statistically insignificant.

Table 3. Questions used for evaluating the acceptance of proposed RA.

Metric	Question
Perceived usefulness	*Rate the unusefulness/usefulness of the COVID-19 related health services provided by the RA.*
Willingness to accept	*Indicate your unwillingness/willingness to accept the proposed RA as an alternative to caregivers/HCPs for non-life-threatening situations during COVID-19.*
Willingness to use	*Indicate your unwillingness/willingness to use the proposed RA during COVID-19.*

Statistically significant differences, however, existed between *perceived usefulness* scores of other groups. Participants ≤ 30 years versus participants above 30 years old (W-statistic $= 979$, P-value $= 0.03285$) were statistically different, with participants above 30 years old showing higher perceived usefulness of the proposed system (mean $= 4.12$ versus 4.45). Second, participants with previous mHealth app experience versus no mHealth app experience also showed statistically significant difference (W-statistic $= 886.5$, P-value $= 0.0238$), with participants without previous mHealth app experience scoring the app higher on perceived usefulness (mean $= 4.47$ versus 4.1). Finally, perceived usefulness scores of infected versus non-infected participants were also significantly different statistically (W-statistic $= 1095$, P-value $= 0.04837$), with infected participants giving a higher score (mean $= 4.46$ versus 4.13).

Willingness to Accept: Overall, the majority (60.00%) of the participants agreed that the proposed RA could be an alternative to caregivers or HCPs for non-life-threatening situations. However, 4.76% of participants declined to accept it as an alternative and the rest (35.24%) were unsure, i.e., neutral.

There was no statistically significant difference between *willingness to accept* scores of females versus males, mHealth app experience versus no mHealth app experience, and COVID-19 mHealth app experience versus no COVID-19 mHealth app experience.

Statistically significant differences, however, existed between *willingness to accept* scores of other groups. Participants ≤ 30 years versus participants above 30 years old (W-statistic $= 1017$, P-value $= 0.04767$) were statistically different, with participants ≤ 30 years old showing higher willingness to accept the proposed system (mean $= 1.52$ versus 1.32).

Willingness to Use: Overall, 78.10% of the participants expressed willingness to use the proposed RA, i.e., they were either willing or very willing in this regard. However, only 0.95% of participants were unwilling to use the RA. Nobody voted for 'Very Unwilling' and 20.95% of participants were neutral.

There was no statistically significant difference between *willingness to use* scores of infected versus non-infected participants, female versus male, and prior mHealth/COVID-19 app experience versus no mHealth/COVID-19 app experience. There was, however, a statistically significant difference between the *willingness to use* scores of participants ≤ 30 years versus participants above 30 years old (W-statistic $= 946$, P-value $= 0.019$), with participants above 30 years showing higher willingness to use the proposed system (mean $= 4.12$ versus 4.45).

Table 4 illustrates the Wilcoxon-Rank Sum test outcomes that are only statistically significant ($p < 0.05$). The Wilcoxon-Rank Sum test were experimented on the participants' votes on metrics used for the evaluation.

Table 4. Statistically significant Wilcoxon-Rank Sum test outcomes that are obtained from participants' votes on metrics used for evaluation (*suggests statistical significance i.e., P-value < 0.05).

	Perceived usefulness		Willingness to accept		Willingness to use	
	W-statistic	P-value	W-statistic	P-value	W-statistic	P-value
Infected vs. non-infected	1095	**0.04837***	1128	0.06308	1151.5	0.1179
Age (18–30 vs. 30–60 years)	979	**0.03285***	1017	**0.04767***	946	**0.019***
Male vs. female	1116.5	0.8183	1038	0.3757	1018	0.3298
mHealth experience (yes vs. no)	886.5	**0.0238***	1064	0.3523	1029	0.2544
COVID-19 mHealth experience (yes vs. no)	785	0.1657	849	0.3691	899.5	0.6853

4   Limitations

There are several limitations of this study. First, our findings can only be viewed as preliminary and indicatory. Although our sample size is large enough to run tests of statistical significance, we do not have a large enough sample size to claim generalizability. Recruiting more participants would have improved the statistical power of our findings. Second, we did not collect any qualitative data to understand the reasoning behind participants' responses to the questions explored in this study. Third, we did not have equal number of participants in each age group to help us conduct more appropriate statistical analysis. The two major groups that we analyzed in this study (i.e. ≤30 years and >30 years) were formed to compare similar sample sizes. Finally, we did not conduct a field trial of our proposed RA, the results were collected based on a one-time interaction with the RA. However, our aim was to understand the acceptability and perceived usefulness of the RA before we conducted a long-term trial, since technology trials are expensive and time consuming.

5   Discussion

The results show that the majority of participants found the proposed RA useful (80.77%) and the majority was willing to use it too (78.29%). The 59.67% majority was willing to accept the RA as a substitute for HCPs but this percentage is smaller compared to percentages of other metrics. Participants who had

COVID-19 infection, those who were >30 years old, and those who had no prior mHealth app experience perceived the RA to be more useful compared to their counterparts. Participants who were >30 years old showed higher willingness to use the RA compared to participants ≤30 years old. Finally, in comparison to their counterparts, participants ≤30 years old were more willing to accept the proposed RA as a HCP substitute for receiving COVID-19-related health services at home.

The acceptability and feasibility of RAs have been established in several studies [5,20,23]. For example, Wang et al. found that an underserved patient population was willing to use and accept an RA that collected their family health histories [23]. Similarly, Thompson et al.'s study showed that the use of behavior change RA by adolescents with diabetes and their patients demonstrated that they found the RA feasible and acceptable [20]. The majority of published studies are concerned with assessing feasibility and acceptability of RAs in patient populations. Our study differs from earlier studies in two ways. First, we investigated and compared the perceived usefulness and acceptability of the proposed RA in both patients and non-patients. Second, we also investigated perceived usefulness and acceptability based on user's prior mHealth experience and demographics (i.e., age and gender). Our findings suggest that RAs can be used by people to handle a broader variety of health issues at home.

The findings show that age may play an important role in the acceptability and perceived usefulness of the proposed RA. The higher willingness to use and perceived usefulness of the RA among individuals >30 years may have been due to infection history. Indeed, there was a higher proportion of infected individuals among participants >30 years old compared to participants ≤30 years (proportions: 0.68 versus 0.38). Moreover, we also found that participants with infection history considered the RA to be more useful as compared to participants with no infection history. This finding suggests that the proposed RA may be suitable for COVID-19 patients before, during, and after the infection. Moreover, we are behooved to explore whether the endorsement of the RA technology by infected participants will encourage the wider uptake of the proposed RA (i.e. among newly infected individuals).

We did not collect any information about participants' health status but it is also possible that participants ≤30 years were healthier as compared to participants >30 years. This may also explain why participants ≤30 years were more comfortable in terms of accepting the RA as a substitute for HCPs. Although we did not have any older adults (≥65 years) in our study, research has shown that older adults are generally accepting of RAs for receiving health related services [3]. Thus, our study may be considered as supporting the hypothesis that participants with advanced ages find RA technology more accepting.

Finally, we found that participants with no prior mHealth experience found the RA more useful compared to participants with prior mHealth experience. There are many important implications of this findings. It is possible that the RA needs additional features in order to be considered more useful by people who had used mHealth before. It is also possible that participants with prior mHealth experience did not have positive experiences with mHealth apps/interventions that they had previously used, or they did not use them long enough to see any positive changes. Several studies indicate that the apps available in the online app stores are often of low quality, compromise or pose a risk to user's private information [8], and are not based on evidence [13]. Unfortunately, we did not collect any information about participants' past experiences with other mHealth apps, e.g. for long they used them, for what purpose, why (and if) they gave up using them, etc. More information about participants' prior experience with mHealth may have shed more light on this issue.

6   Conclusion

We have presented a RA-based health service intervention that can provide essential health services during COVID-19-like pandemic. The preliminary evaluation of the intervention indicates that participants found the proposed intervention useful and there was a general willingness to use the system. Participants also thought that the intervention could be a suitable substitute for HCPs. Perceived usefulness was influenced by age, previous mHealth app experience and infection history. Willingness to accept the RA as a viable alternative to HCPs and willingness to use the RA were also influenced by age. The results suggest that the proposed system may be useful for COVID-19 patients before, during, and after the infection but certain barriers may hinder its uptake. Further research is needed to understand what factors can improve the perceptions of usefulness of the tool among users ≤ 30 years and non-infected participants. Understanding the reasons behind why people with prior mHealth experience are unwilling to use the RA may also help improve the widespread uptake of this useful tool during the pandemic.

References

1. Botsociety. https://botsociety.io/. Accessed 25 Oct 2021
2. Bhattacharyya, O., Mossman, K., Gustafsson, L., Schneider, E.C.: Using human-centered design to build a digital health advisor for patients with complex needs: persona and prototype development. J. Med. Internet Res. **21**(5), e10318 (2019). https://doi.org/10.2196/10318
3. Bickmore, T.W., et al.: A randomized controlled trial of an automated exercise coach for older adults. J. Am. Geriatr. Soc. **61**(10), 1676–1683 (2013)
4. Centers for Disease Control and Prevention: Guidance for COVID-19 (2021). https://www.cdc.gov/coronavirus/2019-ncov/communication/guidance.html. Accessed 25 Oct 2021
5. Dworkin, M.S., et al.: Acceptability, feasibility, and preliminary efficacy of a theory-based relational embodied conversational agent mobile phone intervention to promote HIV medication adherence in young HIV-positive African American MSM. AIDS Educ. Prev. **31**(1), 17–37 (2019)

6. Ferré, F., et al.: Improving provision of preanesthetic information through use of the digital conversational agent "MyAnesth": prospective observational trial. J. Med. Internet Res. **22**(12), e20455 (2020). https://doi.org/10.2196/20455, www.jmir.org/2020/12/e20455

7. Galmiche, S., et al.: Implementation of a self-triage web application for suspected COVID-19 and its impact on emergency call centers: observational study. J Med. Internet Res. **22**(11), e2294 (2020). https://doi.org/10.2196/22924, https://www.jmir.org/2020/11/e22924

8. Han, C., et al.: The price is (not) right: comparing privacy in free and paid apps. Proc. Priv. Enhanc. Technol. **2020**(3), 222–242 (2020)

9. Ishii, E., Winata, G.I., Cahyawijaya, S., Lala, D., Kawahara, T., Fung, P.: Erica: an empathetic android companion for COVID-19 quarantine. arXiv preprint arXiv:2106.02325 (2021)

10. Islam, A., Chaudhry, B.M.: Identifying user personas for engagement with a COVID-19 health service delivery relational agent. In: HAI 2021 pp. 364–366. Association for Computing Machinery, New York (2021)

11. Islam, A., Rahman, M.M., Kabir, M.F., Chaudhry, B.: A health service delivery relational agent for the COVID-19 pandemic. In: Chandra Kruse, L., Seidel, S., Hausvik, G.I. (eds.) DESRIST 2021. LNCS, vol. 12807, pp. 34–39. Springer, Cham (2021). https://doi.org/10.1007/978-3-030-82405-1_4

12. Kabir, M.F., Schulman, D., Abdullah, A.S.: Promoting relational agent for health behavior change in low and middle - income countries (LMICs): issues and approaches. J. Med. Syst. **43**(7), 1–11 (2019). https://doi.org/10.1007/s10916-019-1360-z

13. Knitza, J., Tascilar, K., Messner, E.M., Meyer, M., Vossen, D., Pulla, A., Bosch, P., Kittler, J., Kleyer, A., Sewerin, P., et al.: German mobile apps in rheumatology: review and analysis using the mobile application rating scale (MARS). JMIR mHealth uHealth **7**(8), e14991 (2019)

14. Kramer, L.L., Ter Stal, S., Mulder, B.C., de Vet, E., van Velsen, L.: Developing embodied conversational agents for coaching people in a healthy lifestyle: scoping review. J. Med. Internet Res. **22**(2), e14058 (2020). https://doi.org/10.2196/14058

15. McKillop, M., South, B.R., Preininger, A., Mason, M., Jackson, G.P.: Leveraging conversational technology to answer common COVID-19 questions. J. Am. Med. Inform. Assoc. **28**(4), 850–855 (2021). https://doi.org/10.1093/jamia/ocaa316

16. Miner, A.S., Laranjo, L., Kocaballi, A.B.: Chatbots in the fight against the COVID-19 pandemic. NPJ Digit. Med. **3**(1), 1–4 (2020)

17. Ouerhani, N., Maalel, A., Ghézala, H.B., Chouri, S.: Smart ubiquitous chatbot for COVID-19 assistance with deep learning sentiment analysis model during and after quarantine (2020). https://doi.org/10.21203/rs.3.rs-33343/v1

18. Sillice, M.A., et al.: Using relational agents to promote exercise and sun protection: assessment of participants' experiences with two interventions. J. Med. Internet Res. **20**(2), e48 (2018). https://doi.org/10.2196/jmir.7640, http://www.jmir.org/2018/2/e48/

19. ter Stal, S., Kramer, L.L., Tabak, M., op den Akker, H., Hermens, H.: Design features of embodied conversational agents in ehealth: a literature review. Int. J. Hum.-Comput. Stud. **138**, 102409 (2020)

20. Thompson, D., et al.: Using relational agents to promote family communication around type 1 diabetes self-management in the diabetes family teamwork online intervention: longitudinal pilot study. J. Med. Internet Res. **21**(9), e15318 (2019)

21. Tielman, M.L., Neerincx, M.A., Bidarra, R., Kybartas, B., Brinkman, W.P.: A therapy system for post-traumatic stress disorder using a virtual agent and virtual storytelling to reconstruct traumatic memories. J. Med. Syst. **41**(8), 1–10 (2017). https://doi.org/10.1007/s10916-017-0771-y
22. Tielman, M.L., Neerincx, M.A., Brinkman, W.P.: Design and evaluation of personalized motivational messages by a virtual agent that assists in post-traumatic stress disorder therapy. J. Med. Internet Res. **21**(3) (2019). https://doi.org/10.2196/jmir.9240
23. Wang, C., et al.: Acceptability and feasibility of a virtual counselor (VICKY) to collect family health histories. Genet. Med. **17**(10), 822–830 (2015)
24. Zalake, M., Tavassoli, F., Griffin, L., Krieger, J., Lok, B.: Internet-based tailored virtual human health intervention to promote colorectal cancer screening: design guidelines from two user studies. In: Proceedings of the 19th ACM International Conference on Intelligent Virtual Agents, IVA 2019, pp. 73–80. Association for Computing Machinery, New York (2019). https://doi.org/10.1145/3308532.3329471

The Impact of COVID-19 on LGBTQIA+ Individuals' Technology Use to Seek Health Information and Services

Taylor Schell Martinez$^{(\boxtimes)}$ ⓘ and Charlotte Tang ⓘ

University of Michigan-Flint, Flint, MI 48502, USA
{tschell,tcharlot}@umich.edu

Abstract. Fear of discrimination and stigma has often led many LGBTQIA+ individuals to seek out health information and services online and rely on digital sources. Has the LGBTQIA+ community's heavy reliance on digital use prior to the COVID-19 pandemic lessened the impact on their experience in seeking health information and services compared to the general population? Were the already existing health disparities and inaccessibility issues exacerbated?

An online survey study was conducted with 155 people who self-identified as LGBTQIA+. The goals were to investigate the technologies used by LGBTQIA+ individuals to manage their health and well-being during the COVID-19 pandemic and its impact on how they used technology to find health information, seek health services, and interact with their providers. The challenges and barriers that LGBTQIA+ respondents experienced when accessing health information and services during the pandemic were also identified, along with how these challenges may be alleviated through new or improved technological and non-technological solutions.

Our findings indicate an increased reliance on Internet-based health information seeking, mail order prescriptions, virtual appointments, and telehealth. Most participants were satisfied with the changes in format including the virtual platform used for interacting with healthcare providers. However, a substantial decrease or delay in healthcare and pharmaceutical access have been identified. We also found an increased, recurrent access to mental healthcare for coping with the pandemic. COVID-19 impacted almost every aspect of the LGBTQIA+ community's health.

Keywords: LGBTQIA+ · Health accessibility · COVID-19 pandemic · Virtual appointments

1 Introduction

Discrimination and stigma fears lead many LGBTQIA+[1] individuals to seek out health information and services online and through other digital sources despite the design

---

[1] "LGBTQIA+" is an inclusive umbrella term for all non-heteronormative gender identities and sexualities [43].

© ICST Institute for Computer Sciences, Social Informatics and Telecommunications Engineering 2022
Published by Springer Nature Switzerland AG 2022. All Rights Reserved
H. Lewy and R. Barkan (Eds.): PH 2021, LNICST 431, pp. 53–70, 2022.
https://doi.org/10.1007/978-3-030-99194-4_5

of these avenues not being inclusive of the community [1]. Has the LGBTQIA+ community's heavy reliance on digital use prior to COVID-19 lessen the impact they have experienced? Did the LGBTQIA+ community handle health-related platform transitions and the increased reliance on digital technologies for healthcare better than the general population or were the already documented disparities exacerbated? Could new technologies or improvements to existing ones improve not only LGBTQIA+ individuals' health information seeking experiences and access to health services, but also facilitate the provider-patient relationship?

Our study investigates the COVID-19 pandemics' impact on how LGBTQIA+ individuals use technology to find health information, seek health services, and interact with their medical care professionals. Online surveys were conducted with 155 people who self-identified as LGBTQIA+ to acquire a better understanding of their health information seeking behaviors, their interactions with healthcare providers, and the technologies they used to manage their health and well-being, and how these might have been impacted by the recent COVID-19 pandemic. The goal was to identify possible challenges and barriers LGBTQIA+ individuals experienced during the COVID-19 pandemic when seeking health information and accessing health care services. How these challenges may be alleviated through new or improved technological solutions were also discussed.

2 Background

The Lesbian[2], Gay[3], Bisexual[4], Transgender[5], Queer[6], Intersex[7], and Asexual[8] (LGBTQIA+) community has historically struggled to access LGBTQIA+ related health information, services, and care, forcing them to often seek alternative sources of health care information. Despite the gradually growing acceptance, the LGBTQIA+ community still experiences exclusions, prejudices, and discrimination when seeking health information and services [2–7]. Thus, the Internet has long been considered a safe, accessible, and private way to find health information and services by many LGBTQIA+ individuals of every age category [8–14].

Health disparities between LGBTQIA+ individuals and the general population have been well documented in literature (e.g., references). Long before COVID-19, the LGBTQIA+ community, "especially youth, reported higher rates of anxiety, depression, suicidal ideation and non-suicidal self-injury" [15]. The transgender community is particularly impacted, with nearly 50% reported postponing health care because they

---

[2] "Lesbian" is a woman who is sexually and emotionally attracted to another woman [43].

[3] "Gay" individuals are sexually attracted to the same sex or same gender as themselves [43].

[4] "Bisexual" means to be attracted to two genders, the same gender, and others [43].

[5] "Transgender" or "trans" is a person whose gender is different than the sex they were assigned at birth [43].

[6] "Queer" is an umbrella term to describe anyone who is not heterosexual and/or cisgender [43].

[7] "Intersex" people are "born with variations of sex characteristics that may involve genital ambiguity and/or combinations of chromosomal genotypes and sexual phenotypes other than XY-male and XX-female [43]".

[8] "Asexual" people do not experience sexual attraction or desire [43].

were unable to afford it [16]. Almost 40% of trans reported having at least one negative experience with a medical professional including "being refused treatment, verbal harassment, physical or sexual assault or having to teach the provider about transgender health in order to get appropriate care", 28% had postponed care due to discrimination and 28% had experienced harassment in the medical settings due to their gender identity [6, 16]. Within the transgender community, those of color experience even harsher disparities when attempting to find health professionals who are both LGBTQIA+ friendly and not racist, with feelings that they would be treated better if they were white or cisgender [17].

Despite recommendations from the Institute of Medicine as well as over 150 other health institutions in the United States to collect and document gender identity and sexual orientation information in electronic health records, this information is still not uniformly collected that has led to inaccuracies in statistics and missed opportunities to "assess, track, and combat population-level health disparities" [16, 18–20]. Given the clear lack of inclusion of LGBTQIA+ individuals within the medical setting and health records, they expressed that they often feel invisible. Thus, many internalize and interpret the failure to collect sexual orientation and gender identity information as a way that health professionals reinforce heteronormative, cisgender societal norms or hold possible negative attitudes or beliefs towards the LGBTQIA+ community itself [15].

Prior to the pandemic, LGBTQIA+ individuals were found to more likely use the Internet to find health information, to fill a prescription, and to communicate with their health providers via email [10]. Seeking health information and services online provides a convenient, affordable delivery that also allows privacy and safety from fears of discrimination for many LGBTQIA+ individuals [14]. Online support from social media is commonly reported as a main support mechanism for LGBTQIA+ individuals [14]. LGBTQIA+ individuals even turn to the Internet when experiencing a crisis. For example, 44% of text messages sent to CrisisTextLine, a text message-based crisis support line, were from LGBTQIA+ individuals [13]. Multiple studies have shown a pre-pandemic heavy reliance on the Internet by LGBTQIA+ individuals when seeking health information and services through online LGBTQIA+ communities and social networks [8–14].

The lack of affordable, easily accessible, credible, and representative health information and services for the community without experiencing discrimination or harassment has also caused many to seek out other LGBTQIA+ individuals and their experiences online as their main source of LGBTQIA+ related health information and services [1, 21, 22]. Many use their fellow online community members to find LGBTQIA+ friendly and knowledgeable health information, experiences, providers, and services.

Could this heavier reliance on the Internet for health information have prepared LGBTQIA+ individuals to navigate the new digital workarounds of the pandemic better than the general population? Or were the documented pre-pandemic health disparities already experienced by the LGBTQIA+ community exacerbated by the pandemic [6, 15–17, 19, 22–26]? Our study investigates the impact the COVID-19 pandemic has had on how LGBTQIA+ individuals use technology to seek health information, interact with their health care professionals, and find and access health services.

3 Methodology

3.1 Data Collection

An online survey was conducted using Qualtrics Software between November 2020 and May 2021 to acquire a better understanding of the impact of the COVID-19 pandemic on LGBTQIA+ individuals' use of technology for interacting with their health care professionals and seeking health information and services. Participants were recruited through direct emails and digital flyers posted on local, university, regional, and national LGBTQIA+ organizations', centers', clubs', and support groups' websites, social media platforms and newsletters across the United States. We received 155 completed surveys.

Both qualitative and quantitative data were collected from respondents over the age of 18 and self-identified as LGBTQIA+. There were 70 close-ended questions and 19 short answer, open-ended questions to elicit information about their demographics, LGBTQIA+ identity, health information seeking behaviors, health insurance access, and prescription drug access. Questions related to their mental health and primary care access in relation to the pandemic and technology use were also investigated. Not all questions were answered by each participant; questions may have been skipped based on their earlier responses.

3.2 Data Analysis

Descriptive statistics were used to analyze the quantitative data. Bivariate analysis was then conducted between the general population and our LGBTQIA+ respondents. Affinity diagramming was used to analyze the narrative data to identify emerging themes.

4 Findings

Our findings indicate an increased reliance on Internet-based health information seeking, mail order prescriptions, virtual appointments, and telehealth. Most participants were satisfied with the changes in format including the virtual interaction with their healthcare providers. However, a substantial decrease or delay in healthcare and pharmaceutical access have been identified. We also found an increased, recurrent access to mental healthcare for coping with the pandemic. COVID-19 impacted almost every aspect of the LGBTQIA+ community's health.

Among the participants who were unemployed, 3% were not seeking employment and 2% were unemployed due to a disability. The participants we surveyed were highly educated, significantly higher than the general U.S. population's education attainment rate. Nearly 70% of the survey participants had earned an associate degree or higher, far higher than the general population (45%) [27].

4.1 Demographics

Table 1 shows the participants' demographics: age, race/ethnicity, relationship status, education, pronouns, LGBTQIA+ identification, and employment. Sixty-two percent of

Table 1. Demographics, pronouns, LGBTQIA+ identification, race, and ethnicity

Age		**Pronouns**	
35 and under	62%	She/her/hers	43.15%
36–45	13%	He/him/his	36.99%
46–55	28.1%	They/them/theirs	12.33%
56–65	20.6%	Combination	7.53%
66–75	8.4%	**LGBTQIA+ Identities**	
76–85	2.6%	Bisexual	33.6%
Race & ethnicity		Queer	32.2%
Caucasian	66.7%	Gay	28.1%
Black	6%	Lesbian	20.6%
Asian	9%	Pansexual[a]	16.4%
Hispanic	8%	Demisexual[b]	6.9%
Relationship status		Heterosexual or straight	6.2%
Single (never married)	61%	Asexual	5.5%
Married	24%	Same-gender loving[c]	2.7%
Divorced/separated	9%	Sexual orientation changed	56.9%
Widowed	2.74%	**Employment**	
Registered domestic Partnership	2.74%	Employed	69.5%
Legally recognized Civil Union	0.68%	Retired	7%
Not currently in a relationship	37%	Students	19%
Education		Unemployed	14.3%
Graduate degree	25%	Homemaker/caregiver	1%
Bachelor's degree	40%	Illegal work	1%
Associate degree	5%	Work under the table	1.5%

[a]"Pansexual" a person who is attracted to people of all genders and sexualities [43].
[b]"Demisexual" only experience a sexual attraction to people they have a strong emotional connection with [43].
[c]"Same-gender loving" individuals are attracted to the people of the same gender [43].

the participants were aged 35 and under. This skew is likely due to the use of digital media for recruitment and conduct of the survey.

Sixty-five percent held a bachelor's degree or higher and 25% held a graduate degree. In contrast, the U.S. Census Bureau found in 2020 that the general population's educational attainment was far lower: only 45% of the general population held an Associate degree, 35% held a bachelor's degree and 12.67% held a graduate degree [27].

Despite increased acceptance, inclusion, and representation of LGBTQIA+ individuals nowadays, only 58.9% considered themselves "fully out[9]" in their personal and public lives' while 26% were out to some but "closeted[10]" to others, 11% were out to friends but closeted to family, 10% were out in their private life but closeted in their public or professional life, and 1.4% were fully in the closet.

4.2   A Comparison of Perceived Health Conditions Between LGBTQIA+ participants and General Population in the United States

Physical Health. Our findings, shown in Table 2, indicated that nearly 78% of the LGBTQIA+ participants felt they were in good to excellent health, lower than 84% of the U.S. general population who reported the same perception to the Peterson-KFF Health System Tracker [28]. Only 5.8% of our LGBTQIA+ participants felt they were in excellent health, significantly lower than the 24% of the general population who felt the same, especially considering the LGBTQIA+ population surveyed had a higher percentage covered by health insurance than the general population [28].

Table 2. Self-assessed health

Self-assessed health	General [28]	LGBTQIA+
Poor health	4%	1.65%
Fair health	12%	21%
Good health	27%	44%
Very good health	33%	28%
Excellent health	24%	6%

Nearly 21% of our respondents considered themselves to be in fair health, nearly double the 12% of the general population who felt the same [28]. Notably, 4% of the general population felt they were in poor health, substantially more than the 1.65% of LGBTQIA+ participants who felt that way in our study. The Peterson-KFF Health System Tracker found the general population were more likely to perceive their health status as excellent, very good and poor, placing more of the general population's perceived health status at either ends of the spectrum of health [28]. Our research found LGBTQIA+ individuals are more likely to perceive their health status as fair or good, placing their perceived health status in the middle of the health spectrum despite a higher percentage having insurance coverage.

Mental Health. According to the PRNewswire survey in April 2020, 75% of the general population in the U.S. reported that the COVID-19 pandemic had negatively impacted

---

[9] "Out" refers to being openly and publicly LGBTQIA+, "coming out of the closet" occurs when they publicly begin to announce their LGBTQIA+ identity [43].

[10] "Closeted" refers to not publicly disclosing their LGBTQIA+ identity [43].

their mental health [29]. The mental health of 87% of the LGBTQIA+ individuals we surveyed had been negatively impacted by COVID-19. While the American Psychiatric Association reported 36% of the general population had faced issues with their mental health [30], our study showed that over 40% of our LGBTQIA+ respondents had experienced a great deal of mental health challenges due to COVID-19. Forty percent of the respondents had sought out mental health services to cope with the impact caused by the pandemic. Ten Percent of the LGBTQIA+ respondents seeking mental health services were first timers in seeking mental health assistance. Several respondents indicated that their mental health issues had greatly interfered with their daily lives. For example, *"I am lucky to get anything done these days. Depression has really been holding me back"* (r115).

Three main themes emerged from Costa et al. on the suggested ways to help the mental wellbeing of the general population during the COVID-19 pandemic: 1) the accessibility to mental health care, 2) self-care strategies, and 3) the continued need for community support and relationships [31]. Some of these same themes emerged within our surveyed LGBTQIA+ community as well.

4.3 Health Information Seeking

Strategies Used. COVID-19 impacted health information seeking strategies and accessibility for 27% of our LGBTQIA+ respondents. Due to decreased in-person access to medical providers, libraries, community, and health centers or organizations, some participants had to change the way they sought health information to becoming more heavily reliant on the Internet. In fact, some respondents resorted to solely seeking health information on the Internet, *"Just internet research. No longer going to or contacting doctors, libraries or other in person services."* (r58). In contrast, other respondents have become more reliant on family and friends for health information which was not the case before the pandemic, *"I have discussed medical conditions with friends that I did not discuss such matters before Covid-19"* (r199). Unfortunately, a small number of participants found the health information they needed inaccessible due to the constraints rendered by the pandemic.

Information Sought. The pandemic impacted not only the ways information was sought by LGBTQIA+ respondents but also the types of information sought. General COVID-19 information was the third most searched topic by our LGBTQIA+ respondents, just behind general health information and prescription drug information.

A few LGBTQIA+ respondents mentioned specifically increasing their research on how to stay safe from the COVID-19 virus itself. A few others mentioned the addition of researching in-person appointment safety procedures and protocols instated due to COVID-19, *"I have had to read extensively online about the procedures necessary to set up appointments for my place of testing due to covid which really limited availability for appointments"* (r149). A few of those researching COVID-19 expressed the need for more credible information sources such as official health sites, *"I have been observing more official health sites and offices for information"* (r154).

4.4   Health Care Accessibility

Transportation. The main forms of transportation used by the LGBTQIA+ respondents varied and were considerably different from the general population's main forms reported by the Bureau of Transportation Statistics as shown in Table 3 [32]. Sixty percent of our LGBTQIA+ participants owned their own vehicle considerably less than the 85% of the general population in the U.S. who owns a vehicle [32]. Over twice the number of our LGBTQIA+ respondents relied on public transportation than did the general population: 9.1% of our respondents relied on subway and 2.4% relied on public buses. Another 12% walked, 8.5% relied on rides from family and friends, and 2.4% relied on car hires (e.g., Uber) for their main form of transportation.

Table 3. Main forms of transportation

Transportation type	General [32]	LGBTQIA+
Own vehicle	84.8%	60%
Public transportation	5%	11.5%
Subway	–	9.1%
Public buses	–	2.4%
Family & Friends	–	8.5%
Walking	2.6%	12%
Car hire service	0.2%	2.4%

Transportation has often been cited as a barrier to health care access which undoubtedly was further complicated by the pandemic. A few respondents indicated that they no longer used public transportation or ride shares while others expressed an increased reliance on walking, roommates, and Uber; *"Non-pandemic-NJ transit and subway; pandemic-Walking and uber (because I'm in NJ and not commuting to NYC)"* (r111).

Health Insurance. Slightly more LGBTQIA+ respondents had health insurance coverage (92%) than did the general population (89.2%) [33]. Table 4 illustrates the COVID-19 pandemic's impact on health insurance coverage of our LGBTQIA+ respondents compared to the general population of the U.S. Pre-pandemic, the LGBTQIA+ community had a higher percentage of individuals covered by health insurance, more than the general population, but were experiencing significantly more health disparities including transportation barriers, inaccessible prescriptions, inconvenient appointment times, reductions in health services, poorer perceived health status and their mental health was more negatively impacted [23]. Nearly 21% of the general population had lost their employer-sponsored insurance due to COVID-19 [34], while only 3.4% of the LGBTQIA+ respondents had, significantly less than the general population. It appears that COVID-19 had a lesser impact on health insurance coverage for our LGBTQIA+ respondents than the general population. This may be due to the higher education level of our respondents, thus possibly providing the LGBTQIA+ group with higher job security.

Table 4. COVID-19 pandemic's impact on health insurance

Health insurance	General	LGBTQIA+
Insured	89.2%	92%
Lost due to COVID-19	21%	3.4%

Fourteen percent of LGBTQIA+ participants surveyed stated their insurance plans had changed, premiums had increased, and for some there was a reduction in overall coverage. Others were pleased that COVID-19 related expenses were covered by insurance and COVID-19 testing was free. Some discussed how their insurance began covering telehealth and virtual medical appointments for the first time due to COVID-19, with some insurance companies even waiving copays for virtual appointments to encourage their use during the critical period of the pandemic.

Some respondents had trouble getting prescriptions after losing their health insurance:

"The challenge was once I lost my health insurance, during the pandemic was horrible, and I contacted my local health center after the state opened up and they help me with a prescription patient assistance program, and I got approved or allowed to continue receiving my medication. It was a long process but worth it now that I don't have health insurance just lucky that I had resources with-in my own community." (r137)

Prescriptions. The LGBTQIA+ community experienced a disproportionately higher rate of inaccessibility to prescriptions due to the pandemic, significantly more so than the general population and is shown in Table 5. Nearly a quarter of the LGBTQIA+ respondents had to change how they received their prescriptions due to COVID-19. Of those who changed methods to obtain their prescriptions, three-quarters began to have them delivered via U.S. Postal mail to minimize their risk of exposure to COVID-19 virus. Some LGBTQIA+ individuals had experienced lengthy fights with their insurance companies to get their mail ordered prescriptions covered, sometimes weeks after receiving them.

"I tried to get mail order 90-day supplies for several of my transition-related prescriptions. Initially request was denied, and insurance claimed they needed more info and authorization from my provider, had to go back and forth with them several times and took several weeks to get order to go through. More recently, I was informed via mail that some of my prescriptions were denied - not eligible for mail order apparently. They could've told me that weeks ago." (r102)

A small number of LGBTQIA+ individuals no longer entered the pharmacy to pick up their prescriptions; instead, they took advantage of the pharmacy's drive-thru or curbside pickup options to minimize their chances of exposure to COVID-19. However, the reduced hours of operation of pharmacies during the pandemic increased the difficulty and required better coordination with rides or family members that they already needed pre- pandemic in order to secure their prescriptions. In addition, a few respondents had to switch pharmacies because their previous pharmacy had been near their place of employment, but they had switched to working from home virtually or were no longer employed there.

Table 5. COVID-19 pandemic's impact on health care, mental health and medication

Health care	General	LGBTQIA+
Appointments canceled or postponed due to COVID-19	12.7% [34]	23%
Not seen a doctor due to cost in past 12 months	13.4% [35]	20%
Experienced a platform change for appointments	–	58%
Satisfied with platform change	83% [33]	70%
Mental health care		
COVID-19 pandemic negatively impacted mental health	75% [28]	87%
Had a serious impact on mental health	36% [29]	41.5%
Experienced a platform change for appointments	50% [36]	90%
Satisfied with platform change	–	75%
Prescription medications		
Changed how they received their prescription medication(s)	–	23%
Had difficulty accessing their prescribed medications	3% [28]	18%
Health insurance		
Insured	89.2% [33]	92.5%
Lost insurance due to COVID-19 pandemic	21% [34]	3.4%

Our findings of over 18% of our LGBTQIA+ respondents having difficulties in getting their prescriptions due to COVID-19 was substantially higher than the 3% among the general population according to the National Center for Health Statistics [36]. Of the LGBTQIA+ respondents who had difficulties accessing prescription, 55% were individuals whose gender identity had changed over their lifetime and 35% identified as transgender specifically. The higher percentage was due to increased challenges during the pandemic in getting the unique medications required by these LGBTQIA+ individuals.

"Estradiol valerate vials for injections have been scarce for years now, and this seems to have become even more profound during covid (though this may be happenstance). I spent weeks (without receiving a dose in the meanwhile) attempting to jump through hurdles with my healthcare provider, pharmacies, and online sources trying to get ahold of a vial. Compound pharmacies refused to make it as they claimed there was evidence of stock, while every major pharmacy attempted to order it only to send a notice a few days later that their supplier could not provide any. The only reason I was able to get a vial is one particularly dedicated pharmacist who kept on it throughout looking for sources." (r117)

As such, some alternatives were prescribed as an attempt to work around the inaccessibility issues and prescription shortages. Some of the workarounds included switching from hormone replacement therapy shots to topical testosterone cream, which unfortunately have impacted both the patients' mental and physical health because of the abrupt change that their body had a difficult time adjusting to the new medication. Worse still, such workarounds were not available to some of our respondents forcing them to go without their medication at all for some time until the pharmacy had stock again. One respondent described the multifaceted, unsuccessful attempt in securing their prescriptions and the subsequent physical toll on their body:

"I couldn't get an appointment with a trans clinic to save my soul. I saw an ad on Facebook for Planned Parenthood advertising trans care. I made an appointment. I had to download an app. I couldn't connect because the internet in my area was awful and [an internet provider] couldn't improve it for months. PP had no tech support line. I had to put a message into their portal to get them to call me. They refused to give me a regular phone appointment until I literally screamed at them. What should have been an hour-long appointment was a 20-min appointment. I got T gel instead of shots because if I had wanted to get shots, I would have needed to schedule another appointment and no way in hell was I going to go through that again. I did not get good advice about microdosing. When changes happened too fast, I went off abruptly. A few days later, I almost threw myself off of a highway overpass. At least that got me an appointment with the trans clinic at one of the hospitals in my city. Literally. People just need to a) prioritize the care of the marginalized b) listen to, and believe us, the first time we tell them what we need and c) make themselves easy to access be it by phone, webcam, in person, whatever and d) give us reliable information. Reddit should not be more informative than someone who's spent $300,000+ on med school." (r13)

Some respondents were unable to get their needed prescriptions due to transportation issues. For example, some had been relocated due to COVID-19 which forced them to have to drive to different towns to access their prescriptions. Others could not travel to a pharmacy that would accept their insurance. Others delayed getting their prescriptions until absolutely necessary because of the fear of exposure to the virus. Another respondent, who was forced to move back home with family due to the pandemic, had not filled or taken their prescription since returning home because they worried their family would discover their need for antidepressants. Another participant had been relocated to a different state which required them to get a prescription reconfirmation before they could get their prescriptions in the new state, making it more prone for them to forego their medications.

Care Accessibility. Twenty-five percent of our LGBTQIA+ respondents had trouble seeking health services due to COVID-19. Medical facilities, like LGBTQIA+ health centers, shut down and offered very limited or eliminated access entirely to in-person appointments. For many, in-person appointments were replaced by virtual consultations as safety regulations rendered the facilities to close or reduce their hours.

However, transgender people were negatively affected substantially by the reduction or elimination of in-person appointments because it also changed, reduced, or eliminated their access to their normal hormone replacement therapy. Some ended up with no hormone replacement medications at all. For others, it resulted in prescription changes that often involved transitioning from injectable hormones to an orally or topically administered hormone. As a result, many respondents experienced exceptional stress to the body, both physically and mentally, due to the sudden change or stopping of hormone treatments. Thus, the patients often needed additional care to combat the adverse effects.

Mental Health Care. Twenty-two percent of the general population experienced a reduction in mental health services during the pandemic [37], whereas over one-third of LGBTQIA+ respondents had their mental health appointments postponed or canceled due to the COVID-19 pandemic (Table 5).

Primary Health Care. "Organizations have cancelled, rescheduled or turned away 31.0% of patients" [38]. Nearly a quarter of our LGBTQIA+ survey respondents had their appointments canceled or postponed by their primary care providers (PCPs) due to the COVID-19 pandemic and one-third of our respondents have canceled or postponed appointments themselves with their PCPs to minimize possible exposure to COVID-19. The LGBTQIA+ respondents had experienced a more significant reduction in access to health care than the general population [38] (Table 5).

Appointment Platform Changes. Our LGBTQIA+ respondents experienced an increased platform change with their mental health provider than they were with their primary care providers. In October 2020, 41% of the mental health appointments for the general population were conducted via telehealth after peaking at 50% in May 2020 [38, 39]. Ninety percent of our LGBTQIA+ respondents who received mental health care during the pandemic, experienced a change in the platform for their mental health appointments which was twice the number experienced by the general population [40]. Only 58% of LGBTQIA+ respondents had experienced a platform change with their primary care provider. The platform change rates, satisfaction levels and group comparisons can be found in Table 5.

Satisfaction Level. Over 70% of our respondents were satisfied with their primary care provider's appointment platform change. Over 75% of our respondents who saw a mental health professional were satisfied with the change in platform, slightly less than the 80% satisfaction level of the general population [39, 41]. Eighty-two percent of our LGBTQIA+ respondents were satisfied with how their mental health professional handled the pandemic and 70% were satisfied with how their primary care providers did. Six percent of our LGBTQIA+ respondents were extremely dissatisfied with their mental health platform change and only 2% were extremely dissatisfied with their primary care platform change.

Benefits. Several benefits of telehealth were mentioned by our LGBTQIA+ respondents. Several respondents mentioned not having to commute or "fight traffic", thus reducing their travel time and the time needed off from work. Another respondent pointed out the cost savings from the lack of travel and therefore transportation costs. Others experienced cost savings through waived insurance copays for telehealth and virtual visits.

Some respondents enjoyed maintaining their health through telehealth from the comfort and safety of their own homes. For other respondents, it created a nation-wide pool of virtual LGBTQIA+ friendly and knowledgeable providers. Some LGBTQIA+ respondents felt empowered with the ability to quickly end well-documented condescending, discriminatory, or offensive interactions from both new and seasoned health professionals.

Drawbacks. Not all LGBTQIA+ respondents enjoyed the platform changes. Some respondents struggled with privacy issues, since finding a private space for virtual health appointments was extremely challenging and sometimes impossible. Some sat in their car to ensure privacy from roommates and neighbors during their appointments.

Many LGBTQIA+ respondents felt the telehealth experience was impersonal, uncomfortable, and minimized the ability to read body language. A few respondents even deemed virtual health less productive than in-person:

> *"I experienced a few Tele-Medicine appts and they were okay. It felt like there were more barriers to connect with the physician but once we cleared those it was relatively fine. I flourish in in-person environments, especially when referring to or referencing my body/medical needs so the experiences were lackluster and didn't every really FEEL confident in how to move forward with recovery, etc..."* (r147)

The virtual or telehealth appointment experiences exhausted a few respondents more than their normal in-person appointments did. Our respondents who had experienced technical issues became frustrated as some of their providers, in attempt to improve care, had constantly changed appointment formats, leaving the patient to struggle with new technology at each appointment.

4.5   Recommendations for Improving Healthcare Experiences During Pandemic

Technology Improvements. Despite their relatively young age and high education level, many LGBTQIA+ respondents experienced technology difficulties when interacting with their health care professionals virtually. For some, poor Internet connections and slow speeds affected their ability and experience in the virtual appointment; for others it was the poorly functioning video or telehealth software. In particular, technical support is often absent in these virtual platforms. Thus, timely technical support must be available to healthcare providers and their patients before and during virtual appointments.

In general, patients were not allowed to choose a preferred platform, greatly impacting their comfort level and experience with virtual appointments. Thus, we recommend allowing patients to choose from multiple platforms options for conducting virtual appointments.

Our respondents also criticized how disorganized the online meetings were. Some complained of the long wait times for virtual appointments. A few suggested displaying activities or educational health information pertinent to the patient while they were waiting.

Non-technical Recommendations. Most respondents were satisfied with how both their primary care and mental health providers handled the pandemic making no suggestions for improvements and applauding their providers for keeping them safe. A few LGBTQIA+ respondents offered suggestions on how providers could improve care.

One of the suggestions made by our respondents was to improve health care access for the LGBTQIA+ community during a pandemic since the inability to get an appointment has left some feeling hopeless and desperate. Many respondents also felt that their providers could have improved their outreach to patients. For example, they would like their providers to actively check on how the pandemic was impacting their life and to offer more assistance including increased appointment availability and conveying important information like procedural changes due to COVID-19, hour reduction, staff reduction, change in format, and closures. They also wanted more post-appointment follow-up calls.

5 Discussion

Our study found, as we anticipated, that technology use to seek health information and services was greatly impacted by the COVID-19 pandemic for our LGBTQIA+ respondents, thus further increasing the health disparities they experienced during this vulnerable period. Many of our LGBTQIA+ respondents not only relied on technology for health information but, due to the pandemic, also depended on it for most of their other health needs. Our LGBTQIA+ respondents experienced a significant increase in health disparities due to COVID-19 including increased transportation barriers, inaccessible prescriptions, inconvenient appointment times, reductions in health services, and their mental health was negatively impacted.

Our study found several unexpected findings. Despite a higher percentage of our LGBTQIA+ respondents being covered by health insurance; their self-assessed health statuses were lower than those of the general population. Surprisingly, only few of our LGBTQIA+ respondents had lost their health insurance due to COVID-19. But due to enacted safety protocols and fears of the virus, they were still unable to access health services despite having the coverage. Another surprising finding was the physical and mental trauma some of our LGBTQIA+ respondents suffered when they were unable to access their needed medications and health services.

Other studies have looked at the impact COVID-19 has had on the general population's access to health services and health information [25, 30–32, 36–39]. Several have studied how the pandemic affected the mental health of the general population, but none have focused on the LGBTQIA+ population during the pandemic as ours did [13, 26–28, 34]. Many have studied LGBTQIA+ health and how it could be improved with technology, but that research was conducted before the impact of the pandemic and the new heavy reliance on technology for their health care [5, 8, 11, 21, 40–42]. Unlike earlier research, our study was able to investigate the impact COVID-19 had on LGBTQIA+ respondents' mental health, health services and the experiences they had with increased technology reliance for health needs.

Our study found that the pandemic heavily impacted LGBTQIA+ respondents' technology use to seek health information and health services while simultaneously increasing health disparities within the community. Key findings should be used to improve access to health information and health services for the LGBTQIA+ community and to improve technology design to better serve both the LGBTQIA+ individuals and the general population.

6 Conclusion

Our study had several limitations that should be considered. Our sample was not representative of the population demographics in the U.S. with respect to age, race, ethnicity and education level. The racial and ethnic makeup did not align with the respective ratios in the population. Caucasians and Asians were overrepresented and Black, Hispanics, and Native Americans were underrepresented in our sample, as indicated in [42]. Our study's cohort was very young, 62% of our respondents were under the age of 35 and 77% were under the age of 45, and they were highly educated. These two factors may have increased their comfort level with and use of technology.

Due to the pandemic, respondents were only recruited via digital technology like emails and digital flyers. Therefore, we may have left out those who are less tech-savvy and those who have limited to Internet access. This may also explain why many of our respondents were young, highly educated, and comfortable with technology. Future research should include those who are less tech-savvy such that they may not use technology for their heath needs and those who do not have reliable access to the Internet.

Despite these limitations, our study revealed aggravated health disparities and inaccessibility already experienced by LGBTQIA+ respondents. Our study also identified many areas that the impact of the pandemic was experienced to a greater extent by the LGBTQIA+ respondents than the general population.

References

1. Martinez, T.S., Tang, C.: Design implications for health technology to support LGBTQ+ community: a literature review. In: PervasiveHealth: Pervasive Computing Technologies for Healthcare, pp. 367–370 (2020)
2. Pereira, G.C., Baranauskas, M.C.C.: Supporting people on fighting lesbian, gay, bisexual, and transgender (LGBT) prejudice: a cirtical codesign process. In: IHC 2017: Proceedings of the XVI Brazilian Symposium on Human Factors in Computing Systems, Joinville Brazil (2017)
3. AIChE. AIChE Diversity Report Highlights Gaps in Inclusion, CEP, pp. 4–5, October 2019
4. Subramony, D.P.: Not in our journals - digital media technologies and the LGBTQI community. TechTrends **62**, 354–363 (2018). https://doi.org/10.1007/s11528-018-0266-9
5. Kodadek, L.M., et al.: Collecting sexual orientation and gender identity information in the emergency department: the divide between patient and provide perspectives. Emerg. Med. J. **36**, 136–141 (2019)
6. National Center for Transgender Equality. 2015 U.S. Transgender Survey: Michigan State Report, Washington, DC. (2017)

7. McConnell, E.A., Clifford, A., Korpak, A.K., Phillips, G., II.: Identity, victimization, and support: Facebook experiences and mental health among LGBTQ youth. Comput. Hum. Behav. **76**, 237–244 (2017)
8. Dahlhamer, J.M., Galinsky, A.M., Joestl, S.S., Ward, B.W.: Sexual orientation and health information technology use: a nationally representative study of U.S. adults. LGBT Health **4**(2), 121–129 (2017)
9. Freund, L., Hawkins, B., Saewyc, E.: Reflections on the use of participatory mapping to study everyday health information seeking by LGBTQ youth. Proc. Assoc. Inf. Sci. Technol. **53**(1), 1–10 (2016)
10. Lee, J.H., Giovenco, D., Operario, D.: Patterns of health information technology use according to sexual orientation among US adults aged 50 and older: findings from a national respresentative sample - national health interview survey 2013–2014. J. Health Commun. **22**, 666–671 (2017)
11. Mitchell, K.J., Ybarra, M.L., Korchmaros, J.D., Kosciw, J.G.: Accessing sexual health information online: use, motivations and consequences for youth with different sexual orientations. Health Educ. Res. **29**(1), 147–157 (2014)
12. Perry, G.: Health information for lesbian/gay/bisexual/transgendered people on the internet. Internet Ref. Serv. Quart. **6**(2), 23–34 (2001)
13. Schueller, S.M., Hunter, J.F., Figueroa, C., Aguilera, A.: Use of digital mental health for marginalized and underserved populations. Curr. Treat. Options Psychiatry **6**(3), 243–255 (2019). https://doi.org/10.1007/s40501-019-00181-z
14. Strauss, P., Morgan, H., Toussaint, D.W., Lin, A., Winter, S., Perry, Y.: Trans and gender diverse young people's attitudes towards game-based digital mental health interventions: a qualitative investigation. Internet Interv. **18**, 100280 (2019)
15. Bosse, J.D., Leblanc, R.G., Jackman, K., Bjarnadottir, R.I.: Benefits of implementing and improving collection of sexual orientation and gender identity data in electronic health records. CIN: Inform. Nurs. **36**(6), 267–274 (2018)
16. Donald, C., Ehrenfeld, J.M.: The opportunity for medical systems to reduce health disparities among lesbian, gay, bisexual, transgender and intersex patients. J. Med. Syst. **39**(178) (2015). https://doi.org/10.1007/s10916-015-0355-7
17. Howard, S.D., et al.: Healthcare experiences of transgender people of color. J. Gen. Intern. Med. **10**(34), 2068–2074 (2019). https://doi.org/10.1007/s11606-019-05179-0
18. Cahill, S., Makadon, H.: Sexual orientation and gender identity data collection in clinical settings and in electronic health records: a key to ending LGBT health disparities. LGBT Health **1**(1), 34–41 (2014)
19. Dichter, M.E., Ogden, S.N.: The challenges presented around collection of patient sexual orientation and gender identity information for reduction of health disparities. Med. Care **57**(12), 945–948 (2019)
20. Grasso, C., McDowell, M.J., Goldhammer, H., Keuroghlian, A.S.: Planning and implementing sexual orientation and gender identity data collection in electronic health records. J. Am. Med. Inform. Assoc.: JAMIA **26**(1), 66–70 (2019)
21. Hawkins, B.W., Morris, M., Nguyen, T., Siegel, J., Vardell, E.: Advancing the conversation: next steps for lesbian, gay, bisexual, trans, and queer (LGBTQ) health sciences librarianship. J. Med. Libr. Assoc. **105**(4), 316–327 (2017)
22. Faulkner, S.L., Lannutti, P.J.: Representations of lesbian and bisexual women's sexual and relational health in online video and text-based sources. Comput. Hum. Behav. **63**, 916–921 (2016)
23. Hsieh, N., Ruther, M.: Despite increased insurance coverage, nonwhite sexual minorities still experience disparities in access to care. Health Aff. **36**(10), 1786–1794 (2017)
24. McKay, B.: Lesbian, gay, bisexual, and transgender health issues, disparities, and information resources. Med. Ref. Serv. Q. **30**(4), 393–401 (2011)

25. Price-Feeney, M., Ybarra, M.L., Mitchell, K.J.: Health indicators of lesbian, gay, bisexual, and other sexual minority (LGB+) youth living in rural communities. J. Pediatr. **205**, 236–243 (2019)
26. Trinh, M.-H., Agenor, M., Austin, S.B., Jackson, C.L.: Health and healthcare disparities among U.S. women and men at the intersection of sexual orientation and race/ethnicity: a nationally representative cross-sectional study. BMC Public Health **17**(962), 1–11 (2017)
27. United States Census Bureau. Educational Attainment in the United States: 2020 (2021)
28. Peterson-KFF Health System Tracker. Self-reported health. https://www.healthsystemtracker. org/indicator/health-well-being/self-reported-health-8/. Accessed 6 June 2021
29. Cision PRNewswire. Mental health concerns skyrocket, 75 percent of Americans report negative impact from the pandemic, 01 May 2020. https://www.prnewswire.com/news-rel eases/mental-health-concerns-skyrocket-75-percent-of-americans-report-negative-impact-from-the-pandemic-301050725.html. Accessed 25 May 2021
30. American Psychiatric Association. New Poll: COVID-19 Impacting Mental Well-Being: Americans Feeling Anxious, Especially for Loved Ones; Older Adults are Less Anxious, 25 March 2021. https://www.psychiatry.org/newsroom/news-releases/new-poll-covid-19-imp acting-mental-well-being-americans-feeling-anxious-especially-for-loved-ones-older-adu lts-are-less-anxious. Accessed 25 May 2021
31. Costa, M., Reis, G., Pavlo, A., Bellamy, C., Ponte, K., Davidson, L.: Tele-mental health utilization among people with mental illness to access care during the COVID-19 pandemic. Community Ment. Health J. **57**(4), 720–726 (2021). https://doi.org/10.1007/s10597-021-007 89-7
32. Bureau of Transportation Statistics. Principal Means of Transportation to Work (2020). https:// www.bts.gov/content/principal-means-transportation-work
33. ASPE Office of Health Policy. Trends in the U.S. Uninsured Population, 2010–2020, February 2021. https://aspe.hhs.gov/system/files/pdf/265041/trends-in-the-us-uninsured.pdf. Accessed 25 May 2021
34. Banthin, J., Simpson, M., Buettgens, M., Blumberg, L.J., Wang, R.: Changes in health insurance coverage due to the COVID-19 recession: preliminary estimates using microsimulation. Urban Institute, Washington, DC (2020)
35. Kaiser Family Foundation. Adults Who Report Not Seeing a Doctor in the Past 12 Months Because of Cost by Sex (2019). https://www.kff.org/other/state-indicator/could-not-see-doc tor-because-of-cost-by-sex/?currentTimeframe=0&sortModel=%7B%22colId%22:%22L ocation%22,%22sort%22:%22asc%22%7D
36. National Center for Health Statistics. Reduced Access to Care During COVID-19 (2020)
37. Centers for Medicare & Medicaid Services (CMS). CMS Data Shows Vulnerable Americans Foregoing Mental Health Care During COVID-19 Pandemic, 14 May 2021. https://www.cms.gov/newsroom/press-releases/cms-data-shows-vulnerable-ame ricans-forgoing-mental-health-care-during-covid-19-pandemic. Accessed 21 June 2021
38. Busch, A.B., Sugarman, D.E., Horvitz, L.E., Greenfield, S.F.: Telemedicine for treating mental health and substance use disorders: reflections since the pandemic. Neuropsychopharmacology **46**, 1068–1070 (2021)
39. Orrange, S., Patel, A., Mack, W.J., Cassetta, J.: Patient satisfaction and trust in telemedicine during the COVID-19 pandemic: retrospective observational study. JMIR Hum. Factors **8**(2), 1–13 (2021)
40. Fischer, S.H.: The transition to telehealth during the first months of the COVID-19 pandemic: evidence from a national sample of patients. J. Gen. Intern. Med. **36**, 849–851 (2021)
41. Nelson, H.: COVID-19 Telehealth Delivery Reaps High Patient Satisfaction, 15 April 2021. https://mhealthintelligence.com/news/covid-19-telehealth-delivery-reaps-high-patient-satisf action#:~:text=April%2015%2C%202021%20%2D%20Almost%2080,the%20COVID% 2D19%20Healthcare%20Coalition. Accessed 25 May 2021

42. United States Census Bureau, Quick Facts United States (2019). https://www.census.gov/qui
    ckfacts/fact/table/US/PST045219
43. Davis, C.O.: The Queens' English: The Lgbtqia+ Dictionary of Lingo and Colloquial
    Expressions. Clarkson Potter, New York (2021)

Remote Monitoring

Detecting Bed Occupancy Using Thermal Sensing Technology: A Feasibility Study

Rebecca Hand$^{(\boxtimes)}$ ⓘ, Ian Cleland ⓘ, Chris Nugent ⓘ, and Jonathan Synnott ⓘ

Ulster University, Newtownabbey BT37 0QB, Northern Ireland, UK
hand-r@ulster.ac.uk

Abstract. Measures of sleep and its disturbances can be detected by monitoring bed occupancy. These measures can also be used for alerting of bed exits or for determining sleep quality. This paper introduces an unobtrusive approach to detecting bed occupancy using low resolution thermal sensing technology. Thermal sensors operate regardless of lighting conditions and offer a high level of privacy making them ideal for the bedroom environment. The optimum bed occupancy detection algorithm was determined and tested on over 55,000 frames of 32×32 thermal sensor data. The developed solution to detect bed occupancy achieved an accuracy of 0.997. In this approach the location of the bed and the location of the participant is considered by classification rules to determine bed occupancy. The approach was evaluated using thermal sensor and bed pressure sensor data. Future work will focus on automatic detection of the bed location and improving the system by further reducing the false positives caused from residual heat.

Keywords: Thermal sensor · Bed occupancy detection · Bed pressure sensor · Contactless sleep monitoring · Background subtraction · Residual heat

1 Introduction

Polysomnography (PSG) and Actigraphy are considered the current gold standard in objective sleep monitoring and provide measures of sleep such as total sleep time and sleep quality [1]. PSG requires the physical attachment of obtrusive sensors to the body and is therefore normally conducted within a sleep clinic [1, 2]. Actigraphy is the continuous monitoring of movement levels by a watch-like device worn on the wrist which generates sleep metrics to aid in diagnosis of sleep disorders [3]. Actigraph devices range from medical grade devices to general wellness devices [4]. Medical grade actigraphy devices offer a high level of precision and are therefore very costly, while wellness monitoring actigraphy devices are less accurate and more affordable [4]. There are numerous commercially available unobtrusive sleep monitoring solutions based on Actigraphy such as: the Fitbit Inspire HR, a smartwatch device; Sleep Time: Cycle Alarm Timer, a smartphone app; and Withings Sleep Tracking Mat, a bed pressure sensor, to name but a few [5–7].

© ICST Institute for Computer Sciences, Social Informatics and Telecommunications Engineering 2022
Published by Springer Nature Switzerland AG 2022. All Rights Reserved
H. Lewy and R. Barkan (Eds.): PH 2021, LNICST 431, pp. 73–87, 2022.
https://doi.org/10.1007/978-3-030-99194-4_6

The aim of movement-based sleep monitoring devices, such as the wearables mentioned above, is to generate objective measures of sleep. These measures are typically combined to determine sleep quality and detect sleep disturbances. One such sleep monitoring metric is Bed Occupancy [8, 9]. Developing a metric which can accurately measure the current bed occupancy status can be used to provide a range of measurements in terms of sleep quality and sleep disturbances. In addition to bed occupancy status, many other metrics can be generated from this data such as the total time spent in bed, the timing of bed entry and exits, in addition to the number of bed exits each night. A major cause of bed exits during the night is Nocturia (i.e., waking during the night to urinate), which are recorded causes of sleep disorder and daytime fatigue in elderly [10]. Long-term sleep monitoring generates significant records of data in which patterns can be deduced and therefore deviations from these patterns can be detected as an indication of early illness [11]. Furthermore, a bed occupancy status metric can also be used to issue alerts of bed exits to caregivers, and to sound a bed exit alarm for those most at risk from falls.

The aim of this paper is to evaluate a novel unobtrusive approach to determine bed occupancy duration using low resolution thermal sensing technology. This approach is validated against the gold standard measurement from a pressure sensor and measurement from a human observer. The implementation of logical rules is proposed as a solution to limiting the effects of residual heat on the bed occupancy detection algorithm. The system is designed to produce a bed occupancy log, of which the bed occupancy duration can be determined. The bed occupancy duration determined by the thermal sensor-based system will be compared to that of the bed pressure sensor and the human observer. The contribution of this research is the development a thermal sensor-based system to detect bed occupancy from a ceiling installed thermal sensor. The remainder of this paper is structured as follows: Sect. 2 provides a detailed overview of related work, highlighting the advantages, applications, and challenges, of thermal sensing. Section 3 provides a discussion of the materials (i.e., sensor and dataset) and methods (i.e., data-preprocessing and labelling, background subtraction, and others) used in this approach to detect bed occupancy. Section 4 presents the results from of this approach to detecting bed occupancy and determining bed occupancy duration. Section 5 provides a discussion on the findings and limitations of this approach, while Sect. 6 presents the conclusions.

2   Related Work

Sleep monitoring research has largely focused on the use of actigraphy devices to detect sleep states. The use of actigraphy to detect movement and infer sleep was evaluated against simultaneously collected PSG data [12]. The sleep and wake states determined by the actigraphy device were evaluated and achieved an accuracy and sensitivity of 0.86 and 0.96, respectively, while specificity was 0.32. The low specificity arose from periods spent motionless while awake being determined as time spent asleep due to the absence of movement. Furthermore, several issues have been identified with wearable sleep monitoring technologies. Liu *et al.* discovered that wear discomfort resulted in discontinued use, and that continuous tracking was inhibited by limited battery life [13]. Wearable technologies are not considered appropriate for monitoring those living with certain diseases, such as late-stage dementia.

In recent years, the area of sleep monitoring research has focused on developing automatic, low cost, unobtrusive sensor-based systems suitable for long-term monitoring [14]. Most recent non-wearable movement-based systems designed to monitor sleep and bed occupancy include bed pressure sensors, smartphones, and cameras, including RGB (Red Green Blue), NIR (Near Infrared), and Thermal. Most bed pressure sensors are mats which incorporate a mesh of pressure sensors [15]. Bed pressure sensors can be discretely installed under the mattress out of view. Pouliot et al. developed a clinical user interface to view bed occupancy metrics, such as the number and timing of bed entries and exits, generated using an under-mattress pressure sensor [8]. Similarly, Taylor et al. generated several bed occupancy metrics and observed patterns in bed occupancy, distinguishing days of under sleeping and oversleeping, using an under-mattress pressure sensor [9]. Alternatively, a pressure sensor can be installed under the leg of the bed. Such a set-up detected the activity of lying-in bed with an accuracy of 0.93 [16]. Compared to actigraphy, bed pressure sensors offer the advantage of being an ambient sensor and therefore do not require contact with the user nor do they require being charged. Nam et al. referred to the physical and mental burden of bed pressure sensor users to ensure they are correctly positioned directly on top of the mat [17]. Like wearable devices, bed pressures sensors can also be limited by sensor placement. During an overnight two-subject data collection experiment by Jones et al., one subject did not lie directly on top of the pressure sensor therefore inhibiting the data collection for 5 of the 7.5 h [18].

Ambient sensor types including thermal sensors can overcome these limitations, and therefore researchers have looked at visual sleep monitoring solutions. A near-infrared camera-based solution was developed to detect movement body and determine sleep quality [19]. Activity levels were estimated from high-resolution (640 × 480) images and compared to actigraphy and PSG. The infrared-camera based approach achieved a slightly improved accuracy of 0.921 when compared to the actigraphy achieved accuracy of 0.912. As this approach uses high-resolution images it is fundamentally limited by privacy invasion as the participants can be identified.

To avoid such privacy concerns, Eldib et al. used a low-resolution 10-piece dual 30 × 30 visual sensor network-based system to detect motion patterns to analyze sleep [20]. The visual sensor network was installed into the living space (minus the bedroom) of one elderly participant for 10 months. This system could estimate sleep duration and achieved an accuracy of 0.8 with an absolute error range of 40 min. The ground truth in this study was provided from a sleep diary which is error-prone due to perception and memory. In the given study, the sleep diary was not completed for two weeks of the study as the participant had forgotten. This system's functionality is limited by the lighting conditions, as around 20% of the sleep durations were overestimated due to the participant standing without turning the lights on. Some nightly bathroom visits were also missed due to the participant not using the light. Thermal sensors offer advantages over RGB cameras and IR cameras as they operate regardless of lighting conditions.

Thermal imaging cameras have also been applied to several areas of sleep monitoring. Murthy et al. used a FLIR thermal image camera alongside PSG to monitor airflow and detect sleep apnea events by tracking the nostrils of participants during sleep in a clinical setting [3]. Sleep data were collected from 27 participants for 1–2 h. The thermal imaging system missed 3 of 167 epoch breathing events therefore resulting in a missed detection rate of only 1.8%. Thermal imaging camera systems do provide some user privacy as only humans can be identified as opposed to human individuals.

To further limit invasiveness a very-low resolution thermal sensor (32 × 32) may offer a benefit in terms of human identification, as presented in Fig. 1(a). This study aims to monitor bed occupancy and determine bed occupancy duration using a very-low resolution thermal sensor. Monitoring the temperature data of thermal images, biological temperature readings and a thermal sensor can be used as an alternative to actigraphy [21]. Madrid-Navarro *et al.* found that skin temperature was a good indicator of sleep fragmentation and was therefore presented as a solution to the fundamental limitation of actigraphy [22]. Similarly, Tamura *et al.* concluded that the bed surface temperature data could be used to detect movement and infer sleep duration [23]. Both studies however, used sensors which required contact with the participant or the bed, whereas in the current study a contactless thermal sensor solution is proposed. Such ceiling mounted thermal sensors often have a Field of View (FOV) capable of monitoring activity in and around a double-sized bed, therefore eliminating the need for numerous sensors.

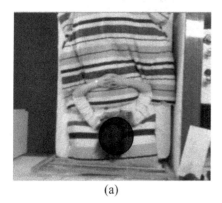
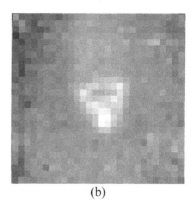

(a)   (b)

Fig. 1. (a) A 320 × 240 RGB frame and (b) the corresponding 32 × 32 greyscale thermal frame.

Contactless thermal sensors have been used for a broad range of human activity monitoring and detection. Shetty *et al.* developed a system to track participants within 8 × 8 thermal sensor data [24]. Taha designed a people counting system to detect participants entering or exiting a room using a 4 × 4 ceiling mounted thermal sensor [25]. Liang *et al.* used a 32 × 32 wall mounted thermal sensor to detect participant movement and falls [26]. The detected movement was then categorized as a fall or non-fall movement. Synnott *et al.* [27] developed a system to detect and monitor sedentary behavior using 16 × 16 thermal sensor data. Burns *et al.* [28] fused two 32 × 31 thermal sensor data to recognize kitchen activities.

Contactless thermal sensing has also been applied to sleep activity detection and monitoring. Taniguchi *et al.* developed a system to detect human posture using two 16 × 16 thermal sensors [29]. One thermal sensor was mounted to the wall and the other mounted to the ceiling. The system was able to detect transitions from 'walking' to 'lying in bed' with an accuracy of 0.889. This study focused on recognizing the transition or microevents between actual events. For example, exiting the bed is made up of four pose transitions: lying on the bed; sitting on the bed; sitting on the edge of the bed; standing beside the bed; walking. The mean accuracy of these four pose transitions is 0.889. Taniguchi *et al.* also detected falling transitions using the same set up [30]. This system was able to detect a transition from 'sitting on the bed' to 'falling from the bed' with a mean accuracy of 0.958 and a transition from 'walking' upon bed exit to 'falling' with a mean accuracy of 0.789. Again, this study focuses on detecting the microevents between actual events.

Asbjørn and Jim used a ceiling mounted 80×60 thermal sensor and ultrasonic sensor to recognize bedside events [31]. Participant location was detected using thermal data, while participant posture was detected using thermal and ultrasonic data (i.e., the number of centimeters to the nearest object). Sitting on the bed achieved a recognition rate of 0.753 while lying on the bed achieved a recognition rate of 0.881. Bed entry and exit events were detected with an accuracy of 0.987 and 0.966, respectively. The bed entry and exits events were recognized by analyzing the participants location and posture, the nearest object distance reading, and the number of changed pixels from the previous frame, across 10 consecutive frames. Our approach to detecting bed entry and bed exit events is designed to be computationally inexpensive while relying on low-resolution thermal data alone. This system was also capable of detecting 'Area Entry' and 'Area Exit' events. Area entry is detected when heat enters the sensor FOV, while area exit is detected when heat leaves the sensor FOV. The area entry events were detected with an accuracy of 0.961, while area exit events were detected with an accuracy of 0.955. Both area entry and exit events suffered from false positive and false negative readings, suggesting the systems performance could have been limited due to thermal noise.

Unlike other visual sensors such as an RGB camera or depth camera, thermal sensor systems must also incorporate a way to reduce or eliminate the effect of residual heat [32]. A study conducted by Lee *et al.*, investigated different types of residual heat, including analyzing the residual heat left from a single fingertip touch visible to a thermal camera [33]. Residual heat is generated from human body heat conducting to the surface it is in contact with and this heat may remain for an extended period of time [32, 33]. For example, after sleeping in bed overnight, the accumulated residual heat could potentially make it more difficult to differentiate the human from the residual heat [32]. Alternatively, after exiting the bed, the residual heat signature could be very similar to that of the participant lying on the bed [31]. Therefore, the effects of residual heat on detecting bed occupancy must be clarified and resolved to prevent false positives [32].

Kuki *et al.*'s system to determine the number of humans in an office environment was susceptible to the effects of residual heat [34]. Once participants had left their chair, the revealed residual heat was inaccurately determined to be a human. Consequently, 7 logical rules based on temperature and change in temperature, and heat source shape and movement were incorporated into the system, to differentiate between humans and residual heat in every frame of thermal data. This system suffered greatly from missed estimations at 51.4%, whereas the over estimation rate was only 7.5%, illustrating a reduction of false positive readings due to residual heat.

In [31] a background subtraction algorithm was designed to incorporate a residual heat disposal algorithm. This algorithm works by tracking the individual temperature of each pixel. If the pixel temperature is reducing at a steady rate, it is detected as residual heat and removed from the foreground. The performance of this algorithm is difficult to analyze due to limited discussion of factors such the time spent in bed to generate residual heat or the number of participants in the study.

This study will investigate the effects of incorporating logical rules to limit false positives resulting from residual heat. Compared to the technique implemented by Kuki *et al.*, this system will be more computationally inexpensive as only one logical rule will be used to determine a 'bed exit' and 'bed landing area exit' [34]. Only once this condition has been met, a logical value will then negate the effects of residual heat, as the heat source within the bed will be ignored by the bed occupancy algorithm. Compared to the technique in [31] this technique has been designed to be computationally inexpensive therefore only one logical value will be tracked across each frame compared to 4,800 pixels.

To summarize, researchers have considered visual bed occupancy and sleep monitoring solutions. In [19] Liao *et al.* used a near-infrared camera-based system to detect body movement and achieved an accuracy higher than actigraphy, when compared to PSG. To limit the invasiveness of such visual solutions a very low-resolution thermal sensor will be evaluated as an approach to monitoring bed occupancy. This study aims to develop a bed occupancy metric which can accurately detect presences within a single bed while participants are using a duvet. This study aims to develop a bed occupancy duration metric, derived from the bed occupancy metric, which accuracy determines bed occupancy duration compared to a bed pressure sensor. This study aims to evaluate the implementation of logical reasoning to distinguish participants from residual heat as an approach to limiting the false positives resulting from residual heat upon bed exit, the implementation of logical reasoning to distinguish humans from residual heat will be evaluated. The contribution of this research is the development a thermal sensor-based system to detect bed occupancy from a ceiling installed thermal sensor.

3   Materials and Methods

This Section details the materials and methods used by the bed occupancy detection algorithm. Firstly, the dataset collection protocol is detailed. Next, the data labelling and data pre-processing methods are presented. Finally, the methods used by the system to determine bed occupancy are explained.

3.1   Thermopile Array Sensor Setup

The thermal sensor used in the current study was a Heimann HTPA32 × 32 Infrared Thermopile Array Sensor, which has a 32 × 32 resolution, a 90-degree FOV and an ambient temperature range of −20 to 85 °C. The thermal sensor, power cable and ethernet cable were installed onto a frame, providing a birds-eye view of the bed area. The frame height was set to the standard ceiling height of 240 cm. The sensor generated temperature data with a frame rate of 7.8 Hz which is transmitted via UDP using Heimann Sensor HTPA ArraySoft v.1.28 and stored in a. txt file.

3.2 Data Collection

Ethical approval of this research was granted by Ulster University Research Ethics Filter Committee. The experiment involved collecting 20 examples of bed occupancy data from 5 participants. The participants were made up of both male and female aged 24–45. Each participant performed the activity with a target bed occupancy duration of 1 min, 3 min, 5 min, and 10 min. The data collection resulted in a total of 55,529 frames of thermal data. The participants were instructed to follow the experimental protocol: Enter the room, closing the door behind them; approach the bed; pull back the duvet, get into the bed, and cover up with the duvet; on alarm, pull back the duvet, get out of the bed replacing the duvet; exit the room and close the door. The participants were free to move within the bed throughout the bed occupancy. A researcher was present inside the room and started the timer for the specified time once the participants had entered the bed.

To provide a reference for comparison of the determined bed occupancy duration, a Tynetec bed pressure sensor (Model No. ZCS844) was installed between the mattress and bed frame. The pressure sensor creates a bed occupancy log, providing timestamped logical values representing either an "in bed" or "not in bed" status. The first instance of each status is noted, and the duration of bed occupancy is calculated.

3.3 Data Pre-processing

The thermal sensor data were imported into MATLAB and each instance was manipulated into a 32×32 matrix of temperature readings. To remove any fisheye distortion around the edge of the frame, the matrix of temperature readings was cropped with a 5 pixel-width perimeter, resulting in a resolution of 22×22. This matrix is converted into an intensity image (i.e., a greyscale image) containing values ranging from 0 (i.e., black) to 1 (i.e., white) before being rescaled by a factor of 10, resulting in a 220×220 matrix, as illustrated in Fig. 2. A bicubic interpolation method was used as it resulted in smoother and more defined images compared to the nearest-neighbor or bilinear interpolation methods.

3.4 Data Labelling

Each frame of thermal data was manually labelled 'in bed' or 'not in bed' by the researcher to provide ground truth values to measure the classification performance. The thermal data were visualized as a greyscale image with the bed location superimposed, as depicted in Fig. 3. The thermal frames were labelled 1 if the participant's blob, or more than 50% of the participant's blob, was within the location of the bed. Conversely, thermal frames were labelled 0 if the participant's blob, or more than 50% of the participant's blob, was outside the location for the bed.

3.5 Background Subtraction

The greyscale image is then segmented using a determined temperature threshold value for heat source identification. The aim of the background subtraction algorithm is to segment the hottest pixels within the frame of thermal data which may be representative

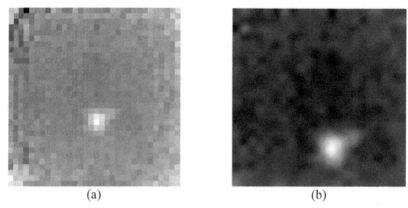

Fig. 2. A 32 × 32 greyscale image of thermal data (a). White represents the hottest pixels while black represents the coldest. The image is rescaled to a 220 × 220 greyscale thermal image (b).

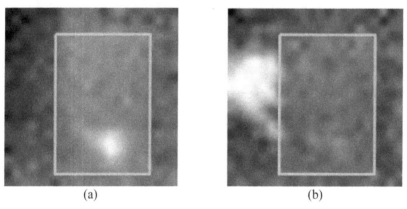

Fig. 3. Thermal frames used in the labelling processing - visualized as greyscale images with the bed location superimposed. Labels include 'in bed' (a) and 'not in bed' (b).

of a human heat source, while any other undesired sources of heat (such as from radiators, hot water bottles, or temperature drifts) are discarded and remain within the background. The temperature difference between the human body and the background reading is used for successful image segmentation.

Pixels with a value larger than the selected threshold are determined to be foreground pixels and are assigned the logical value of 1, which make up a white blob representing the participant. Pixels with a value smaller than the set threshold are determined to be background pixels and are assigned the logical value of 0. The resulting image is called a binary mask, presented in Fig. 4 (right).

3.6 Blob Detection and Tracking

The remaining white blobs within the binary mask are detected and properties are calculated for each. Blobs with a surface area of less than 20 pixels are filtered out of the

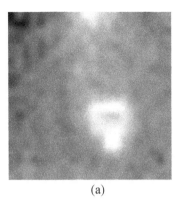 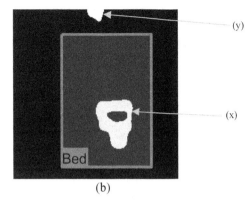

(a)   (b)

Fig. 4. A 220 × 220 greyscale thermal frame (a) and corresponding binary mask (b). The participant (x) and researcher (y) heat signatures are segmented using thresholding. The bed location is predefined and labelled. The participant is in the bed with their arms folded above the blanket. (Color figure online)

foreground and removed from the binary mask. A surface area of 20 pixels or more was determined as it allowed for successful segmentation of blobs representing a human head while preventing minor noise (e.g., a radiator) from being segmented. The centroid of each detected blob is determined, returning an x- and y-coordinate of the centre of mass of the blob within the binary image. The blob centroids are calculated and stored so that the participant's current location and previous location can be determined.

3.7 Region of Interest Identification

The location of the bed is predefined using a rectangular Region-Of-Interest (ROI). To determine the bed position within the frame of thermal data, heat emitting elements were placed on each corner of the mattress and the defined ROI encompassed these pixels. This was performed during the setup phase. The bed location is illustrated in Fig. 4 as a red rectangle.

3.8 Logical Reasoning

Logical reasoning is applied to distinguish residual heat from the participant. Using the bed ROI, bedside events such as entering the bed and exiting the bed can be identified. Including an ROI encompassing the area along the side of the bed where participants enter and exit the bed as the "landing area", means bedside events of entering the bed landing area and exiting the bed landing area can also be identified. The bed "landing area" is illustrated in Fig. 5 (right) as a blue rectangle. Once the logical steps of exiting the bed and exiting the bed landing area is identified, any remaining heat in the bed is assumed to be residual heat. The logical reasoning algorithm was designed so that is could be included or excluded in the bed occupancy algorithm for performance evaluation.

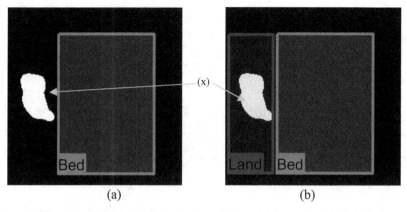

(a)   (b)

Fig. 5. Two binary masks of thermal data. The participant (x) has approached the bed. The bed location is predefined with a red rectangular ROI (a) while the bed "landing area" location is predefined with a blue rectangular ROI (b). (Color figure online)

3.9 Bed Occupancy Detection

The information obtained from both objects (i.e., ROI and blob) is used to determine if the participant is in or is not in bed. To detect presence within the bed, a timestamped logical value is returned for each frame of the timeseries data depending on if the blob's centroid coordinates are within the ROI or not. Timestamps of the first instance of an "in bed" status and the first instance of an "not in bed" status are recorded, and the bed occupancy duration is calculated for each sample of data. The bed occupancy duration determined by the system is compared to the gold stand measurement from the bed pressure sensor and the measurement from the human observer. To assess the performance of the bed occupancy detection algorithm evaluation metrics of accuracy, precision and recall are calculated.

4 Results

This Section presents the finding from this study. The performance of the bed occupancy detection algorithm with and without logical reasoning is provided in Table 1.

The measured bed occupancy duration for each target duration determined by the thermal sensor, pressure sensor and human observer is provided in Fig. 6.

4.1 Bed Occupancy Detection

The bed occupancy detection algorithm susceptible to the effects of residual heat achieved an accuracy of 0.969 and a precision of 0.964. The precision is affected by false positives, in this case, resulting from the residual heat in the bed. With logical reasoning incorporated to limit the effects of residual heat, the bed occupancy detection algorithm achieved an improved accuracy of 0.997 and a precision of 0.997.

Table 1. Performance statistics of the bed occupancy detection algorithm.

Performance measures	Bed occupancy detection	
	Without LR[*]	With LR
Accuracy	0.969	0.997
Precision	0.964	0.997
Recall	1	1

[*]Logical Reasoning

4.2 Bed Occupancy Duration

A comparison between the bed occupancy duration determined from using a thermal sensor, pressure sensor and human observer is shown in Fig. 6. Mean occupancy time refers to the mean (average) duration of which bed occupancy was detected across each sample of data, for each set target duration. A one-way ANOVA ($F(2, 57) = 0.0024$, $p = 0.9975$) determined there were no statistically significant differences amongst the methods, therefore illustrating that the system performed closely to gold standard measure from the bed pressure sensor.

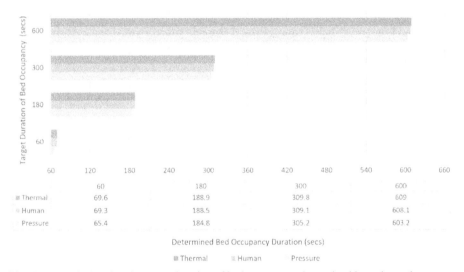

	60	180	300	600
Thermal	69.6	188.9	309.8	609
Human	69.3	188.5	309.1	608.1
Pressure	65.4	184.8	305.2	603.2

Determined Bed Occupancy Duration (secs)

■ Thermal   ■ Human   Pressure

Fig. 6. A graph showing the mean duration of bed occupancy determined by a thermal sensor, a pressure sensor and human observer. The data table is included.

5 Discussion

The bed occupancy detection algorithm with and without logical reasoning achieved a recall of 1 as no false positives were returned. This result illustrates the effectiveness of the thermal sensor data pre-processing methods, as only the human heat signatures are segmented as the foreground in images. The system only suffered from the false positives resulting from the residual heat, as was to be expected. Without logical reasoning, the system returned 1,968 false positives, reducing to 185 frames with the inclusion of the logical rules. Without the rules, the system returned false positives on all frames with residual heat after the participant exited the bed, until the residual heat temperature was less than that of the temperature threshold in the background subtraction algorithm. Whereas, with the rules, the system only returned false positives until the participant remained in contact with the residual heat on the blanket and/or mattress.

The thermal sensor consistently provided a longer duration of detected occupancy time by an average of 0.6 s (±0.24 s), compared to the human observer. This increased duration can be explained due to the residual heat on the blanket. Once the blanket becomes the same temperature as the participant it is therefore segmented as foreground pixels on the binary mask and merges with the blob of the participant. Therefore, as the participant is replacing the blanket after they have exited the bed and entered the landing area, the heat source from the participant and the heat signature from the residual heat are combined into one large foreground blob, in turn returning a false "in bed" status until the participant drops the blanket (i.e., approximately 0.6 s).

The thermal sensor consistently provided a longer duration of detected occupancy time by an average of 4.7 s (±0.68 s), compared to the pressure sensor. A large portion of this duration can be explained as the thermal sensor returns an "in bed" status once the centroid of a given heat source is within the bed location, whereas the pressure sensor returns an "in bed" status once weight has been registered on the centre of the bed. Similarly, on exiting the bed, the pressure sensor returns a "not in bed" status once body weight has been removed from the centre of the bed, whereas the thermal sensor returns a "not in bed" status once the blanket has been replaced on the bed and the heat source centroid is outside of the bed location. This variation in operation is also illustrated by the duration difference determined by the human observer. The pressure sensor consistently provided a longer duration of detected occupancy time by an average of 4.1 s (±0.47 s), compared to the human observer.

5.1 Limitations

Whilst the results are promising, this study is not without limitations. The data on which the system was tested was collected in one environment, therefore all participants used the same bed and blanket, in the same location of the room. Consequently, uncertainty remains regarding the system's performance across other sleeping environments and with varied blanket tog/thickness. Similarly, each sample of data contained the same scenario which consisted of only one bed enter and one bed exit with a short bed occupancy duration, thus the system's performance cannot be inferred for detecting bed occupancy long-term, for example, across a number of nights incorporating many bed entry and exits. The logical reasoning algorithm is also currently limited to a single occupant environment as the performance has not been evaluated in situations where another participant approaches and leaves the bed, such as in a caring situation.

The performance of this system may also be limited across different climates and weather conditions as all data were collected over a short time frame in which the weather conditions remained similar. Likewise, the system has not been tested on a range of clothing and therefore the performance may differ when very thick clothing is worn. With thicker clothing the surface temperature of the participant may appear cooler. Finally, the most fundamental limitation to the use of thermal sensing to detect bed occupancy is that heat sources can be obscured by blankets. Therefore, if the blanket is pulled up to cover the face and whole body, the system would result in a false negative as the human heat source cannot be detected.

6   Conclusions

This paper has presented a contactless approach to detecting bed occupancy using low-resolution thermal sensing timeseries data. This approach achieved the highest accuracy of 0.997 and precision of 0.997 in detecting bed occupancy. The algorithm developed in this study was capable of producing a bed occupancy log to determine the overall bed occupancy duration. The thermal sensor system consistently provided a longer duration of detected bed occupancy by an average of 4.7 s when compared to a pressure sensor and 0.6 s when compared to a human observer. The finding of this study demonstrates that the inclusion of logical reasoning to differentiate participants from residual heat improved the accuracy of the bed occupancy algorithm by 0.28, from 0.9694 to 0.9974. This study demonstrates the capabilities of a low-resolution ceiling-mounted thermal sensor to detect bed occupancy and determine occupancy duration within a bedroom environment.

It is thought that this approach could be integrated as part of a movement-based sleep monitoring system within care homes, in which bed exits and periods of restfulness can be detected for the purpose of caregiver alerts. To facilitate this, numerous metrics (such as 'bed enter time' or 'number of bed-exits') must be generated from the thermal binary images. Therefore, the focus of the future work is creating accurately represented foregrounds within the binary images.

The future work begins with updating components of the background subtraction algorithm as the current algorithm was designed to work on the collected bed occupancy data. Currently the average background temperature reading, used in the background subtraction algorithm to determine the threshold value, updates where no humans are detected in the frame. The longest example of bed occupancy recorded lasts 10 min whereas bed occupancy in the real world could be expected to be the typical sleep time of 8 h. Therefore, to ensure real world viability the background average background temperature should be closely tracked, and the threshold value continually updated. A residual heat detection and removal algorithm will also be integrated into the background subtraction algorithm. Finally, future work focuses on investigating a machine learning approach to detecting bed occupancy on a larger and more diverse dataset.

References

1. Guarnieri, B., Sorbi, S.: Sleep and cognitive decline: a strong bidirectional relationship. It is time for specific recommendations on routine assessment and the management of sleep disorders in patients with mild cognitive impairment and dementia. Eur. Neurol. **74**, 43–48 (2015)

2. Ooms, S., Ju, Y.: Treatment of sleep disorders in dementia. Curr. Treat Options Neurol. **18**, 18–40 (2016)
3. Murthy, J., et al.: Thermal infrared imaging: a novel method to monitor airflow during polysomnography. Sleep **32**(11), 1521–1527 (2009)
4. Scott, J., et al.: Can consumer grade activity devices replace research grade actiwatches in youth mental health settings? Sleep Biol. Rhythms **17**, 223–232 (2019)
5. Fitbit, Fitbit Inspire and Fitbit inspire HR Health and Fitness Trackers. https://www.fitbit.com/uk/shop/inspire. Accessed 10 May 2019
6. Apple, Sleep Time: Cycle Alarm Timer. https://apps.apple.come/us/sleep-time-cycle-alarm-timer/id555564825. Accessed 15 Jun 2020
7. Withings, Sleep Tracking Mat. www.withings.com/us/en/sleep. Accessed 20 Jun 2019
8. Pouliot, M., et al.: Bed occupancy monitoring: data processing and clinician user interface design. In: IEEE EMBS Proceedings, pp. 5810–5814 (2012)
9. Taylor, M., et al.: Bed occupancy measurements using under mattress pressure sensors for long term monitoring of community-dwelling older adults. In: IEEE MeMeA 2013 Proceedings, pp. 130–134 (2013)
10. Umlauf, M.J., et al.: Obstructive sleep apnea, nocturia and polyuria in older adults. Sleep **27**(1), 139–144 (2004)
11. Popescu, M.: Early illness detection in elderly using sensor networks: a review of the TigerPlace experience. In: IEEE EHB 2015 Proceedings, pp. 1–6 (2015)
12. Marino, M., et al.: Measuring sleep: accuracy, sensitivity, and specificity of wrist actigraphy compared to polysomnography. Sleep **36**(11), 1747–1755 (2013)
13. Liu, W., et al.: In bed with technology: challenges and opportunities for sleep tracking. In: OzCHI 2015 Proceedings, pp. 142–151 (2015)
14. Pan, Q., et al.: Current status and future challenges of sleep monitoring systems: systematic review. JMIR Biomed. Eng. **5**(1), e20921 (2020)
15. Enomoto, M., et al.: Newly developed waist actigraphy and its sleep/wake scoring algorithm. Sleep Biol. Rhythms **7**, 17–22 (2009)
16. Oguntala, G., et al.: Unobtrusive mobile approach to patient location and orientation recognition for elderly care homes. In: IWCMC 2017 Proceedings, pp. 1517–1521 (2017)
17. Nam, Y., et al.: Sleep monitoring based on a tri-axial accelerometer and a pressure sensor. Sensors **16**(5), 1–14 (2016)
18. Jones, M., et al.: Identifying movement onset times for a bed-based pressure sensor array. In: MeMeA 2006 Proceedings, pp. 111–114 (2006)
19. Liao, W.-H., Yang, C.-M.: Video-based activity and movement pattern analysis in overnight sleep studies. In: Pattern Recognition Proceedings, pp. 1–4 (2008)
20. Eldib, M., Deboeverie, F., Philips, W., Aghajan, H.: Sleep analysis for elderly care using a low-resolution visual sensor network. In: Salah, A.A., Kröse, B.J.A., Cook, D.J. (eds.) HBU 2015. LNCS, vol. 9277, pp. 26–38. Springer, Cham (2015). https://doi.org/10.1007/978-3-319-24195-1_3
21. Seba, D., et al.: Thermal-signature-based sleep analysis sensor. Informatics **4**(4), 37 (2017)
22. Madrid-Navarro, C., et al.: Validation of a device for the ambulatory monitoring of sleep patterns: a pilot study on Parkinson's disease. Front. Neurol. **10**, 1–15 (2019)
23. Tamura, T., et al.: Monitoring bed temperature in elderly in the home [ECG/body movements]. In: IEEE EMBS 1996 Proceedings, pp. 57–58 (1996)
24. Shetty, A., et al.: Detection and tracking of a human using the infrared thermopile array sensor - 'Grid-EYE'. In: ICICICT 2017 Proceedings, pp. 1490–1495 (2017)
25. Taha, A., et al.: Design of an occupancy monitoring unit: a thermal imaging-based people counting solution for socio-technical energy saving systems in hospitals. In: CEEC 2019 Proceedings, pp. 1–6 (2019)

26. Liang, Q., et al.: Activity recognition based on thermopile imaging array sensor. In: IEEE EIT 2018 Proceedings, pp. 770–773 (2018)

27. Synnott, J., et al.: Detection of workplace sedentary behavior using thermal sensors. In: IEEE EMBS 2016 Proceedings, pp. 5413–5416 (2016)

28. Burns, M., et al.: Fusing thermopile infrared sensor data for single component activity recognition within a smart environment. Sens. Actuator Netw. **8**(1), 1–16 (2019)

29. Taniguchi, Y., et al.: Estimation of human posture by multi thermal array sensors. In: IEEE SMC 2014 Proceedings, pp. 3930–3935 (2014)

30. Taniguchi, Y., et al.: A falling detection system with plural thermal array sensors. In: SCIS 2014 Proceedings, pp. 673–678 (2014)

31. Asbjørn, D., Jim, T.: Recognizing bedside events using thermal and ultrasonic readings. Sensors **17**(6), 1342 (2017). (Switzerland)

32. Larson, E., et al.: HeatWave: thermal imaging for surface user interaction. In: CHI 2011 Proceedings, pp. 2565–2574 (2011)

33. Lee, K., Lee, S.H., Park, J.-I.: Hands-free interface using breath residual heat. In: Yamamoto, S., Mori, H. (eds.) HIMI 2018. LNCS, vol. 10904, pp. 204–217. Springer, Cham (2018). https://doi.org/10.1007/978-3-319-92043-6_18

34. Kuki, M., et al.: Multi-human locating in real environment by thermal sensor. In: IEEE SMC 2013, no. 2, pp. 4623–4628 (2013)

Sensor-Based Measurement of Nociceptive Pain: An Exploratory Study with Healthy Subjects

Mevludin Memedi[1]([✉]) [ID], Adriana Miclescu[2] [ID], Lenka Katila[2] [ID],
Marianne Claesson[3], Marie Essermark[2], Per Holm[3], Gunnar O. Klein[1] [ID],
Jack Spira[3] [ID], and Rolf Karlsten[2] [ID]

[1] Informatics, Örebro University, Örebro, Sweden
mevludin.memedi@oru.se
[2] Pain Center, Uppsala University, Uppsala, Sweden
[3] Sensidose AB, Stockholm, Sweden

Abstract. Valid assessment of pain is essential in daily clinical practice to enhance the quality of care for the patients and to avoid the risk of addiction to strong analgesics. The aim of this paper is to find a method for objective and quantitative evaluation of pain using multiple physiological markers. Data was obtained from healthy volunteers exposed to thermal and ischemic stimuli. Twelve subjects were recruited and their physiological data including skin conductance, heart rate, and skin temperature were collected via a wrist-worn sensor together with their self-reported pain on a visual analogue scale (VAS). Statistically significant differences ($p < 0.01$) were found between physiological scores obtained with the wearable sensor before and during the thermal test. Test-retest reliability of sensor-based measures was good during the thermal test with intraclass correlation coefficients ranging from 0.22 to 0.89. These results support the idea that a multi-sensor wearable device can objectively measure physiological reactions in the subjects due to experimentally induced pain, which could be used for daily clinical practice and as an endpoint in clinical studies. Nevertheless, the results indicate a need for further investigation of the method in real-life pain settings.

Keywords: Pain · Sensors · Physiological data · Healthy subjects

1 Introduction

Pain is a common physical sensation, and its perception is highly subjective, based on personal experience [1]. Pain is accompanied by many elements that will modify its expression including fear, anxiety, and depression [2]. The demand for high quality postoperative pain relief has increased partly based on the goal of delivering an efficacious healthcare to reduce lengths of hospital stay and to reduce associated healthcare costs [3]. Therefore, there is a need for valid measurement of pain that can be used in routine clinical practice as primary and secondary endpoints [4] and for enhancing the patients' quality of life by suggesting an individualize treatment plan.

H. Lewy and R. Barkan (Eds.): PH 2021, LNICST 431, pp. 88–95, 2022.
https://doi.org/10.1007/978-3-030-99194-4_7

Opioids such as morphine, oxycodone, and fentanyl, commonly used in postoperative care, act on opioid receptors in the brain. Nevertheless, prolonged use of opioids postoperatively is one of the reasons for both increased opioid use and addiction development in many patients [5]. In today's healthcare, pain treatment occurs initially during the hospitalization phase. However, a large part of pain treatment and rehabilitation occur at home [6]. Where unsupervised use of opioids leads to side effects such are respiratory insufficiency and opioid addiction [7].

Pain is difficult to measure because of its multifaceted and subjective nature. Pain can be either nociceptive or neuropathic. Nociceptive pain is usually acute and is developed in response to external stimuli whereas neuropathic pain refers to damages in the nervous system that are not because of external stimuli. In routine clinical practice, Visual Analogue Scale (VAS) and Numeric Rating Scale (NRS) measure the intensity or frequency of various symptoms related to pain. However, self-rating instruments are highly subjective, based on previous experience of pain [8] and depend on many factors other than pain, e.g. mood [9].

Therefore, it is challenging to measure pain in an objective manner. Moreover, adequate pain control as well as tools to monitor dose consumption of the opioids prescribed at home are lacking. Coupling objective nociceptive pain assessment methods based on physiological indicators with dose monitoring devices enable collection of information that will reduce the risk associated with opioid treatment. It could reduce the prolonged postoperative opioid use and the effect of postoperative exposure to opioids such as misuse among high-risk patients.

The aim of this study was to develop an objective method for nociceptive pain assessment using wearable sensors. The pain-related information expressed as physiological signals was collected from healthy subjects exposed to experimental pain stimuli using sensor devices. We also investigated if multimodal physiological data could be used to identify pain-related and no pain-related episodes.

2   Methods

2.1   Study Subjects

Twelve healthy subjects were recruited in an open, single site exploratory study conducted at the Multidisciplinary Pain Centre at Uppsala University Hospital, Sweden (Table 1). All the research subjects provided, after they have been informed about the study, a written informed consent to participate. The study was approved by the Swedish Ethical Review Authority.

Table 1. Subject characteristics, mean ± standard deviation.

Variable	Value
Gender	8 males, 4 females
Mean age (years)	24.8 ± 6.8
Mean length (cm)	177.8 ± 8.4
Mean weight (kg)	75.2 ± 13.2
Mean BMI	23.6 ± 3.2

2.2 Data Collection

2.2.1 Collection of Physiological Data

To evaluate and induce pain in controlled settings, two human experimental pain models including thermal (cold) stimuli and ischemic pain were employed.

The subjects immersed their non-injured hand up to the wrist in a cold-water bath at 4 °C cooled by a refrigerated water circulator (Somedic, 2015, Sweden), for 2 min. The water level was set at a height of 7 cm to keep the stimulated area consistent. Participants were told that they would be informed by the researcher when this time period had elapsed. They were also told that they could remove their hand from the bath before 2 min if the examination become too painful. Time to withdrawal of the hand (Cold-Pressor Tolerance - CPT, seconds) from the cold water was recorded. The subjects continuously rated the pain intensity during the test stimulation and the conditioning stimulus. Pain intensity was measured using a computerized visual analog scale which ranged from 0 (no pain) to 100 (most intense pain tolerable).

During the Ischemic Block Test (IBT) the subjects were comfortably lying in a reclined position with their neck and head supported and the right forearm resting comfortably on a table in a semi-pronated position, with the elbow slightly flexed. A well-padded tourniquet was applied on the forearm, just below the elbow and inflated to 100 mm Hg above the subject's systolic blood pressure. The tourniquet was inflated for a maximum of 30 min.

Each subject performed both tests and the order of the tests was randomized, using a paper-based, sealed envelope technique. The subjects had a minimum of 45 □ 15 min between the two tests and they were instructed to tolerate the cold or the painful pressure for as long as they possibly could, but that they can terminate the trial at any time.

While performing the tests the patients wore a wrist-worn sensor (Empatica E4) on the other arm to collect physiological data including skin conductance, skin temperature, movement, and heart rate. The Empatica E4 sensor [10] was equipped with a photoplethysmography (PPG) sensor, which collected blood volume pulse used to calculate heart rate variability, a 3-axis accelerometer, which collected acceleration and physical activity, a galvanic skin response (GSR) sensor, which collected electrodermal activity (EDA), and a sensor to measure peripheral skin temperature. The EDA data was extracted by using two electrodes connected to the palm of the subjects. The sampling frequency was fixed at 64 Hz for PPG, 4 Hz for EDA, 4 Hz for temperature, and 32 Hz for acceleration signal. The data were stored locally and then transferred to a secure cloud service.

2.2.2 Self-assessed Pain

During CPT the VAS pain was collected using an electronic device. During the test the subjects were asked to slide a horizontal bar in the device using their free arm. The VAS pain score ranged from 0 mm (no pain, lower anchor) to 100 mm (unbearable pain, upper anchor). Subjects rated the intensity of cold test-stimulus continuously until they became pain free. The pain scoring during ischemic test continued minimum 3 min after the test or until pain and physiological signals have normalized.

During IBT the pain was reported orally on the NRS scale (0-no pain, 10-maximal pain) every minute during the first 10 min of the test and then every second minute till the 30 min interval. The reporting of pain continued till maximum 15 min after the tourniquet pressure was released and physiological signals have normalized.

2.3 Data Analysis

2.3.1 Feature Extraction

The recorded signals of the sensor were processed to extract clinically relevant information related to pain. The acceleration data were omitted since the subjects were specifically asked to move during the tests. During the thermal stimuli the body temperature might have influenced the results and due to this fact, the peripheral skin temperature signal was omitted when analyzing the data collected during the CPT.

For the IBT test, a window of 3 min was used to extract the features. For the CPT test, the signals were separated into two windows: before the test (baseline) and during the test (intervention). In total, 58 features were calculated: 17 from the EDA of the PPG sensor, 17 from blood volume pulse (BVP) and 12 from heart rate (HR) of the PPG sensor, and 12 features from peripheral skin temperature signal.

For each of the four signals: EDA, BVP, skin temperature, and HR, the following 12 features were calculated: (1) mean of the signal, (2) standard deviation of the signal, (3) skewness of the signal, (4) mean of low-frequency coefficients extracted from first level Discrete Wavelet Transform (DWT), (5) standard deviation of first level low-frequency DWT coefficients, (6) mean of first level high-frequency DWT coefficients, (7) standard deviation of first level high-frequency DWT coefficients, (8) mean of second level high-frequency DWT coefficients, (9) standard deviation of second level high-frequency DWT coefficients, (10) mean of third level high-frequency DWT coefficients, (11) standard deviation of third level low-frequency DWT coefficients, and (12) Approximate Entropy of the signal. Ten additional features were calculated for EDA and BVP based on the study performed by Nabian et al. [11]. For EDA the following additional features were calculated: mean duration of skin conductance response, mean amplitude of skin conductance response, mean rise-time skin conductance response, mean skin conductance, and number of detected skin conductance responses. For BVP, mean diastolic pressure, mean systolic pressure, mean dicrotic peak pressure, mean dicrotic notch pressure, and mean arterial pressure were calculated and used in the feature set.

To reduce the dimensions of the 58 extracted features from the different modalities a Principal Component Analysis (PCA) was applied. After PCA, the first 4 principal components (PCs) were used in subsequent analysis. All the feature extraction analysis were performed with MATLAB 9.6.

2.3.2 Statistical Analysis

All statistical analysis was performed with Minitab 19. Descriptive statistics are presented as means and standard deviations for continuous variables and absolute numbers and percentages for categorical variables. To assess if the PCs (principal components) were coherent with subjective, perceived pain, VAS correlation coefficients were calculated. To assess differences in mean PCs between the baseline (no stimuli) and intervention periods one-way ANOVA was applied. Test-retest reliability of the PCs was assessed by calculating their intraclass correlation coefficients (ICC) between the baseline (before applying tourniquet pressure) and the first window that is the first 3 min of the IBT test.

3 Results

3.1 Self-assessed Pain

For the IBT, the mean NRS increased from the first 3 min window till the end of the test (Fig. 1) and was significantly different ($p < 0.05$). For the CPT test, the mean VAS was significantly different ($p = 0$) between the baseline and intervention windows (Fig. 2).

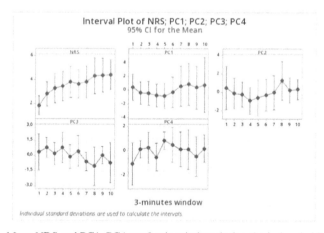

Fig. 1. Mean NRS and PC1–PC4 per 3 min window during the ischemic block test.

3.2 Sensor-Based Measures of Pain

For the CPT test, only mean PC3 was significantly different between the baseline and intervention windows ($p < 0.01$, Fig. 2).

For the IBT test, there were weak correlations between NRS and the four PCs with correlation coefficients ranging from 0.067 to 0.217. After comparing the NRS and PC scores between the baseline window (3 min before the IBT test) and the last window (last 3 min before tourniquet pressure release) it was shown that the duration of tourniquet application corresponds with increased pain scores, demonstrated by significant differences NRS pain (p = 0) and PC4 (p < 0.005) (Fig. 1). All four PCs, except PC2, demonstrated good test-retest reliability (Table 2).

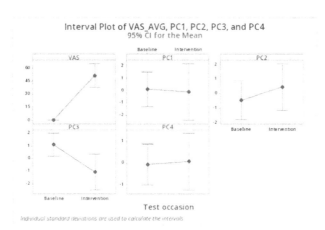

Fig. 2. Mean VAS and PC1–PC4 during the baseline and intervention test occasions during the cold pressor test.

Table 2. Intra-class correlation coefficients of VAS and PC1–PC4 between the baseline and follow-up test windows during the ischemic block test.

Variable	ICC
VAS	1
PC1	0.84
PC2	0.22
PC3	0.89
PC4	0.8

4 Discussion and Conclusion

In this study a multimodal sensor-based method for quantification of experimental, nociceptive pain intensity induced by two pain stimuli models (thermal CPT and ischemic IBT tests) is proposed. The method used information related to pain collected from multiple sensors (temperature, PPG, and GSR). The data were obtained from healthy subjects exposed to experimental pain stimuli of different intensities and durations.

A weak correlation between the PCs and self-assessments of pain using VAS and NRS was found. Correlating objective measures of pain to self-assessed pain remains controversial [12]. When no correlation is found the assumption is that the objective method is not valid. On the other hand, when good correlation is demonstrated the objective method does not add any value in the assessment of nociceptive pain, which could indicate that the easy-to-use pain rating scales could be preferred in daily clinical practice. As suggested by Wagemakers et al. [12] an additional measure to validity is test-retest reliability to assess the reproducibility of the sensor-based scores. From Table 2, the PCs, except PC2, had good test-retest reliability indicating that the scores show consistent values associated with the healthy subjects.

The results indicated that the mean PC3 was significantly different between the baseline and intervention windows of the CPT test (Fig. 2). The PCs were not derived by mapping them to self-assessed pain scores but instead they were obtained in a data-driven manner by fusing information from multiple sensors through reduction of individual features in a new data space using PCA, which can be seen as strength of the proposed methodology. The findings from this study suggested that the proposed method of collecting data from multiple devices could be used to detect and differentiate episodes of experimental-induced pain from periods with no pain. This could lead to a low-cost method to determine and quantify a patient's pain more objectively. Similar results were obtained by Chu et al. [13] using a multiple physiological signal method. Their method was developed in healthy volunteers subjected to an externally induced pain by an electrical simulator. The method could correctly classify pain intensity during different electrical stimulus levels.

The results from this study indicate that combining multiple physiological markers can be used to objectively measure pain, which is complex in nature. This multimodal approach seems to provide a good prediction of pain intensity [14]. In the study it can be noticed that the subjective pain sensation measured by VAS and NRS in healthy subjects does not truly follow the physiological measurements. For instance, some patients scored high pain on the VAS and NRS scales without having any visible sign of pain and viceversa [12]. It was a priori understood that experimental pain reflected only a part of the multidimensional, complex pain experience that could not be compared directly to clinical pain. To overcome confounders of the experimental system in healthy volunteers and to validate the results from this study it is necessary to collect data from patients experiencing real life pain. In the future, a new study with postoperative pain patients will be performed. The new study design will focus on continuous collection of physiological data in a non-invasive way from patients and their opinions on their pain.

One limitation of the study is the low number of healthy subjects and observations, which in turn limits the generalizability of the method. Due to this limitation, we could not compute correlations during the CPT since we had two observations (baseline and intervention) per subject. Additionally, this limited us to employ machine learning on the data and to try to relate features extracted from the multiple sensors with the VAS and NRS.

In conclusion, the results from this study indicated that the method could objectively detect pain periods in subjects with experimentally induced pain by a thermal stimulus.

Further evaluation is needed to assess its validity and reliability for continuous and personalized assessment and treatment of pain with opioids.

Acknowledgment. The study has been supported by the Swedish Agency for Innovation (VIN-NOVA) under the project "Controlled treatment of opiate-requiring pain using biosensors - SEN-SOP" in collaboration between the Multidisciplinary Pain Centre and Rehabilitation Medicine at Uppsala University Hospital, Sensidose AB, and Örebro University.

References

1. Bhardwaj, P., Yadav, R.J.: Measuring pain in clinical trials: pain scales, endpoints, and challenges. Int. J. Clin. Exp. Physiol. **2**, 151–156 (2015)
2. Michaelides, A., Zis, P.: Depression, anxiety and acute pain: links and management challenges. Postgrad. Med. **131**, 438–444 (2019)
3. Rawal, N.: Current issues in postoperative pain management. Eur. J. Anaesthesiol. **33**, 160–171 (2016)
4. Triano, J.J., McGregor, M., Cramer, G.D., Emde, D.L.: A comparison of outcome measures for use with back pain patients: results of a feasibility study. J. Manipulative Physiol. Ther. **16**, 67–73 (1993)
5. Lanzillotta, J.A., Clark, A., Starbuck, E., Kean, E.B., Kalarchian, M.: The impact of patient characteristics and postoperative opioid exposure on prolonged postoperative opioid use: an integrative review. Pain Manag. Nurs. **19**, 535–548 (2018)
6. Chou, R., et al.: Management of postoperative pain: a clinical practice guideline from the American pain society, the American society of regional anesthesia and pain medicine, and the American society of society of anesthesiologists' committee on regional anesthesia, executive committee, and administrative council. J. Pain **17**, 131–157 (2016)
7. Hah, J.M., Bateman, B.T., Ratliff, J., Curtin, C., Sun, E.: Chronic opioid use after surgery: implications of perioperative management in the face of the opioid epidemic. Anesth. Analg. **125**, 1733–1740 (2017)
8. Angelini, E., Wijk, H., Brisby, H., Baranto, A.: Patients' experiences of pain have an impact on their pain management attitudes and strategies. Pain Manag. Nurs. **19**, 464–473 (2018)
9. Taenzer, P., Melzack, R., Jeans, M.E.: Influence of psychological factors on postoperative pain, mood and analgesic requirements. Pain **24**, 331–342 (1986)
10. Empatica Homepage. https://www.empatica.com/en-eu/research/e4/. Accessed 2 Sept 2021
11. Nabian, M., Yin, Y., Wormwood, J., Quigley, K.S., Barret, L.F., Ostadabbas, S.: An open-source feature extraction tool for the analysis of peripheral physiological data. IEEE J. Trans. Eng. Health Med. **6**, 1–11 (2018)
12. Wagemakers, S.H., van der Velden, J.M., Gerlich, A.S., Hindriks-Keegstra, A.W., van Dijk, J.F.M., Verhoeff, J.J.C.: A systematic review of devices and techniques that objectively measure patients' pain. Pain Physician **22**, 1–13 (2019)
13. Chu, Y., Zhao, X., Han, J., Su, Y.: Physiological signal-based method for measurement of pain intensity. Front. Neurosci. **11**, 279 (2017)
14. Cowen, R., Stasiowska, M.K., Laycock, H., Bantel, C.: Assessing pain objectively: the use of physiological parameters. Anaesthesia **70**, 828–847 (2015)

Dynamics Reconstruction of Remote Photoplethysmography

Lin He$^{(\boxtimes)}$, Kazi Shafiul Alam, Jiachen Ma, Richard Povinelli,
and Sheikh Iqbal Ahamed

Marquette University, Milwaukee, WI, USA
lin.he@marquette.edu

Abstract. Photoplethysmography based medical devices are widely used for cardiovascular status monitoring. In recent years, many algorithms have been developed to achieve cardiovascular monitoring results comparable to the medical device from remote photoplethysmography (rPPG). rPPG is usually collected from the region of interest of the subject face and has been used for heart rate detection. Though there were many works on the study of chaos dynamics of PPG, very few are on the characteristics of the rPPG signal. The main purpose of this study is to discover rPPG dynamics from nonlinear signal processing techniques, which may provide insight for improving the accuracy of cardiovascular status monitoring. Univ. Bourgogne Franche-Comté Remote PhotoPlethysmoGraphy dataset is used for the experiment. The results show rPPG is considered as chaotic. The best-estimated embedding dimension for the rPPG signal is between 3 to 4. The time delay is 10 for an interpolated 240 Hz rPPG signal. The interpolation process will increase the complexity level and reduce the correlation dimension of the rPPG. The bandpass filtering process will reduce the complexity level and the correlation dimension of the rPPG. Introducing the features derived from reconstructed phase space such as Lyanpunov exponent, correlation dimension and approximate entropy, could improve the accuracy of heart rate variability detection from rPPG.

Keywords: Remote photoplethysmography · Phase space reconstruction · Heart rate · Heart rate variability

1 Introduction

Cardiovascular disease is one of the most prevalent diseases for adults over 20 years old in the United States [1]. Photoplethysmography (PPG) based medical devices are widely used for cardiovascular health monitoring in clinical settings. PPG is a typical noninvasive method that measures subtle changes in the light reflection from human skin due to the blood volume variations through the cardiovascular pulse cycle [2]. Professional PPG measurement devices are expensive

Published by Springer Nature Switzerland AG 2022. All Rights Reserved
H. Lewy and R. Barkan (Eds.): PH 2021, LNICST 431, pp. 96–110, 2022.
https://doi.org/10.1007/978-3-030-99194-4_8

and uncomfortable to use. In recent years, several algorithms have been developed to achieve heart rate (HR) and heart rate variability (HRV) results similar to professional devices through remote PPG (rPPG), which uses a camera to collect a video of the region of the skin from a distance instead of using near-infrared light for PPG recording. The rPPG signals could be extracted from the video recordings and provide similar health monitoring results to PPG signals.

There are many works about nonlinear analysis of the PPG signals to improve the detection accuracy and discover underlying characteristics of the PPG signals. PPG signals collected from healthy young human subjects is consistent with the definition of chaos movement [3]. The method of phase space reconstruction has been applied to PPG signals and shows PPG can provide an earlier warning of deterioration based on PPG signals because it provides a similar trend for the parameters derived from arterial blood pressure (ABP) [4]. There are also studies on PPG signals collected not from near-infrared light. The experiment results show the PPGs collected under the red or green light is chaotic [5].

In addition to PPG, nonlinear signal processing techniques also apply to the rPPG. It is possible to use phase space reconstruction on the rPPG signals collected from the skin of the wrist. The interpolated and filtered signals can be considered as noise-contaminated deterministic signals [6]. However, the previous studies are based on PPG signals with a high sampling rate, mostly 200 Hz or the study of the rPPG collected in an area with little noise and motion. There has been little work on rPPG chaotic analysis based on video collected from the face, which has a lower sampling rate 30 Hz and large noise due to the distance and the motion of the body. In this paper, we present the analysis of the chaotic dynamics of rPPG collected from human face videos.

The contribution of this paper is as follows:

- We compared the chaotic dynamics for different PPG and rPPG signals.
- We use the phase space reconstruction method to discover the underlying characteristics of rPPG.
- We showed introducing the features derived from reconstructed phase space could improve the accuracy of HRV detection.

The structure of the remaining parts of the paper is as follows: In Sect. 2, we present the method we used for rPPG extraction. Section 3 evaluates the results of the dynamics of PPG and rPPG signals. In Sect. 4, we present conclusions.

2   Related Works

2.1   rPPG Extraction Methods

PPG signals can be collected from fingertips positioned on a smartphone camera [7]. However, this method still requires the subject to stay in a fixed position, which has the same disadvantage of traditional methods. Poh et al. [8] proposed a new non-contact method, which is known as remote PPG (rPPG). The method uses the front face of the phone camera to extract PPG signals and heart rate measurements has a $RMSE < 5bpm$ and a correlation of 0.95. [9] extends the work by using CHROM for rPPG extraction for heart rate detection. This method is further implemented by [10], which provides an algorithm with improvement in the detection accuracy for heart rate and heart rate variability for low-resolution videos. [11] proved the Plane orthogonal to the Skin-tone method (POS) can generate a better quality signal than CHROM for heart rate measurement. It also compared the signal to noise ratio (SNR) of different rPPG extraction approaches and proved the rPPG from POS has an average SNR of 5.16, which is larger than all the other approaches. Table 1 shows the different related works on rPPG extraction algorithm developed over the years.

Table 1. Algorithms on rPPG extraction

Ref.	ROI	Algorithm	Parameter	Year
Poh et al. [8]	Face	BSS	HR	2010
Lewandowska et al. [12]	Forehead	ICA	HR	2012
de Haan et al. [9]	Face	CHROM	HR	2013
de Haan et al. [13]	Face	PBV	HR	2014
Wang et al. [14]	Face	2SR	HR	2016
Huang et al. [10]	Face	CHROM	HR, HRV	2016
Wang et al. [11]	Face	POS	HR	2017

2.2 Dataset Used for rPPG Testing

Many efforts have been made in recent years on studying the rPPG algorithms on heart rate with existing public datasets such as MAHNOB and MMSE-HR. However, these videos are under strong compression making valuable information impossible to extract [15]. Normally heart rate estimation requires a lower quality video than heart rate variability. An uncompressed video data set is required to derive the best results of heart rate variability. We developed the algorithms and compared the performance on the public data set UBFC-rPPG.

Univ. Bourgogne Franche-Comte Remote PhotoPlethysmoGraphy (UBFC-rPPG) is a data set proposed for remote PPG (rPPG) studies [16]. Subject faces were recorded using a webcam (Logitech C920 HD Pro) at 30fps and a resolution of 640 × 480. The video file is an avi file in an uncompressed 8-bit RGB format. The ground truth PPG signal wave was recorded using the CMS50E transmissive pulse oximeter. It is a popular data set used for the validation of different rPPG approaches. The video files and ground truth data are used in this research.

3 rPPG Extraction Method

Our approach mainly follows the method proposed by Huang et al. [10]. Some recent enhancements such as amplitude selective filtering [20] and plane orthogonal to skin tone method [11] are included. The flowchart of the whole method is in Fig. 1.

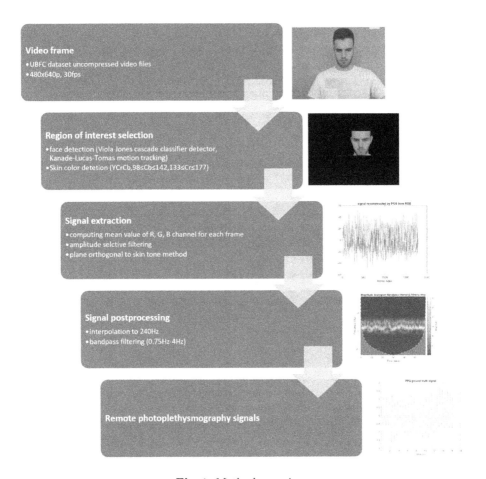

Fig. 1. Method overview

3.1 Region of Interest Selection

The region of interest (ROI) is first selected by the face detection algorithm using Viola-Jones detection [17] and Kanade-Lucas-Tomasi [18] for motion tracking. After the face detection algorithm locates the position of the face in a rectangular bounding box, the skin detection algorithm is applied to the ROI to select the skin pixels in the YCrCb color space [19]. As provided, a pixel is detected as skin if $98 \leq Cb \leq 142, 133 \leq Cr \leq 177$.

3.2   Signal Extraction

After the skin pixels are selected from the ROI, the mean value of the RGB channels of each frame is calculated to form a series of raw signals of R, G, B channel. Then, amplitude selective filtering [20] is used to eliminate noise distortions from the signals. The plane orthogonal to the Skin-tone method [11] is used to extract pulse signals from the RGB signals. It assumes the RGB signals are the mixture result from three different source signals. One of them is the pulse signal and the others are light sources or background noise. The algorithm is based on the study of the optical and physiological model of the skin reflection and can separate the pulse signal that is independent of the skin tone and the light source. The result from [11] shows rPPG from POS has an average SNR of 5.16, which is larger than all the other extraction methods.

3.3   Signal Postprocessing

After the pulse signal is extracted, postprocessing steps are used for denoising. Because the signal is sampled 30 Hz, interpolation 240 Hz is needed to smooth the signal.

There are many approaches for post-processing the rPPG signal. The most widely used approach is bandpass filtering, which is to select only the magnitude of the signal within the pulse rate range (0.75 Hz 4 Hz) and to use inverse wavelet transformation to reconstitute the signal.

4   Chaotic Dynamics Analysis of PPG and rPPG

4.1   PPG and rPPG Signals

UBFC-rPPG is a dataset containing video data of an average length of 1 min. Logitech C920 HD Pro is used to collect the video of the frontal face at a distance of about 1 m from the camera. All experiments are conducted indoors with varying amounts of sunlight and indoor illumination. The recordings have an uncompressed AVI format at 30 fps and a resolution of 640 × 480. The ground truth PPG signal was recorded simultaneously using the CMS50E transmissive pulse oximeter. An example of the ground truth PPG signal is in Fig. 2.

Based on the data provided by the UBFC-rPPG data set, we extract 4 signals for phase space reconstruction. The ground truth PPG signal is not uniformly sampled. To apply the approach, we interpolate the ground-truth signal 240 Hz by linear spline (PPG 240 Hz). The rPPG signal is extracted from the video files at an original frequency 30 Hz (rPPG 30 Hz) and interpolated 240 Hz (rPPG 240 Hz). Then the signal is bandpass filtered by the continuous wavelet transformation (rPPG filtered).

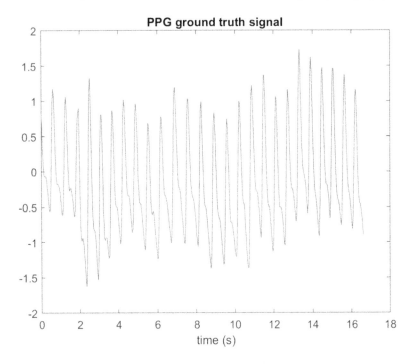

Fig. 2. Ground truth PPG signal

4.2   Phase Space Reconstruction

A uniformly sampled time series signal with a single variable $X =$ $(x_1, x_2, x_3 \ldots x_n)$ can be reconstructed a phase space which has m-dimension. If the embedding method uses time lag τ, the delayed reconstruction has coordinates as $X_r = (x_j, x_{j+\tau}, \ldots x_{j+(m-1)\tau})$.

The time delay τ can be estimated by finding the first minimum value of the average mutual information (AMI), which is computed as

$$AMI(t) = \sum_{i=1}^{N} p(x_i, x_{i+t}) log_2 [\frac{p(xi, x_{i+t})}{p(x_i)p(x_{i+t})}]$$ (1)

where N is the length of the signal and t is the time lag.

The embedding dimension m can be estimated using the false nearest neighbor algorithm. For a dimension m, the points X_i^r and nearest point X_i^{r*} are false neighbors if

$$\sqrt{\frac{D^2(m+1) - D^2(m)}{D^2(m)}} > Threshold$$ (2)

where $D^2(m) = ||X_i^r - X_i^{r*}||^2$.

The result for the estimation of the time delay τ and embedding dimension are in Figs. 3 and 4.

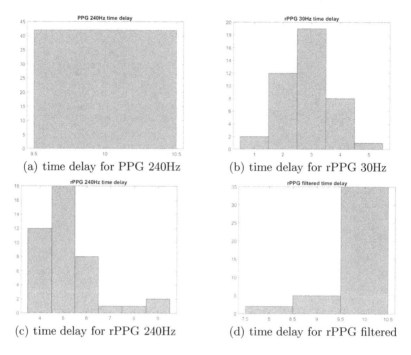

(a) time delay for PPG 240Hz

(b) time delay for rPPG 30Hz

(c) time delay for rPPG 240Hz

(d) time delay for rPPG filtered

Fig. 3. The estimated time delay τ for 4 signals. Histogram x-axis: the value range of the τ. Histogram y-axis: frequency

The estimated time delay for rPPG 30 Hz is centered and 3. The estimated time delay for PPG 240 Hz and rPPG filtered is mostly at $\tau = 10$ and for rPPG 240 Hz is centered at $\tau = 5$. It shows after the filtering step, the estimated time delay change from 5 to 10. The bandpass filtering for rPPG signal is required to keep the time delay τ similar to the PPG signal after interpolation. The embedding dimension for all signals is either $m = 3$ or $m = 4$. And PPG 240 Hz, rPPG 30 Hz, and rPPG 240 Hz have the majority of the signal from 42 subjects at embedding dimension $m = 4$. After bandpass filtering by continuous wavelet transformation, the rPPG filtered has a majority of embedding dimension $m = 3$. It shows that the postprocessing of the signal by bandpass filtering reduces the complexity of the signal.

An example of the phase space reconstruction result is shown in Fig. 5. The phase space reconstruction result is based on the 4 signals collected and extracted from Subject No. 10. The embedding dimension is $m = 3$ for data visualization purposes. The time delay $\tau = 10$ for PPG 240 Hz and rPPG filtered and $\tau = 3$ for rPPG 30 Hz and $\tau = 5$ for rPPG 240 Hz. The example shows there are similarities between the PPG 240 Hz and the rPPG filtered signal.

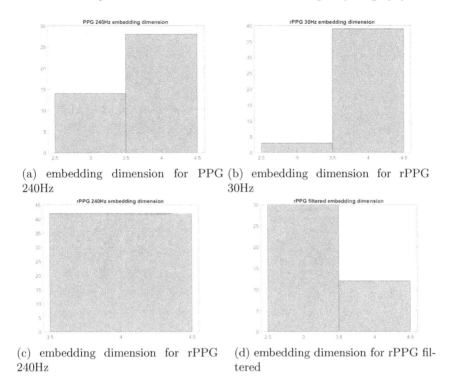

(a) embedding dimension for PPG 240Hz

(b) embedding dimension for rPPG 30Hz

(c) embedding dimension for rPPG 240Hz

(d) embedding dimension for rPPG filtered

Fig. 4. The estimated embedding dimension m for 4 signals. Histogram x-axis: the value range of the m. Histogram y-axis: frequency

4.3 Lyapunov Exponent

A chaotic system is sensitive to initial conditions. The chaotic level can be quantified by the Lyapunov exponent, which is used to characterize the trajectories in the phase space to measure the rate of divergence of neighboring trajectories. Any chaotic system must have at least one positive Lyapunov exponent. So the largest Lyapunov exponent (LLE) can be used to determine whether a system is chaotic. The algorithm for computing LLE mainly follows [21]. The LLE of all signals is positive, indicating the PPG and rPPG signals are consistent with the definition of a chaos dynamic system.

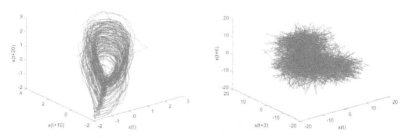

(a) reconstructed trajectories for PPG (b) reconstructed trajectories for rPPG
240Hz   30Hz

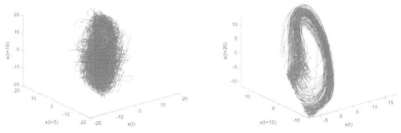

(c) reconstructed trajectories for rPPG (d) reconstructed trajectories for rPPG
240Hz   filtered

Fig. 5. An example of reconstructed trajectories in $m = 3$ for 4 signals

4.4 Correlation Dimension

The correlation dimension is usually refers to a type of fractal dimension, which measures the dimension of the space occupied by random points. It can be used to separate the chaos from random noise. The correlation dimension is the slope of $C(R)vs.R$, where R is the radius of similarity and $C(R)$ is given by

$$C(R) = \frac{2\sum_{i=1}^{N} N_i(R)}{N(N-1)} \tag{3}$$

where $N_i(R)$ is the number of the points within the range R of point i. The statistical distribution for correlation dimension is in Fig. 6.

The average value for correlation dimension is 2.5022 for ground truth PPG 240 Hz signal. The correlation dimensions are 4.1118 and 3.2700 for rPPG 30 Hz and rPPG 240 Hz respectively. In general rPPG contains more noise from the illumination and the motion of the subject than PPG signals, thus the correlation dimension should be higher. The result rPPG 240 Hz has less correlation dimension than rPPG 30 Hz also indicates the interpolation process reduces the correlation dimension. rPPG filtered has an average correlation dimension value of 2.908, which is less than the unfiltered signal. It means the filtering process

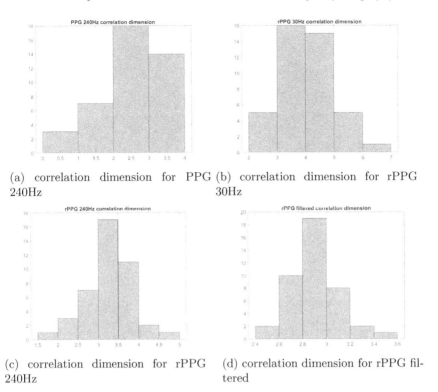

(a) correlation dimension for PPG 240Hz

(b) correlation dimension for rPPG 30Hz

(c) correlation dimension for rPPG 240Hz

(d) correlation dimension for rPPG filtered

Fig. 6. The estimated correlation dimension for 4 signals. Histogram x-axis: the value range of the correlation dimension. Histogram y-axis: frequency

significant reduces the noise in the rPPG signals. The reduce in the correlation dimension also means the filtered rPPG signal is more close to the ground truth signal.

4.5   Approximate Entropy

The unpredictability of the time series data can be quantified by approximate entropy. A higher value of approximate entropy indicates a higher irregularity and more fluctuations in the uniformly sampled time series data. If more repetitive patterns of a signal is observed, the signal is more predictable and thus has a smaller value of approximate entropy. The complexity level can be quantified by the approximate entropy derived from a time series.

The approximate entropy is calculated as $\phi_m - \phi_{m+1}$, where,

$$\phi_m = \frac{\sum_{i=1}^{N-m+1} log(N_i)}{N - m + 1} \qquad (4)$$

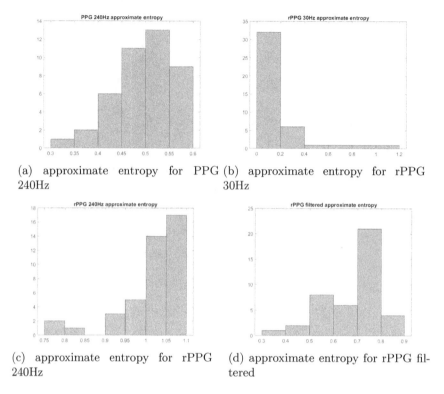

(a) approximate entropy for PPG 240Hz

(b) approximate entropy for rPPG 30Hz

(c) approximate entropy for rPPG 240Hz

(d) approximate entropy for rPPG filtered

Fig. 7. The estimated approximate entropy for 4 signals. Histogram x-axis: the value range of the approximate entropy. Histogram y-axis: frequency

where m is the embedding dimension, N is the number of data points, N_i is s the number of the points within the radius of similarity R of point i. The statistical distribution for approximate entropy is in Fig. 7.

5 Results

The average value for approximate entropy is 0.4963 for ground truth PPG 240 Hz signal. The approximate entropy are 0.2315 and 1.0156 for rPPG 30 Hz and rPPG 240 Hz respectively. The result rPPG 240 Hz has higher approximate entropy than rPPG 30 Hz indicating the interpolation process increases the approximate entropy and introduces more complexity into the signal. rPPG filtered has an average approximate entropy value of 0.6885, which is less than the unfiltered signal. It means the filtering process will significantly reduce the complexity of the signal. It also means the filtered rPPG signal is more close to the ground truth signal.

The signal properties derived from the reconstructed phase space include Lyanpunov exponent, correlation dimension and approximate entropy. These

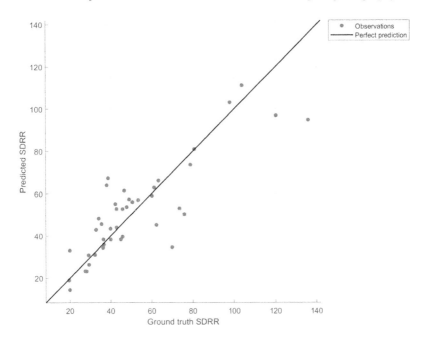

Fig. 8. SDRR results derived from the rPPG filtered (RMSE = 13.72)

properties can be used to improve the current HRV detection method accuracy based on rPPG as an addition feature for a regression model.

After the rPPG signal is derived from the face video (rPPG 30 Hz), interpolated (rPPG 240 Hz), and bandpass filtered (rPPG filtered), the signal is reconstructed by inverse CWT. The peak detection algorithm is used to detect peaks of the signal.

RR interval is defined as the time interval of the consequent peaks.

$$RR_i = PP_i - PP_{i-1} \qquad (5)$$

where RR_i is the ith RR interval and PP_i is the time for the ith peak.

We use HRV time domain definitions SDRR. SDRR is defined as standard deviation of all RR intervals, that is

$$SDRR = \sqrt{\frac{\sum_i (RR_i - mean(RR))^2}{N-1}} \qquad (6)$$

The HRV result derived from the ground truth signal and rPPG filtered is shown in Fig. 8. With RMSE = 13.72. We can improve the accuracy by building a regression model using 4 features, including the HRV detection results derived from the rPPG, Lyanpunov exponent, correlation dimension and approximate entropy. The HRV result derived from the ground truth PPG240 Hz signal and Gaussian process regression model is shown in Fig. 9 with RMSE = 12.19.

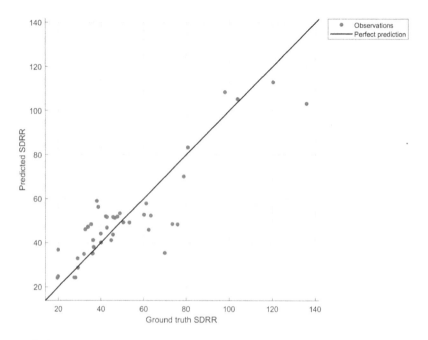

Fig. 9. SDRR results derived from the regression model using HRV detection results derived from the rPPG, Lyanpunov exponent, correlation dimension and approximate entropy (RMSE = 12.19)

6   Conclusion

The main purpose of this study is to investigate rPPG dynamics from non-linear signal processing techniques. The PPG and rPPG signals obtained from UBFC-rPPG dataset are used for the experiment. The phase space reconstruction methods are applied to test the chaotic characteristics of rPPG dynamics. The obtained results provided strong evidence that rPPG is considered as deterministic chaotic after interpolation and bandpass filtering. Additionally, we discovered the best embedding dimension for the rPPG signal is between 3 to 4. The time delay is 10 for 240 Hz rPPG signal. The phase space reconstruction shows bandpass filtering is required to preserve the topological similarities of the rPPG signal and the PPG signals. The interpolation process will increase the complexity level and reduce the correlation dimension of the rPPG. The bandpass filtering process will reduce the complexity level and the correlation dimension of the rPPG. Including the features such as Lyanpunov exponent, correlation dimension and approximate entropy could reduce the RMSE of HRV detection.

This result provides some insight into the feasibility of using rPPG signal for cardiovascular state monitoring. Nonlinear approaches may become a potential method used to evaluate the quality of different rPPG extraction algorithms. The applications of nonlinear signal methods may also contribute to future studies of human mental and physiological health detection.

Acknowledgement. This project is partially supported by a number of grants from the Ubicomp lab at Marquette University.

References

1. Benjamin, E.J., Muntner, P., Bittencourt, M.S.: Heart disease and stroke statistics-2019 update: a report from the American Heart Association [Internet]. Circulation **139**(10), e56–e528 (2019). https://doi.org/10.1161/CIR.0000000000000659
2. Verkruysse, W., Svaasand, L., Nelson, J.: Remote plethysmographic imaging using ambient light. Opt. Express **16**, 21434–21445 (2008)
3. Sviridova, N., Sakai, K.: Human photoplethysmogram: new insight into chaotic characteristics. Chaos, Solitons Fractals **77**, 53–63 (2015)
4. Charlton, P.H., et al.: Measurement of cardiovascular state using attractor reconstruction analysis. In: 2015 23rd European Signal Processing Conference (EUSIPCO), pp. 444–448. IEEE (2015)
5. Sviridova, N., Zhao, T., Aihara, K., Nakamura, K., Nakano, A.: Photoplethysmogram at green light: where does chaos arise from? Chaos, Solitons Fractals **116**, 157–165 (2018)
6. Sviridova, N., Savchenko, V., Savchenko, M., Aihara, K., Okada, K., Zhao, T.: Reconstructed dynamics of the imaging photoplethysmogram. In: 2018 40th Annual International Conference of the IEEE (2018)
7. Peng, R.-C., Zhou, X.-L., Lin, W.-H., Zhang, Y.-T.: Extraction of heart rate variability from smartphone photoplethysmograms. Comput. Math. Methods Med. **2015**, 516826 (2015)
8. Poh, M.-Z., McDuff, D.J., Picard, R.W.: Non-contact, automated cardiac pulse measurements using video imaging and blind source separation. Opt. Express **18**(10), 10762–10774 (2010)
9. de Haan, G., Jeanne, V.: Robust pulse rate from chrominance-based rPPG. IEEE Trans. Biomed. Eng. **60**(10), 2878–2886 (2013)
10. Huang, R.-Y., Dung, L.-R.: Measurement of heart rate variability using off-the-shelf smart phones. Biomed. Eng. Online **15**(11), 1–16 (2016)
11. Wang, W., den Brinker, A.C., Stuijk, S., de Haan, G.: Algorithmic principles of remote-PPG. IEEE Trans. Biomed. Eng. **PP**(99), 1 (2016). (Posted 13 September 2016, in press)
12. Lewandowska, M., Ruminski, J., Kocejko, T., Nowak, J.: Measuring pulse rate with a webcam - a non-contact method for evaluating cardiac activity. In: Proceedings of Federated Conference on Computer Science and Information Systems, pp. 405–410. IEEE (2011)
13. de Haan, G., van Leest, A.: Improved motion robustness of remote-PPG by using the blood volume pulse signature. Physiol. Meas. **35**(9), 1913–1922 (2014)
14. Wang, W., Stuijk, S., de Haan, G.: A novel algorithm for remote photoplethysmography: spatial subspace rotation. IEEE Trans. Biomed. Eng. **63**(9), 1974–1984 (2016)
15. Unakafov, A.M.: Pulse rate estimation using imaging photoplethysmography: generic framework and comparison of methods on a publicly available dataset. Biomed. Phys. Eng. Express **4**(4), 045001 (2018)
16. Bobbia, S., Macwan, R., Benezeth, Y., Mansouri, A., Dubois, J.: Unsupervised skin tissue segmentation for remote photoplethysmography. Pattern Recogn. Lett. **124**, 82–90 (2017)

17. Viola, P.A., Jones, M.J.: Rapid object detection using a boosted cascade of simple features. In: IEEE CVPR (2001)
18. Lucas, B.D., Kanade, T.: An iterative image registration technique with an application to stereo vision. In: International Joint Conference on Artificial Intelligence (1981)
19. Vezhnevets, V., Sazonov, V., Andreeva, A.: A survey on pixel-based skin color detection techniques. In: Proceedings of Graphicon, vol. 3, pp. 85–92, Moscow (2003)
20. Wang, W., den Brinker, A.C., Stuijk, S., de Haan, G.: Amplitude-selective filtering for remote-PPG. Biomed. Opt. Express **8**, 1965–1980 (2017)
21. Rosenstein, M.T., Collins, J.J., De Luca, C.J.: A practical method for calculating largest Lyapunov exponents from small data sets. Physica D **65**(1–2), 117–134 (1993)

Remote Care

Iris: A Low-Cost Telemedicine Robot to Support Healthcare Safety and Equity During a Pandemic

Sachiko Matsumoto[1]([✉]), Sanika Moharana[1], Nimisha Devanagondi[1],
Leslie C. Oyama[2], and Laurel D. Riek[1,2]

[1] Computer Science and Engineering, UC San Diego, San Diego, USA
smatsumo@eng.ucsd.edu
[2] Emergency Medicine, UC San Diego, San Diego, USA

Abstract. The COVID-19 pandemic exacerbated problems of already overwhelmed healthcare ecosystems. The pandemic worsened long-standing health disparities and increased stress and risk of infection for frontline healthcare workers (HCWs). Telemedical robots offer great potential to both improve HCW safety and patient access to high-quality care, however, most of these systems are prohibitively expensive for under-resourced healthcare organizations, and difficult to use. In this paper, we introduce *Iris*, a low-cost, open hardware/open software telemedical robot platform. We co-designed *Iris* with front-line HCWs to be usable, accessible, robust, and well-situated within the emergency medicine (EM) ecosystem. We tested *Iris* with 15 EM physicians, who reported high usability, and provided detailed feedback critical to situating the robot within a range of EM care delivery contexts, including under-resourced ones. Based on these findings, we present a series of concrete design suggestions for those interested in building and deploying similar systems. We hope this will inspire future work both in the current pandemic and beyond.

Keywords: Healthcare Robotics · Telemedicine · Healthcare management · Human robot interaction · Emergency medicine

1 Introduction

The COVID-19 pandemic is exacerbating many societal inequities, including burdening already-overwhelmed healthcare ecosystems, putting millions of healthcare workers (HCWs) at high risk of occupational harm due to severe stress and the looming risk of infection [1]. The pandemic also worsened long-standing

Work supported by the National Science Foundation under Grant No. IIS-1527759 and the Institute for Engineering and Medicine (IEM).

H. Lewy and R. Barkan (Eds.): PH 2021, LNICST 431, pp. 113–133, 2022.
https://doi.org/10.1007/978-3-030-99194-4_9

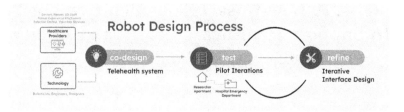

Fig. 1. To build *Iris*, we engaged in an iterative co-design process with stakeholders.

health disparities, with many groups now at an even higher risk of adverse mental, physical, and socioeconomic health outcomes due to a lack of access to high-quality care [2].

Telemedical robots offer great potential to improve HCWs' safety and patient access to high-quality care, but most commercial systems are prohibitively expensive for under-resourced healthcare organizations, and difficult for stakeholders to use.

Also, most commercial telemedical robots are not well-suited (nor designed) for COVID-19 treatment contexts. Most hospitals are busy, noisy, and crowded, some so full of COVID-19 cases that patients are housed in hallways, ambulance bays, or tents, creating difficulties for teleoperators (people driving robots), interactants (people speaking to the teleoperator), and bystanders (people physically near the robot but not directly using it), including: situational awareness (SA), visibility, audiblity, and presence.

Since the pandemic began, our team has been working to address these gaps by partnering closely with key stakeholders to create *Iris*, a low-cost, open hardware/open software telemedical robot platform (Fig. 1). We co-designed *Iris* with front-line HCWs to be usable, accessible, robust, and well-situated within the emergency medicine (EM) ecosystem (the "front door" for COVID-19 treatment). We tested *Iris* with 15 EM physicians who used it to conduct patient interviews and exams. They reported high usability, provided detailed feedback critical to situating the robot within a range of EM care delivery contexts, and provided insights on supporting longitudinal robot deployments.

Based on these findings, we present concrete design suggestions for those in the robotics community interested in building and deploying similar systems, including the importance of supporting: (1) system durability, given the unique needs of the emergency department (ED) environment, (2) adaptability, so users can easily adjust the system to fit their unique clinical settings, and (3) familiarity, trust, and presence, so the operators and interactants feel comfortable with remote care delivery.

Our code, designs, and research instruments are publicly available at https://github.com/UCSD-RHC-Lab/IRIS. We hope this work will inspire roboticists to utilize *Iris's* open source/open hardware platform and deploy similar systems to support their local communities.

2   Background

Even before the COVID-19 pandemic, most healthcare systems worldwide were in a precarious state. In the US, HCWs were overburdened, overworked, stressed, and chronically under-funded, leading to high rates of adverse mental health outcomes, including suicide [1,3]. Many hospitals experienced overcrowding, particularly in the ED representing a public health crisis [4]. This is all exacerbated by the pandemic; HCWs now have the added worry about contracting or spreading the disease, leading to stress, anxiety, depression, and insomnia [1]. EM HCWs have been particularly negatively affected, because most COVID-19 patients first present in the ED [5].

The pandemic also brought to light substantial health disparities in how patients access care and their treatment. In the US, African Americans, Latinos, and Native Americans experience a disproportionate risk of adverse health outcomes compared to other groups [2]. Many of these individuals are likely to seek care at under-resourced facilities, which were already operating in poor conditions or closing pre-pandemic.

Pre-pandemic, some healthcare systems explored telemedicine to help address these issues, often in the form of video teleconference (e.g., Zoom) [6,7], and many increased their use with the pandemic. Unfortunately, this requires patients to have access to technology, knowledge of how to use it, and broadband internet access, which a large percentage do not [8]. For HCWs, the rapid deployment of telemedical technology also increased their cognitive burden and workload, both due to needing to themselves receive training and provide it to patients and their families [9].

In both the research community and commercial sector, many have explored the use of mobile telemedical robots over the years, even more so recently, including performing telerounds in hospitals, remote teaching, and monitoring patients at home [10]. They have seen multiple new clinical uses since the start of the pandemic, including patient admissions, social support, etc. [11–15], and use in prior pandemics [16].

Telepresence robots provide several advantages over static telemedicine devices. They offer operators more independence, since the operator can move on their own, which can also increase their field of view and social presence [10,17]. They are also safer for HCWs, since operators do not need to expose themselves to infectious diseases by going into the patient's room to deliver a telemedicine device.

However, many telepresence robots currently on the market have significant barriers to use. Few were designed for hospitals or were co-designed with stakeholders, which can make them more difficult to use in hospital settings. Additionally, many are prohibitively expensive, and ones designed for hospitals tend to be even more costly (e.g., the RP-VITA costs between $4,000 and $6,000 a month). Furthermore, such robots often are not easily customizable to different settings, which can be problematic given that HCWs need systems to fit within their unique care delivery setting [18].

EDs are a particularly difficult environment to situate robots because they are fast-paced and chaotic. For instance, codes, in which a patient needs resuscitation, occur frequently and require quick response and complex team dynamics [19]. Additionally, ED patients often have high levels of acuity, so robots must be particularly well-designed to avoid causing mistakes that could lead to injury or death [20,21].

3   Designing Telepresence Robots for Overwhelmed HCWs

To design a successful system that addresses issues commonly faced by frontline HCWs, we must consider what is affordable, familiar, and usable to them. We engaged in an iterative design process, where we co-designed our system with HCWs, ran remote studies with them, and used feedback to continue to refine our system.

3.1   Design Requirements

Researchers have co-designed robotics technology with ED clinicians for the past few years, including characterizing their workflow and physical space [3,19–21]. We drew on this work to understand how the ED ecosystem changed in the pandemic, which helped us understand the challenges they face, driving our design decisions.

Many members of the hospital's ecosystem represent key stakeholder groups in the robot design space. These include: (1) HCWs, who seek alternative safe methods for conducting patient consults instead of donning and doffing personal protective equipment (2) Patient experience practitioners, who seek to ensure that patients still experience a high quality of care (3) Volunteers, who seek to provide support services to patients and staff, including isolated patients experiencing loneliness, (4) Infection control practitioners, who seek to ensure all staff and patients are safe from the spread of COVID-19 and other diseases. Across all these groups, perhaps the most important design consideration was to ensure any technology we introduced did not add to an overly-burdened workforce [3]; it was critical the system was easy to learn and use.

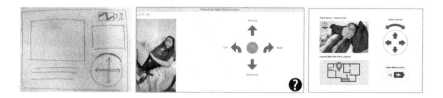

Fig. 2. An iterative evolution of the *Iris* control interface.

3.2   Software and Hardware Requirements

Software Requirements: As the pandemic placed additional pressure on existing stressors of ED staff, our software had to be rooted in addressing these realities. Designing an effortless system meant prioritizing learnability, ease of use, ease of adoption, and accessibility. These design values determined how the user flow, user control, and the screen's UI materialized into the system's visual display and controls for the robot.

We did not want healthcare providers to spend time learning new programs or intricacies of robot control. We took into account technology literacy (can be low among HCWs [3,9]), so it was important our robot had a very short onboarding, setup, and tutorial process for users of all backgrounds and levels of familiarity with technology.

To simplify the number of elements and interactions, while maximizing control screen real estate, we implemented only three components: navigation controls, the robot's video feed, and troubleshooting assistance (see Fig. 2). Arrows on the screen indicate movement in four directions, with a button for an immediate stop. A wide-angle webcam attached at the top of the robot captured the video feed. We added a help button that led users to a short FAQ to aid in troubleshooting. We later removed this troubleshooting button, as several HCWs mentioned they did not find it helpful.

With this minimalistic UI approach, the robot's video feed had the highest importance as its content determined users' driving decisions. The directional control buttons changed to a bright color on selection for clear feedback. Keeping the video and controls side-by-side aimed to keep the users' focus in the same area. We did not want them to have to turn their head or switch their frame of reference when operating the robot.

Hardware Requirements: In designing *Iris*, we focused on five considerations: affordability, ease of sanitation, hospital network integration, physical design considerations, and ease of replicability by other roboticists.

Affordability: We wanted the system to be inexpensive to increase its accessibility for under-resourced health systems, including rural health systems and austere environments. Thus, with *Iris*, we sought to keep costs as low as possible.

Sanitation: We required *Iris* to be composed of materials that were easy to sanitize to reduce the risk of infection and decrease the burden on HCWs. To fulfill this requirement, we consulted a hospital's infection control team.

Hospital Network Integration: We did not want *Iris* to interfere with a hospital's existing network infrastructure, so we designed it to only use a local network. This provides additional security by reducing risks of Internet-based attacks.

Physical Design Considerations: We ensured the tablet and camera mounts were easily adjustable, so HCWs could change their positions to better suit their needs. Furthermore, we made sure the mounts were stable when the robot moved.

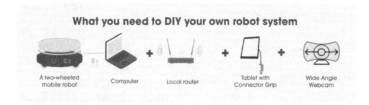

Fig. 3. *Iris's* hardware design is straightforward: a two-wheeled mobile robot with a computer, a local router, a tablet, and a wide-angle camera mounted four feet high on the robot.

Ease of Replication: We selected readily-available hardware components which are easily interchangeable. For example, developers could easily change the type of camera, tablet, or robot base. This allows developers to customize the system to their needs and potentially reduce costs by using components they already have.

4   Implementation

We developed a web-based control interface using Python's Flask framework on the backend, and a webpage with a CSS-styled HTML template on the front-end.

We designed the start up and shut down procedures to be easy for users and require no knowledge of the Robot Operating System (ROS) or Linux. To startup, users turn on the robot and laptop then click an icon that automatically starts the robot's ROS programs. They then turn on the tablet and open a browser, which opens the control interface webpage. The shutdown procedure is simply to turn off the laptop/robot.

We wanted our system to be robust to failures. For instance, if the camera was disconnected or not working the robot would still respond to commands. Also, if the webpage crashed or froze, or if the robot became unresponsive, we created recovery procedures to enable HCWs to simply turn the robot's laptop off and on to restart the system. This is a fairly straightforward procedure that enables people without deep technical knowledge to recover from most problems with the system.

We wanted our system to be low-cost, so we chose low-cost hardware from our lab. The components of our system included a Turtlebot 2 with a Kobuki base, three tablets (one for robot control, two for the hospital's telemedical platform), a computer, a portable router, a wide angle camera, a tablet mount, and a camera mount, as shown in Fig. 3. In total, all components can be acquired for less than $1000.

Additionally, the components of our system are easily interchangeable. For example, a Turtlebot 2 could be swapped out for another ROS-based mobile robot. Similarly, any machine capable of running Ubuntu 18.04 with ROS Melodic may be used; this includes industrial/embedded systems, as well as small form-factor consumer systems.

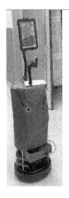 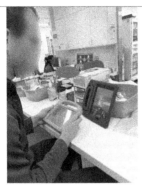 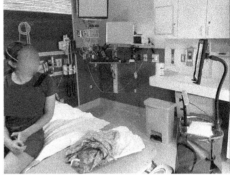

Fig. 4. Left: The *Iris* platform. Center/Right: A HCW remotely interviews a patient using *Iris*.

We wanted the hardware to be robust to the demands of hospital operation. We securely mounted the tablet and camera to the robot, and put the tablet in a case. The laptop is in a box attached to the robot. This provides protection if the robot crashes or is knocked over. Also, all parts fit within the robot's footprint-nothing sticks out.

Finally, we wanted to ensure all interactants and bystanders could easily determine the purpose of the robot, so made the robot a "costume" (see Fig. 4). We printed a banner that looked similar to scrubs commonly worn by ED HCWs with the words "Telemedicine Robot" prominently displayed and wrapped it around the robot.

5 Evaluation

We ran two studies to evaluate *Iris*. The first was conducted at a researcher's apartment, in which a HCW controlled the robot to remotely conduct a mock patient exam (referred to as *APS*). This was while we waited for approval from infection control before deploying the robot in a hospital. The second was at a suburban ED (referred to as *EDS*).

Study Design *APS:* We used inspiration from pre-pandemic visits to our local ED and patient-room photos sent from stakeholders, to re-envision the researcher's 1-bedroom apartment. Similar to an actual ED, the *APS* set up consisted of a patient room with a bed and an area in the kitchen that we designated as the nurses' station. *EDS:* We conducted the study in patient rooms at the ED.

Procedure: Participants were recruited opportunistically via word of mouth and email by our EM collaborators. All participants gave written informed consent.

APS: After the study's introduction, participants could ask questions. They then practiced driving the robot. The robot started in the kitchen. From there, participants drove the robot to the head of the bed in the experimenter's bed-room. The experimenter laid on the bed, wearing a mask, and used a simulation case script, provided by an EM physician. The participant conducted a patient interview taking this history about the patient's physical state then conducted an examination by having a patient follow instructions. After the patient exam, the participant drove back to the kitchen, and engaged in a short interview and survey.

EDS: The design was similar to *APS*. Participants practiced driving the robot, then drove it from the physicians' work area to a patient room and conducted a patient history and exam with a researcher using the same script. For five participants, the tablet had a low quality microphone, resulting in garbled audio, so they stood near the door where they could hear but not see the patient to do the exam; we addressed this for other participants by using a different tablet. Participants drove the robot back to the work area, and engaged in a short interview and survey.

Measures: We conducted semi-structured interviews to gather feedback about how the robot might work for HCWs in the ED, especially during a pandemic. The interview was split into five categories: patient interview experience, robot experience, system improvements, situating the robot in the ED, and comparisons to existing systems.

We followed our interview with a survey. We used the System Usability Scale (SUS) questionnaire, a validated and effective questionnaire for usability [22]. We also asked demographic questions concerning their medical specialty, experience, age, type of hospital they worked in and comfort level working with robots and technology.

Participants: A total of 15 HCWs participated across both pilots (*APS:* 6, *EDS:* 9; 28–59 years old; three did not provide their age). Participants had one to more than thirty years of experience (mean = 7.2 years); one did not provide this information. Our participants had experience working in a variety of hospitals. In the health system they work for, there are three EDs: one located in a suburban area (referred to as Suburban ED), one in an urban area (City ED), and one in a rural area (Rural ED). All three hospitals have overflow tents constructed on outdoor parking lots to accommodate COVID-19 patients. To preserve participant identities, we use the pseudonyms shown in Table 1.

6   Results

6.1   Situating Robots in the ED

EDs are dynamic environments with unique factors that need to be considered when introducing robots [16,20,21]. Here, we discuss the factors our participants brought up.

Providing Awareness to the Operator, Interactant, and Bystanders in the ED: The physical environment in the ED can make navigation difficult for operators. 8/15 participants (*APS:* 3/6, *EDS:* 5/9) discussed how the hallways in the ED are narrow and can be cluttered with carts and equipment. Dominique expressed concern about how "There is often stuff on the ground, so I worry that [...] if it got under the wheel, would that stop [the robot]?" Trevor was concerned about navigating around people standing in the hallways who might not hear the robot coming up behind them. 10/15 participants (*APS:* 3/6, *EDS:* 7/9) indicated their need for situational and spatial awareness in order to navigate around these obstacles.

The ED is also a very dynamic environment. 7/15 participants (*APS:* 3/6, *EDS:* 4/9) described gurneys, which often house patients in hallways or quickly move down the hallways transporting patients. Daniel described how he often checks over his shoulder to see if a gurney is behind him in case he needs to get out of the way. Luna said patients in hallways can make it "much harder to navigate." Navigating around such obstacles with little warning could be challenging for a robot. Participants also described how there are a lot of people rushing around. To drive the robot, they would need enough SA and visibility to avoid collisions with quickly moving obstacles and people.

Some participants also discussed the benefits of alerting others of the robot's presence. Dominique suggested having a light, flag, or audio signal on the robot so people would notice *Iris* more when it moved. She thought this might help avoid collisions, particularly around corners, where people might not know the robot is coming.

Patients Act in Unexpected Ways Towards Robots: According to Yuri, robots in the ED would have to deal with unexpected patient behavior, "[be]cause [there are] always patients moving, and [you need to be prepared for] patient possibly attacking robot." Trevor described some additional unexpected ways patients may interact with the robot. "There are patients who will urinate on the robot, [and] patients who are very intoxicated [are] just wandering through hallways." For the robot to operate in the ED, it must be robust to these types of interactions with patients.

Infection Control: Participants discussed the importance easily cleaning the robot, especially during a pandemic. Mandy suggested using a cover that could be disposed of between visits to infectious patients. Trevor discussed how the robot would need to endure frequent cleanings. He remembered an ultrasound machine that "broke after three days" because cleaning solution got inside of it. Thus, the robot would need to be easy to clean, durable, and have a clear protocol for how and when to clean it.

Table 1. Participant demographic information and pseudonyms. The abbreviations for Hospital Type are: T: Teaching, NT: Non-Teaching, U: Urban, R: Rural. The abbreviations for Location are: A: Apartment, ED: Emergency Department

Pseudonym	Experience	Role	Hospital type	Study location
Daniel	1–5 years	EM resident	T, NT, U, R	A
Yuri	1–5 years	EM resident	T, R	A
Trevor	1–5 years	EM resident	T, NT, U, R	A
Xavier	1–5 years	EM resident	T, NT, U, R	A
Dominique	11–15 years	EM attending	T, U	A
Nitya	1–5 years	EM attending	T, NT, U, R	A
Aaron	6–10 years	EM attending	T, NP, U	ED
Tobi	1–5 years	EM attending	T, NT, U, R	ED
Mandy	6–10 years	EM attending	T, NT, U	ED
Dennis	16+ years	Physician assistant	T	ED
Luna	16+ years	EM attending	T	ED
Jay	1–5 years	EM resident	T, U, R	ED
Nia	1–5 years	Medical student	T, NP	ED
Rita	1–5 years	EM attending	T, U, R	ED
Neil	–	EM attending	T, NT, U, R	ED

Different ED Care Settings Exist: Participants also told us that there are variations in ED care settings that may affect the robot's effectiveness. 8/15 participants (*APS:* 2/6, *EDS:* 6/9) noted that there are significant differences between the EDs in their health system, and at each location the robot could face different challenges.

One aspect in which EDs differ from one another is their physical environment. Rural ED has narrow hallways, while Suburban ED is comparatively spacious. Participants said other hospitals, such as City ED, are more chaotic and have more obstacles than Suburban ED. Rita also observed that City ED's WiFi is not as reliable. Nitya said the temperatures in Rural ED's overflow tents can reach 115 °F, so they often run air conditioning units, making the environment very loud. She "had to literally scream at people for them to hear me." This suggests the noisy environment could make it difficult for the robot to operate in the tents, since it could be hard for patients and HCWs to hear each other over a video call. In contrast, 5/6 *APS* participants thought the overflow tents in City ED would be a setting where the robot might be useful.

Patients at different EDs may also have different expectations about their care. Nitya speculated that a patient's age and familiarity with their doctor may play a role in these expectations, and how a robot factors into that care. "Specifically out in [Rural ED], [...] people mostly get all of their healthcare from four internal medicine doctors [...They are] used to knowing [their] doctors, having face to face contact. And if [they] come into ER and [are] not just seeing an unfamiliar face [but] also seeing a robot, [it] might be a shock...[younger people] would probably think it's not so far fetched."

Different EDs also have different patient demographics, which may affect how a robot is used. For instance, Nitya described how patients at Suburban ED are generally older, and many have difficulty hearing. She was concerned they might have difficulty hearing the HCW over the video call. Alternatively, Nitya noted that at Rural ED over 50% of patients speak Spanish, and they might benefit from a robot that could "loop in interpreter services." Meanwhile, at City ED, there are sometimes "patients [who] are intoxicated," and some might intentionally or unintentionally bump into the robot.

6.2   Integrating Robots Within HCW's Existing Workflow

High cognitive load is well documented among HCWs [3]. Our participants' experiences reinforced this; many recounted how they were often very busy and everyone in the ED always rushes around. To avoid contributing to HCWs' high cognitive load, any robotic system must be easily integrable into the existing HCW workflow.

Seamlessly Integrating into Existing ED Practices: Physical space management is a concern when introducing robots to EDs. 5/9 *EDS* participants thought *Iris's* small footprint was suitable for an ED environment so it could be easily stored and avoid obstacles (*APS* were not able to see *Iris's* size). However, Aaron was concerned it might not have enough presence in patient rooms and would get lost if it was too small. Trevor discussed how "desk space is real estate" in the ED. In the "doc box," where physicians work when not seeing patients, computers are in high demand. Thus, Trevor suggested the robot be accessible via a tablet, so as to not interfere with people using computers.

Two participants suggested it might be difficult to locate the robot in the ED. Trevor compared it to finding the portable ultrasound machine, saying he could walk around the ED three times without finding it. He noted that "people will forget the robot in the patient's room," making it hard to find. Dennis expressed concern that the control tablet we used in *EDS* would get separated from the robot and lost.

Participants were also concerned about the battery life of the robot. 4/15 participants (*APS:* 3/6, *EDS:* 1/9) mentioned this, saying, "things are always running out of battery" (Xavier). Two participants drew parallels to the portable ultrasound machine, noting that if someone does not charge it, whoever wants to use it next needs to plug it in and "come back half an hour later," which Trevor described as a "huge waste of time." Because of these issues, two participants suggested automatic docking might be a nice feature, and Aaron suggested a "very rigorous plan" around the robot might be necessary.

Pandemic-Specific Workflow: All *APS* participants felt the overflow tents were inefficient and did not adequately support their workflow, suggesting ways robots might help (no *EDS* participants talked about the tents, as they were not using them). One reason Nitya thought "something like [Iris] would be useful [was because HCWs need to] run back and forth [and] keep track of both" tents and inside the ED. Trevor described "almost miss[ing] a stroke patient in the department because [he was] in the tent." He also thought it "defeats the purpose [of the tents]" if he is in person with Covid patients.

Nearly all *APS* participants (5/6) felt that the tent was a setting in which a telemedicine robot could be particularly useful. Xavier observed that "most of the patients" at the tent are "pretty healthy," so he would be "more comfortable" just seeing the patient over a video call, whereas patients in the ED typically need "more of an assessment." Trevor described how a system like ours would enable him to check on patients in the tents, but if something more critical came up inside the ED, he could tell the patient in the tent, "Hey, hold on a minute," and quickly switch his focus to the situation in the ED. Similarly, Tobi imagined that she could drive the robot to a patient while on the phone with a consultant and talk to the patient as soon as the phone call was over.

6.3 Robots Supporting HCWs' Ability to Evaluate Patients

Especially in a pandemic, it is important to know if HCWs felt they could thoroughly assess patients remotely. 8/15 *APS* participants (*APS: 3/6, EDS: 5/9*) said they got the information needed to assess the patient via *Iris* (though two had slight audio/video issues). Although robot exams were similar to existing telemedical calls conducted over a tablet, participants thought *Iris* gave them increased mobility, letting them get different views of the patient to examine them better, an ability utilized by seven participants (*APS: 3/6, EDS: 4/9*). Some *EDS* participants (3/9) also noted advantages of not having patients hold the tablet, such as reduced errors and better visibility of the patient's body.

Being able to see different angles of the patient was especially important when the operator wanted to conduct a physical examination of the patient. 10/15 participants (*APS: 4/6, EDS: 6/9*) felt comfortable conducting aspects of a physical exam via the robot. In addition to asking questions verbally, these participants often asked the patient to move their eyes, head, arms, or stick out their tongue. A few participants even asked the patient to stand up and walk in a straight line. However, 9/15 participants (*APS: 3/6, EDS: 6/9*) expressed wanting to conduct further physical exams than was possible through the current robot. "A light would have been nice to assess her pupil function. [I would have liked to] look into her throat, and probably in this case would need to listen to her [breathing], but that could also be hard [through the robot]" (Xavier).

6.4 Physical Interaction Is Important

As a result of our study, we noticed how important physical interaction was for patient evaluation. 9/15 participants (*APS: 1/6, EDS: 8/9*) said a way to physically interact with the patient could be useful. Daniel said, "[I] would like to have a way to physically interact with [the] patient. Physical exams [are] typically very hands on. [After the virtual interview, I'm] not one hundred percent certain in [the] neurologic exam because I couldn't physically interact [with the patient]." Increasing physical interaction, e.g. by using a telemanipulator, could impact the accuracy of patient evaluations via a robot.

Physical interaction is also important for the patient experience. Based on their experiences, participants speculated that physical interaction with HCWs makes patients feel seen and cared for. Trevor mentioned using a robotic arm to provide more sympathy. He also recounted an experience where he had to stand outside the patient's room. "As long as someone is in there physically with them they appreciate it more. [We] tried [...] call[ing the patient] from outside the room, [...] prison style on phone, but they can see you. They don't like it because you're 10 ft away. [The robot] might be better than that, [but] they still appreciate when there's actually someone there."

6.5 Physicians' Perspectives on Patient Experience

Though a majority of participants saw robots as having the potential to improve patient care, two participants had concerns about the quality of patient experience when using a robot. One concern was the lack of physical presence or interaction with the HCW. Trevor mentioned how facial expressions and body language, such as shrugging, are also limitations that may impact patient experience.

Participants also helped outline current patient experience, with regards to the pandemic. In addition to the "prison-style call" (see Sect. 6.4), nurses facilitate telemedicine calls via an tablet on wheels. However, this method still puts them at risk of exposure to COVID-19. Dennis recalled a colleague who called patients to ask preliminary questions before an exam to reduce exposure, and Dominique described another telemedicine method: "[Having an] intercom [is like a] 'voice of god' into the patient room. [...][It's] alarming [because] you can't see [the person]." Designers must consider the patient experience during telemedicine to avoid alarming patients, which could detract from their care, while still ensuring the patients feel seen and HCWs are protected.

6.6 Use Cases Ideated by Participants

Participants often ideated new uses for systems like *Iris* we had not considered. These ideas provide inspiration for ways we can make our system more useful for HCWs.

Providing More Compassionate Care: Dominique highlighted that a robotic system could help HCWs provide more compassionate care for patients while minimizing exposure to infectious diseases. She described how "there's that stigma, like if you're a physician and you're there with someone who's infectious, you want to get the f- out of there." Yuri shared how while working in a pandemic, he has had to consider jeopardizing patient experience for the sake of minimizing his exposure, thinking "Do I need to see this person less or do I need to expose myself more?" Using telemedicine would help HCWs feel more comfortable spending time with patients because there is less risk, which would provide more support for isolated patients.

Integrating with Translators: As mentioned in Sect. 6.1, 3/15 participants (*APS:* 3/6, *EDS:* 0/9) discussed integrating translation services with our system to assist with communicating with non-native and sign language speakers. Yuri noted this might affect using a robot: "Using an interpreter and robot at the same time would be challenging. Like if [you're] speaking to a patient who doesn't speak English or uses sign language." Integrating the robot with pre-existing interpreter services or offering the ability for a translator to join the call would be beneficial to the robot's functionality. This also can have an impact on health equity and access.

Assisting ED Flow: Two participants also envisioned using the robot for delivering medication and supplies. For instance, Trevor suggested, "if you could have grooves for medication cups, [that] would be useful because then [nurses] can send in meds." Using the robot to deliver items to the patient reduces HCW's' risk of exposure.

Additionally, implementing some autonomous care delivery tasks on the robot could support HCWs providing more compassionate care. For instance, Dominique discussed needing to make sure a patient can walk and eat before discharge, but this is often neglected for more important tasks. Tobi also suggested using the robot for discharge instructions. Having a robot complete delivery tasks would be useful in an ED's hectic environment, as it could speed up patient discharge and save time for the HCW.

6.7 *Iris*-Specific Feedback

Generally, participants found *Iris* easy to use. 12/15 participants (*APS:* 5/6, *EDS:* 7/9) had little to no robotic experience, but ten stated that the system was easy or straightforward to use. On SUS, our system scored a mean of 76.67 (s.d. = 15.79) among *APS* participants and 78.33 (s.d. = 12.2) among *EDS* participants, implying *Iris* is usable [22].

Participants generally said navigation was intuitive and the controls were easy to use. All participants were able to complete the task. The controls had a small learning curve; participants expressed no concerns navigating after a few initial button clicks.

11/15 participants (*APS:* 5/6, *EPS:* 6/9) reported no difficulty seeing and hearing the patient, who was wearing a mask. There were a few times where the speaker had to repeat what they were saying; however, this can happen normally in face to face conversations, especially ones involving masks.

Nearly all participants wanted the video on the interface to be wider to aid with navigation and provide a better view of the patient. Many participants indicated that they had limited situational awareness, saying they were concerned about crashing the robot or thought they might have been able to get closer to the patient but were not sure.

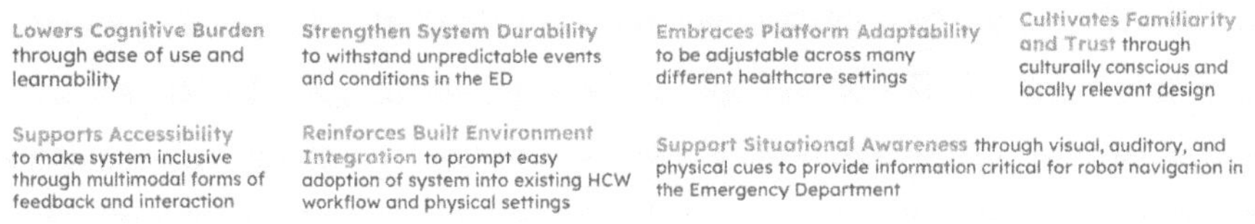

Lowers Cognitive Burden through ease of use and learnability	Strengthen System Durability to withstand unpredictable events and conditions in the ED	Embraces Platform Adaptability to be adjustable across many different healthcare settings	Cultivates Familiarity and Trust through culturally conscious and locally relevant design
Supports Accessibility to make system inclusive through multimodal forms of feedback and interaction	Reinforces Built Environment Integration to prompt easy adoption of system into existing HCW workflow and physical settings	Support Situational Awareness through visual, auditory, and physical cues to provide information critical for robot navigation in the Emergency Department	

Fig. 5. Design recommendations for situating a telehealth robot in the ED.

Participants also wanted a camera that could pan, tilt, and zoom without moving the robot, and some requested a rear view camera.

7 Discussion

Our results provide important considerations for deploying telehealth robots in the ED during a pandemic. Based on these findings, we provide seven design recommendations, including situational awareness, accessibility, and familiarity and trust (see Fig. 5). We also briefly explore the implications of our findings with regard to health equity and access. Finally, we discuss ideas for future work.

7.1 Design Recommendations

Co-designing with key stakeholders in the ED ecosystem and running a remote apartment study with *Iris* yielded additional insights and considerations for telehealth robot design, as described in our findings. Here, we present what we have learned to be the most integral parts of situating a teleoperated robot in the ED. The following design suggestions discuss various aspects of human-robot interaction (HRI) crucial to the operator, interactants, and others around the ED.

Situational Awareness: In the ED, SA is critical for all key stakeholders (teleoperators, interactants, and bystanders). Most prior work focuses on teleoperators' SA and information the robot acquires to carry out the commands or activities. However, interactant and bystander SA are equally important.

Interactants and bystanders may be alarmed by seeing a robot. To mitigate this, the robot should clearly convey its purpose. Emphasizing the presence of the operator, as discussed below, could also be helpful. Bystanders also include HCWs, who will be engaged in safety critical tasks. Because HCWs already have high cognitive load, the system should not place the burden of attention on HCWs. Therefore, we must account for the bystanders' awareness of the robot for successful deployment in ED settings.

Making the robot more visible and audible is critical to operator, interactant, and bystander SA, and can be realized through non-verbal communicative cues. Designers should consider employing a combination of cue types to support patients with hearing and vision loss (common among the majority of older patients).

Visual Cues can help direct attention to the robot, especially when in motion, helping bystanders avoid colliding with it. Multiple cues may be helpful, both via the robot's features (e.g., lights or gaze cues to indicate directionality), and physical indicators on the robot (e.g., paper photographs of teleoperators affixed to the rear of the robot, flags). *Physical Cues*, such as motion and/or haptics, can also be helpful for supporting SA.

Finally, *Audio Cues* can be integral in supporting SA, and can alert people to the presence of the robot and what task state it is in. For the ED, it is important to carefully consider how to design sound, as both a noisy robot and a quiet one could add to HCWs' cognitive burden, and interactant/bystanders' discomfort.

System Durability: The robot needs to be robust for use in safety critical functions. The robot may encounter environmentally austere conditions, including extreme temperatures (e.g., inside COVID tents). Inside the ED, there may be many obstacles, including: uneven surfaces and debris, crowded hallways, etc. The robot also has to endure frequent decontamination required for repeated use, especially during a pandemic. Additionally, from Yuri and Trevor's experiences we learned that the robot needs to withstand patients who might be under the influence and attack the robot.

Additionally, the robot system must be robust to failures to maintain people's trust. Trust is often primarily influenced by robot performance [23], so the system must perform as expected for people to use it. This is especially important because we do not want to compound the high stress of HCWs by also making them worry about a robot.

Accessibility: The system needs to be accessible for all stakeholders. For example, most hospitals are populated with older adults, who experience high levels of hearing loss. Since hearing aids are expensive and easily lost, many will not bring them to the hospital. All staff and patients wearing masks has also made communication difficult for many, as it's difficult to read lips and infer expressions. Unfortunately, due to social stigma, many individuals will not admit they cannot hear well, causing them to miss important instructions, impacting their ability to make informed medical decisions. Having the robot support textual feedback and subtitles could help address these issues. This can help support deaf interactants of all ages, as well as non-native English speakers, who can be supported through interpretation/translation services.

External sound design should be embedded to provide visual accessibility. The system needs to relay audio reinforcement and feedback for those who may be blind, experience low vision, or color blindness to indicate the robot's presence.

Trust, Familiarity, and Presence: The robot should be perceived as acceptable and trustworthy, as this will affect its ultimate adoption [23]. Technology familiarity can play a role, as embodying new concepts within older ones can help build familiarity [24]. Familiarity can also be cultivated by technology being locally, culturally, and socially relevant to an individual's lived experiences, e.g., as created via stakeholder-centered, co-design processes [19]. Additionally, robot designers can add images to robots to reassure patients, similarly to how HCWs displayed pictures of themselves to patients who could not see their faces due to PPE.

In the case of using telemedical robots to provide care in a pandemic, cultural awareness is particularly important for designers. Many groups have deep distrust of healthcare in general, where it is already a struggle to have them seek care, and thus may be particularly discouraged to learn their care is being delivered via a robot.

Finally, conveying presence [17] is an important aspect of creating trust and necessary for successful robot-mediated telehealth, which can be conveyed via mobility and spatial awareness. This helps the operator feel comfortable in the remote space, and that interacting remotely is not a barrier to providing care.

It is also crucial for the interactant to sense the presence of the teleoperator, so they feel they are being seen and receiving quality care, a factor our participants felt was important to cultivating trust. Highlighted by Trevor's prison-style phone call experience with a patient, visibility of the HCW alone might not be enough to express presence-patients still highly value physical presence. As seen in previous research [17], the physical embodiment of the robot can help more closely mimic face-to-face interaction and enrich the operator-interactant communication.

Platform Adaptability: The robot needs to have the ability to be adaptable for different operators and interactants, and for different contexts [3,18,19,21, 25,26]. It needs to be flexible and adaptable to the various use cases discussed by participants.

The system should exhibit adjustable software and hardware capabilities. This will allow the system to be personalized to various ED needs depending on the physical conditions such as light and sound. Additionally, the system should be adjustable to the various types of exams HCWs might need to conduct. For instance, HCWs might add a light to the robot to better conduct neurological exams, as participants mentioned.

Robots need to be adaptable to different types of healthcare delivery, hospital settings, and locations of care. This can mean urban or rural hospitals, crowded or uncrowded, noisy or quiet, etc. They should also be adaptable to different interactants, such as populations of non-native speaking groups needing translation capabilities.

Built Environment Integration: Locating the robot within physical space is a critical part of effectively using it within the ED. The system should not add more burden for HCWs by making the robot difficult to find and recharge. In a busy ED, HCWs need an easy way to track and locate the robot and its connected interface. For example, designating a physical docking location is a simple but pivotal aspect of integrating the robot into the ED that can ease anxiety and streamline system management [27].

Cognitive Burden: It is important that the system reduces cognitive burden. The control interface should have a short learning curve, fulfilled through recognizable and familiar UI controls. The operator should not have to manage multiple programs nor spend time troubleshooting. The robot should be designed to reduce the cognitive load of interactants/bystanders, such as by including aforementioned communicative cues.

An interesting design tension which came up in our findings was Trevor's desire to use the robot to support task switching. This was already a substantial patient safety problem in the profession pre-pandemic, with EM HCWs being interrupted every six seconds, leading to many adverse events [16,20,21]; we certainly had not forseen the possibility that the robot could exacerbate this problem. Designers should consider this possible dual-use of the robot and consider ideas for mitigation.

7.2 Implications for Health Equity

One of our goals in designing *Iris* was to support health equity; many of our decisions were made with accessibility and community engagement in mind. We ensured our system was low cost and easy to use, made our hardware and software open source, and designed the system to be adaptable to different contexts. We hope this approach can help build broader community support and involvement, such as from local hobbyists and makers [28], many who want to support their local healthcare systems during a pandemic but might not know where to start.

Additionally, people can adapt the system to their unique local contexts, which is critical for the system to be well-contextualized to and adopted across different healthcare environments [18,29]. Developers can add, remove, or adjust features to best fit the environment in their healthcare setting. For instance, some might add a speaker to amplify the call volume if the robot is in a noisy ED, whereas those using the robot in a quiet ward at night may not want the robot disturbing others. They also could build a robot using systems they already have to decrease costs, for example, adding a boon with a camera and mini-screen to an old Roomba. Or they might add culturally-relevant "costumes" to their robot to help improve patient experience.

7.3 Limitations and Future Work

Our work had several limitations. First, no patients participated, so our feedback is centered on the physician's (teleoperator's) experience, and their interpretation of the patient's experience. Also, most of our HCW participants were EM physicians, who have different needs and expectations than other HCWs (e.g., nurses, technicians, volunteers). This is something we plan to address in our future work, by including patients, family members, and other stakeholders in the co-design and evaluative process [24,30–32], as we have in other projects [24,32].

In this study, *Iris* was entirely teleoperated. While we one day would like to have a system which supports shared autonomy, due to how crowded hospitals currently are, our stakeholders required a fully teleoperated system. However, in the future, we plan to design a shared control system for *Iris* to further reduce the cognitive load on HCWs, such as by supporting low-level navigation and obstacle avoidance tasks.

Our work raises many open questions for future HRI research. For instance, how can designers improve the quality of robot-mediated interaction in healthcare? What are key ways to convey presence and provide SA to operators providing and interactants receiving remote care, particularly given potentially challenging environments (e.g., noise, crowdedness)? Additionally, these questions may be informed by exploring increasingly active research areas in robotics, including soft robotics, haptic feedback, and virtual/augmented reality-based interfaces, all of which could improve care delivery. Finally, more work needs to be done to determine how robots can best support health equity, an emerging area of research in HRI and Healthcare Robotics [32].

We hope our work inspires others to design accessible, equitable, open hardware, open software systems. Our study provides valuable insights into situating telemedicine robots into the ED, particularly during a pandemic. We hope others in the robotics community can leverage these insights to improve healthcare in their communities.

References

1. Spoorthy, M.S., Pratapa, S.K., Mahant, S.: Mental health problems faced by healthcare workers due to the COVID-19 pandemic–a review. Asian J. Psychiatry **51**, 102119 (2020)
2. Hooper, M.W., Nápoles, A.M., Pérez-Stable, E.J.: COVID-19 and racial/ethnic disparities. JAMA - J. Am. Med. Assoc. **323**(24), 2466–2467 (2020)
3. Riek, L.D.: Healthcare robotics. Commun. ACM **60**(11), 68–78 (2017)
4. McKenna, P., Heslin, S.M., Viccellio, P., Mallon, W.K., Hernandez, C., Morley, E.J.: Emergency department and hospital crowding: causes, consequences, and cures. Clin. Exp. Emerg. Med. **6**(3), 189–195 (2019)
5. Whiteside, T., Kane, E., Aljohani, B., Alsamman, M., Pourmand, A.: Redesigning emergency department operations amidst a viral pandemic. Am. J. Emerg. Med. **38**(7), 1448–1453 (2020)
6. Kane-Gill, S.L., Rincon, F.: Expansion of telemedicine services: telepharmacy, telestroke, teledialysis, tele-emergency medicine. Crit. Care Clin. **35**(3), 519–533 (2019)
7. Hayden, E.M., et al.: Telehealth in emergency medicine: a consensus conference to map the intersection of telehealth and emergency medicine. Acad. Emerg. Med. **28**, 1452–1474 (2021)
8. Benda, N.C., Veinot, T.C., Sieck, C.J., Ancker, J.S.: Broadband internet access is a social determinant of health! Am. J. Public Health **110**(8), 1123–1125 (2020)
9. Zhai, Y.: A call for addressing barriers to telemedicine: health disparities during the COVID-19 pandemic. Psychother. Psychosom. **90**(1), 64–66 (2021)
10. Kristoffersson, A., Coradeschi, S., Loutfi, A.: A review of mobile robotic telepresence. Adv. Hum.-Comput. Interact. **2013**, 1–17 (2013)
11. Shen, Y., et al.: Robots under COVID-19 pandemic: a comprehensive survey. IEEE Access **9**, 1590–1615 (2020)

12. Sierra Marín, S.D., et al.: Expectations and perceptions of healthcare professionals for robot deployment in hospital environments during the COVID-19 pandemic. Front. Robot. AI **8**, 102 (2021)
13. Esterwood, C., Robert, L.: Robots and COVID-19: re-imagining human-robot collaborative work in terms of reducing risks to essential workers. ROBONOMICS: J. Autom. Econ. **1**, 9 (2021)
14. Chai, P.R., et al.: Assessment of the acceptability and feasibility of using mobile robotic systems for patient evaluation. JAMA Netw. Open **4**(3), e210 667 (2021)
15. Fossati, M.R., et al.: LHF connect: a DIY telepresence robot against COVID-19. Strateg. Des. Res. J. **13**(3), 418–431 (2020)
16. Kraft, K., Smart, W.D.: Seeing is comforting: effects of teleoperator visibility in robot-mediated health care. In: Proceedings of the 2016 ACM/IEEE International Conference on Human-Robot Interaction, pp. 11–18. IEEE Computer Society (2016)
17. Rae, I., Mutlu, B., Takayama, L.: Bodies in motion: mobility, presence, and task awareness in telepresence. In: Human Factors in Computing Systems (CHI), pp. 2153–2162 (2014)
18. Gonzales, M.J., Cheung, V.C., Riek, L.D.: Designing collaborative healthcare technology for the acute care workflow. In: Proceedings of the 9th International Conference on Pervasive Computing Technologies for Healthcare, PervasiveHealth, pp. 145–152 (2015)
19. Taylor, A., Lee, H.R., Kubota, A., Riek, L.D.: Coordinating clinical teams: using robots to empower nurses to stop the line. In: Proceedings of the ACM on Human-Computer Interaction, vol. 3, no. CSCW, pp. 1–30 (2019)
20. Taylor, A.M., Matsumoto, S., Xiao, W., Riek, L.D.: Social navigation for mobile robots in the emergency department. In: IEEE International Conference on Robotics and Automation (ICRA), pp. 3510–3516 (2021)
21. Taylor, A., Matsumoto, S., Riek, L.D.: Situating robots in the emergency department. In: AAAI Spring Symposium on Applied AI in Healthcare: Safety, Community, and the Environment (2020)
22. Bangor, A., Kortum, P., Miller, J.: Determining what individual SUS scores mean: adding an adjective rating scale. J. Usability Stud. **4**(3), 114–123 (2009)
23. Washburn, A., Adeleye, A., An, T., Riek, L.D.: Robot errors in proximate HRI: how functionality framing affects perceived reliability and trust. ACM Trans. Hum.-Robot Interact. (THRI) **9**(3), 1–21 (2020)
24. Moharana, S., Panduro, A.E., Lee, H.R., Riek, L.D.: Robots for joy, robots for sorrow: community based robot design for dementia caregivers. In: ACM/IEEE International Conference on Human-Robot Interaction (HRI), pp. 458–467 (2019)
25. Ahumada-Newhart, V., Olson, J.S.: Going to school on a robot: robot and user interface design features that matter. ACM Trans. Comput.-Hum. Interact. (TOCHI) **26**(4), 1–28 (2019)
26. Fitter, N.T., Strait, M., Bisbee, E., Mataric, M.J., Takayama, L.: You're wigging me out! Is personalization of telepresence robots strictly positive? In: Proceedings of the 2021 ACM/IEEE International Conference on Human-Robot Interaction, pp. 168–176 (2021)
27. Cesta, A., Cortellessa, G., Orlandini, A., Tiberio, L.: Long-term evaluation of a telepresence robot for the elderly: methodology and ecological case study. Int. J. Soc. Robot. **8**(3), 421–441 (2016). https://doi.org/10.1007/s12369-016-0337-z

28. Hofmann, M., Lakshmi, U., Mack, K., Hudson, S.E., Arriaga, R.I., Mankoff, J.: The right to help and the right help: fostering and regulating collective action in a medical making reaction to COVID-19. In: Proceedings of the 2021 CHI Conference on Human Factors in Computing Systems, pp. 1–13 (2021)

29. Jang, S.M., Hong, Y.J., Lee, K., Kim, S., Chiên, B.V., Kim, J.: Assessment of user needs for telemedicine robots in a developing nation hospital setting. Telemed. e-Health **27**(6), 670–678 (2021)

30. Kubota, A., Peterson, E.I., Rajendren, V., Kress-Gazit, H., Riek, L.D.: Jessie: synthesizing social robot behaviors for personalized neurorehabilitation and beyond. In: Proceedings of the 2020 ACM/IEEE International Conference on Human-Robot Interaction, pp. 121–130 (2020)

31. Kubota, A., Riek, L.D.: Methods for robot behavior adaptation for cognitive neurorehabilitation. Annu. Rev. Control Robot. Autonom. Syst. **5**, 1–27 (2021)

32. Guan, C., Bouzida, A., Oncy-Avila, R.M., Moharana, S., Riek, L.D.: Taking an (embodied) cue from community health: designing dementia caregiver support technology to advance health equity. In: Proceedings of the 2021 CHI Conference on Human Factors in Computing Systems, pp. 1–16 (2021)

Wireless Sensor Networks for Telerehabilitation of Parkinson's Disease Using Rhythmic Auditory Stimulation

Stephen John Destura$^{(\boxtimes)}$ ⓘ, Glorie Mae Mabanta ⓘ, John Audie Cabrera ⓘ, and Jhoanna Rhodette Pedrasa ⓘ

University of the Philippines Diliman, Quezon City, Philippines
stephen.john.destura@eee.upd.edu.ph

Abstract. Parkinson's Disease (PD) is a neurodegenerative disease affecting mainly the elderly. Patients affected by PD may experience slowness of movements, loss of automatic movements, and impaired posture and balance.

Physical therapy is highly recommended to improve their walking where therapists instruct patients to perform big and loud exercises. Rhythmic Auditory Stimulation (RAS) is a method used in therapy where external stimuli are used to facilitate movement initiation and continuation.

Aside from face-to-face therapy sessions, home rehabilitation programs are used by PD patients with mobility issues and who live in remote areas. Telerehabilitation is a growing practice amid the COVID-19 pandemic.

This work describes the design and implementation of a wireless sensor network to remotely and objectively monitor the rehabilitation progress of patients at their own homes. The system, designed in consultation with a physical therapist, includes insole sensors which measure step parameters, a base station as a phone application which facilitates RAS training sessions and communication interface between the therapist and patients, and an online server storing all training results for viewing. Step data from the system's real-time analysis were validated against post-processed and reconstructed signals from the raw sensor data gathered across different beats. The system has an accuracy of at least 80% and 72% for the total steps and correct steps respectively.

Keywords: Parkinson's disease · Wireless sensor network · Rhythmic auditory stimulation

1 Introduction

Parkinson's Disease (PD) is a neurodegenerative disorder which targets the nerve cells in the area of the brain for controlling movement. It mostly affects the

H. Lewy and R. Barkan (Eds.): PH 2021, LNICST 431, pp. 134–146, 2022.
https://doi.org/10.1007/978-3-030-99194-4_10

elderly population. Symptoms can start to manifest for people ages 60 and above, and have a mean age diagnosis of 70.5 years [1]. In the United States alone, 60,000 people are diagnosed per year and at the present, about 10 million people in the world have this condition [2].

People affected by this disease may experience a variety of symptoms. In the early phases, noticeable changes in basic functional movements like the swinging motion of the arms while walking or the person's speech patterns can be observed. As time progresses, more gradual symptoms like tremors in the limbs, usually at the hand and fingers; slowness of movements (also known as bradykinesia); stiffness in different muscle groups; speech changes; loss of automatic movements like blinking; and impaired posture and balance can be observed [1]. The manner of walking of people with PD is described as having small and narrow steps (gait festination), slow movements, freezing of gait, and loss of balance [3].

Physical rehabilitation is a highly recommended step in order to improve and increase mobility, strength, balance and most importantly, independence of these patients [4]. In physical therapy of patients with this disease, therapists structure rehabilitation programs aimed to target and improve the patients' movements, most importantly, their manner of walking. They train patients to be able to walk safely, walk with independence, and walk on leveled and non-leveled surfaces.

Several studies have shown the role of auditory cues in improving a person's motor and predictive processes. Rhythm auditory stimulation (RAS) uses external temporal or spatial stimuli to facilitate movement initiation and continuation [5,6]. Therapists use RAS as a pacemaker in order to improve the coordination and walking of patients with PD or with similar conditions.

Aside from face-to-face sessions between patients and therapists, home rehabilitation programs are also being used. Recent advancement in technology gave way to different telerehabilitation systems. Telerehabilitation involves the use of electronic devices in order to remotely monitor and rehabilitate different kinds of patients [7]. It is practical to use especially for patients with mobility impairments such as limb amputations and patients living in remote and far places which make their access to rehabilitation clinics limited. Furthermore, amidst the Coronavirus Disease (COVID-19) pandemic where limiting time spent outside and social distancing are enforced, telerehabilitation can prove to have a lot of potential.

2   Related Work

2.1   Telerehabilitation

Telerehabilitation is a growing technology which aims to deliver evaluation, consultation, and therapy to patients remotely through information and communication technology as opposed to face-to-face delivery of rehabilitation in clinics. Even before the pandemic, the uptake of telerehabilitation from 2012 has increased, compelled by a more accessible mode of rehabilitation in rural areas [8]. Moreover, health precautions made from the COVID-19 pandemic pushed for telerehabilitation systems which are found effective for patients with musculoskeletal conditions, targeting the improvement of motor functions [9].

Despite the growing trend, telerehabilitation methods are prone to error due to its subjective nature and can, therefore, yield unreliable results. Other challenges of telerehabilitation include: lack of knowledge and skills in mobile health, lack of policies, laws and support for this method, and internet connectivity problems [7]. Given these challenges, there is a need to implement a system which can give objective evaluation to assess progress, and to prioritize ease of use and convenience for both patient and therapist.

2.2 Rhythmic Auditory Stimulation

Studies have shown the effectiveness of Rhythmic Auditory Stimulation (RAS), a method of using rhythm and music in improving the motor functions of patients with Parkinson's Disease and other related conditions [10]. It shows that motor learning is preserved after training with RAS for PD patients [5]. However, a more recent study during the COVID-19 pandemic shows that there is a lower uptake of RAS for telerehabilitation. Considerations in patient's conditions in the remote set-up, including safety, access to a caregiver and technological challenges influenced this result [11]. While RAS is an effective method for rehabilitation, efforts must be made to address patient's conditions in patient-therapist interpersonal connection, technological, safety, and health aspects.

2.3 System Design for Telerehabilitation

Walking assessment in telerehabilitation is an emerging application of wireless sensor networks (WSN). For the purposes of home programs classified under telerehabilitation, WSN is used to monitor human motion and activities to supervise rehabilitation. Hadjidj et al. discusses applications for WSN in continuous rehabilitation monitoring which cannot be done with current management and economic issues. Design considerations for WSN were divided into its 4 components: sensor node, communication protocols, signal processing, and framework [12].

Given the remote applications of the system, the system's ease of set-up and use, sensor functionality, and communication aspects were focused similar to the following studies [6,13,14] to cater to the elderly population.

3 System Design

The system is a supplement for the rehabilitation programs of people diagnosed with PD. It can be used during days where the patient and the therapist won't meet or even after the whole rehabilitation period to keep the patients engaged in physical therapy. It monitors the patient's progress throughout the rehabilitation period and gives objective assessment for their performance in the home setting.

The system has three major parts: the sensor node, the base station node, and the server. The sensor node is responsible for gathering and computing data for every training session. It connects wirelessly to the base station node (phone) and sends the computed data through Bluetooth connection. The Android phone application facilitates rhythmic auditory stimulation training and serves as an interface for both the patient and therapist to communicate and visualize training results. Through a Wireless Fidelity (WiFi) connection, it sends data to the server where data is stored and accessed by both users (Fig. 1).

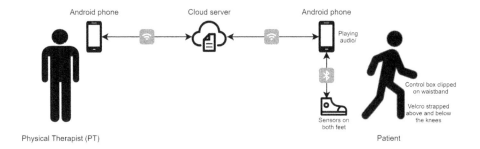

Fig. 1. Full system set-up

3.1   Sensor Node

The sensor node is composed of the insole sensors and the microcontroller. The insole sensors can be placed on slides and they are wired directly to the microcontroller. On the other hand, the microcontroller, the power supply and the insole sensor circuit are housed in a casing that are clipped to the waistband of the clothing of users. Velcros are used to strap the wires on each leg of the user to keep them in place when trainings are executed.

Insole Sensor. The insole sensor approach was adopted from the researches [15–17]. The insole sensor model, ZNX-01, is made out of eight force sensitive resistors placed in different areas of the foot. The body itself is laminated on a plastic material shaped as an insole which prevents air bubbles and unwanted contamination from dirt, affecting the readings of the sensors. Its tail, composed of the pins, is separated from the insole body so that it prevents bending during walking and thus, prolongs the usability of the device.

Both feet had one insole sensor each. The insoles can be placed on different footwears but it is highly recommended to use footwears with open backs to exclude the sensor tail from the bending stress during walking. This is essential since the sensors can produce unnecessary readings when stress is applied on the tails. The insole sensors were able to identify steps when weight is applied on the toe area.

Arduino Nano. Arduino Nano was used in this project because of its small size. The microcontroller was responsible for performing necessary calculations for the step parameters which are cadence (steps per minute), total steps, and correct steps.

3.2   Bluetooth Module and Communication

Bluetooth was used for short-range data transmission, from the sensor node to the phone. Bluetooth was the chosen network technology since it ensures interoperability and compatibility with other devices to fit end user's gadgets, transmission of data, and communication with other services such as the Internet so that information can be relayed to therapists remotely [18]. To provide the communication between the microcontroller and the phone, a Bluetooth module (HC-06) was used to transmit the training data once training is completed.

3.3   Base Station Node

Since patients perform training sessions remotely, android phones, an easily accessible item, serve as the base station of the system. From the sensor nodes, it receives the computed data which are presented in the Android application. Furthermore, it serves as the gateway to the cloud server where all past training session data are stored and accessed anytime.

The application facilitates the RAS training of the patient by playing the mp3 files of generated metronome sounds which the patients follow per training session. It provides options for the beat pace which are 49, 55, and 60 beats per minute [20]. Training durations of 10, 15, and 20 min were also implemented in the application. Both the beat pace and training duration will be based on the instruction of the therapist.

On the physical therapist's side, they have access to data of all their patients for the ease of progress monitoring and provide feedback afterwards. They can also schedule training sessions, view the schedules and give feedback for each of their patients.

Used in many health applications [21,22], Android Studio is chosen as the IDE for developing the Android-based application because it is a free and open source platform with many online libraries and resources. Furthermore, Samsung Galaxy S7 and Samsung Galaxy A7 were the Android phones used to run the application due to their similarities and availability.

3.4   Server

Database and Authentication. To connect the therapist and patient remotely, a cloud server is made with the use of Firebase. All computed training data from the phone is uploaded and stored on the database for online access. A user database was set-up to manage user profiles and login. From the gateway, the server obtains this data. Both the online database and authentication heavily rely on the internet since the server is online.

4   Testing

Testing was done on each of the system's components: sensor node, Bluetooth communication, base station node, and server, and the integrated system functionality, focusing on the sensor node's accuracy on counting correct and total steps.

4.1   Sensor Node

The behavior of the insole circuit was tested for no load and when load is applied. Different known weights with 1 kg increments were placed on cell C to identify their effect on the data reading displayed in the serial monitor of the Arduino IDE. 2 kg was used as the trigger point of the system. A step was only counted if this minimum weight was applied into the sensor and registered into the microcontroller. Moreover, filtering was done to implement the minimum step duration for the total step counter in the code. A step must be held for a specified amount of time in order for it to be counted (Table 1).

Table 1. RAS training step parameter

Step parameters	Conditions
Total steps	Minimum stepping duration achieved
	Minimum trigger point reached
Total correct steps	Minimum stepping duration achieved
	Minimum trigger point reached
	Where $T_{beat-start} \leq t_{step} \leq T_{beat-end}$

The minimum step durations for total steps and correct steps are shown below (Table 2):

Table 2. Minimum step duration filters

BPM	Total step duration	Correct step duration
49	$475\,\mathrm{ms} \leq t_{step}$	$175\,\mathrm{ms} < t_{step}$
55	$450\,\mathrm{ms} \leq t_{step}$	$175\,\mathrm{ms} < t_{step}$
60	$425\,\mathrm{ms} \leq t_{step}$	$175\,\mathrm{ms} < t_{step}$

Data computations were made in the microcontroller while the results were initially displayed on the Arduino serial monitor on a computer for easier debugging. After the sensor node prototype was completed, it was tested on the phone for connectivity and data transfer testing.

4.2   Base Station Node

Bluetooth Protocol. For the purpose of checking the functionality of the Bluetooth connection, received computed training data from the sensor node were printed on the application. At the same time, received instructions from interfacing with the application were printed on the serial monitor of the Arduino IDE. This was to ensure that the application is able to control the functions of the microcontroller especially when starting the data polling for training sessions.

Android Application. The Android application was tested separately for the patient and the therapist sides. Given the functions for patients and therapists, user interface testing and database testing were conducted to test the frontend and the backend functions of the application.

User Interface Testing includes validating buttons, dropdowns, page navigation, and the overall look and feel of the application. It must be readable and interactions with buttons and clickable elements must function properly. Database Testing on the other hand, includes validating the fields of the database, and queries.

The application's capability to facilitate RAS training sessions was also tested by simulating training sessions. User-friendliness and convenience were also ensured to address the users' remote situation.

4.3   Server Node

To test the server, the Android phone application sent dummy data based on the fields set-up on the database. The database includes the user information, training schedule, step parameters such as the total step count, correct step count, and the cadence. The dummy data must be reflected on the mobile application after uploading.

4.4   Integrated Testing

To simulate the use of the system in a remote set-up, it was divided into 2 parts: the patient and the physical therapist side. Both parts were integrated into one system with the common point of integration being the Android phone application and Bluetooth module. With this, the interactions by the users with the phone application were fully tested.

The full system was subjected to tests varying in bpm and duration to ensure every component was working. The accuracy for the computed step parameters were tested by simulating multiple complete training sessions and validating against baseline results from the reconstructed and post-processed plots of the sampled data using a python script.

The application functionalities for different user roles were also checked. Lastly, the system's capability to handle multiple users were simulated to ensure that data sent in the database corresponds to each user properly.

5   Results and Discussion

5.1   Sensor Node Tests

Considering that the majority of users are in the elderly population, it was ensured that the system is comfortable to wear and easy to use. From the rubber shoe insoles, to the wire, velcros and control box placements, the physical therapist confirmed at online consultations its ease of wearing the device and use in walking, so that the patient would not trip from the wires.

Highly sensitive FSRs utilized filters implemented on the microcontroller to identify and count steps based on the specified conditions. Moreover, since conditions for total steps and correct steps are not dependent on each other, any direct calculations between the two parameters such as a wrong step parameter, defined as the difference between the total step and correct step, were not possible.

5.2   Base Station Node Test

The application's User Interface was validated by interacting with each of the buttons of the application on Android Studio's emulator, then installed on Samsung Galaxy A7. Moreover, since the application has a function to start training sessions, its Bluetooth communication with the sensor node was also tested.

Bluetooth Communication. A Bluetooth serial application was used to initially test sending and receiving of data of 1s and 0s from the microcontroller to the phone. The data sent would contain the start command, BPM, and duration. These values for bpm are: 49, 55 and 60 while the values for the duration are: 10, 15, 20.

Similar to the function of the Bluetooth serial application, sending and receiving of data was added into the application in development to test the sending and receiving of commands. The serial monitor of the Arduino was monitored alongside the terminal for the phone application. With the Bluetooth communication coded into the application, data was sent in json format, processed and uploaded into the database.

Time Synchronization. For earlier testing of synchronization between audio sending data, it was observed that there was a noticeable delay between the time the audio starts playing and the time the start command is received by the Arduino. Since synchronization of both devices is important in the function of the system, round trip times were measured. The round trip time was assumed to be uniform for the Bluetooth communication. One-way trip time or half the round-trip time of 536 ms was the delay coded onto the application to ensure data has reached the Arduino before playing the audio.

5.3   Server Tests

To test reading data from Google's Cloud Firestore platform, test data were manually inputted and verified on the Firebase console in order to be read by the application [13].

5.4   No Load Test

The first test for accuracy done was the no load test. The system was run for three 10 min tests where no load was applied on the insole sensors. This was done to check if the system detects stray signals and unwanted values and counts them as steps.

An average accuracy of 100% was obtained for the three tests performed which shows that the system was able to filter out noise properly for cases where no load was applied on the sensors.

5.5   Correct Step Test

To characterize the performance of the system during training sessions, three 10 min tests were conducted for the 49, 55, and 60 bpm options. The researcher walked through a walkway with minimal obstruction and the beats played through the phone application were followed as much as possible. The 10 min duration option was chosen since it was long enough to produce sufficient data points needed for the results.

After each training session, the sampled data from the microcontroller were saved in a CSV file which was processed by analyzing the graphs of the signals from the CSV file automated using a Python script with a recreated filtering and step counting algorithm based from the microcontroller code. The baseline data was set to be the ideal performance of the system since it utilizes the raw and actual readings from the sensors without the effects of the real time filtering and step counting algorithm from the microcontroller (Fig. 2).

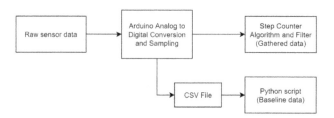

Fig. 2. Gathered and baseline values

The errors from each test came from the difference between the gathered and the baseline values. These differences came from the delays caused by the off synchronization between the microcontroller and the phone application due

Table 3. Gathered and baseline results for 49 BPM, 10 min

Test	Parameter	Gathered	Baseline	Difference
1	Total steps	352	382	30
	Correct steps	212	321	109
	Cadence	35.2	–	–
2	Total steps	496	436	60
	Correct steps	258	243	15
	Cadence	49.6	–	–
3	Total steps	573	432	141
	Correct steps	332	227	105
	Cadence	57.3	–	–

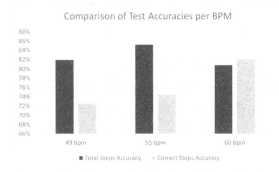

Fig. 3. Comparison of test accuracies per BPM

to the beat generation in the microcontroller. The microcontroller has its own process of beat generation independent from the phone application. The beats in the microcontroller were run sequentially within a single loop. The delays caused the off synchronization between the microcontroller and the phone, which affects the performance of the system especially for longer training durations. Synchronization is critical since the microcontroller and phone application work independently in terms of generating the beats. Thus, beats heard by the patient can differ significantly from the generated beat by the Arduino (Table 3 and Fig. 3).

5.6   System Functionality

Multiple user accounts were made to verify the functionality of the system in receiving and transmitting data properly. 3 patient accounts along with 1 therapist account were created to test the start training, view results, and calendar functions for the patient, and to view and access all the training results of every patient and calendar functions for the therapist.

6   Conclusion

A wireless sensor network was designed and implemented to aid Parkinson's Disease patients and therapists to objectively assess and monitor rehabilitation progress during telerehabilitation. The system was composed of a sensor node, a base station node, and cloud server. Considering the age demographic of users, ease of use and comfortability were considered in the design.

The sensor node was able to gather data and compute for the step parameters which were the cadence, total step count, and correct step count. It was found that delays, which became more evident on longer training durations, were present in the system and affected its accuracy and overall performance.

The base station node in the form of a phone application was able to communicate with the sensor node using Bluetooth at every start and end of a training session. To facilitate rhythmic auditory stimulation training, auditory cues with 49, 55 and 60 bpm frequencies were played through the phone. The application displayed the results of every training session as well as serve as an interface for both the patients and therapists.

The server was used as an online authentication and database where data such as user information, training schedules, results and feedback gathered every session are uploaded and requested for viewing for both patients and therapists.

An accuracy of at least 80% and 70% for the total step and correct step parameters respectively were measured for a 10 min training session. These are favorable results given that the system is still in its first stages of prototype development.

References

1. Mayo Clinic Staff: Parkinson's disease. Mayo Clinic, blog, December 2020 (2020). https://www.mayoclinic.org/diseases-conditions/parkinsons-disease/symptoms-causes/syc-20376055
2. Ratini, M.: Parkinson's disease: what to know. WebMD, blog, 7 January 2020 (2020). https://www.webmd.com/parkinsons-disease/ss/slideshow-parkinsons-overview
3. Han, S., Hersh, E.: Understanding Parkinsonian gait. Healthline, blog, 18 September 2018 (2018). https://www.healthline.com/health/parkinsons/gait
4. N.A.: Physical therapy for Parkinson's disease. John Hopkins Medicine, blog, N.A. https://www.hopkinsmedicine.org/health/conditions-and-diseases/physical-therapy-for-parkinsons-disease
5. Nieuwboer, A., et al.: Cueing training in the home improves gait-related mobility in Parkinson's disease: the rescue trial. J. Neurol. Neurosurg. Psychiatry **78**(2), 134–140 (2007)
6. Aholt, K., et al.: A mobile solution for rhythmic auditory stimulation gait training. In: 2019 41st Annual International Conference of the IEEE Engineering in Medicine and Biology Society (EMBC), pp. 309–312 (2019)
7. Leochico, C.F.D., Espiritu, A.I., Ignacio, S.D., Mojica, J.A.P.: Challenges to the emergence of telerehabilitation in a developing country: a systematic review. Front. Neurol. **11**, 1007 (2020)

8. Cowper-Ripley, D.C., et al.: Trends in VA telerehabilitation patients and encounters over time and by rurality. Fed. Pract. **36**(3), 122–128 (2019). For the health care professionals of the VA, DoD, and PHS
9. Prvu Bettger, J., Resnik, L.J.: Telerehabilitation in the age of COVID-19: an opportunity for learning health system research. Phys. Ther. **100**(11), 1913–1916 (2020). https://doi.org/10.1093/ptj/pzaa151
10. McIntosh, G.C., Brown, S., Rice, R.R., Thaut, M.: Rhythmic auditory-motor facilitation of gait patterns in patients with Parkinsons disease. J. Neurol. Neurosurg. Psychiatry **62**, 22–26 (1997)
11. Cole, L.P., et al.: Neurologic music therapy via telehealth: a survey of clinician experiences, trends, and recommendations during the COVID-19 pandemic. Front. Neurosci. **15**, 347 (2021)
12. Hadjidj, A., Souil, M., Bouabdallah, A., Challal, Y., Owen, H.: Wireless sensor networks for rehabilitation applications: challenges and opportunities. J. Netw. Comput. Appl. **36**, 1–15 (2013)
13. Pepita, A.G., Juhana, T.: User interface, creation and retrieval of user health information with Google firebase, and delivery of automatic emergency SMS for ambient assisted living system: monitoring of elderly condition using smart devices. In: 2018 4th International Conference on Wireless and Telematics (ICWT), pp. 1–4 (2018). https://doi.org/10.1109/ICWT.2018.8527794
14. Nawka, N., Maguliri, A.K., Sharma, D., Saluja, P.: SESGARH: A scalable extensible smart-phone based mobile gateway and application for remote health monitoring. In: 2011 IEEE 5th International Conference on Internet Multimedia Systems Architecture and Application (IMSAA), Bangalore, Karnataka, India, 12 December 2011–13 December 2011, pp. 1–6 (2011). https://doi.org/10.1109/imsaa.2011.6156341
15. Howell, A.M., et al.: Kinetic gait analysis using a low-cost insole. IEEE Trans. Biomed. Eng. **60**(12), 3284–3290 (2013)
16. Lin, F., Wang, A., Zhuang, Y., Tomita, M.R., Xu, W.: Smart insole: a wearable sensor device for unobtrusive gait monitoring in daily life. IEEE Trans. Industr. Inf. **12**(6), 2281–2291 (2016). https://doi.org/10.1109/TII.2016.2585643
17. Kawanami, T., Josen, R., Sato, S.: Proposal of easily distributable insole type gait sensor for health promotion of elderly people. In: 2019 Joint 8th International Conference on Informatics, Electronics and Vision (ICIEV) and 2019 3rd International Conference on Imaging, Vision and Pattern Recognition (icIVPR), pp. 130–133 (2019). https://doi.org/10.1109/ICIEV.2019.8858549
18. Nguyen, A.: How Bluetooth 5.0 is changing the medical industry. Symmetry Blog, blog, 26 April 2018 (2018). https://www.semiconductorstore.com/blog/2018/How-Bluetooth-5-0-is-Changing-the-Medical-Industry-Symmetry-Blog/3167
19. Michaud, T.C.: Human Locomotion: The Conservative Management of Gait-Related Disorders. Newton Biomechanics (2011)
20. Schlachetzki, J.C.M., et al.: Wearable sensors objectively measure gait parameters in Parkinson's disease. PLoS ONE **12**(10), e0183989 (2017). https://doi.org/10.1371/journal.pone.0183989
21. Goh, V.H., Wen Hau, Y.: Android-based mobile application for home-based electrocardiogram monitoring device with Google technology and Bluetooth wireless communication. In: 2018 IEEE-EMBS Conference on Biomedical Engineering and Sciences (IECBES), pp. 205–210 (2018). https://doi.org/10.1109/IECBES.2018.8626603

22. Mamoun, R., Nasor, M., Abulikailik, S.H.: Design and development of mobile healthcare application prototype using flutter. In: 2020 International Conference on Computer, Control, Electrical, and Electronics Engineering (ICCCEEE), pp. 1–6 (2021)
23. Soushine. Final Insole Sensor Product Parameters

"We're Not Meant to Deal with Crisis for a Year": Supporting Frontline Healthcare Providers' Wellness During a Pandemic

Kazi Sinthia Kabir[1]([⊠]), Alexandra Flis[2], Melody Mickens[3], Stephen K. Trapp[4], and Jason Wiese[1]

[1] School of Computing, University of Utah, Salt Lake City, USA
{sinthia.kabir,jason.wiese}@utah.edu
[2] Division of Physical Medicine and Rehabilitation,
University of Utah, Salt Lake City, USA
alexandra.flis@hsc.utah.edu
[3] Department of Physical Medicine and Rehabilitation, School of Medicine,
University of Pittsburgh, Pittsburgh, USA
mickensmn@upmc.edu
[4] Salt Lake City Veterans Affairs Medical Center, University of Utah,
Salt Lake City, USA
stephen.trapp@va.gov

Abstract. The newly discovered respiratory disease, COVID-19, has caused significant physical and psychological strain for frontline healthcare providers (HCPs). Researchers have found higher levels of anxiety, stress, depression, and poor sleep quality in HCPs during this time. It is crucial to ensure the well-being of HCPs to secure a functioning health system amid a pandemic. This work explores how HCPs might interact with a Just-in-Time Adaptive Intervention (JITAI) system that collects their biopsychosocial metrics using off-the-shelf fitness trackers and ecological momentary assessments (EMAs) for providing actionable interventions in real-time. We found that different healthcare-related life factors influenced our participant HCPs' engagement with the technological tools in the study. HCPs also expressed the need for better tools to help them convey their emotional exhaustion from a year-long pandemic. We also observed that HCPs sometimes could not maintain their psychological well-being due to other external factors, especially workload. These findings point to important design requirements for JITAIs to support frontline providers' psychological well-being, both within healthcare and beyond.

Keywords: COVID-19 · Healthcare providers · Stress · Sleep · Psychological well-being · JITAI · Fitness tracker · EMA

A. Flis and M. Mickens—Both authors had equal contribution.

H. Lewy and R. Barkan (Eds.): PH 2021, LNICST 431, pp. 147–163, 2022.
https://doi.org/10.1007/978-3-030-99194-4_11

1   Introduction

On March 11, 2020, the outbreak of the disease caused by the novel virus SARS-CoV-2, COVID-19, was declared a global pandemic by the World Health Organization (WHO) [7]. Since that time, the pandemic has been a constant strain on healthcare systems globally. Frontline healthcare providers (HCPs) have been dealing with overwhelming stress at work due to this disease's highly contagious and lethal nature, and the increased demands on the overall healthcare system. Researchers found higher levels of anxiety, stress, depression, and poor sleep quality in HCPs [41,47] during this pandemic. COVID-19-related HCP suicides have also been reported across the world [32]. Amid a global pandemic, HCPs provide the most critical service of ensuring quality treatment for patients battling the novel disease, and the demands of the pandemic also impact their ability to maintain the broad array of normal medical services. Therefore, to ensure a functioning health system, it is critical to ensure the physical and psychological well-being of these HCPs.

A Just-in-Time Adaptive Intervention (JITAI) [27] has the potential to provide wellness resources for HCPs under unusual strain associated with a pandemic. However, designing a JITAI to provide support in this context is resource-intensive. Deploying JITAIs also requires the integration of technology in users' everyday lives, which might be especially burdensome for the HCPs who are now asked to modify their practice to accommodate the needs novel to the pandemic (e.g., wearing personal protective equipment throughout their day). Therefore, in this paper, we set out to explore how HCPs might interact with a JITAI that collects their biopsychosocial metrics using off-the-shelf fitness trackers and ecological momentary assessments (EMAs). We collected these metrics from the users every day, monitored them, and offered professional support as an intervention if the measurements were out of a normal range. Our goal was to understand how the HCPs perceive a JITAI-like system designed to provide psychological support. We asked 12 HCPs to track their sleep with an off-the-shelf fitness tracker (*Garmin Vivosmart 4*) and report their psychosocial measures with regular EMA questionnaires for seven days as a baseline period followed by a 40-day intervention period. After the baseline week, we conducted semi-structured interviews with the participants to understand their experiences with the tools.

This study found that lifestyle factors related to being HCPs influenced how the HCPs engage with the fitness tracker and the EMAs. HCPs also mentioned that the tools provided by the study did not fully capture their emotional exhaustion. We also found that even though HCPs are aware of the importance of sound psychological health, they are sometimes unable to act to support their psychological well-being due to other external factors (e.g., extensive workload, family responsibilities). Drawing from these findings, we argue that automation and context-sensing are more crucial for effective intervention delivery of a JITAI for frontline service providers. We also suggest deploying micro-interventions in a JITAI to balance the burden of HCPs amid a pandemic. We conclude our discussion with a call for alternative measurements to capture the emotional exhaustion of HCPs, especially during periods of high demand, such as the current pandemic. We believe these opportunities will facilitate the design of supportive technology for frontline providers who dedicate their careers to supporting the well-being of others.

2   Related Work

Coronavirus disease (COVID-19) is an infectious respiratory disease caused by a newly discovered coronavirus named SARS-CoV-2 [48]. As of July 28, 2021, there have been 195,266,156 confirmed cases of COVID-19 infection globally and 4,180,161 confirmed deaths from this disease [49]. On March 11, 2020, the WHO declared the COVID-19 outbreak as a global pandemic [7]. While the entire world is fighting to end this pandemic, frontline HCPs are particularly affected because they face a range of new demands on their jobs novel to this disease.

The range of psychosocial stressors associated with the global pandemic of COVID-19 caused significant psychological distress and disturbances for the frontline HCPs. Several articles on the impact of COVID-19 on HCP wellness found that healthcare workers had elevated levels of fear, anxiety, and depression [41,47]. Liu et al. showed that 50.7%, 44.7%, 36.1%, and 73.4% of epidemiologists and healthcare workers experienced depression, anxiety, sleep disorder, and stress, respectively [24]. Many researchers have started investigating methods for supporting the psychological health of HCPs during global pandemics like COVID-19. Greenberg et al., for instance, suggested that HCPs are at risk of moral injury during a pandemic, and that their well-being should be actively monitored and they should be provided with necessary support [16]. Krystal et al. suggested that digital applications, ranging from actigraphs to mobile phone-based heart rate monitors, could be used to provide feedback on the stress levels of the HCPs [20]. Fessell et al. suggested that 'micro-practices' such as deep breathing during hand washing might help to strengthen burnout prevention of HCPs [9]. Cai et al. reported positive attitude and support from friends and family as a common coping mechanism for stress [3]. These considerations are important for supporting the wellbeing of HCPs, however they lack timely and adaptive components necessary to tailor intervention qualities at the most effective time.

Many hospitals provided their HCPs with online educational programs and online counseling to cope with this global health crisis [24]. Sasangohar et al. called out the need for feasible and practical methods to assess HCP fatigue and burnout [38]. They also mentioned the potential of wearable sensors to monitor fatigue, stress, and sleep biomarkers noninvasively and then integrate this information for timely interventions. In addition, they mentioned that mobile health (mHealth) tools might guide simple methods such as breathing exercises, biofeedback, and mindfulness to mitigate acute episodes of stress and anxiety. Furthermore, telehealth services can enable peer support and occupational counseling. However, they also caution that integration of new technologies with current workflows may present an additional burden and needs to be further examined

[38]. Among others, the benefits and burdens have been well documented in the literature examining workplace wellness programs [25,30,39]. Together, these studies collectively suggest the importance of workplace wellness programs and that mHealth technologies have clear potential to support the psychological well-being of HCPs. Accordingly, the first research question of this study is:

RQ1: How does the integration of new technologies interact with the lives, both professional and personal, of healthcare providers?

Literature suggests value in implementing tailored psychological interventions based on the needs of individual staff to mitigate the risk of deteriorated psychological health [35,36]. Since the COVID-19 pandemic is a relatively recent situation, we do not have evidence of tailored psychological interventions for supporting the needs of HCPs. However, HCI literature has focused on tailored interventions and technology to support psychological well-being in other conditions. Liang et al. found that tracking sleep behaviors with a *Fitbit* device increased users' awareness; however, it did not result in improved sleep behaviors [23]. *SleepCoacher* is a system that monitors the users' sleep behavior with mobile sensors and provides tailored recommendations to improve their sleep behaviors [8]. Levin et al. designed a skills training app that assessed users' sadness and anxiety using EMAs and automatically provided tailored skills training based on the EMA responses [22]. Similarly, other JITAIs focus on providing relevant interventions for reducing their users' stress [15,28,43]. However, assessing psychosocial measures (e.g., stress, anxiety) with EMAs requires significant effort from users. It is also unclear how the HCPs would interact with the EMAs amid a global pandemic when they already have an increased workload. Therefore, our second set of research questions includes:

RQ2a: How do HCPs interact with the burden of standard EMA questionnaires?

RQ2b: How effective are EMAs in capturing their psychosocial measures?

In addition, we also need to understand what interventions might be helpful for the HCPs. Therefore, to better understand the HCPs' current practices for coping with stress, we also explore the following research question:

RQ3: What are our participants' current approaches to stress management?

The next section describes our study, the "HCP Wellness" study, designed to answer the aforementioned research questions. We will then discuss our observations from this study and reflect on those observations.

3   Methods

We designed and deployed the "HCP Wellness" study in 2020. We recruited participants on a rolling basis from the university hospital, and the data collection for this study continued from December 2020 to March 2021. We asked participants to track their health metrics (e.g., sleep, stress, heart rate). For this purpose, participants received a *Garmin Vivosmart 4* fitness tracker from the study team. We asked them to wear the tracker as much as possible, but most importantly, when they sleep. We also collected psychosocial measures from the participants, including perceived stress, anxiety, and burnout through EMAs. We did not collect any information that may identify the participants individually.

During recruitment, the research coordinators reviewed study procedures with participants and obtained informed consent prior to enrollment. Participants completed baseline surveys that assessed demographics, adverse childhood experiences (ACE) [26], resilience (Brief Resilience Scale; BRS) [42], work-related burnout (Copenhagen Burnout Inventory Work subscale; CBI) [18], anxiety symptoms (General Anxiety Disorder-7; GAD-7) [45], depressive symptoms (Patient Health Questionnaire-9; PHQ-9) [19], current stress (Perceived Stress Scale; PSS) [6], sleep quality (Pittsburgh Sleep Quality Index; PSQI) [2], coping resources (Brief COPE) [5], social support (Social Support Questionnaire; SSQ-6) [37], and pandemic stress (Pandemic Stress Index; PSI) [17]. Participants also completed daily EMAs using Likert scale ratings to assess perceived sleep quality and stress in addition to a daily administration of the State-Trait Anxiety Scale (STAI-S) [44]. HCPs were screened weekly for depression using the Center for Epidemiological Studies Depression Scale (CES-D) [31] and monthly for burnout and pandemic stress using the CBI and PSI. We collected data from the fitness tracker and the EMAs for seven days without any interventions to collect baseline data. After the baseline week, we collected data for 40 days where we observed the participants' biopsychosocial metrics and offered support if the metrics were outside of the normal range (see Fig. 1). Note that initially, we planned to collect data for 90 days after the baseline week; however, we had to adjust the duration to 40 days based on participant feedback. We discuss this further in Sect. 4.

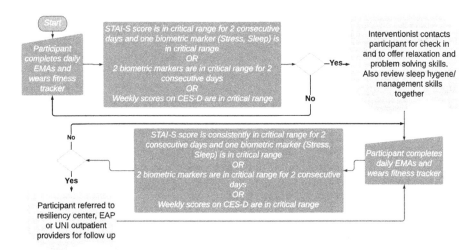

Fig. 1. Flow chart for intervention decision for the "HCP Wellness study."

After the baseline week, we conducted semi-structured interviews with participants to understand their experience with the wearable fitness tracker and EMAs. The first author conducted the interviews with the participants over video calls. The average duration of the interviews was 20 min. The interviews were recorded with the participant's consent and transcribed verbatim. The transcripts were de-identified and stored in a password-protected computer.

Table 1. A summary of participants' demographic information.

Participant	Age	Gender	Professional role	Years in current role
P1	28	F	Nurse	2
P2	30	F	Physician (resident)	2.5
P3	28	F	Physician (resident)	2.5
P4	38	F	Physician with administrative duties	1
P5	35	F	Physician (fellow)	4
P6	50	M	Physician (surgeon)	10
P7	30	F	Physician (resident)	3
P8	28	F	Physician (resident)	1.5
P9	32	M	Physician (resident)	2.5
P10	58	F	Physical therapist	15
P11	31	F	Speech pathologist	4
P12	35	F	Physician (resident)	4.5

3.1 Study Participants

The purpose of the study is to use biometric data collection via fitness trackers and psychosocial assessments to identify HCPs in need of psychological interventions during their work shifts and to utilize brief interventions designed to increase provider wellness. Therefore, we invited HCPs (e.g., residents, surgeons) working at the university hospital over email to participate in the study. Eligible participants included HCPs from a range of specialties providing care to patients in the hospital during the COVID-19 pandemic. Considering how the pandemic has caused strain across medical specialties, not simply those serving individuals infected with COVID-19, the breadth of sampling was intended to capture a range of data associated with provider wellness across medical specialties. We excluded medical staff who were not HCPs or not providing care to patients during this global pandemic of COVID-19.

We screened 16 potential participants; however, one did not meet the inclusion criteria. Two HCPs did not consent to participate. One HCP signed the informed consent form; however, they never responded to further contact attempts. Ultimately, 12 HCPs participated in the study (P1–P12); however, one participant did not participate for the entire duration of the study. The demographic information of the participants is summarized in Table 1.

We invited all the enrolled participants for the interviews after the baseline week. However, only five (P4–P6, P8, P10) agreed to participate in the interviews with the first author. Therefore, we analyzed fitness tracker data and EMA responses from 11 participants and interview responses from 5 participants. In the next section, we discuss our data collection and analysis.

3.2   Data Collection and Analysis

During the baseline week and active intervention period, participants wore *Garmin Vivosmart 4* fitness trackers to monitor their health metrics and used their personal smartphones to respond to EMA questionnaires delivered via text messages. *Garmin Vivosmart 4* data were collected using the *Fitabase* platform [10] and exported for analysis. We administered the EMA questionnaires through *RedCap* [33]. To send the *RedCap* survey links through automated text messages, we integrated *Twillio* [46] with the *RedCap* project. We then exported the EMA responses from *RedCap* for further analysis. The semi-structured interviews after the baseline week were conducted over video calls. We recorded the interviews with participants' permission and transcribed them verbatim using a paid transcription service.

We conducted a thematic analysis with the data collected from the post-baseline week interviews. The first author analyzed the transcripts of the five interviews and extracted 245 codes from them. However, we disregarded 21 codes from our analysis that were not relevant to the study's technology-related aspects (e.g., "taking melatonin for better sleep"). Therefore, we continued our analysis with the remaining 224 codes and merged similar codes. We then iteratively grouped codes to identify themes. By the end of this process, nine themes emerged, which we then carefully considered in the context of the above-mentioned research questions to identify findings and implications for designing similar interventions. In the next section, we discuss our findings based on the data we collected in this study.

4   Findings

This study revealed that the off-the-shelf fitness tracker we used was not well-suited to capture the desired health metrics of the HCPs. We also found that participants felt the standard EMA questionnaires we used did not effectively capture the accumulated emotional burden of HCPs over the previous year. We also gained insights into the different sources of stress for the HCPs amid a global pandemic and their different coping strategies.

4.1   Challenges for HCPs Integrating Technology into Daily Life

As we mentioned earlier, the HCPs were asked to wear a *Garmin Vivosmart 4* fitness tracker and responded to regular EMA questionnaires administered through automated text messages. Overall, we found that participants were interested in interacting with their health data and found the data helpful. For instance, P5 mentioned that she looked at her heart rate variability (represented as the 'stress' measure by *Garmin Vivosmart 4*) and observed how her health behaviors impact them, which she found interesting. She said,

> *"it's looking at my heart rate variability... I just tried to calm myself down. And then I could watch my body battery increase. I was like, Oh, that's kind of cool!"*

Note that *Garmin Vivosmart 4* analyzes heart rate variability and uses that to infer the user's overall stress [13]. Users can only see their stress level from the device, not their heart rate variability. P5 had prior knowledge about the measurement process, and therefore, she mentioned looking at the heart rate variability while she was actually looking at her stress measures. P5 further mentioned that since she is an HCP and had a Ph.D., she had the background knowledge, and interacting with the health data was especially interesting to her. As found in literature [12], our participants learned about their health behaviors by tracking their behaviors with the fitness tracker.

However, participants also indicated that the integration of technology needs to consider the specific lifestyle of the HCPs. For instance, P6 is a transplant surgeon, and he is usually on-call at night. If he receives a call from the hospital, he must commute to the hospital and perform his job function. Surgeons do not stay in the hospital for the night if they are not assigned surgery or are not called. There can be situations where the surgeon goes back home in the morning and sleeps, as P6 described. In contrast, medical resident physicians may stay the entire night at the hospital and balance between sleeping and working. Residents are usually given some space to rest at the hospital. However, the duration of night shifts varies based on which year of residency they are in, as P5 and P8 explained. Overall, we observed that HCPs' sleep schedules are nuanced and can vary significantly between HCPs, and even within the same person, it varies by day. The *Garmin Vivosmart 4* we used in our study takes input from the user about their expected bedtime and starts measuring sleep metrics around that preset time. It cannot detect a sleeping session automatically. From our experience in this study, we realized that while a non-HCP population might be able to maintain a specific bedtime considering standard sleep hygiene, the professional demands of being an HCP might prevent a similar level of regularity in sleeping times. Therefore, a technology that requires a preset time might not be practical to capture their health metrics.

Similarly, participants reported that a preset time for the EMAs was not helpful since they could be on duty and, therefore, unable to respond to the EMAs when they were sent. While they could respond later, which some participants did, this may compromise the quality of the data since the responses to the assessments are no longer *'momentary'*. In the interviews, participants also mentioned that tracking their biopsychosocial metrics for 90 days seemed burdensome. As a result, we had to reduce the post-baseline duration to 40 days. We also note that when participants' EMA responses indicated they should receive an intervention, several participants were unable to schedule a meeting with the psychologist on our team due to the participant's already overwhelmed schedule. These observations help to address RQ1. Specifically, the integration of technology needs to consider both the existing professional burden of the HCPs and the expected burden of using the integrated technological tools. For successful integration, the technology needs to be context-aware for this population.

4.2   Capturing Emotional Burden

We included EMA questionnaires in this study to capture momentary psychosocial measures of the participants. We also collected sleep metrics of the participants through the fitness tracker to observe the impact of stress on their sleep quality. However, when we spoke with participants about this data, they reported that these measures do not reflect their perceived emotional burden. For instance, P4 commented,

> "it's emotional exhaustion. It's not physical exhaustion... I feel like I sleep great. I feel like I get up well-rested. But then it's like, once I get to work, and when stuff just keeps happening, I just feel like my bandwidth just shrinks."

Even when she sleeps well, P4 is emotionally exhausted due to the pandemic circumstances. In this case, the sleep metrics do not represent her emotional condition. Similarly, P4 further commented that,

> "I don't think that the surveys measure burnout well... in my last week on service, it was exhausting. I felt terrible at the end. But none of the survey questions measure that. They basically just asked how I felt every morning and every evening. I'm like, Well, I think I'm better right now than I [was] last night. But I don't think it takes that perfect account. And I think that really where we are is burnout, is surviving in a crisis for a year."

Even though we administered the Copenhagen Burnout Inventory at the baseline and every month, it was unable to capture what P4 called "burnout of surviving in a crisis for a year." Cao et al. used the Maslach Burnout Inventory-Medical Personnel (MBI) to measure burnout and emotional distress in 37 HCPs [4]. However, they did not find elevated levels of burnout and emotional distress within their sample either. P4 explains this in her own words:

> "we are not meant to deal with crisis for a year. We're meant to deal with crises for hours, days, maybe weeks. But to continue to just have everything look differently in your life and worry all the time. We're not, as humans, meant to do that."

Other participants (P5, P6) also expressed a similar opinion that current questionnaires were not sufficient to capture their perceived emotional burnout. These comments help to answer RQ2b, that the current surveys for psychosocial measures that capture momentary emotional conditions might not be enough to capture long-term emotional exhaustion that may arise from a global pandemic.

Concerning RQ2a, our participants had a mixed opinion about the burden of the EMAs. While some were okay with the EMA frequency and did not consider them burdensome, others mentioned them as burdensome and repetitive. They explained that after surviving a pandemic for a year, their emotional status does not change every day. For instance, P5 said that,

> "I always am answering roughly the same. So then to me, it's like, I don't need to be answering this often. Because my answers don't change that often."

Again, P4 commented that,

> "it's also like a little bit of like a salt in the wound, where it's like, yeah, this week I've been isolating for, or I've been socially distancing for 360 days instead of 330, or whatever."

Participants suggested that the system should not send the EMAs every day since their responses do not change much at this point. Even though the psychologists on our research team expressed the importance of capturing the momentary measures of the participants' emotional condition to provide immediate support, the participants expressed a different opinion. This perspective of the participants indicate a need for advanced adaptiveness in the JITAI; while it should be able to identify the user's momentary needs, it should also adapt to users' willingness to engage with an intervention.

4.3 HCPs' Approach to Emotional Well-Being

To address RQ3, we also explored the sources of emotional burdens for the HCPs and their different coping mechanisms. Participants explained that the pandemic impacted their family life, social interactions, healthy lifestyle behaviors, and increased workload. P6 talked about moral injury, saying that,

> "there's an ethical dilemma that we're having between, you know, should you die of liver failure and kidney failure? Or should you get a transplant and then have the potential risk of COVID. And I think that liver and kidney failure is worse than COVID. However, it's very nuanced, and it's created a lot of anxiety and stress."

[16] also mentioned that moral injury is expected for HCPs during the global pandemic of COVID-19. Again, P4 explained the burden of multiple responsibilities and the lack of decompression time. She said,

> "I was here [in the hospital] from seven to four, I got home at four, and immediately, like, get home, and my house is a disaster. My kids are crazy. And I just like jump right in. And it's not like I have an easy job. So there is no decompression time until, like, nine o'clock at night, when my kids are in bed. And by then, I'm exhausted. And so it's like, there's just no, there's no downtime ever."

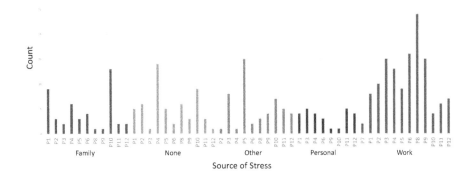

Source of Stress for Each Participant

Fig. 2. Source of stress for reported by the participants everyday through the EMA responses at the end of the day.

The participants claimed in the interviews that they have now acclimatized with the increased stress of the pandemic. However, the EMA data unsurprisingly shows that their stress still largely comes from their work (See Fig. 2).

In response to the daily evening EMAs, the participants reported their coping mechanisms for the most stressful part of the day. We observed that participants frequently reported having to face stressful moments and could not do anything to minimize them. Even though, as HCPs, these participants are aware that psychological well-being is essential to function properly and provide the frontline service, they could not do anything to reduce stress in many situations. P4, for instance, mentioned in the interview that,

> "I've been anxious, but that's not going to change anything. So you have to just live with it, deal with it, and move on, and we manage ourselves because if I am an anxious disaster, everyone around me is an anxious disaster. And that does not help any of us."

Participants sometimes sought support from family, friends, and peers, which was helpful for them. Cai et al. reported that support from family and friends could be effective for the psychological well-being of the HCPs [3]. We also found that some participants felt better thinking that they were not alone in this.

5   Discussion

With more profound insights into how HCPs might interact with an intervention that involves self-tracking technology and EMAs, we now discuss how these findings inform our understanding of the needs and constraints of HCPs interacting with technology for self-care.

5.1 Automation and Context-Sensing

The target participants for this study were HCPs. Unsurprisingly, this population lacks healthy sleep behaviors due to their work shifts [14]. Wearable fitness trackers and automated EMA surveys assume a specific routine for a user's life that might work for most other study populations. However, our study unfolded that this approach might not be practical for frontline service providers (e.g., healthcare providers, firefighters, policemen) who adapt to the irregular lifestyle due to their occupations. Considerations for the range of sleep hygiene indices, such as total sleep time, sleep efficiency, wake after sleep onset, and sleep latency, are critical to consider in aggregation or combination to better measure sleep in this group. Moreover, along with poor sleep hygiene, their services may contribute to increasing their stress (e.g., a global pandemic for HCPs, life losses during a fire incident). Therefore, the technology we design to support them should accommodate their heterogeneous needs, which differ both between individuals and also from day to day and week to week within the same individual.

Sleep monitors, for instance, should be able to detect sleep sessions automatically rather than asking the user about the expected bedtime. Some wearable devices (e.g., *Fitbit versa* [11]) can detect sleep sessions automatically without input from the users. Again, we administered the EMAs in the morning, and the evening, where morning EMA asked about their sleep quality and night EMA asked about the perceived stress for that day. However, a frontline provider may work during the night shift and go to sleep at a different time. In such cases, the perceived stress EMA should be administered at the end of the work shift, and the sleep quality EMA should be administered when they wake up. Standard rules for administering the EMAs might not be meaningful for these participants.

To summarize, the technology should collect data more automatically and be context-aware to balance the burden for frontline providers. Currently available technology for implementing these studies does not support this flexibility, significantly increasing the barrier to running a study that accommodates these participants. While automation and context-sensing can benefit any user, this is especially significant for the frontline providers since they have minimal control over their schedule and are more vulnerable to work-related stress.

5.2 Deployment of Micro-interventions

As mentioned earlier, HCPs are overwhelmed with their schedules and duties, especially amid a global pandemic. Even prior to this pandemic, the significant prevalence of burnout and its critical consequences had been widely reported in the literature [29,40]. As we observed, sometimes HCPs could not make the time to schedule a call with the study-provided therapists for support. This indicates an additional burden associated with the digital intervention or limited awareness of the HCPs' needs and contextual barriers. Many hospitals around the world have made online counseling and educational materials available for their HCPs [24]. However, as we mentioned earlier, participants frequently reported that they simply had to face stressful situations and could not do anything to reduce their stress. Even though HCPs are aware of the significance of psychological well-being, some of them perceived that they could not improve their situations. Digital interventions need to account for these barriers to provide optimal access to important therapeutic solutions.

Micro-practices [9] could be helpful in such situations since they require only a few seconds to a minute to execute. For instance, a JITAI could automatically collect a user's contextual data and offer micro-interventions (e.g., deep breathing) while they are carrying out other activities that do not require their full attention (e.g., using hand sanitizer, washing hands). However, the JITAIs would also need to consider the 'state of receptivity' [21] of the HCPs while offering such micro-interventions since there can be activities that may not be suitable for micro-interventions (e.g., while performing care for a patient or in the middle of a conversation).

5.3   Explore Alternative Paths for Measurements

In this study, we administered commonly used validated survey instruments to capture the psychosocial measures of participants. However, the participants perceived that these questions did not capture the mental exhaustion or emotional burnout they were experiencing. This could be explained by a misunderstanding of the construct being measured or that the design did not account for constructs pertinent to the HCPs' experience. They also mentioned that a fitness tracker could capture their physical stress (e.g., when exercising) but could not capture their emotional stress. Moreover, the participants wanted more adaptiveness in the frequency of the EMA surveys, which they found burdensome and not worth their effort. Further, alternate forms of measures could be used to reduce the burden or sense of repetitiveness. Some constructs might have been most effectively measured using quick visual analog scales rather than lengthy self-report measures. Together, these observations indicate we should pursue alternate options for measurements to capture these psychosocial measures.

One opportunity to adapt the frequency of the EMAs is to observe the stress measured by the fitness trackers when the participant is sleeping since they represent emotional stress more than physical stress [34]. On the one hand, the stress-level data provided by the *Garmin Vivosmart 4* does not provide an overall estimation of participants' stress during sleep-time. On the other hand, the *Fitbit API* does not allow exporting the heart rate variability data for researchers. As a result, we could not incorporate this optimization in our study regardless of the device we used.

Some fitness trackers or smartwatches (e.g., *Fitbit Versa* [11]) do measure heart rate variability, heart rate, and sleep patterns and translate into stress management scores during the users' sleep-time, and use this data internally. In an ideal world, a JITAI could integrate this data to estimate the users' stress levels. However, currently, fitness trackers alone cannot measure emotional burnout accurately since they cannot integrate other external context information (e.g., an exercise session right before sleeping; psychotherapeutic practices, such as exposure therapy, that elicit a stress response). A JITAI might ask further check-in questions through EMAs for more accurate estimation if the stress measurements are elevated in the fitness trackers. If they are not elevated, the JITAI might skip administering the EMAs on that day or randomly decide whether to send the EMA survey or not in a microrandomized fashion [1]. This approach might help to reduce participants' response fatigue from daily EMAs.

The participants mentioned that their responses to many of the EMA questions might not change every day because of cognitive worries and coping patterns established across the duration of the pandemic (e.g., if they are worried about their family). Specifically, the participants pointed out that the presence of a global pandemic made some factors persistent for them (e.g., risk of a COVID-19 infection for their family members). Therefore, there was limited variation in some of the EMA responses. For such questions, as the participants suggested, the JITAI might first ask if their perceived level of stress changed or not. For instance, the JITAI could show the participants their previous responses and ask if their perception has changed in the last 24 h. Alternatively, it could ask them if their perceived mental condition changed in the last 24 h without showing their previous responses. However, we do not have a 'one-size-fits-all' solution to what question format might work best for the participants, and different ways of asking this question may bias or prime participants in different ways that would require further investigation. Regardless, if they respond in the affirmative, a JITAI could follow up with further questions for better measurements and other contextual information.

6 Study Limitations

Since this study was conducted amid a global pandemic, the frontline HCPs who participated in this study were already experiencing longitudinal stress due to increases in expected clinical duties. This snapshot of their experience is, therefore, contextually bound and does not include a pre-pandemic baseline. Further, the additional burdens of being a clinician in a pandemic context likely resulted in limited recruitment. Additionally, the conditions of the pandemic have been shown to vary over time by geographic location (e.g., higher incidence due to spread, clinical resources taxed due to population demands). The participants were all employees of the same healthcare system in the same location and a relatively small sample size, thus limiting generalizability. In the future, we plan to study a wider and greater number of frontline HCPs to understand their experience with tracking biopsychosocial measures and design technology to better support their overall well-being.

7 Conclusion

A global pandemic causes significant psychological strain for the world population, especially for frontline health care providers. These providers are especially critical to population health during global health events like the current

COVID-19 pandemic. To maintain optimal functioning, it is critical to support their physical and psychological well-being. This paper explored how HCPs might interact with a JITAI-like system that collects biopsychosocial metrics using off-the-shelf fitness trackers and EMAs to implement a JITAI to support their mental health. Our findings indicated that contextual variables, like work demands, influenced the HCPs' engagement with the technology integration. We also identified a need for better tools to capture emotional exhaustion over the long term. Finally, we argue for advanced automation and context-sensing to fuel a JITAI targeted towards frontline service providers and suggest integrating micro-interventions in JITAIs to reduce the response burden further. We believe our contribution would help future research in designing better supportive technology for the many frontline providers who dedicate their professional lives to caring for all people in difficult times.

Acknowledgment. This research was supported by an award from the Immunology, Inflammation and Infectious Diseases Initiative and the Office of the Vice President for Research at the University of Utah. The authors would like to acknowledge Heidi Hansen and Alyssa Louise Duenes for their support in coordinating with different stakeholders of this study.

References

1. Battalio, S.L., et al.: Sense2Stop: a micro-randomized trial using wearable sensors to optimize a just-in-time-adaptive stress management intervention for smoking relapse prevention. Contemp. Clin. Trials **109**, 106534 (2021)
2. Buysse, D.J., Reynolds, C.F., III., Monk, T.H., Berman, S.R., Kupfer, D.J.: The Pittsburgh sleep quality index: a new instrument for psychiatric practice and research. Psychiatry Res. **28**(2), 193–213 (1989)
3. Cai, H., et al.: Psychological impact and coping strategies of frontline medical staff in Hunan between January and March 2020 during the outbreak of coronavirus disease 2019 (COVID-19) in Hubei, China. Med. Sci. Monit. Int. Med. J. Exp. Clin. Res. **26**, e924171-1 (2020)
4. Cao, J., et al.: A study of basic needs and psychological wellbeing of medical workers in the fever clinic of a tertiary general hospital in Beijing during the COVID-19 outbreak. Psychother. Psychosom. **89**(1) (2020)
5. Carver, C.S.: You want to measure coping but your protocol' too long: consider the brief cope. Int. J. Behav. Med. **4**(1), 92–100 (1997). https://doi.org/10.1207/s15327558ijbm0401_6
6. Cohen, S., Kamarck, T., Mermelstein, R.: Perceived stress scale. In: Measuring Stress: A Guide for Health and Social Scientists (1994)
7. Cucinotta, D., Vanelli, M.: WHO declares COVID-19 a pandemic. Acta Bio Medica: Atenei Parmensis **91**(1), 157 (2020)
8. Daskalova, N., et al.: SleepCoacher: a personalized automated self-experimentation system for sleep recommendations. In: Proceedings of the 29th Annual Symposium on User Interface Software and Technology, pp. 347–358 (2016)
9. Fessell, D., Cherniss, C.: Coronavirus disease 2019 (COVID-19) and beyond: micro-practices for burnout prevention and emotional wellness. J. Am. Coll. Radiol. **17**(6), 746 (2020)

10. Fitabase. https://www.fitabase.com/. Accessed 4 Aug 2021
11. Fitbit. https://www.fitbit.com/global/us/products/smartwatches/versa. Accessed 1 Sept 2021
12. Fritz, T., Huang, E.M., Murphy, G.C., Zimmermann, T.: Persuasive technology in the real world: a study of long-term use of activity sensing devices for fitness. In: Proceedings of the SIGCHI Conference on Human Factors in Computing Systems, pp. 487–496 (2014)
13. Garmin: Heart rate variability and stress level. https://www8.garmin.com/manuals/webhelp/vivosmart4/EN-US/GUID-9282196F-D969-404D-B678-F48A13D8D0CB.html. Accessed 1 Sept 2021
14. Ghalichi, L., Pournik, O., Ghaffari, M., Vingard, E.: Sleep quality among health care workers. Arch. Iran. Med. **16**(2), 100–103 (2013)
15. Gracey, C.D.: Anxiety and Asperger's syndrome: an investigation into the delivery of a novel real-time stress management approach. The University of Manchester, United Kingdom (2011)
16. Greenberg, N., Docherty, M., Gnanapragasam, S., Wessely, S.: Managing mental health challenges faced by healthcare workers during COVID-19 pandemic. BMJ **368**, m1211 (2020)
17. Harkness, A.: The pandemic stress index (2020)
18. Kristensen, T.S., Borritz, M., Villadsen, E., Christensen, K.B.: The Copenhagen Burnout Inventory: a new tool for the assessment of burnout. Work Stress. **19**(3), 192–207 (2005)
19. Kroenke, K., Spitzer, R.L.: The PHQ-9: a new depression diagnostic and severity measure. Psychiatr. Ann. **32**(9), 509–515 (2002)
20. Krystal, J.H.: Responding to the hidden pandemic for healthcare workers: stress. Nat. Med. **26**(5), 639–639 (2020)
21. Künzler, F., Mishra, V., Kramer, J.N., Kotz, D., Fleisch, E., Kowatsch, T.: Exploring the state-of-receptivity for mHealth interventions. Proc. ACM Interact. Mob. Wearable Ubiquit. Technol. **3**(4), 1–27 (2019)
22. Levin, M.E., Haeger, J., Cruz, R.A.: Tailoring acceptance and commitment therapy skill coaching in the moment through smartphones: results from a randomized controlled trial. Mindfulness **10**(4), 689–699 (2019). https://doi.org/10.1007/s12671-018-1004-2
23. Liang, Z., Ploderer, B.: Sleep tracking in the real world: a qualitative study into barriers for improving sleep. In: Proceedings of the 28th Australian Conference on Computer-Human Interaction, pp. 537–541 (2016)
24. Liu, S., et al.: Online mental health services in china during the COVID-19 outbreak. The Lancet Psychiatry **7**(4), e17–e18 (2020)
25. Madison, K.M.: The risks of using workplace wellness programs to foster a culture of health. Health Aff. **35**(11), 2068–2074 (2016)
26. Murphy, A., Steele, H., Steele, M., Allman, B., Kastner, T., Dube, S.R.: The clinical adverse childhood experiences (ACEs) questionnaire: implications for trauma-informed behavioral healthcare. In: Briggs, R.D. (ed.) Integrated Early Childhood Behavioral Health in Primary Care, pp. 7–16. Springer, Cham (2016). https://doi.org/10.1007/978-3-319-31815-8_2
27. Nahum-Shani, I., Hekler, E.B., Spruijt-Metz, D.: Building health behavior models to guide the development of just-in-time adaptive interventions: a pragmatic framework. Health Psychol. **34**(S), 1209 (2015)
28. Nguyen-Feng, V.N.: A randomized controlled trial of a mobile ecological momentary stress management intervention for students with and without a history of emotional abuse. Ph.D. thesis, University of Minnesota (2019)

29. Panagioti, M., et al.: Controlled interventions to reduce burnout in physicians: a systematic review and meta-analysis. JAMA Intern. Med. **177**(2), 195–205 (2017)
30. Pomeranz, J.L.: Participatory workplace wellness programs: reward, penalty, and regulatory conflict. Milbank Q. **93**(2), 301–318 (2015)
31. Radloff, L.S.: The CES-D scale: a self-report depression scale for research in the general population. Appl. Psychol. Measur. **1**(3), 385–401 (1977)
32. Rahman, A., Plummer, V.: COVID-19 related suicide among hospital nurses; case study evidence from worldwide media reports. Psychiatry Res. **291**, 113272 (2020)
33. REDCap. https://redcap01.brisc.utah.edu/ccts/redcap/. Accessed 4 Aug 2021
34. Ring, O.: What is heart-rate variability? https://ouraring.com/blog/what-is-heart-rate-variability/. Accessed 2 Aug 2021
35. Rose, S.C., Bisson, J., Churchill, R., Wessely, S.: Psychological debriefing for preventing post traumatic stress disorder (PTSD). Cochrane Database Syst. Rev. (2), 1–39 (2002). https://doi.org/10.1002/14651858.CD000560. John Wiley & Sons, Ltd. ISSN 1465-1858
36. Ruzek, J.I., Brymer, M.J., Jacobs, A.K., Layne, C.M., Vernberg, E.M., Watson, P.J.: Psychological first aid. J. Ment. Health Couns. **29**(1), 17–49 (2007)
37. Sarason, I.G., Levine, H.M., Basham, R.B., Sarason, B.R.: Assessing social support: the social support questionnaire. J. Pers. Soc. Psychol. **44**(1), 127 (1983)
38. Sasangohar, F., Jones, S.L., Masud, F.N., Vahidy, F.S., Kash, B.A.: Provider burnout and fatigue during the COVID-19 pandemic: lessons learned from a high-volume intensive care unit. Anesth. Analg. **131**, 106–111 (2020)
39. Schmidt, H., et al.: Carrots, sticks, and health care reform problems with wellness incentives. N. Engl. J. Med. **362**(2), 192 (2010)
40. Shanafelt, T.D., Noseworthy, J.H.: Executive leadership and physician well-being: nine organizational strategies to promote engagement and reduce burnout. In: Mayo Clinic Proceedings, vol. 92, pp. 129–146. Elsevier (2017)
41. Shreffler, J., Petrey, J., Huecker, M.: The impact of COVID-19 on healthcare worker wellness: a scoping review. West. J. Emerg. Med. **21**(5), 1059 (2020)
42. Smith, B.W., Dalen, J., Wiggins, K., Tooley, E., Christopher, P., Bernard, J.: The brief resilience scale: assessing the ability to bounce back. Int. J. Behav. Med. **15**(3), 194–200 (2008). https://doi.org/10.1080/10705500802222972
43. Smyth, J.M., Heron, K.E.: Is providing mobile interventions "just-in-time" helpful? An experimental proof of concept study of just-in-time intervention for stress management. In: 2016 IEEE Wireless Health (WH), pp. 1–7. IEEE (2016)
44. Spielberger, C.D.: State-trait anxiety inventory. In: The Corsini Encyclopedia of Psychology, p. 1 (2010)
45. Spitzer, R.L., Kroenke, K., Williams, J.B., Löwe, B.: A brief measure for assessing generalized anxiety disorder: the GAD-7. Arch. Intern. Med. **166**(10), 1092–1097 (2006)
46. Twillio: https://www.twilio.com/. Accessed 4 Aug 2021
47. Wang, N., Li, Y., Wang, Q., Lei, C., Liu, Y., Zhu, S.: Psychological impact of COVID-19 pandemic on healthcare workers in china Xi'an central hospital. Brain Behav. **11**(3), e02028 (2021)
48. W.H.O.: Coronavirus. https://www.who.int/health-topics/coronavirus. Accessed 28 July 2021
49. W.H.O.: Who coronavirus (COVID-19) dashboard. https://covid19.who.int/. Accessed 28 July 2021

Therapist-Informed Design Directions for Mobile Assistive Technologies for Anxiety

Hashini Senaratne[1]([✉]), Glenn Melvin[2], Sharon Oviatt[1], and Kirsten Ellis[1]

[1] Monash University, Melbourne, Australia
{hashini.senaratne,sharon.oviatt,kirsten.ellis}@monash.edu
[2] Deakin University, Melbourne, Australia
glenn.melvin@deakin.edu.au

Abstract. Anxiety is increasingly becoming a global burden. Although several mobile anxiety assistive technologies have been designed and developed aiming to support the increasing demands, it is not well understood how the design can be improved to aid better regulation outcomes for patients while providing therapists with useful and timely data to make better clinical decisions in assessments and treatments. We explore this area through fifteen interviews with specialist therapists treating anxiety disorders. The uniqueness of this exploration lies in its special attention to therapists' knowledge on inter-and intra- patient differences in anxiety. This focus enabled the identification of novel therapists-informed, therefore, clinically meaningful customization approaches that could be automated and integrated into the future assistive technologies for anxiety. The therapists' notion of unintended adverse consequences of envisioned technologies is also revealed and discussed. Overall, this paper contributes to the future design of in-the-moment digital interventions and digital diaries for anxiety, an understudied area in the literature.

Keywords: Anxiety · Digital diaries · Digital interventions · Mobile assistive technologies · Personalization · Temporal adaptations

1 Introduction

Designing mobile mental health technologies is a rapidly emerging branch of interest for human-computer interaction (HCI) researchers [54]. Research in this area increasingly collaborates with mental healthcare professionals to understand the prerequisites for future design [29,38,52]. The aim is to aid the development of mobile technologies with improved effectiveness and accessibility in the treatment of several mental health conditions. Anxiety is one such condition that has gained attention recently, as COVID and its related quarantines have almost doubled the prevalence of anxiety disorders and imposed barriers for traditional face-to-face therapy [59].

© ICST Institute for Computer Sciences, Social Informatics and Telecommunications Engineering 2022
Published by Springer Nature Switzerland AG 2022. All Rights Reserved
H. Lewy and R. Barkan (Eds.): PH 2021, LNICST 431, pp. 164–182, 2022.
https://doi.org/10.1007/978-3-030-99194-4_12

Anxiety is a set of physiological, behavioral, and cognitive responses to a perceived threat that is usually future-oriented and uncertain [11,16,17]. Pathological anxiety leads to a variety of anxiety disorders, impairing the daily functioning of affected people and contributing significantly to global non-fatal health loss [50,60]. Although the prevalence of anxiety disorders is increasing at a rate of 14.9% per year [2,60], only one-fourth of the affected are estimated to receive any treatment [2]. To remedy this situation, rethinking and improving the design of mobile assistive technologies for anxiety is important, given the great potentials associated with these technologies (e.g., access to patients outside therapy).

Existing mobile technologies that assist anxiety mainly act either as digital interventions (e.g., [21,45]) or digital diaries (e.g., [30,39]), whereas some have overlapping roles (e.g., [7,49,53]). Existing digital interventions aim to facilitate the self-regulation of anxiety, and digital diaries collect mostly subjective data related to anxiety experiences aiming to support later reflections by patients or with therapists. Three of the compelling limitations of these technologies can be related to lack of (1) inclusion of evidence-based interventions [19], (2) customization to accommodate patient-specific (inter-individual) differences, and (3) adaptations to temporal (intra-individual) differences in anxiety [25]. Research has not adequately investigated how to address these limitations motivated by traditional therapy practices. Further, other areas for improvement targeting mobile usage are yet under-explored. Examples include capturing useful information about in-the-moment anxiety experiences without burdening patients and accommodating common concerns around stigmatizing mobile interactions.

To expand this limited knowledge, this paper attempts to (1) explore challenges arising due to limitations of current mobile assistive digital technologies for anxiety and (2) identify design directions to overcome such challenges and potentially improve treatment effectiveness, based on therapists' expertise. A special focus has been laid on challenges related to adapting to inter- and intra-patient differences in anxiety, capturing useful information on anxiety experiences outside the therapy, and mitigating unintended adverse consequences that assistive technology can raise. We explored the above areas, with a focus on five common anxiety presentations. We initiated this exploration by reviewing HCI, psychology, and psychiatric literature. Then we conducted fifteen interviews with therapists specialized in anxiety disorders to explore further and refine the high-level concepts recognized in reviewing related work.

2   Background and Related Work

Anxiety disorders often begin in early adolescence or young adulthood [22]. Some common DSM-5 classified anxiety disorders that are prevalent in these populations are social anxiety disorder (i.e., excessive anxiety about social interactions and situations), specific phobia (i.e., excessive anxiety about a specific object or situation), generalized anxiety disorder (i.e., excessive anxiety and worry about numerous events or activities perceived to be difficult to control), panic disorder (i.e., excessive anxiety about having additional panic attacks), and agoraphobia (i.e., excessive anxiety about a range of situations where escape is difficult) [4,20]. Therapists use diverse pharmacological and psycho-social interventions to treat them, depending on their educational background, practice and judgments.

According to a meta-analysis conducted on clinical randomized control trials of psychosocial interventions, mindfulness, relaxation and cognitive-behavior therapy approaches are found to be the three most effective interventions for anxiety disorders [6]. Cognitive-behavior therapy (CBT) is a widely accepted and practiced treatment for anxiety due to its extensive evidence base [24,44]. Some primary treatment components of these approaches include psychoeducation (i.e., educating about anxiety, including etiology, progression, consequences, prognosis, and treatment), relaxation (i.e., training to achieve a state of decreased arousal), mindfulness (i.e., regulating attention and orienting towards the present moment), exposure (i.e., encouraging to confront triggers), cognitive restructuring strategies (i.e., reframing anxious thoughts to have positive emotional impacts), and later reflection (i.e., after-thinking about anxiety experience and learning from them) [32]. However, a recent review suggests that most freely available mobile apps marketed toward assisting anxiety and highly rated by users were largely inconsistent with such components [19].

2.1   Design Approaches for Anxiety Mobile Assistive Technologies

The approaches taken to design currently highly available commercial mobile apps for anxiety are not clear. Existing HCI or psychology research-based mobile technologies, on the other hand, often attempt to base them on traditional evidence-based psychosocial approaches [25,45,53,58]. While many of them are designed with a focus on promoting general mental health, only a few have been designed with specific attention to anxiety [39,53]. Mental health professionals have often been involved in the design process of research-based technologies. Examples include using their expertise to translate the content of training manuals of psychotherapy approaches to mobile or online app formats [45,53,58] and receiving their feedback on initial prototypes of technologies such that the designers can refine them before presenting to patients [25].

A few designs are also implemented or envisioned considering the literature evidence on advances of physiological and behavioral analytics that provide means to detect anxiety. Some technologies are designed as wearable or handheld devices that can record heart rate like signals continuously or as needed, so patients can visualize representations of those signals and attempt to regulate anxiety to reach a relaxed state (i.e., biofeedback technique) [14,21]. Some are envisioned (but not implemented) as wearables that can continuously record physiological signals, request users' subjective inputs, and trigger other objective recordings (e.g., audio-visual and location data) when an anxious state is detected, so recorded data can support patients and clinicians in identifying actual triggers later on [39].

The existing design approaches that involve therapists have not attempted to explore areas such as how to make the assistive technologies adaptive for inter-individual and temporal differences in anxiety. Therapists' extensive experiences with a range of patients can potentially be useful in understanding such under-explored areas. Further, the design that incorporates literature-based knowledge of objective anxiety analytics lacks therapists' perspectives and expectations.

2.2   Underexplored Design Directions

Accommodating Individual Differences in Anxiety Regulation. Different patients (and even the same patient) respond to different interventions depending on various factors related to their in-the-moment anxiety experiences. However, only a very few technologies provide several options of interventions [45,53,58]. Other technologies usually offer only a couple of treatment components [3,5,13,25,30,37], sometimes supporting limited anxiety presentations [39,43,56], leading patients to rely on multiple technologies. Further, due to limitations in clinically meaningful adaptations within interventions, diverse regulation outcomes occur from one patient to another (e.g., [25]). Although it is not evaluated for regulation outcomes of one particular patient at different times of use, closely similar regulation outcomes at each time point are unlikely to expect.

Intending to improve interventions' effectiveness for a variety of patients, related technologies often allow a level of customizability [7,25,45,53]. One such approach is interface-specific customizations, for example, allowing users to choose a color to incorporate in a relaxation exercise [7], or a surface-material of a biofeedback device [25]. However, these superficial interface changes of generic nature have little or no clinical impact compared to customizing actual interventions. Limited technologies use the customization approach of providing choices of interventions to choose from [45,49,53] and the option to adjust some therapy-specific parameters within an intervention (e.g., adjusting breathing-in/out duration within a relaxation exercise [53]). Such approaches have a better clinical validity, as they closely align with tailoring techniques used in clinics [44,48].

Guiding Suitable Interventions. The technologies that provide customizations in interventions rely on patients' judgments and make patients decide which intervention to use, when, and with what adjustments. On the other hand, people with anxiety often face challenges in making the right decisions, as they are prone to avoidant decision making [8]. Also, they usually find it challenging to generate insights about their own anxiety experience (e.g., whether they are anxious, what is triggering anxiety) due to poor emotional awareness [51]. Therefore, relying only on their judgment to customize cannot be counted on to improve regulation outcomes. Very few technologies attempt to understand how the user is feeling based on subjective inputs and then suggest some interventions [5,13]. However, their criteria for suggesting an intervention are not clear. Further, they can only guide an intervention if the user initiates the technology use or has set up reminders for regular check-ins, so patients still need to determine when to use an intervention. Therefore, before any detailed design, it is vital to explore clinically meaningful adaptation techniques to be incorporated.

Psychology or psychiatric literature has not yet derived establishments on how to match patients to suitable treatments for anxiety. In fact, personalized psychotherapy is still a growing body of interest that explores which interventions work for whom, considering various mental health conditions [12,44]. Related work in the anxiety domain mainly involves analyzing randomized controlled trials to understand the pre-treatment characteristics of patients that are influencing the treatment outcomes [10,33,44]. The characteristics that are under consideration for moderating treatments vary and can be categorized into classes such as clinical factors (e.g., symptom severity, anxiety presentations, treatment history), cognitive and behavioral factors (e.g., stigma of treatment, capacity for participation, avoidance tendency), non-cognitive traits (e.g., personality, motivation), sociodemographic factors, and biological factors.

There is some emerging evidence of treatment components that are suitable for different anxiety presentations [18]. Further, patient-centered baseline severity of symptoms is identified to be correlated with treatment outcomes in some clinical studies [33]. These two factors, i.e., anxiety presentations and baseline severities, have a clear relation to anxiety experiences, vary considerably among different patients, and could also change within the same patient from time to time. Hence, it would be useful to explore whether (and how) therapists tailor the interventions depending on these factors while exploring other potential factors. Such exploration would support deriving potential criteria to guide interventions within mobile assistive technologies.

Capturing In-the-Moment Anxiety Experiences. The existing digital diaries for anxiety either provide a platform to manually enter subjective anxiety levels from time to time with or without notes on triggers and thoughts (as in [30,49]). Subjective recordings within these technologies need to be initiated by the user, which would be problematic for those facing challenges in developing insights on their anxiety experience. As detailed earlier, a few technologies have envisioned triggering subjective recordings through objective anxiety detection [39]. While this approach can potentially address this limitation, relying on indicative metrics for objective detection of anxiety is vital. Otherwise, many false positives may occur, resulting in unwanted interruptions for patients (e.g., elevated heart rates may also trigger instances of high-intense physical activities). On the other hand, triggering patients on the detection of brief and common high-anxious states is not meaningful (e.g., increase of anxiety level in a driver for a short duration due to an unexpected crossing of a pedestrian).

The knowledge on user's anxiety experience based on objective metrics could support technologies to understand when a user requires intervention, and then to guide a suitable intervention, as envisioned for assistive technologies for other mental health conditions [9]. For this purpose, relying on rapidly fluctuating levels of anxiety would not be suitable. A more realistic approach would be guiding interventions based on momentary but somewhat prolonged phases. The psychology literature points to some phases specific to social anxiety (e.g., anticipation, confrontation, and termination in social anxiety disorder) [31]. However, there is a limited understanding of regular temporal phases encountered by patients in daily field contexts, maybe because of the lack of attention paid to symptom variations that occur in between therapy sessions. Some recent analytic research has shown the interest in objectively exploring anxiety patterns that arise relating to certain anxiety presentations such as panic disorder without providing interpretations or benefits of any observable patterns [28, 40, 41]. Exploration with therapists could be helpful in this area, as they can support identifying a set of phases that could potentially contribute to the future design of in-the-moment interventions for anxiety, given their broad experience with patients.

Unintended Adverse Consequences of Assistive Technologies. A major challenge faced by users of any kind of assistive technologies is stigmas around using mobile technology in public settings [36]. This issue is more prominent when it comes to anxiety due to stigmas surrounding mental health issues [27], and can lead to obsessive preoccupation, inducing anxiety further. Current technologies seem to have paid limited attention to these types of sensitive concerns in their designs. For example, although tangible interface-based digital interventions and diaries [7, 21, 49] can produce rich interactions, it is unclear whether users would tend to use them in mobile settings due to their high tendency to draw others' attention. Further, limited attention has been paid to privacy concerns for sensitive information that these technologies collect and long-term effects of usage (e.g., effects resulting from high reliance on devices [36]). Attention to these areas before the detailed design is vital, and it can support mitigating unintended adverse consequences that new technologies can raise.

Overall, the above-identified gaps of related work point to some high-level design directions for future assistive technologies for anxiety. Those are the needs for (1) delivering a set of carefully-chosen interventions based on evidence-based psychosocial approaches, (2) facilitating clinically meaningful customizations (e.g., guiding suitable interventions based on patients' anxiety experience), (3) incorporating appropriate mechanisms to identify factors that would support deciding suitable customizations, and (4) careful consideration of unintended adverse consequences that new technologies can raise and plan to mitigate them.

3   Method

To further investigate the design directions identified through gaps in related work, we interviewed therapists who are specialized in treating anxiety disorders based on a few reasons. We realized that approaching therapists prior to patients is appropriate because: (1) therapists are more likely to offer rich insights on patients' differences in anxiety based on their broad experiences, which individual patients are not able to provide [51, 57], (2) although the therapists' knowledge on anxiety experiences in between therapy sessions is limited, they are likely to have a reconstructed knowledge based on patients' retrospective reports, and (3) therapists' expertise in psychotherapy can support identifying suitable intervention based customizations. Further, similar studies conducted in other mental health domains have demonstrated the discovery of well-grounded design directions through involving high-level informants like therapists [38,45].

3.1 Participants

Fifteen therapists volunteered for this study (female = 9; years of experience: [M = 14.13 (2–40)]; practicing hours per week: [M = 23.80 (2–50)]), in response to email invitations that we distributed to publicly available email addresses of therapists who were identified to be treating anxiety disorders in a major city of Australia. Twelve were psychologists, and others were a psychiatrist (P6), counselor (P8), or social worker (P1). Seven held doctoral degrees (P2–5, P11, P13, P15), six held master's degrees (P1, P6–7, P9, P12, P14), one a graduate diploma (P10), and one was studying for the master's (P8). All used cognitive behavioral therapy (CBT) to treat anxiety. Other approaches used in treating anxiety are relaxation-based therapies (P1–2, P5–10, P12–14), mindfulness-based therapies (P1–2, P4, P7–9, P11, P13), acceptance and commitment therapy (P4–5, P7, P9–10, P12), and dialectical behavior therapy (P2, P12, P14).

3.2 Data Collection

The principal researcher (first author) conducted face-to-face hour-long semi-structured interviews over three months in compliance with the institutional ethical requirements. Each interview was conducted in person, except for one as a remote video interview. This highly interactive setting allowed us to ask follow-up questions to improve the clarity of responses. All the interviews were audio-recorded. We also used an online questionnaire prior to interviews to collect therapists' professional demographics. Based on the review of related work, we used five questions to primarily guide the interviews:

Q1. Which treatment components have you identified as the most effective for anxiety disorders in general?
Q2. How do you customize treatments depending on patients' anxiety presentation (social anxiety, specific phobic anxiety, panic-inducing anxiety, agoraphobic anxiety and generalized anxiety) and severity?
Q3. Can you identify different temporal phases of anxiety experienced by patients?
Q4. What are your preferred treatment components to be used during those phases?
Q5. What are the challenges you and your patients face due to the limitations of digital or non-digital assistive tools used, and how can those be improved?

These broader questions (without specifics) were used to minimize biasing the responses. However, we provided some examples whenever a clarification was needed. For instance, the concept of general anxiety phases in Q3 was often clarified by providing an example from the literature [31]: "*literature on social anxiety shows that patients go through phases related to anticipation, confrontation, and termination. Have you identified any phases that are applicable for different anxiety presentations?*". This clarification was always presented as an example for social anxiety not to influence participants' insights on general phases.

Follow-up questions and some visual prompts were used as interview probes. The researcher asked follow-up questions when clinicians did not relate to some insights extracted from literature (e.g., *"Do your patients share that they stigmatize usage of mobile apps for anxiety in public?"*). Further, clinicians were presented with some images of recent research-based assistive tools as prompts to extract more insights on Q5 (e.g., the researcher presented those images, briefly explained those and asked *"what modifications would you like to have before recommending these technologies to your clients?"*).

3.3   Analysis

The fully transcribed interviews were analyzed using a thematic analysis method similar to the one suggested by Nowell et al. [34]. This method is recognized as useful for examining various perspectives while capturing similarities and differences and generating unanticipated insights. Using the NVivo software, coding was started with a deductive approach focusing on the themes around the main question areas. As the familiarization with the data improved, coding was performed, taking an inductive approach, resulting in novel themes. One researcher performed the analysis; others engaged in verification and revisions during weekly team meetings. During the analysis stages, we further utilized a design process framework, which focuses on generating prerequisites for personalized mobile mental health technologies, as a guide for deriving design directions [46]. The results and discussions are categorized into final codes.

4   Results and Discussions

4.1   Supporting a Variety of Effective Treatment Components

As responses to Q1, the therapists suggested psychoeducation (13/15), exposure (13/15), mindfulness (12/15), relaxation (11/15), cognitive restructuring (9/15), cognitive defusion (4/15) (i.e., encouraging to defuse thinking related to false or irrational beliefs), self-soothing or distraction strategies (2/15) (i.e., coping behaviors which provide a sense of safety), and later-reflection (1/15), as the most effective treatment components for anxiety in general. Note that each therapist pointed to more than one component. The components suggested by more than half of the therapists echoed the core components of cognitive-behavioral therapy [32], except for the later reflection, which seemed to be ignored as a treatment component because it is a common exercise practiced in every therapy session.

One-third of therapists preferred cognitive defusion over cognitive restructuring strategy, saying that it is *"more suitable for patients who are not ready to directly accept that their thoughts are not valid"* (P5). Similarly, about two-thirds of therapists discouraged self-soothing and distraction components, as they do not contribute to developing skills in overcoming fears, others who work with vulnerable populations (e.g., P2: *"autism"*, P14: *"self-harm tendencies"*) claimed that those are useful to calm down patients. They provided options to interact with fidgeting devices, carry around soothing items, and play with therapy dogs. However, since *"high-demand for comfort is a common anxiety symptom that needs to be overcome"* (P15), all the therapists agreed that these strategies should only be provided through technologies for highly vulnerable patients or as a last option for less vulnerable patients.

The above results point to the need for different interventions by different patients. Although therapists agreed that technology needs to support a range of interventions, they also raised the concern that technology should not overwhelm patients with too many options. They suggested implementing a digital *"toolbox of interventions"* with add or remove capabilities (P6, P9, P14) (as in [53]), providing a *"default set of interventions at set-up"* (P11), and *"sorting"* mechanism to categorize interventions (P6, P13).

4.2   Anxiety Condition Specific Customizations of Interventions

Baseline Severity Based Customizations. Aligned to the customization suggested above for highly vulnerable patients, in responding to Q2, three therapists stated that they start therapy with direct and easy-to-follow components for people with higher baseline anxiety severities. Since they are *"anxious most of the time"* (P12), therapists used mindfulness-like components prior to complex cognitive restructuring strategies. Further, those therapists claimed not using interoceptive exposure (i.e., engage in activities that deliberately bring on the feared physical sensations [32]) component with emotionally sensitive patients, as *"it require skills to control reactions to bodily sensations"* (P14).

These results point out that patients' severity level-based customizations (related to the order of interventions and interventions to filter out) need to be incorporated into technology design to enhance engagement and mitigate risks.

Anxiety Presentations Based Customizations. Related to Q2, almost all therapists suggested that psychoeducation, exposure, and cognitive restructuring interventions are effective for all types of anxiety. Psychoeducation on *"what anxiety is"* (P3), *"what common symptoms are"* (P6), and *"how therapy can be supportive"* (P15), is identified as an early preparation step for treatment by all therapists. Many therapists preferred the combination of cognitive restructuring and exposure, as those contribute directly to *"addressing the underlying problems"* (P8) of avoidant behavior [8] and maladaptive thoughts (i.e., thinking related to false or irrational beliefs) [55]. For all anxiety types except generalized anxiety, many therapists indicate that much focus should be on exposure compared to cognitive strategies. However, practicing exposure component for generalized anxiety is identified to be not straightforward as *"intentional creation of triggers is difficult"* (P12), as they closely relate to the *"uncertainty of various situations"* (P15) and *"frequent worry"* (P3).

Therapists also related to specific customizations within treatment components. For example, many therapists claimed to alter the content of psychotherapy according to patients' anxiety *"triggers"* (P9, P12, P15) and *"reactions"*

(P7, P9, P14). Some therapists also provided examples of using customized experiments that combine exposure and cognitive restructuring interventions. For example, P3 explained an experiment involved in asking a patient to hold a fully filled glass of water while delivering a speech, intending to invalidate the patient's particular belief of shaking a lot when anxious. Further, the type of exposure techniques used by therapists also varied for different anxiety types. For social anxiety and specific phobia, imaginal exposure (i.e., vividly imagine being in the presence of feared circumstances), stimulated exposure (e.g., using virtual reality or video), in-vivo exposure (i.e., real-life confrontation with triggers) were commonly used. For generalized anxiety, some therapists claimed to use uncertainty-based in-vivo exposure. For panic and agoraphobic anxiety, imaginal exposure was used to reduce sensitivity before interoceptive exposure.

Based on these results, we can hypothesize that the regulation outcomes would be more effective if future technologies could be designed to guide the most appropriate interventions with customized content considering patients' anxiety presentations. Some of the above results also point to customizations required in order of interventions to reduce risks to the users.

4.3   A Conceptual Framework for Regular Phases of Anxiety

In responding to Q3, many therapists required clarifications such as whether the researcher is referring to phases that are "cyclic" (P4), occurring "across the life span" (P13), or "related to therapy work" (P3). This result confirmed that the concept of anxiety phases is less established in clinical practice. However, given an example from literature [31] and conveying that we are interested in phases recurrently occurring in daily context during anxiety experiences and generic to different anxiety presentations, everyone provided useful insights, leading to tentative classes of regular and generic phases of anxiety. Figure 1 illustrates a conceptual framework of temporal phases of anxiety that we derived based on therapists' responses to this question.

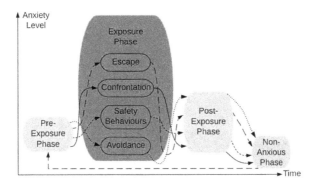

Fig. 1. Conceptual illustration of cyclic class of regular anxiety phases

We named the four identified phases as pre-exposure phase (i.e., occurs when anticipating negative outcomes before exposing to a trigger), exposure phase (i.e., occurs when or closer to exposing to a trigger), post-exposure phase (i.e., occurs after exposing to a trigger), and non-anxious phase (i.e., occurs when the maladaptive thoughts are inactive) aligned to terms used by some therapists. While the exposure phase was assumed to reflect a confrontation response to the trigger, some alternative phases were also identified: avoidance (i.e., when decided not to face the trigger at all), escape (i.e., fleeing from the trigger), safety behaviors (i.e., facing the trigger with the support that provides a sense of safety). These three alternative phases can potentially contribute to creating vicious cycles of anxiety [1], which are discerned to bring short-term relief and reinforce anxiety in the long term.

Overall, this class of phases can be better explained using an example given by P3: "*A person who has a fear of driving will anticipate well in advance if they need to drive somewhere* (pre-exposure). *Deciding not to drive and use an alternative transport mode can give them short-term relief* (avoidance). *However, later on, there is a chance that they will ruminate about their inability* (post-exposure with increasing anxiety levels). *Choosing to drive on their own can make them feel extremely anxious once they start driving* (confrontation). *Afterward, their success will give them a sense of confidence* (post-exposure with decreasing anxiety levels)". Similarly, one can imagine the outcomes of driving by having a supporter nearby (safety behavior) or deciding to stop halfway through and return without completing the trip (escape).

Rough approximates of anxiety level fluctuations across the phases, which are based on the examples given by therapists, are represented with arrows in Fig. 1. The duration of phases is not illustrated, as it was identified as highly subject to inter- and intra-patient differences; "*people with severe conditions quickly get into anxious phases, and stay most of the time in anxious phases*" (P11). An example provided by P2 clarifies this: "*a patient who only used to get anxious during lectures [...] felt anxious once got to the university, eventually became anxious while driving to the university, then started to become anxious as soon as got in the car, then got anxious as soon as woke up in the morning*". Similarly, anxiety levels and frequency of phases were also identified to vary depending on patients' triggers and baseline severity (P12, P15). Further, the four phases were identified to be occurring mostly in order for many anxiety experiences that include an apparent trigger. However, when no anticipation is involved (e.g., uncued panic attacks), therapists presumed that the pre-exposure phase is likely to be "*skipped*" (P2, P11). Also, distinguishing these phases for generalized anxiety was identified to be difficult as anxiety itself is the trigger (i.e., "*worrying that they are worrying too much*") (P5), "*anticipation is a habit*" (P7); and "thought switching" happens quickly and frequently (P7, P9, P11).

4.4   Anxiety Phases Based Customizations of Interventions

In response to Q4, therapists acknowledged that they "do not usually ask patients to involve particular interventions in certain phases of anxiety" (P3).

However, almost every therapist indicated their preferred components for identified phases with some rationale. Many therapists recommended using relaxation
during the pre-exposure phase to minimize the increase in anxiety levels. Relaxation, self-soothe or distraction, and mindfulness were perceived to support the
confrontation in the exposure phase (P3, P9, P14–15). However, all therapists
agreed that priority should be given to *"ride out fear"* (P15) without using those
strategies when direct confrontation is not highly risky. No preferences were suggested for alternative phases, as those phases should not be the goal. Aligned
to face-to-face therapy, many therapists suggested using later reflection during
the post-exposure phase. Psychoeducation and cognitive restructuring components, which require high concentration levels, were preferred for the non-anxious
phase. Moreover, a majority of therapists suggested using mindfulness, relaxation
and cognitive restructuring components regularly, regardless of patients' anxious
state. Those components were assumed to promote disorders *"prevention"* (P3,
P6, P8, P11–12, P15) and *"provide a chance to use interventions frequently for
those who report being anxious most of the time"* (P11).

These results indicate that future assistive technologies can attempt to objectively detect identified phases and guide interventions as above criteria, without
leaving patients to decide when to use which intervention.

4.5   Design Directions Motivated by Current Challenges

Through initiating discussions on Q5, we could collect therapists' insights on (1)
how the future assistive technologies can support overcoming common challenges,
as well as (2) what unintended consequences can be introduced through these
novel technologies and how we can plan to potentially mitigate them.

Practicing Environment Based Customizations. Many therapists identified stigmatization as a common challenge faced by their patients. They assumed
that their patients' lack of digital diary usage might have relations to their
concerns about whether technology usage would reveal to others that they are
experiencing a mental health condition and engaging in therapy. Therapists highlighted the need to customize interventions to users' context; designing to mini-
malize technology usage when in public by promoting non-technology activities,
such as *"socializing with friends"* (P3) or *"mindfully eating a meal"* (P7), and
designing the interventions to be practiced in public with *"hard-to-recognize"*
(P4, P13) form factors and interactions may be by integrating them into "everyday products" (P14). "Games" (P6), "mindful painting" (P4), "non-visual" feedback (P13) were among suggested technology components.

Flexible Practicing Times. Our interviews also revealed a failed method used
by current mobile technologies to involve users in interventions. The therapists,
who often review existing mobile applications aiming to select ones to recommend for their patients, claimed that frequent reminders implemented to promote engagement in interventions often do not use "gentle and encouraging language" (e.g., *"you have not used it for three months"*) (P7, P9). Such reminders

were identified to *"induce patients' anxiety"* (P7). They suggested facilitating patients' autonomy by implementing *"flexible scheduling"* (P6) for interventions to be practiced regularly, considering patients' *"anxiety states"* (P11) and *"other schedules"* (P3). Facilitating *"supporting for rescheduling"* was also identified to be important. Moreover, some therapists highlighted that technology needs to pace the frequency of interventions to avoid being over *"interruptive"* (P3, P12) and to discourage *"long-term reliance"* on technology (P4, 5). Their suggestion was to *"reduce the frequency of interventions"* (P3) as patients show progress.

Fostering Awareness and Insights on Anxiety Experience. Many therapists claimed to face the challenge of not receiving precise and sufficient information about the anxiety experiences of their patients that occur outside therapy through the recommended traditional thought and behavioral records or digital diaries. This was identified as affecting therapists' decisions, therefore, effectiveness in treatments and assessments. Many therapists linked this challenge to patients' lack of awareness and insights on their anxiety experiences. Improved awareness can support *"realizing anxiety triggers"* (P7) and also indirectly support *"understanding how much they are impaired due to anxiety"* (P1). Therefore, therapists showed their interest in digital diaries, which can (1) automatically record longitudinal behavioral analytic data related to anxiety for later reflection and (2) carefully trigger users in the real-time to record needed information based on experiencing anxiety phase.

Monitoring Progress. A majority of therapists reported spending a lot of time filling assessment questionnaires frequently with patients and comparing the results over time to understand patients' progress because that information is imperative to decide the next steps for treatment. The absence of objective evaluation metrics in current therapy was identified to *"waste a lot of time that could have been used for deep therapy work"* (P10). Therapists agreed that if future technology could at least roughly estimate and keep track of regular phases experienced by patients, those estimated could support detecting the direction and rate of progress. Some patterns that were identified as indicative of positive progress are: *"reduced frequency"* of phases corresponding to avoidance, escape and safety behavior responses (demonstrating greater *"tendency to confront"*) (P2, P4, P6, P10); *"reduced duration"* of pre-exposure (demonstrating reduced resistance to exposure) and post-exposure (demonstrating ability to quickly settle down); and *"reduction in anxiety levels"* within phases (P6, P7). Recognition of these three patterns would be possible through longitudinal objective monitoring of anxiety phases. Further, some therapists pointed to subjective ways to estimate patients' positive progress; improved ability to *"challenge negative or anxious thoughts"* (P4). This measure reflects the patient's progress in developing new skills and needs to be supported by subjective data collected during repeated cognitive restructuring interventions over time (P8).

Selecting Interventions that Work Best. In selecting an intervention out of various options to suit patients' learning styles and other preferences, therapists claimed to "*collaborate with patients*" (P1) as they are the "*experts of themselves*" (P5). For this purpose and to validate the appropriateness of selected interventions, usage history on different interventions could support. Measures such as: (1) whether there was a significant anxiety level change from prior-to-after usage of an intervention, and (2) how much the user liked using an intervention were identified to be relevant to understand which interventions worked best in the past. Some therapists also shared experiences of patients who got bored and less reactive to certain intervention options that were used repeatedly. Based on this observation, clinicians suggested that future technologies can guide different intervention options at the detection of reduced progress.

Not Inducing Anxiety Through Careful Presentation. Despite the benefits of fostering awareness regarding anxiety, therapists presumed that presenting anxiety detection data too often or to a patient who is not ready for it could generate obsessive preoccupation. They suggested that technologies should not be designed to make users "*overattentive to their anxiety patterns*" (P7). They pointed that "*guidance from a therapist is important for sensitive users when reviewing such information*" (P5), as they may over-ruminate due to the "*lack the ability to process information*" (P12) and "*use it for their benefit*" (P10).

Therapists also provided insight into the idea that technologies can use carefully designed data presentation to find a balance between improving awareness and mitigating the related risks. One such mechanism is reflecting on areas that need improvement while emphasizing positive progress. For example,"*without presenting that the user had x number of panic attacks since beginning, present facts such as: earlier you had one attack every day, but now it is five days a week; and you do not stay in panic state for 15 min anymore, but only 10 min*" (P7). Another approach is not directly reporting detected adverse phases or negative progress without reconfirming, as algorithms are not always accurate. To gain further insights, a questioning approach can be used: "*for most people when they display a similar pattern, they feel quite anxious, and for some people, it might mean* (involving in an intense physical activity) *or* (excitement), *are any of these apply to you right now?*" (P11). Part of this strategy is to inform users that they are not the only ones with anxiety problems and not upset them when technology produces false anxiety reports. Further, technology can present neutral or negative progress "*with recommendations to act upon*" (P13); e.g., see a therapist. These strategies can reduce the risk for users who require additional support in interpreting information from technology. Therapists suggested that they can play a role in this process by communicating information to patients in appropriate forms while making important clinical decisions (e.g., modifying therapy or "*referring patients to new therapists that suit them better*") (P13).

Overall, in order to convert therapist-guided customizations into automated adaptations envisioned in this section, the technologies need to gain the ability to detect the user-specific, context-specific, and time-specific factors that rule those customizations. The potential factors that we discovered include patients' anxiety presentations, their baseline severity, the experiencing phase of anxiety, whether they have completed prerequisite interventions, and timeliness to practice interventions. Objective anxiety assessment research could potentially support automating the detection of these anxiety-related factors [15, 23, 26, 35, 42, 47]. Further, the technology can keep track of previously practiced interventions by the user and use that data to check whether the user has completed prerequisite interventions. Moreover, the technology can use anxiety phase detection data and subjective data from other applications like calendar apps to check the timeliness to practice interventions.

5   Limitations and Future Work

The validity of the reported results can be supported by the literature evidence, therapists' expertise, and the empirically validated interventions that they use. However, involving potential end-users (i.e., patient and general public populations) is vital to perform refinements in future work. The tentative phases and customizations suggested in this paper can be used as a starting point to investigate further and needs to be done through the collection and analysis of subjective and objective data from potential end-user populations in future research. An initial attempt towards this goal is presented in [47]. Further analysis of longitudinal data collected in the wild could yield more rigorous discoveries (e.g., modified phases, new measures to estimate patients' progress).

Achieving all the design directions indicated in this paper in a single design would not be straightforward because some of the suggested goals cannot be achieved without extensive research work. Examples include analytically detecting the factors that rule the suggested customizations; implementing various interventions, customization criteria and other design considerations; validating them through user studies over extended periods; and refining to accommodate individual differences of anxiety experience. Such efforts require collaborations in HCI, data-analytic, and psychology areas, encouraged in this paper to achieve envisioned benefits to the patient, therapists, and general public populations.

6   Conclusion

This paper contributes to a unique area of knowledge; design directions for more effective and personalized mobile assistive technologies for anxiety. As major contributions, it identifies a rich set of literature-driven and expert therapist-informed design directions for future digital intervention and digital diary technologies, including (1) a set of user's anxiety experience-specific and context-specific factors, which can be considered in guiding suitable interventions for a user, (2) preliminary directions for detecting those factors, including a conceptual framework for regular phases of anxiety; (3) potential intervention-based customizations considering those factors, which could accommodate inter- and intra-individual differences in anxiety; and (4) directions for overcoming current challenges faced by patients and therapists using proposed capabilities and for mitigating unintended adverse consequences that new adaptive technology can raise. These contributions can draw the attention of human-computer interaction researchers to critical design directions, which incorporate clinical knowledge and analytic capabilities beyond the traditional user-interface design.

Acknowledgments. We thank our participants for their time and valuable insights. We also thank Swamy Ananthanarayan, Jarrod Knibbe, Patrick Olivier and Kim Marriott for providing feedback at different stages to improve this manuscript.

References

1. Albano, A.M., Barlow, D.H.: Breaking the vicious cycle: cognitive-behavioral group treatment for socially anxious youth. In: Psychosocial Treatments for Child and Adolescent Disorders: Empirically Based Strategies for Clinical Practice, pp. 43–62 (1996)
2. Alonso, J., et al.: Treatment gap for anxiety disorders is global: results of the world mental health surveys in 21 countries. Depress. Anxiety **35**(3), 195–208 (2018)
3. Aslan, I., Burkhardt, H., Kraus, J., André, E.: Hold my heart and breathe with me: tangible somaesthetic designs. In: Proceedings of the 9th Nordic Conference on Human-Computer Interaction, NordiCHI 2016, pp. 92:1–92:6. ACM, New York (2016)
4. American Psychiatric Association, et al.: Diagnostic and statistical manual of mental disorders (DSM-5®). American Psychiatric Publishing, Arlington (2013)
5. Bakker, D., Kazantzis, N., Rickwood, D., Rickard, N.: Development and pilot evaluation of smartphone-delivered cognitive behavior therapy strategies for mood-and anxiety-related problems: moodmission. Cogn. Behav. Pract. **25**(4), 496–514 (2018)
6. Bandelow, B., Reitt, M., Röver, C., Michaelis, S., Görlich, Y., Wedekind, D.: Efficacy of treatments for anxiety disorders: a meta-analysis. Int. Clin. Psychopharmacol. **30**(4), 183–192 (2015)
7. Barker, M., Van der Linden, J.: Sprite catcher: a handheld self-reflection and mindfulness tool for mental healthcare. In: Proceedings of the Eleventh International Conference on Tangible, Embedded, and Embodied Interaction, TEI 2017, pp. 419–425. ACM, New York (2017)
8. Beckers, T., Craske, M.G.: Avoidance and decision making in anxiety: an introduction to the special issue. Behav. Res. Ther. **96**, 1–2 (2017)
9. Boukhechba, M., Baglione, A.N., Barnes, L.E.: Leveraging mobile sensing and machine learning for personalized mental health care. Ergon. Des. **28**(4), 18–23 (2020)
10. Brandenburg, A.: Cognitive behavioral therapy for anxiety disorders: predictors of outcome. Master's thesis, University of Twente (2017)
11. Chen, C., George, S., Liberzon, I.: 4.13 - stress and anxiety disorders. In: Pfaff, D.W., Joëls, M. (eds.) Hormones, Brain and Behavior, 3rd edn, pp. 251–274. Academic Press, Oxford (2017)
12. Cuijpers, P., Ebert, D.D., Acarturk, C., Andersson, G., Cristea, I.A.: Personalized psychotherapy for adult depression: a meta-analytic review. Behav. Ther. **47**(6), 966–980 (2016)
13. Fitzpatrick, K.K., Darcy, A., Vierhile, M.: Delivering cognitive behavior therapy to young adults with symptoms of depression and anxiety using a fully automated conversational agent (Woebot): a randomized controlled trial. JMIR Ment. Health **4**(2), e19 (2017)

14. Frey, J., Grabli, M., Slyper, R., Cauchard, J.R.: Breeze: sharing biofeedback through wearable technologies. In: Proceedings of the 2018 CHI Conference on Human Factors in Computing Systems, pp. 1–12 (2018)
15. Giannakakis, G., et al.: Stress and anxiety detection using facial cues from videos. Biomed. Sig. Process. Control **31**, 89–101 (2017)
16. Grupe, D.W., Nitschke, J.B.: Uncertainty and anticipation in anxiety: an integrated neurobiological and psychological perspective. Nat. Rev. Neurosci. **14**(7), 488–501 (2013)
17. Hobfoll, S.E.: Conservation of resources: a new attempt at conceptualizing stress. Am. Psychol. **44**(3), 513 (1989)
18. Kaczkurkin, A.N., Foa, E.B.: Cognitive-behavioral therapy for anxiety disorders: an update on the empirical evidence. Dialogues Clin. Neurosci. **17**(3), 337–346 (2015)
19. Kertz, S.J., MacLaren Kelly, J., Stevens, K.T., Schrock, M., Danitz, S.B.: A review of free iPhone applications designed to target anxiety and worry. J. Technol. Behav. Sci. **2**(2), 61–70 (2017). https://doi.org/10.1007/s41347-016-0006-y
20. Kessler, R., Petukhova, M., Sampson, N., Zaslavsky, A., Wittchen, H.: Twelve-month and lifetime prevalence and lifetime morbid risk of anxiety and mood disorders in the United States. Int. J. Methods Psychiatr. Res. **21**(3), 169–184 (2012)
21. Liang, R.H., Yu, B., Xue, M., Hu, J., Feijs, L.M.G.: BioFidget: biofeedback for respiration training using an augmented fidget spinner. In: Proceedings of the 2018 CHI Conference on Human Factors in Computing Systems, CHI 2018, pp. 613:1–613:12. ACM, New York (2018)
22. de Lijster, J.M., et al.: The age of onset of anxiety disorders: a meta-analysis. Can. J. Psychiatry **62**(4), 237–246 (2017)
23. Liu, H., Wen, W., Zhang, J., Liu, G., Yang, Z.: Autonomic nervous pattern of motion interference in real-time anxiety detection. IEEE Access **6**, 69763–69768 (2018)
24. Loerinc, A.G., Meuret, A.E., Twohig, M.P., Rosenfield, D., Bluett, E.J., Craske, M.G.: Response rates for CBT for anxiety disorders: need for standardized criteria. Clin. Psychol. Rev. **42**(C), 72–82 (2015)
25. Macik, M., et al.: Breathing friend: tackling stress through portable tangible breathing artifact. In: Bernhaupt, R., Dalvi, G., Joshi, A., K. Balkrishan, D., O'Neill, J., Winckler, M. (eds.) INTERACT 2017. LNCS, vol. 10516, pp. 106–115. Springer, Cham (2017). https://doi.org/10.1007/978-3-319-68059-0_6
26. Martinez, H., Bengio, Y., Yannakakis, G.: Learning deep physiological models of affect. IEEE Comput. Intell. Mag. **8**(2), 20–33 (2013)
27. Martinez, S.G., Badillo-Urquiola, K.A., Leis, R.A., Chavez, J., Green, T., Clements, T.: Investigation of multimodal mobile applications for improving mental health. In: Schmorrow, D.D.D., Fidopiastis, C.M.M. (eds.) AC 2016. LNCS (LNAI), vol. 9744, pp. 333–343. Springer, Cham (2016). https://doi.org/10.1007/978-3-319-39952-2_32
28. Meuret, A.E., et al.: Do unexpected panic attacks occur spontaneously? Biol. Psychiatry **70**(10), 985–991 (2011)
29. Mohammedali, M., Phung, D., Adams, B., Venkatesh, S.: A context-sensitive device to help people with autism cope with anxiety. In: CHI 2011 Extended Abstracts on Human Factors in Computing Systems, CHI EA 2011, pp. 1201–1206. Association for Computing Machinery, New York (2011)
30. Mood tracker (2020). https://www.moodtracker.com

31. Morrison, A.S., et al.: Anxiety trajectories in response to a speech task in social anxiety disorder: evidence from a randomized controlled trial of CBT. J. Anxiety Disord. **38**, 21–30 (2016)
32. Nezu, C.M., Nezu, A.M., Bullis, J.R., Hofmann, S.G.: Adult anxiety and related disorders. In: The Oxford Handbook of Cognitive and Behavioral Therapies, 1 edn. Oxford University Press (2015)
33. Niles, A.N., et al.: Advancing personalized medicine: application of a novel statistical method to identify treatment moderators in the coordinated anxiety learning and management study. Behav. Ther. **48**(4), 490–500 (2017)
34. Nowell, L.S., Norris, J.M., White, D.E., Moules, N.J.: Thematic analysis: striving to meet the trustworthiness criteria. Int J Qual Methods **16**(1), 1–13 (2017)
35. Özseven, T., Düğenci, M., Doruk, A., Kahraman, H.İ.: Voice traces of anxiety: acoustic parameters affected by anxiety disorder. Arch. Acoust. **43**(4), 625–636 (2018)
36. Parette, P., Scherer, M.: Assistive technology use and stigma. Educ. Train. Dev. Disabil. **39**(3), 217–226 (2004)
37. Poon, S.K.: Pacifica: stressed or worried? An app to help yourself (mobile app user guide). Br. J. Sports Med. **50**(3), 191–192 (2016)
38. Qu, C., Sas, C., Doherty, G.: Exploring and designing for memory impairments in depression. In: Proceedings of the 2019 CHI Conference on Human Factors in Computing Systems, CHI 2019, pp. 510:1–510:15. ACM, New York (2019)
39. Rennert, K., Karapanos, E.: Faceit: supporting reflection upon social anxiety events with lifelogging. In: CHI 2013 Extended Abstracts on Human Factors in Computing Systems, CHI EA 2013, pp. 457–462. ACM, New York (2013)
40. Richter, J., Hamm, A.O., Pané-Farré, C.A., et al.: Dynamics of defensive reactivity in patients with panic disorder and agoraphobia: implications for the etiology of panic disorder. Biol. Psychiatry **72**(6), 512–520 (2012)
41. Rosenfield, D., Zhou, E., Wilhelm, F.H., Conrad, A., Roth, W.T., Meuret, A.E.: Change point analysis for longitudinal physiological data: detection of cardio-respiratory changes preceding panic attacks. Biol. Psychol. **84**(1), 112–120 (2010)
42. Rubin, J., Abreu, R., Ahern, S., Eldardiry, H., Bobrow, D.G.: Time, frequency & complexity analysis for recognizing panic states from physiologic time-series. In: Proceedings of the 10th EAI International Conference on Pervasive Computing Technologies for Healthcare, PervasiveHealth 2016, pp. 81–88. ICST (Institute for Computer Sciences, Social-Informatics and Telecommunications Engineering), Brussels (2016)
43. Sanchez, A.Y.R., Kunze, K.: Flair: towards a therapeutic serious game for social anxiety disorder. In: Proceedings of the 2018 ACM International Joint Conference and 2018 International Symposium on Pervasive and Ubiquitous Computing and Wearable Computers, UbiComp 2018, pp. 239–242. ACM, New York (2018)
44. Schneider, R.L., Arch, J.J., Wolitzky-Taylor, K.B.: The state of personalized treatment for anxiety disorders: a systematic review of treatment moderators. Clin. Psychol. Rev. **38**(C), 39–54 (2015)
45. Schroeder, J., et al.: Pocket skills: a conversational mobile web app to support dialectical behavioral therapy. In: Proceedings of the 2018 CHI Conference on Human Factors in Computing Systems, CHI 2018, pp. 398:1–398:15. ACM, New York (2018)
46. Senaratne, H., Ellis, K., Oviatt, S., Melvin, G.: Designing efficacious mobile technologies for anxiety self-regulation. In: Extended Abstracts of the 2019 CHI Conference on Human Factors in Computing Systems, CHI EA 2019, pp. 1–6. ACM, New York (2019)

47. Senaratne, H., Kuhlmann, L., Ellis, K., Melvin, G., Oviatt, S.: A multimodal dataset and evaluation for feature estimators of temporal phases of anxiety. In: Proceedings of the 2021 International Conference on Multimodal Interaction, ICMI 2021, pp. 52–61. Association for Computing Machinery, New York (2021)
48. Silfvernagel, K., Wassermann, C., Andersson, G.: Individually tailored internet-based cognitive behavioural therapy for young adults with anxiety disorders: a pilot effectiveness study. Internet Interv. **8**, 48–52 (2017)
49. Simm, W., Ferrario, M.A., Gradinar, A., Whittle, J.: Prototyping 'clasp': implications for designing digital technology for and with adults with autism. In: Proceedings of the 2014 Conference on Designing Interactive Systems, DIS 2014, pp. 345–354. ACM, New York (2014)
50. Steimer, T.: The biology of fear-and anxiety-related behaviors. Dialogues Clin. Neurosci. **4**, 231–249 (2002)
51. Summerfeldt, L.J., Kloosterman, P.H., Antony, M.M., McCabe, R.E., Parker, J.D.: Emotional intelligence in social phobia and other anxiety disorders. J. Psychopathol. Behav. Assess. **33**(1), 69–78 (2011)
52. Thieme, A., et al.: Challenges for designing new technology for health and well-being in a complex mental healthcare context. In: Proceedings of the 2016 CHI Conference on Human Factors in Computing Systems, CHI 2016, pp. 2136–2149. ACM, New York (2016)
53. Topham, P., Caleb-Solly, P., Matthews, P., Farmer, A., Mash, C.: Mental health app design: a journey from concept to completion. In: Proceedings of the 17th International Conference on Human-Computer Interaction with Mobile Devices and Services Adjunct, MobileHCI 2015, pp. 582–591. ACM, New York (2015)
54. Torous, J., Wolters, M.K., Wadley, G., Calvo, R.A.: 4th symposium on computing and mental health: designing ethical emental health services. In: Extended Abstracts of the 2019 CHI Conference on Human Factors in Computing Systems, CHI EA 2019, pp. Sym05:1–Sym05:9. ACM, New York (2019)
55. Watt, M.C., Stewart, S.H., Conrod, P.J., Schmidt, N.B.: Personality-based approaches to treatment of co-morbid anxiety and substance use disorder. In: Stewart, S.H., Conrod, P.J. (eds.) Anxiety and Substance Use Disorders. SARD, pp. 201–219. Springer, Boston (2008). https://doi.org/10.1007/978-0-387-74290-8_11
56. Wehbe, R.R., et al.: Above water: an educational game for anxiety. In: Proceedings of the 2016 Annual Symposium on Computer-Human Interaction in Play Companion Extended Abstracts, CHI PLAY Companion 2016, pp. 79–84. ACM, New York (2016)
57. Williams, C., Garland, A.: Identifying and challenging unhelpful thinking. Adv. Psychiatr. Treat. **8**(5), 377–386 (2002)
58. Wilson, C., Draper, S., Brereton, M., Johnson, D.: Towards thriving: extending computerised cognitive behavioural therapy. In: Proceedings of the 29th Australian Conference on Computer-Human Interaction, OZCHI 2017, pp. 285–295. ACM, New York (2017)
59. Winkler, P., et al.: Increase in prevalence of current mental disorders in the context of COVID-19: analysis of repeated nationwide cross-sectional surveys. Epidemiol. Psychiatr. Sci. **29**(e173), 1–8 (2020)
60. World Health Organization: Depression and other common mental disorders: global health estimates (2017). Licence: CC BY-NC-SA 3.0 IGO

Queering E-Therapy: Considerations for the Delivery of Virtual Reality Based Mental Health Solutions with LGBTQ2IA+ Communities

Adrian Bolesnikov[✉], Aryan Golshan, Lauren Tierney, Ashi Mann, Jin Kang, and Audrey Girouard

Carleton University, Ottawa, ON K1S 5B6, Canada
{adrian.bolesnikov,aryan.golshan,lauren.tierney,ashi.mann,
jin.kang,audrey.girouard}@carleton.ca

Abstract. Virtual Reality (VR) has emerged as a rapidly advancing technology with substantial attention from scientific disciplines including Psychology and Human-Computer Interaction. It has become an attractive tool that can offer healthcare support. Marginalized groups like lesbian, gay, bisexual, transgender, queer/questioning, two-spirit, intersex, and asexual/aromatic (LGBTQ2IA+) adults are at increased risk of poor mental health outcomes. The design of digital mental health tools, including VR, often overlook queer adults. In this study, we investigate the experience and the potential of digital mental health services for queer adults and mental health practitioners (MHP) that may inform future designs and implementation. We deployed an online survey and collected responses from 12 queer participants and 7 MHP. We found five themes that address general digital mental health for queer adults and MHP: (1) simple delivery, (2) flexible use, (3) seamless interactivity, (4) personalization, and (5) support. In addition, we noted six themes for VR-specific design considerations: (1) low cost (2) research, training, and education, (3) usability, (4) safety and privacy, (5) immersion, and (6) provider control and customization. Our findings highlight a series of actionable design considerations for digital mental health tools, and emphasize the importance of factors such as usability and accessibility when designing digital mental health tools for the queer community.

Keywords: Support technology · Mental health · LGBTQ+ · E-therapy

1 Introduction

Lesbian, gay, bisexual, transgender, queer/questioning, two-spirit, intersex, and asexual/aromantic (LGBTQ2IA+, hereinafter referred to as *queer*) adults are more likely to have negative mental health experiences and may struggle with anxiety, depression, or suicidal thoughts [1–4]. Although queer individuals are as diverse as the general Canadian population with regards to their experiences of mental health and well-being, they

H. Lewy and R. Barkan (Eds.): PH 2021, LNICST 431, pp. 183–203, 2022.
https://doi.org/10.1007/978-3-030-99194-4_13

face higher risks for some mental health issues because of discrimination and the social determinants of health [5–8]. There are three significant determinants of positive mental health and wellbeing as outlined by a report from the Centre for Addiction and Mental Health [9] including: social inclusion, freedom from discrimination and violence, as well as access to economic resources. All three factor LGBTQ2IA+ individuals and communities; Bisexual and trans people are over-represented among low-income Canadians and the average personal incomes of LGBTQ2IA+ income earners are significantly less than those of non-LGBTQ2IA+ people [10, 11].

Queer individuals experience stigma and discrimination across their life spans, and are often targets of hate crimes, sexual and/or physical assault and harassment [7]. In Canada, hate crimes motivated by sexual orientation were deemed the most violent of all hate crimes and more than doubled between 2007 and 2008 [8]. Furthermore, trans people in both Canada and the US have reported high levels of violence, harassment, and discrimination when seeking services such as stable housing, employment, health, or even social services [12]. These are but a few of many factors that may impact the mental health and well-being for queer adults [5].

In line with what has been seen historically, queer individuals face various social, structural, and behavioural barriers to adequate healthcare services [13–15]. Barriers include a lack of adequately trained healthcare professionals on queer health needs, high costs, and systemic discrimination [3, 4].

Human-Computer Interaction (HCI) researchers and healthcare professionals have long been interested in employing digital mental health services to overcome barriers of access and address psychological impacts [16–18]. Digital services have proven to be effective for the delivery of various mental health interventions such as counselling, mindfulness, and therapy [19, 20]. The growing effectiveness of video-conferencing tools (e.g., Zoom, Jane.app, Doxy.me, Microsoft Teams, etc.) for the delivery of mental health services opens the door for other emerging technologies, such as Virtual Reality (VR), to be further explored for practicality [21–23].

While often debated, the definition of VR is an umbrella term for the real-time presentation of a computer-generated environment that users may interact with through multisensory stimulation capable of triggering emotional and physiological responses [24, 25]. These technologies have beneficial applications with decreasing costs of hardware and increased availability of open-access software [24–30]. The primary consideration for applying VR in healthcare, and more specifically within the mental health context (Clinical VR), is due to the level of immersion enabled by the technology and the level of presence experienced by the user [31]. This is vital as highly immersive virtual experiences have proven to improve users' cognitive and affective abilities when participating in a variety of situations, particularly in anxiety reduction through therapy [32]. However, clinical rehabilitation requires further exploration, particularly for the potential VR has when addressing certain challenges faced by queer adults [1, 4, 14, 15, 19, 33–35].

Our study contributes a unique perspective into the use of current digital mental health tools for the delivery of mental health services and focuses on the needs of queer adults and Mental Health Practitioners (MHP) alike. Furthermore, this study explores their attitudes of VR for the use in clinical mental health care and can inform the future design of digital mental health tools and VR systems for queer adults and MHP. We offer design considerations that can be applied to both mainstream and queer-specific contexts, which can address concerns of both inequality and inequity of mental health services provided to queer individuals [36–38].

We conducted a qualitative survey with a group of queer adults and MHP to address the following two research questions:

Our objective was to answer the following research questions:

Research Question 1 (RQ1): What is the experience of modern digital mental health tools for queer adults and mental health practitioners?
Research Question 2 (RQ2): What do queer adults and MHP think about the use and implementation of clinical VR as a tool for mental health services?

2 Related Work

Recent HCI research has played a large role in examining the effectiveness and design implications for technologies designed to address the broad spectrum of complex mental health needs [22, 39–42]. These technologies, referred to as *digital mental health services* in this paper, include a vast array of mediums from web and mobile-based applications for mood tracking, to VR simulations to address phobias [19, 39]. We now discuss a myriad of design consideration for the queer community followed by a discussion on the current state of VR as a digital mental health service.

2.1 HCI and VR Considerations for the Queer Community

Prominent user experience discussions for queer communities often focus on the creation of inclusive websites, graphic design, and surveys [43–46]. DeVito et al. [34], however, label Queer HCI as "research in HCI by, for, or substantially shaped by the queer community itself and/or queering methods and theory, regardless of application subdomain" (p. 2).

As a field in design, Queer HCI has largely focused on topics of queer social media usage [47] and has only recently begun to branch into popular topics of identity and trans technology [48, 49]. The use of VR for queer adults, however, has begun to be explored further and has shown to provide positive user experiences, particularly when expressing evolving queer identities [50–53]. Jones et al. [51] explored queer avatars in the video game *Second Life*. They found the in-game feature of finding "virtual bodies" (i.e., representation of one's presence in a digital context) and configuration options lend to heightened agency via gender and sexual expression granting opportunities for interpersonal connection and experiential immersion [51]. Similarly, Pare et al. [50] explored how VR can support the development of critical literacies on gender and sexuality. Their analysis showed that the figured worlds of the participants (i.e., a simulated environment based on particular worldviews and effective thinking) were emergent and dynamically constructed through creative and collaborative efforts and that engagement with others enabled participants to find affirmation on their identities.

HCI researchers have also incorporated VR to support queer individuals in other ways. For instance, Muessig et al. [54] created an artificial intelligence-based VR system designed to aid queer HIV+ men practise disclosing their status in a variety of scenarios. They found that 81% of participants felt the system was easy to use and found the system effective to practise holding difficult discussions regarding HIV status. This finding highlights the potential of VR as a tool for addressing complex and difficult personal situations for queer adults.

2.2 VR for Digital Mental Health

HCI and psychology literature has explored VR as a tool for digital mental healthcare, notably in the treatment of anxiety disorders. This is largely due to the increased subjective perceptions of safety and control over how the stimuli are presented [25]. While not meant to replace the need for trained therapists, VR offers a tool that can augment the access and effectiveness of techniques such as exposure therapy through subtle and gradual progression protocols [28]. Similarly, patients living with social anxiety may benefit from the opportunity to enhance and train their skills with virtual exposure [54]. A patient can use computer designed environments to experience triggering situations [26].

One particular affordance of VR makes this technology an effective mental healthcare tool for queer adults; this affordance can alleviate some of the psychosocial barriers that discourage queer adults from utilizing mental healthcare services. In VR, the patient and the healthcare provider interact in a multidimensional computer-generated environment in real time and both participants can represent themselves in the form of virtual avatars [55, 56]. This digital representation adds a layer of anonymity (e.g., the patient does not need to reveal their physical appearance and even adopt a pseudonym), encouraging the patient to fear less about the healthcare provider's evaluation and also encouraging the patient to express their thoughts more openly and honestly [56, 57].

Main psychosocial barriers that discourage queer adults from seeking out mental healthcare services are their experience of past discrimination [58] and their fear of being negatively evaluated and stigmatized by others, including healthcare providers [59, 60]. VR's affordance of anonymity and the resulting sense of safety and control can alleviate these unique barriers experienced by queer adults.

VR technology does present barriers to implementation. Not only does cyber-sickness pose a potentially negatively impact to a user's experience [25, 28], acquisition of VR technologies in a clinical setting is often expensive and requires training for therapists to become familiar with the use of these tools [25, 33]. Questions remain as to how users will cope with extended treatments through VR as VR is not being readily implemented for interventions such as "talk therapy," and it remains a relatively unexplored area.

Despite these limitations, VR is becoming accessible to the general population due to it being increasingly affordable and accommodating for individuals with various abilities (including those with temporary or chronic disabilities) through virtual deployment [26, 28]. The current research and design efforts are geared towards non-queer individuals. It is important to investigate the potential of VR as a mental healthcare tool for queer adults with the ultimate goal of creating inclusive design and implementation guidelines that incorporate the needs of as many user populations as possible.

3 Study Methodology

We distributed two online Qualtrics surveys to queer participants and MHP to address our two RQs. We created two surveys; one for queer participants, and another for MHP. We obtained approval from the Carleton University Research Ethics Board.

3.1 Data Collection and Analysis

The survey collected both qualitative and quantitative information, included 38 questions for MHP and 32 questions for queer participants, and explored demographic information, mental healthcare experiences, and perceptions of VR. We piloted both surveys to ensure clarity and functionality. We collected survey responses during a one-week period between March 23 and March 30, 2021.

MHP and queer participants responded to long form survey questions including questions such as the following: (1) Describe the aspects about the services/tools that worked well, or could use improvement; (2) Describe the most significant barriers to providing/receiving mental health services/tools; (3) Describe the necessary criteria when choosing/providing a mental health service or tool; (4) Describe and expand on whether or not you are interested in using VR technologies for providing/receiving mental health service; and (5) Describe the necessary features and resources required for VR-based technology to provide effective mental health services.

We analyzed participant responses using a collaborative, inductive approach to thematic analysis through Microsoft Excel and Miro. We downloaded the survey responses from Qualtrics and separated the responses into respective qualitative and quantitative spreadsheets. One researcher further broke down qualitative responses into meaningful segments prior to coding while another created a pivot table of quantitative responses for quick processing. We systematically and iteratively coded the collected qualitative survey data using primarily emotion and value coding techniques [35, 61, 62]. Due to the length of the surveys, all researchers were able to participate in the coding process by establishing meaning units to ascribe both condensed meanings and the initial code frame prior to working as a team towards refining codes and establishing a codebook that highlighted the final major themes using Miro digital whiteboarding.

3.2 Participants and Recruitment

We recruited participants (N = 19) through online special interest groups (e.g., Queer Design Club and Psychology Today Canada), social media, word of mouth, and snowballing techniques. We recruited queer participants who were 18 years of age or older, comfortable with the English language and self-identified as queer. We also recruited MHP who were 18 years of age or older, comfortable with the English language and actively practising and registered with a Canadian regulatory body. We did not require either participant group to have experience using digital mental health services or VR but deemed it beneficial. We assigned unique pseudonyms to both groups (MHP as PM#, queer participants as PL#).

For the MHP survey, we had a total of 7 participants. All participants were from the province of Ontario and most of them had over 3 years of working experience and held positions as Clinical Psychologists or Psychotherapists (see Table 1 for a full summary of demographic information related to MHP).

Table 1. Mental health professional participant demographics

Participant	Age range (Years)	Gender	Sexual orientation	Race	Clientele
PM02	26–35	Woman/womxn	Straight/Heterosexual	White/Caucasian	Adolescents, Adults, Students, Young adults
PM03	26–35	Woman/womxn	Straight/Heterosexual	Middle Eastern	Adolescents, Children, Families
PM04	26–35	Woman/womxn	Straight/Heterosexual	White/Caucasian	Adolescents, Adults, Students, Young adults
PM05	26–35	Woman/womxn	Straight/Heterosexual	White/Caucasian	Adolescents, Adults, Children, Families, Students, Young adults
PM06	36–45	Woman/womxn	Straight/Heterosexual	White/Caucasian	Adolescents, Adults, Children, Families, LGBTQ+ community, Students, Young adults
PM07	36–45	Woman/womxn	Straight/Heterosexual	White/Caucasian	Adolescents, Adults, Students, Young adults

(*continued*)

Table 1. (*continued*)

Participant	Age range (Years)	Gender	Sexual orientation	Race	Clientele
PM08	36–45	Woman/womxn	Straight/Heterosexual	White/Caucasian	Adolescents, Adults, Children, Seniors, Students, Young adults

For the queer participants' survey, we had a total of 12 responses. Participants were from Canada ($n = 8$) and the United States ($n = 4$), mostly White or Caucasian, and between 18 and 35 years of age. Only one participant identified as transgender. See Table 2 for a full summary of demographic information related to queer participants.

Table 2. Queer participant demographics

Participant	Age range (Years)	Gender	Sexual orientation	Race	Digital mental health services/Tools
PL01	18–25	Woman/womxn	Queer	Hispanic/Latinx	Yes (virtual counselling, meditation app)
PL02	18–25	Man	Gay/Homosexual	White/Caucasian	Yes (meditation app)
PL03	26–35	Man	Gay/Homosexual	White/Caucasian	Yes (virtual therapy, meditation app)
PL04	18–25	Woman/womxn	Lesbian	White/Caucasian	Yes (virtual counselling, meditation app)
PL05	18–25	Woman/womxn	Bisexual, Pansexual, Queer	White/Caucasian	Yes (meditation app)
PL06	26–35	Man	Gay/Homosexual	Multiracial or Biracial	No

(*continued*)

Table 2. (*continued*)

Participant	Age range (Years)	Gender	Sexual orientation	Race	Digital mental health services/Tools
PL07	18–25	Woman/womxn	Bisexual, Queer	Asian	No
PL08	26–35	Man	Gay/Homosexual	White/Caucasian	Yes (virtual counselling, virtual therapy)
PL09	18–15	Man	Gay/Homosexual	White/Caucasian	No
PL10	18–25	Woman/womxn	Bisexual	White/Caucasian	Yes (meditation app)
PL11	26–35	Man	Gay/Homosexual	White/Caucasian	Yes (virtual counselling, meditation app)
PL12	18–25	Genderfluid, Woman/womxn	Lesbian	White/Caucasian	No

4 Findings

4.1 Descriptive Information on Mental Health Services

4.1.1 Barriers of Digital Mental Health Services

Four queer participants did not use mental health services. Two participants indicated not requiring these services, while two participants highlighted a lack of locally available resources and felt uncomfortable with seeking out said services. The most significant barriers to accessing mental health services and tools for queer participants were high cost ($n = 9$), limited availability ($n = 7$), and lack of queer-friendly resources ($n = 7$). Four queer participants stressed the importance of making digital mental interventions readily available and accessible to clients.

Four MHP indicated a lack of queer-friendly resources as a potential barrier to accessing mental health services, while three indicated limited availability, stigma from friends and family, and lack of culturally sensitive/representative resources as prominent barriers. They identified the need for accessibility and availability of services for their clients. Equity of these services, due to cost and wait times, were the most common barriers associated with accessibility ($n = 6$). These participants identified the cost of mental health services and tools, and the need for additional funding support for both clients and therapists as a major barrier.

4.1.2 Use of Digital Mental Health Tools

Most queer participants with experience using digital mental health services indicated having done so either from a recommendation (friends or family [$n = 6$]; an MHP [$n = 1$]) or due to a required shift to online services because of the COVID-19 pandemic ($n = 3$). Queer participants showed no steady trend in how frequently they use devices (daily ($n = 2$), weekly ($n = 1$), biweekly ($n = 1$), "when I need it" ($n = 1$)) in relation to factors such as the services they use. We found, however, that most queer participants with previous experience ($n = 6$) access their respective services and tools via their mobile device (smartphones) as opposed to a desktop computer or laptop ($n = 3$).

The majority of MHP had provided mental health services digitally ($n = 6$), while one had not due to confidentiality concerns. All MHP who had used digital services indicated that the ongoing pandemic required the shift online or the use of the digital platforms were recommended by a client or fellow MHP ($n = 1$). The digital services and tools used to provide mental health services included mental-health questionnaires (via q-global, MHS online assessment centre, etc.), video-conferencing platforms (Jane.app, Zoom, Microsoft Teams, Doxy.me, Virtual Care, etc.), and telerehabilitation. These services were used daily ($n = 4$), or weekly ($n = 2$) with clients.

Seven queer participants had experience with VR technologies with all but one having used it for entertainment purposes such as digital gaming. Only one MHP had experience using VR to provide mental health services. This participant used VR for exposures therapy to simulate experiences such as phobias.

4.2 Experiences with Digital Mental Health Services

We found five considerations for the delivery of a digital mental health services (Fig. 1).

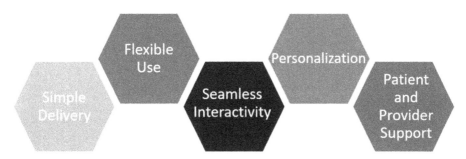

Fig. 1. An overview of five considerations in response to RQ1.

Requirement 1: Simple Delivery. Queer participants highlighted a need for these systems to operate simply and consistently ($n = 5$). A "low-pressure environment" (PL08) was vital to creating positive experiences that aligned with goals of clinical care. However, it remains crucial that this did not impact the tool's ability to address the user's needs.

For MHP, the most significant barrier for using digital tools for the delivery of mental health services was a lack of familiarity ($n = 4$). To address this, they indicated the delivery of care worked well when the product was visually appealing ($n = 1$), easy to navigate and user-friendly (thus requiring minimal need for technological skills, $n = 4$), simple to troubleshoot ($n = 2$) and integrate smoothly with other tools ($n = 3$). PM04 highlighted simplicity, requiring few steps to avoid frustrating experiences. A virtual platform may be as "simple as copying and pasting the zoom link into their web browser" (PM03). They further explained that "it is tricky for clients to navigate, who are not as tech savvy … you are then faced with navigating frustration on top of your client's goals for the session." PM03 also expressed the importance of considering that MHP are "working with individual's impacted by potentially poor mental health, [so] asking them to navigate systems that are multi-stepped needs to be factored in advance by the clinician."

Requirement 2: Flexible Use. Four MHP described flexible delivery as the integration of services and tools with current technology (i.e., smartphones, computers, tablets), and providing flexible service that can address geographic, transportation, physical and mental barriers. Furthermore, they desire a digital service that could be a multi-use tool. PM02 and PM04 gave examples where the integration of "scheduling appointments," "encompasses everything that is required," and a system that allows for "forms/scales/questionnaires to be completed."

Requirement 3: Seamless Interactivity. MHP mentioned poor internet connection ($n = 4$) and changes in service providers ($n = 3$) as common issues. This caused connection delays, and internet unreliability such as freezing, delays in connection, losing access to video stream, and dropped calls. PM05 captured the impact of technology issues on client comfort in the following statement: "Sometimes the call drops or the device battery dies, seemingly always in the most critical point of the session." Furthermore, privacy ($n = 4$) was another concern for MHP.

Requirement 4: Personalization. Queer participants emphasized the importance to have personalized experiences that were highly customizable and client-focused ($n = 5$). PL01 provided an example in a comparison of their experiences with two leading meditation apps: "Headspace has become a bit generic in all their meditations, but Balance is a great customized experience for meditation." Similarly, ensuring a sense of agency and control, particularly for when and how users navigate a system, was vital to the queer experience. Certain MHP noted that digital services and tools may provide the opportunity to interact in a sensory flexible environment or opportunity for increased privacy or anonymity. PM05, for instance, described that "for some clients…participating over the phone or through zoom with cameras off, opens the door for them." For PL04, functionality that enabled users to see their progress over time was particularly beneficial when measuring the efficacy of digital mental health solutions.

Requirement 5: Patient and Provider Support. Adequate support networks are a vital aspect for queer adults when they select digital mental health services and tools. Four queer participants discussed the reputability of the service and the provider to provide adequate care that research has verified. Four queer participants shared that the ethos of the clinicians must also align with their own personal beliefs, such as feminism (PL10) and secularism (PL03). For PL02 and PL11, it was important that clinicians are educated on queer topics and implement services using gender-neutral language. PL12 summarized conversations about the ethos of mental health providers when discussing the importance of empathy versus sympathy: "There is a fine line between providers being educated on LGBTQ+ topics and… being condescending towards us. I don't want to be babied because of my gender and sexuality, just be respectful and try to empathize." MHP identified support for the client through access to the necessary tools, and understanding the stigma associated with mental healthcare. PM06 exemplified this process as providing adequate "compassion, empathy, open-mindedness, [and] collaboration with [the] client." PM05 highlighted client support to be dependent on the client's commitment to therapy, including their readiness and willingness to participate and engage in various interventions. MHP identified community support through mental health training for teachers, and other community members as a necessity to support the client. They also discussed reduced wait times and cost as areas of support.

4.3   Impressions and Considerations for the Use of VR as a Tool for Digital Mental Health Services

We found six considerations for VR as a tool for digital mental health services (Fig. 2).

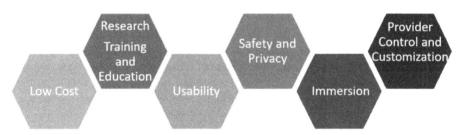

Fig. 2. An overview of six considerations in response to RQ2.

Requirement 1: Low Cost. Queer participants highlighted cost ($n = 8$) and availability of technology ($n = 7$) as significant barriers to the use of VR. Despite these barriers, ten queer participants indicated that they would be interested in using VR as a specialized mental health service. One of the two that indicated otherwise shared the disinterest as not wanting to spend money on a large head mounted display. Similarly, one MHP who had previous experience using VR identified cost of implementation as a major barrier when using VR. MHP identified further funding resources to support VR. All MHP expressed that VR must be cost-effective ($n = 2$).

Requirement 2: Research, Training and Education. Queer participants highlighted lack of familiarity ($n = 8$) as significant barriers to the use of VR; six shared that they perceive VR technologies as niche. PL01 exemplified this perceived niche as relating solely to gaming or entertainment experiences: "It's not really common... It always feels like some experimental gamer experience." Three other queer participants echoed this perception as they felt VR applications for mental health as unimaginable before completing the study. MHP identified a need for evidence-based training and treatment for both digital services ($n = 5$) with PM03 expressing that the successful VR implementation requires more research, as it "needs time for it to be considered evidence-based."

Requirement 3: Usability. Five queer participants shared that aesthetics, relating particularly to calming audio and visuals, are key components of ensuring VR interventions remain engaging and realistic. As such, two queer participants shared that graphical issues such as drops in frame rates negatively impact immersion. Certain MHP felt difficulties associated with using VR for mental healthcare exist. PM03 shared that there may exist a "complexity in learning and implementing it," which may contribute to a disinterest in the use for mental health services. For successful VR implementation, MHP desired limited steps, efficiency, and simplicity of the tools.

Requirement 4: Safety and Privacy. When discussing VR implementations, two queer participants expressed concerns regarding the safety of such systems. PL07 shared worries of undue mental influence, while PL06 was uneasy regarding risks of motion sickness. Three queer participants also signified concerns for the data privacy. PL12 mentioned that data privacy was in fact a greater concern with digital mental health solutions, not just potential VR implementations.

Requirement 5: Immersion. Five queer participants highlighted the immersive benefits of VR-based digital mental health solutions. Two suggested that a VR-based solution would afford extremely realistic and engaging opportunities that current mobile application-based services and tools lack. In the PL09's case, the major disadvantage of contemporary digital mental health solutions is that they are widely screen-based and lack the social connection that physical services offer. Four queer participants signified that VR would provide a unique opportunity to circumvent the impersonal nature of modern digital solutions by potentially allowing clients to interact with an avatar version of their therapist.

Requirement 6: Provider Control and Customization. Four   queer   participants addressed a concern of user control. PL11 shared that it would be useful to not only allow users to see their therapist but also allow them to control the avatar's location to ease any potential discomfort that comes with talking to a professional head-on. MHP echoed this idea as they identified that VR technology must be able to customize the use to a specific experience and needs of the client ($n = 3$). They highlighted flexible scenarios as a requirement for the use of VR in exposure therapy. PM02 explained that "a lot of different situations [are required] to address particular phobias." Both MHP and queer participants alike felt providing control to the mental health professionals to help guide the patient through the experience offered a greater sense safety and control, with PM02 classifying it as a particular boon for exposure therapy.

5   Discussion

Clinical VR presents itself as a viable approach with the potential to address mental health needs that disproportionately affect the queer community. As such, we explored the current state of digital mental health tools, particularly with VR systems, and how it addresses the needs of queer adults and MHP. Using the data collected from 12 queer participants and 7 MHP, we observed key design considerations from each participant group's unique experiences to address our two research questions.

Our study highlights the varied design needs and considerations that both queer adults and MHP have for digital mental health services (see Fig. 1 and Fig. 2). These considerations can specifically address unique psychosocial stressors faced by queer adults, which prevent them from seeking mental healthcare services. We now offer the interpretation, and discuss the implications of our findings.

5.1   Considerations for Improved Experiences with Digital Mental Health Tools

MHP converted to offering mental health services digitally due to the COVID-19 pandemic, however, both groups benefitted from accessing mental health services digitally. This was grounded in the reduced need for geographic proximity to mental health services, as well as the improved access to sensory flexible experiences. Although digital mental health tools may have improved access to services, financial costs proved to be the most prominent barrier to access. Lack of funding allocations introduce an increased cost to service and equity of services for MHP and queer clients alike. This supports the notion for greater government subsidies and funding resources and make digital mental health services and tools readily available and accessible to queer clients [1, 63].

The usability of the digital mental health tools implicated the overall experience of digital mental health services for both queer participants and MHP. It is vital for designers to create services that limit the steps required by clinicians and patients using these tools to provide a flexible delivery of care.

Furthermore, these systems often lack a level of customization, thereby not providing opportunities for MHP and clients to customize the experience to a specific context. This is a notable oversight when working with queer clients whose queer experiences fall short in the proper education of queer needs. Queer participants highlighted a need for customization, bringing attention to the importance for digital services that have a personalized element that is client-focused and offering a sense of agency and control when using the system. MHP can personalize inclusive language based on queer adults' preference (e.g., how a queer adult would like their gender identity to be addressed while receiving a mental healthcare service intervention). Personalization can build trust with queer clients, whom have expressed mistrust towards healthcare systems [64].

This design consideration also aligns with the specific demand for tools and services that address their unique queer ethos and personal beliefs. To address both client and clinician needs, the design of digital mental health tools requires collaboration between medical and IT experts and end users by their feedback and comments to provide effective content and increase the likelihood of successful implementation [33].

We also found modern digital mental solutions to be largely impersonal. The screen-based nature of mental health applications lends itself to the common misconception that these services are simply products meant for consumption than mental healthcare enabled by the unique properties that technology can offer [65]. Modern digital solutions present the inability to properly perceive client comfort. While thought of as a barrier for MHP, it also makes it difficult for queer people to be able to experience an enhanced sense of self-awareness and trust. Due to the unavailability of substantial technological training, MHP have a limited understanding on how to personalize therapeutic use based on the context and client's specific needs and abilities. Dissemination of knowledge in this area would be beneficial for queer adults so that MHP can customize interventions for varying sexual orientations and gender experiences.

Privacy and confidentiality were highlighted concerns for queer participants and MHP concerning digital mental health tools. Queer participants requested agency control, while MHP requested safeguards to protect themselves and the client. In considering 'apps' (mobile applications) that clients may use, threats to data privacy are increasing, with clients reporting privacy concerns and may inhibit and discourage their use of possible health-related apps [66–68]. This is important, as when clients use these apps various data points are frequently shared with the developers. Information such as an individual's username, password, contact information, age, gender and phone number are often monitored by app companies, and this information is even sometimes sold to third parties [69].

MHP's who encourage the use of these tools with their clients should acknowledge these limits of confidentiality and encourage their clients to use these apps with caution and limit their personal disclosure if possible. However, it is important to consider how the experience using these apps may change (i.e. customizability of app experience). In the event that a client loses their device, utilizing tools that can remotely wipe data may be hlepful [70, 71].

5.2 Considerations for Clinical VR as a Tool for Digital Mental Health

From our results, it is apparent that there needs to be evidence-based training and research for a VR to become a credible mental health service tool. This will make the technology more approachable and reduce perceived niche of this technology, as expressed by our queer participants. When it comes to MHP, training and education have various overlapping elements with MHP's comfort using VR technology and their respective need to have support through collaboration with industry experts, co-workers and ultimately their clients. The adoption of VR across mental healthcare is seemingly limited, and insufficient training that encompasses technological onboarding results in a worsened comfort level using this technology. Professional education on evidence-based research must ensure MHP are educated on queer issues, mental health needs, and available resources before creating or administering VR e-therapy simulations for queer adults [33, 72].

Beyond technology, we found that the success of the service is dependent on many factors. First, the success somewhat depends on the support of clinicians and the client's willingness to participate and improve (PM05). VR mental healthcare tools that appropriately address previously mentioned design considerations, including a system that provides personalization and that ensures privacy and consideration, can alleviate queer adults' fear of being negatively evaluated and stigmatization, which in turn can encourage them to actively participate during interventions, Also, providing MHP with the necessary support, may in-turn support their clients. This notion demonstrates a foundational need to support MHP through collaboration and providing the necessary resources prior to implementing a novel technology such as VR.

Second, the success of the service needs to consider accessibility needs in the domains of cost and stigmatization. The cost of administering virtual services and procuring necessary VR technology appear to be of great significance to both MHP and queer participants. Despite a recent decrease in price [30], their cost is still comparably higher than video-conferencing tools and make VR an expensive alternative for MHP. Similarly, some queer participants did not appear interested in spending money purchasing the required VR equipment when market applications are available to download for substantially less. The current perception of VR technologies being niche and only intended for certain audiences, such as video game players, makes this even more evident. MHP and alike can consider adopting cost-effective and publicly known alternatives that are commercially available such as Google Cardboard, Samsung Gear VR, and Merge VR Goggles. To this end, VR gathering tools such as Hubs by Mozilla or ALtspace VR may also be viable alternatives to the standard HMD interaction with VR that can be costly. Hubs by Mozilla and AltspaceVR are designed for almost every headset and browser, and are open-source projects, that are built on principles of flexibility, privacy and scalability and present a unique opportunity for further investigation as a Clinical VR tool.

Third, the success of the service depends on the usability and immersion. Usability principles are currently at a crossroads with the technical limitation of VR. For some, the size of VR systems limits their use in certain clinical settings. For others, mobile VR platforms can only provide so much immersion with a pocket-size computer. Computer specifications and the resolution of available VR devices can be limiting for some private clinics. Providing immersive experience is especially important for queer adults. The experience of immersion and the resulting emotional and cognitive engagement [73] and enjoyment [74] can motivate queer adults to continuously utilize mental healthcare services and change their negative attitude towards healthcare providers.

Fourth, a successfully VR-based service should craft individualized experiences that can easily be controlled and adjusted mid-use [75]. With this in mind, customizable digital mental health solutions will ensure an individual's therapy program is the most comfortable for them with gradual progression based on their needs, level of growth, and commitment to the program. For example, VR in exposure therapy requires the use of flexible scenarios. With proper VR implementation providing MHP control to help guide patients through experiences, both parties obtain a greater sense of safety and control.

6   Limitations and Future Work

We identified several limitations of our study. First, barring unpredicted technical issues with the software, participants may have felt inclined to progress through a survey as quickly as possible which results in less rich data when compared to other qualitative methodologies such as interviews [76]. While we did provide opportunities to provide open-ended text answers, long-text answers are often a deterrent to study participants in research surveys [77]. Second, many participants had limited experience using VR, while having prominent experiences with digital tools due to the COVID-19 pandemic. In certain cases, this contributed to an emphasis of insights from digital services and tools in general and less on specific VR potential. However, these insights are important contributions to consider in the development of VR tools to promote the usability and accessibility of these tools. Third, our survey results provide a very limited but generalized perspective of VR use and the factors influencing their adoption at a broader health system level. Repeat evaluations in different countries and practise settings over time will enable comparisons to understand more clearly the dynamics of VR adoption in these differing contexts. Likewise, repeat evaluations should also consider reaching out to a greater number of participants with a wider variety of demographic makeup, particularly in the case of MHP.

While we acknowledge these limitations, we similarly discuss several noteworthy future works. Primarily, future work should consider incorporating additional research methods in tandem with a survey, such as qualitative interviews. This would provide MHP and queer participants to expand on the themes identified and potentially introduce new ideas.

Future studies should consider conducting controlled studies to evaluate the feasibility regarding customizable, scenario-based VR mental health therapy. They may consider assessing the usability of VR tools in the teletherapy setting for client and clinician use. Evaluating user experience will provide further justification for use of VR in teletherapy settings and help support the lack of evidence-based research for MHP to provide appropriate services for queer clients.

Finally, to follow human-centred design principles [78], an evaluation of the themes found from the survey responses would be an effective follow-up study to this paper. Researchers would accurately inform and verify future design with the appropriate stakeholders by having both MHP and queer individuals critique our findings. A useful method of conducting such would make use of experience or journey map to highlight design scenarios for both queer adults and MHP's. Participants would be able to use the contextual nature of a journey map to evaluate the validity of our conclusions. Furthermore, future work could complete a Wizard of OZ or similar methods to pilot VR within the context of a clinical counselling.

7   Conclusion

Throughout our study, we simultaneously investigated the experiences and opinion of queer individuals and mental health professionals with digital mental health services and the potential for VR technology as a medium for digital mental health. We distributed two surveys and collected insight from both groups; these insights demonstrate the potential VR-based digital mental health solutions for addressing the unique needs of the queer community when designed with considerations such as safety, customizability, and immersion. We highlight the importance of user-centred design principles and the importance of creating tools that balance being technologically innovative while understanding complex and unique user needs. We then presented a series of design considerations for digital mental health and VR-based mental health tools that leverage our user-informed findings.

Acknowledgments. We would like to thank all of our participants for their time, expertise, and insights.

References

1. Green, A., Price-Feeney, M., Dorison, S.: Implications of COVID-19 for LGBTQ Youth Mental Health and Suicide Prevention. https://www.thetrevorproject.org/2020/04/03/implic ations-of-covid-19-for-lgbtq-youth-mental-health-and-suicide-prevention/
2. Mitchell, K.M., Lee, L., Green, A., Skyes, J.S.: The gaps in health care of the LGBT community: perspectives of nursing students and faculty. Pap. Publ. Interdiscip. J. Undergrad. Res. **5**, 21–30 (2016)
3. Pike, D.: Creating Positive Space for the LGBTQ Community in Hamilton, Hamilton, ON (2008)
4. Casey, B.: The Health of LGBTQIA2 Communities in Canada: Report of the Standing Committee on Health (2019)
5. Russell, S.T., Fish, J.N.: Mental health in lesbian, gay, bisexual, and transgender (LGBT) youth. Annu. Rev. Clin. Psychol. **12**, 465–487 (2016). https://doi.org/10.1146/annurev-cli npsy-021815-093153
6. Bauer, G.R., Scheim, A.I., Deutsch, M.B., Massarella, C.: Reported emergency department avoidance, use, and experiences of transgender persons in Ontario, Canada: Results from a respondent-driven sampling survey. Ann. Emerg. Med. **63**, 713-720.e1 (2014). https://doi. org/10.1016/j.annemergmed.2013.09.027
7. Meyer, I.H.: Prejudice, social stress, and mental health in lesbian, gay, and bisexual populations: conceptual issues and research evidence. Psychol. Bull. **129**, 674–697 (2003). https:// doi.org/10.7202/101747
8. Dauvergne, M.: Police-reported hate crime in Canada. Juristat **30**, 15–16 (2008)
9. Centre for Addiction and Mental Health Canadian Mental Health Association Ontario, Centre for Health Promotion, Nexus Health, Ontario Public Health: Mental Health Promotion in Ontario: A Call to Action (2008)
10. Tjepkema, M.: Health care use among gay, lesbian and bisexual Canadians. Heal. Rep. **19**, 53–64 (2008)
11. Statistics Canada: A statistical portrait of Canada's diverse LGBTQ2+ communities (2021)
12. Bauer, G.R.B., Pyne, J., Francino, M.C., Hammond, R.: Suicidality among trans people in Ontario: implications for social work and social justice. J. Serv. Soc. **59**, 35–62 (2013). https:// doi.org/10.7202/1017478
13. Rapid Response Service: Rapid Response: Facilitators and barriers to health care for lesbian, gay and bisexual (LGB) people, Toronto, ON (2014)
14. Roland, C.B., Burlew, L.D.: Counseling LGBTQ Adults Throughout the Life Span (2017)
15. King, M., Semlyen, J., Killaspy, H., Nazareth, I., Osborn, D.: A systematic review of research on counselling and psychotherapy for lesbian, gay, bisexual & transgender people (2007)
16. Vigo, D., et al.: Mental health of communities during the COVID-19 pandemic. Can. J. Psychiatry. **65**, 681–687 (2020). https://doi.org/10.1177/0706743720926676
17. Brooks, S.K., et al.: The psychological impact of quarantine and how to reduce it: rapid review of the evidence. Lancet **395**, 912–920 (2020). https://doi.org/10.1016/S0140-6736(20)304 60-8

18. Hawryluck, L., Gold, W.L., Robinson, S., Pogorski, S., Galea, S., Styra, R.: SARS control and psychological effects of quarantine, Toronto Canada. Emerg. Infect. Dis. **10**, 1206–1212 (2004). https://doi.org/10.3201/eid1007.030703
19. Wiederhold, B.K.: CyberTherapy & rehabilitation. In: Wiederhold, B.K. (ed.) 21st Annual CyberPsychology, CyberTherapy & Social Networking Conference. The Virtual Reality Medical Institute (2016)
20. Morin, A., Blackburn, S.: Best Online Therapy Programs. https://www.verywellmind.com/best-online-therapy-4691206#best-for-access-to-a-psychiatrist-mdlive
21. Torous, J., et al.: Towards a consensus around standards for smartphone apps and digital mental health. World Psychiatry **18**, 97–98 (2019). https://doi.org/10.1002/wps.20592
22. Hankala, P.M., Kankaanranta, M., Kepler-Uotinen, K., Rousi, R., Mehtälä, S.: Towards a scenario of virtual mental health environments for school-aged children (2017). https://doi.org/10.1145/3131085.3131100
23. Tal, A., Torous, J.: The digital mental health revolution: opportunities and risks. Psychiatr. Rehabil. J. **40**, 263 (2017). https://doi.org/10.1037/PRJ0000285
24. Krohn, S., et al.: Multidimensional evaluation of virtual reality paradigms in clinical neuropsychology: application of the VR-check framework. J. Med. Internet Res. **22** (2020). https://doi.org/10.2196/16724
25. Eichenberg, C.: Application of "Virtual Realities" in psychotherapy: possibilities, limitations and effectiveness. In: Virtual Reality, pp. 469–484. InTechOpen, Cologne (2011). https://doi.org/10.5772/12914
26. Dey, P., Rukshshan, S.: Virtual reality therapy in clinical psychology-a conceptual paper. Indian J. Ment. Heal. **6**, 213–224 (2019)
27. Zeng, N., Pope, Z., Lee, J.E., Gao, Z.: Virtual reality exercise for anxiety and depression: a preliminary review of current research in an emerging field. J. Clin. Med. **7**, 42 (2018). https://doi.org/10.3390/jcm7030042
28. Boeldt, D., McMahon, E., McFaul, M., Greenleaf, W.: Using virtual reality exposure therapy to enhance treatment of anxiety disorders: identifying areas of clinical adoption and potential obstacles. Front. Psychiatry. **10**, 773 (2019). https://doi.org/10.3389/fpsyt.2019.00773
29. Dellazizzo, L., Potvin, S., Phraxayavong, K., Dumais, A.: Exploring the benefits of virtual reality-assisted therapy following cognitive-behavioral therapy for auditory hallucinations in patients with treatment-resistant schizophrenia: a proof of concept. J. Clin. Med. **9**, 3169 (2020). https://doi.org/10.3390/jcm9103169
30. Headset technology is cheaper and better than ever. https://www.economist.com/technology-quarterly/2020/10/01/headset-technology-is-cheaper-and-better-than-ever. Accessed 27 Apr 2021
31. McGlynn, S.A., Rogers, W.A.: Design recommendations to enhance virtual reality presence for older adults. In: Proceedings of the Human Factors and Ergonomics Society Annual Meeting, pp. 2077–2081 (2017). https://doi.org/10.1177/1541931213602002
32. Winkler, N., Röthke, K., Siegfried, N., Benlian, A.: Lose Yourself in VR: Exploring the Effects of Virtual Reality on Individuals' Immersion (2020)
33. Baniasadi, T., Ayyoubzadeh, S.M., Mohammadzadeh, N.: Challenges and practical considerations in applying virtual reality in medical education and treatment. Oman Med. J. **35**, e125 (2020). https://doi.org/10.5001/omj.2020.43
34. Devito, M.A., et al.: Queer in HCI: supporting LGBTQIA+ researchers and research across domains. In: CHI EA 2020: Extended Abstracts of the 2020 CHI Conference on Human Factors in Computing Systems, pp. 1–4. Association for Computing Machinery, New York (2020). https://doi.org/10.1145/3334480.3381058
35. Glaser, B., Strauss, A.: The Discovery of Grounded Theory: Strategies for Qualitative Research. AldineTransaction, Piscataway (1999)

36. Strategies for Reducing Health Disparities. https://www.cdc.gov/minorityhealth/strategie s2016/index.html. Accessed 17 Nov 2021
37. Equity vs. Equality: What's the Difference. https://onlinepublichealth.gwu.edu/resources/equ ity-vs-equality/. Accessed 17 Nov 2021. https://doi.org/10.1080/13561820400011750
38. Visualizing Equality vs. Equity. https://risetowin.org/what-we-do/educate/resource-module/ equality-vs-equity/index.html. Accessed 17 Nov 2021
39. Zhang, R., Ringland, K.E., Paan, M., Mohr, D.C., Reddy, M.: Designing for Emotional Well-being: Integrating Persuasion and Customization into Mental Health Technologies (2021). https://doi.org/10.1145/3411764.3445771
40. Khwaja, M., Pieritz, S., Faisal, A.A., Matic, A.: Personality and Engagement with Digital Mental Health Interventions; Personality and Engagement with Digital Mental Health Interventions (2021). https://doi.org/10.1145/3450613.3456823
41. Lattie, E.G., Kornfield, R., Ringland, K.E., Zhang, R., Winquist, N., Reddy, M.: Designing Mental Health Technologies that Support the Social Ecosystem of College Students (2020). https://doi.org/10.1145/3313831.3376362
42. Bergin, A.D., et al.: Preventive digital mental health interventions for children and young people: a review of the design and reporting of research. https://doi.org/10.1038/s41746-020-00339-7
43. Ellice: How to Design an LGBTQ-Inclusive Website. https://www.dreamhost.com/blog/how-to-design-lgbtq-inclusive-website/
44. Johnson, J.: LGBT graphic design: the art of logo and print design from a queer perspective. https://99designs.ca/blog/creative-inspiration/lgbt-graphic-design/
45. Ke, M.: How to make an LGBTQ+ inclusive survey. https://uxdesign.cc/how-to-make-an-lgbtq-inclusive-survey-bfd1d801cc21. Accessed 08 Mar 2021
46. Sethfors, H.: LGBTQ-inclusive web design. https://axesslab.com/lgbtq-inclusive-web-des ign/. Accessed 08 Mar 2021
47. Spiel, K., et al.: Queer(ing) HCI: moving forward in theory and practice. In: CHI EA 2019: Extended Abstracts of the 2019 CHI Conference on Human Factors in Computing Systems, pp. 1–4. Association for Computing Machinery (2019). https://doi.org/10.1145/3290607.331 1750
48. Haimson, O.L., Brubaker, J.R., Hayes, G.R.: DDF seeks same: sexual health-related language in online personal ads for men who have sex with men. In: CHI 2014: Proceedings of the SIGCHI Conference on Human Factors in Computing Systems, pp. 1615–1624. Association for Computing Machinery (2014). https://doi.org/10.1145/2556288.2557077
49. Argüello, S.B., Wakkary, R., Andersen, K., Tomico, O.: Exploring the potential of apple face ID as a drag, queer and Trans technology design tool. In: Designing Interactive Systems Conference 2021 (DIS 2021), pp. 1654–1667. Association for Computer Machinery (2021)
50. Paré, D., Sengupta, P., Windsor, S., Craig, J., Thompson, M.: Queering virtual reality: a prolegomenon. In: Sengupta, P., Shanahan, M.-C., Kim, B. (eds.) Critical, Transdisciplinary and Embodied Approaches in STEM Education. ASE, pp. 307–328. Springer, Cham (2019). https://doi.org/10.1007/978-3-030-29489-2_17
51. Jones, D.: Queered Virtuality: The Claiming and Making of Queer Spaces and Bodies in the User-Constructed Synthetic World of Second Life (2007). https://repository.library.geo rgetown.edu/bitstream/handle/10822/551594/etd_jonesd3.pdf?sequence=1&isAllowed=y
52. Acena, D., Freeman, G.: "In My Safe Space": Social Support for LGBTQ Users in Social Virtual Reality; "In My Safe Space": Social Support for LGBTQ Users in Social Virtual Reality (2021). https://doi.org/10.1145/3411763.3451673
53. McKenna, B., Chughtai, H.: Resistance and sexuality in virtual worlds: an LGBT perspective. Comput. Human Behav. **105** (2020). https://doi.org/10.1016/J.CHB.2019.106199

54. Muessig, K.E., et al.: "I didn't tell you sooner because I didn't know how to handle it myself." developing a virtual reality program to support HIV-status disclosure decisions. Digit Cult Educ. **10**, 22–48 (2018)
55. Wilson, P.N., Foreman, N., Tlauka, M.: Transfer of spatial information from a virtual to a real environment in physically disabled children. Disabil. Rehabil. **18** (1996). https://doi.org/10.3109/09638289609166328
56. Falconer, C.J., Davies, E.B., Grist, R., Stallard, P.: Innovations in practice: avatar-based virtual reality in CAMHS talking therapy: two exploratory case studies. Child Adolesc. Ment. Health. **24** (2019). https://doi.org/10.1111/camh.12326
57. Kang, R., Brown, S., Kiesler, S.: Why do people seek anonymity on the Internet? Informing policy and design. In: Conference on Human Factors in Computing Systems - Proceedings (2013). https://doi.org/10.1145/2470654.2481368
58. Facilitators and barriers to health care for lesbian, gay and bisexual (LGB) people
59. Russell, S.T., Toomey, R.B., Ryan, C., Diaz, R.M.: Being out at school: the implications for school victimization and young adult adjustment. Am. J. Orthopsychiatry **84** (2014). https://doi.org/10.1037/ort0000037
60. Mays, V.M., Cochran, S.D.: Mental health correlates of perceived discrimination among lesbian, gay, and bisexual adults in the United States. Am. J. Public Health. **91** (2001). https://doi.org/10.2105/AJPH.91.11.1869
61. Braun, V., Clarke, V.: Successful Qualitative Research: A Practical Guide for Beginners. SAGE Publications Inc., London (2013)
62. Maria Rosala: How to Analyze Qualitative Data from UX Research: Thematic Analysis. https://www.nngroup.com/articles/thematic-analysis/. Accessed 01 Feb 2021
63. Ussher, J.M.: Heterocentric practices in health research and health care: implications for mental health and subjectivity of LGBTQ individuals. Fem. Psychol. **19**, 561–567 (2009). https://doi.org/10.1177/0959353509342933
64. Alpert, A.B., CichoskiKelly, E.M., Fox, A.D.: What lesbian, gay, bisexual, transgender, queer, and intersex patients say doctors should know and do: a qualitative study. J. Homosex. **64**, 1368–1389 (2017). https://doi.org/10.1080/00918369.2017.1321376
65. Mohr, D.C., Weingardt, K.R., Reddy, M., Schueller, S.M.: Three problems with current digital mental health research. Technol. Ment. Heal. **68**, 427–429 (2017). https://doi.org/10.1176/appi.ps.201600541
66. Crowther, A., et al.: The impact of Recovery Colleges on mental health staff, services and society. Epidemiol. Psychiatr. Sci. **28**, 481–488 (2019). https://doi.org/10.1017/S20457960 1800063X
67. Martínez-Pérez, B., de la Torre-Díez, I., López-Coronado, M.: Privacy and security in mobile health apps: a review and recommendations. J. Med. Syst. **39**(1), 1–8 (2014). https://doi.org/10.1007/s10916-014-0181-3
68. Vonholtz, L.A.H., et al.: Use of mobile apps: a patient-centered approach. Acad. Emerg. Med. **22** (2015). https://doi.org/10.1111/acem.12675
69. Martinez-Martin, N., Kreitmair, K.: Ethical issues for direct-to-consumer digital psychotherapy apps: addressing accountability, data protection, and consent. JMIR Ment. Heal. **5** (2018). https://doi.org/10.2196/mental.9423
70. Jones, N., Moffitt, M.: Ethical guidelines for mobile app development within health and mental health fields. Prof. Psychol. Res. Pract. **47** (2016). https://doi.org/10.1037/pro0000069
71. Karcher, N.R., Presser, N.R.: Ethical and legal issues addressing the use of mobile health (mHealth) as an adjunct to psychotherapy. Ethics Behav. **28** (2018). https://doi.org/10.1080/10508422.2016.1229187
72. Gromala, D., Rose, H., Ayalasomayajula, F.: VR health care: best practices for clinical implementation. https://ai-med.io/mental-health/virtual-reality-health-best-practices-clinical-implementation/

73. Molinillo, S., Aguilar-Illescas, R., Anaya-Sánchez, R., Vallespín-Arán, M.: Exploring the impacts of interactions, social presence and emotional engagement on active collaborative learning in a social web-based environment. Comput. Educ. **123** (2018). https://doi.org/10.1016/j.compedu.2018.04.012

74. Lin, J.J.W., Duh, H.B.L., Parker, D.E., Abi-Rached, H., Furness, T.A.: Effects of field of view on presence, enjoyment, memory, and simulator sickness in a virtual environment. In: Proceedings - Virtual Reality Annual International Symposium (2002). https://doi.org/10.1109/vr.2002.996519

75. Rizzo, A.S., Kim, G.J.: A SWOT analysis of the field of virtual reality rehabilitation and therapy. Presence **14**, 119–146 (2005). https://doi.org/10.1162/1054746053967094

76. Jones, T.L., Baxter, M., Khanduja, V.: A quick guide to survey research. Ann. R. Coll. Surg. Engl. **95**, 5–7 (2013). https://doi.org/10.1308/003588413X13511609956372

77. Why We Need to Avoid Long Surveys. https://www.relevantinsights.com/articles/long-surveys/. Accessed 27 Apr 2021

78. Maguire, M.: Methods to support human-centred design. Int. J. Hum. Comput. Stud. **55**, 587–634 (2001). https://doi.org/10.1006/ijhc.2001.0503

FatigueSet: A Multi-modal Dataset for Modeling Mental Fatigue and Fatigability

Manasa Kalanadhabhatta[1]([✉]), Chulhong Min[2], Alessandro Montanari[2], and Fahim Kawsar[2]

[1] College of Information and Computer Sciences,
University of Massachusetts Amherst, Amherst, USA
manasak@cs.umass.edu
[2] Nokia Bell Labs, Cambridge, UK
{chulhong.min,alessandro.montanari,fahim.kawsar}@nokia-bell-labs.com

Abstract. A comprehensive understanding of fatigue and its impact on performance is a prerequisite for fatigue management systems in the real world. However, fatigue is a multidimensional construct that is often poorly defined, and most prior work does not take into consideration how different types of fatigue collectively influence performance. The physiological markers associated with different types of fatigue are also underexplored, hindering the development of fatigue management technologies that can leverage mobile and wearable sensors to predict fatigue. In this work, we present FatigueSet, a multi-modal dataset including sensor data from four wearable devices that are collected while participants are engaged in physically and mentally demanding tasks. We describe the study design that enables us to investigate the effect of physical activity on mental fatigue under various situations. FatigueSet facilitates further research towards a deeper understanding of fatigue and the development of diverse fatigue-aware applications.

Keywords: Fatigue · Multi-modal sensing · Cognitive performance

1 Introduction

Fatigue is a complex psychophysiological condition that is characterized by experiential feelings of tiredness or sleepiness, suboptimal performance, and a broad range of physiological changes [33]. Fatigue has a detrimental effect on physical and mental performance, leading to reduced decision making and planning abilities, reduced alertness and vigilance, loss of memory, increased risk-taking and errors in judgment, and increased sick time, incident rates, and medical costs [5]. Therefore, fatigue management systems have received much attention for managing potential risks from fatigue in organizations and for promoting individual wellbeing [6,15,38]. In common, they aim to detect individuals' fatigue in time and intervene to mitigate any resulting lapses in performance.

© ICST Institute for Computer Sciences, Social Informatics and Telecommunications Engineering 2022
Published by Springer Nature Switzerland AG 2022. All Rights Reserved
H. Lewy and R. Barkan (Eds.): PH 2021, LNICST 431, pp. 204–217, 2022.
https://doi.org/10.1007/978-3-030-99194-4_14

There have been extensive efforts to study the causes and temporal dynamics of fatigue in the domain of physiology, medicine, and neuroscience [39,42,43]. However, since these attempts have been mostly made with medical devices in a clinical setting, it is difficult to adopt the findings from these studies into ubiquitous computing for healthcare and wellbeing. While there have been attempts to computationally model fatigue using physiological signals from wearable sensors in the mobile computing domain [15,26], they have mostly been limited to the consideration of a single type of fatigue. However, different types of fatigue have been shown to influence each other in significant ways [20,27,41].

Motivated by these observations, we present FatigueSet[1], a multi-modal dataset for modeling the interplay between physical and mental fatigue and its impact on cognitive performance. As a first step for computationally modeling this interplay, in this paper, we collect and introduce a dataset for exploring the impact of physical activity on mental fatigue and associated cognitive performance; we leave the impact of mental fatigue on physical fatigue to be explored in future work. We recruit 12 participants and collect multi-modal sensor data while inducing different levels of neuromuscular burden as well as cognitive load, and observing their physiological responses and performance on cognitive tasks. To enable a comprehensive study, we include a variety of physiological sensors – electroencephalography (EEG), photoplethysmography (PPG), electrocardiography (ECG), electrodermal activity (EDA), skin temperature sensor, accelerometer, and gyroscope – on four different wearable devices (an earable prototype based on Nokia eSense [2], Empatica E4 wrist band [1], Muse S EEG headband [3], and Zephyr BioHarness 3.0 ECG chestband [4]). We hope this dataset will expedite studies towards a deeper understanding of fatigue in the research community as well as facilitate the development of diverse fatigue-relevant applications.

2   Background and Related Work

2.1   Defining Fatigue

Fatigue is a multifaceted construct that lacks a single clear definition. Prior work has attempted to define fatigue in terms of at least three sets of characteristics – experiential, behavioral, and physiological [33].

Experiential definitions of fatigue emphasize feelings of tiredness, exhaustion, and lack of energy, along with low levels of motivation and a disinclination to continue a task. Fatigue as an experiential construct is measured in terms of individuals' self-reported feelings, often on one of many standardized fatigue measurement scales (see [11] for a review). Targeting an experiential measure of fatigue can be a valid treatment goal for clinically fatigued individuals and is also a desirable outcome for fatigue management technologies for the general population. However, there may be a gap between an individual's perception of tiredness and exhaustion and the external consequences resulting from it.

---

[1] https://www.esense.io/datasets/fatigueset.

Behavioral definitions of fatigue focus on these consequences, emphasizing decline in performance as a fundamental indication of fatigue. Prior work has conceptualized fatigue as decrements measured either on a *primary* task or a *probe* task. Performance measures on primary tasks are those that are recorded as participants engage in the fatiguing task of interest. For instance, fatigue-related effects of time on task have been measured in terms of reaction times or lapses on the psychomotor vigilance test (PVT) [42]. On the other hand, *probe* tasks are interspersed with the primary task and used to obtain momentary performance levels at different points in time. A probe task such as the PVT or the Mackworth Clock Test can be administered several times between trials of a different fatiguing task, or at regular intervals throughout a workday [23].

Prior work has also operationalized fatigue in terms of the neurophysiological changes that occur either to cause it, or as a response to a fatigued condition. This provides an opportunity to objectively measure fatigue in terms of its physiological markers, which is necessary for fatigue management systems based on wearable or environmental sensors. The exact physiological responses depend on the type of fatigue under consideration, and will be discussed Sect. 2.3.

2.2 Operationalizing Fatigue for Fatigue Management Technologies

From the above discussion, it is clear that attempts to define fatigue solely in terms of either experiential, behavioral, or physiological variables present an incomplete view. Prior research has also shown dissociation between fatigue measurements across two or more dimensions (no change in physiological responses even as individuals report higher levels of fatigue, or dissociation between experiential and performance measures, for example) [33]. This has led to increased interest in a dynamic, multidimensional definition of the concept of fatigue.

We adopt the taxonomy proposed by Kluger et al. [19] to define this concept in terms of two complementary constructs – *fatigue* and *fatigability*. For the remainder of this paper, we use the term "fatigue" to refer to the subjective sensations and perceptions of tiredness and exhaustion. We use the term "fatigability" to refer to objective changes in performance resulting from fatigue and the underlying mechanisms driving it.

Based on the adopted taxonomy, fatigue and fatigability are often co-occurring and are accompanied by associated neurophysiological responses. An ideal fatigue management system should target both these constructs separately as well as consider how they influence each other. Also, physiological measures should be closely monitored and their relationship with both fatigue and fatigability must be individually assessed. FatigueSet is an attempt in this direction, measuring both fatigue and fatigability along with physiological sensor data.

2.3 Types of Fatigue

Prior work has identified two primary types of fatigue based on its causes, physiological markers, and symptomatology: physical and mental fatigue. *Neuromuscular* or *physical fatigue* is fatigue induced by physical exercise, which leads to a decline in muscle power or exerted force [43]. Physical fatigue is associated with changes in EMG activity in the muscles [14]. Other potential indicators of physical fatigue include biomarkers related to the metabolism of adenosine triphosphate, oxidation, or inflammation in the body [43].

Mental fatigue is in turn experienced during and after prolonged periods of demanding cognitive activity. Mental fatigue is characterized by feelings of tiredness, lack of concentration, and performance decline on cognitive tasks [40]. It is associated with increased EEG alpha and theta wave activity in all regions of the cortex, and an increase in beta activity in frontal sites as individuals attempt to maintain vigilance under fatigue [9].

While a majority of prior studies have focused exclusively on either physical or mental fatigue, there is evidence that the two processes influence each other. Studies investigating physical fatigability following mental fatigue have found that mental fatigue or time on task led to less adequate preparation for new tasks and more errors [24]. Mental fatigue significantly reduced time to physical fatigue during a cycling task, though physiological responses to exercise remained unchanged. It was also associated with higher subjective perception of effort [27]. On the other hand, studies have observed both a decline and improvement in different cognitive functions after different physical exercises. The type of physical activity and the level of physical fatigue (low-to-medium activity vs maximal exertion), duration of activity, type of mental fatigability investigated, and initial levels of physical fitness are all thought to be deciding factors [20]. A variety of theories have been proposed to explain this relationship, but prior works lack consensus on how this effect is manifested on various cognitive tasks. In this work, we study this relationship with a focus on two tasks that require different levels of attentional and processing resources.

2.4   Datasets for Fatigue Detection

While a few datasets for fatigue modeling are currently available, most of these are inadequate for deeply understanding the interplay between physical and mental fatigue and between fatigue and fatigability. Luo et al. presented a dataset for the assessment of fatigue using wearable sensors [25]. While they collected longitudinal sensor data from 27 subjects with various sensors, they lack fatigability measures which are essential to understand changes in performance resulting from fatigue and its underlying mechanisms. Other fatigue-related datasets are extremely domain-specific, e.g., Gjoreski et al. presented datasets [13] to infer cognitive loads on mobile games and physiological tasks on a PC using wearable sensors. Elshafei et al. presented a dataset [12] for modeling bicep fatigue during gym activities. Our dataset focuses on task-independent, lower-level cognitive performance and how it is influenced by physical *and* cognitive activity.

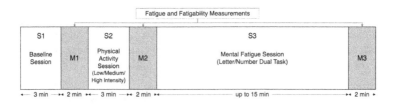

Fig. 1. Study protocol

3   Methodology

3.1   Study Design

Twelve participants (9 male, 3 female) between the ages of 21 and 40 (mean age: 30.75 years, SD: 5.78 years) completed the present study. One participant had mild asthma and another had seasonal asthma, while none of the others had any current or past health conditions. All participants completed an informed consent before the study and were compensated with a £30 gift card upon completion.

The study consisted of three sessions conducted on three different days, with a gap of up to 19 days between sessions. Figure 1 shows the protocol for each session. All sessions for a participant were conducted at roughly the same time of the day whenever possible in order to control for circadian effects. Before the first session, participants were asked to fill a preliminary demographic questionnaire. We assessed participants' personality on the short Big Five Inventory (BFI-10) scale [34] and their chronotype (early bird or late owl-ness) using the Munich Chronotype Questionnaire (MCTQ; [35]). Participants also reported the impact of fatigue on their daily functioning using the Fatigue Severity Scale (FSS; [21]) and their general fitness levels on the International Fitness Scale (IFIS; [30]).

Participants began each session by reporting their current sleepiness levels on the Stanford Sleepiness Scale (SSS; [37]) and their baseline vigor and affect on the Global Vigour and Affect Scale (GVAS; [28]). The SSS gives a score between 1 to 7, with 1 corresponding to minimal sleepiness and 7 to highest sleepiness. The GVAS requires participants to rate various aspects of vigor, mood, and affect on visual analogue scales (VAS), which are then converted to separate scores for vigor and affect. Our implementation of the GVAS used a 10-point rating instead of a VAS for easier administration and scoring.

Participants were then fitted with four wearable devices to monitor physiological signals, each of which are described in Sect. 3.5. They were seated at rest in a comfortable position for three minutes while baseline physiological data was recorded ($S1$). Following the baseline recording period $S1$, participants completed a survey to measure physical and mental fatigue and completed two cognitive tasks to measure baseline cognitive performance for mental fatigability at later stages in the experiment (henceforth referred to as $M1$). This was followed by a 3-min physical activity session ($S2$), where participants were assigned to one of three conditions (low, medium, or high intensity activity) on a given day. Our study followed a within-subjects design, with all participants completing one session corresponding to each condition. The order in which these conditions are performed was counterbalanced across participants using a balanced Latin Square design.

The period of physical activity in each session was followed by a second measurement of mental fatigue and cognitive performance, $M2$, as shown in Fig. 1. Subsequently, participants completed a mental fatigue-inducing task that lasted approximately 15 min ($S3$), followed by a third fatigue and fatigability measurement ($M3$). In total, each session lasted up to 30 min, and physiological data was recorded for this entire duration. The following subsections provide more details about each part of the study session.

3.2   Physical Activity Protocol

Based on prior research that theorizes an inverted-U relationship between physical activity and cognitive performance [8], we were interested in investigating the effect of low, medium and high intensity physical activity on the development of mental fatigue. We use the metabolic equivalent of task (MET) as an objective indicator of the intensity of physical activity. A MET is defined as the resting metabolic rate, or the amount of oxygen consumed while sitting at rest [16]. The amount of energy required to perform a given physical activity can be quantified in terms of METs, e.g., work requiring twice the resting metabolism is said to be 2 METs. Activities demanding 1–4 METs, 5–8 METs, and >8 METS, are considered light, medium, and high intensity activities, respectively.

We therefore selected walking at 5 km/hr (3.2 METs), jogging at 7 km/hr (5.3 METs), and jogging at 9 km/hr (8.8 METs) as our low, medium, and high intensity physical activities respectively [16]. During $S2$, participants were asked to walk or run at the given speed on a treadmill without incline for three minutes. Activity sessions were ended early if participants reported a rating equal to or above 10, 14, and 16 on Borg's Rating of Perceived Exertion (RPE) scale [7] during low, medium, and high intensity conditions respectively [29] to avoid overexertion and ensure the safety of the participants.

3.3   Inducing Mental Fatigue

Following the physical activity session $S2$, we used the well-validated dual letter/number task switching paradigm [36] to induce cognitive fatigue in $S3$. Switching between dual tasks has been shown to require additional cognitive overhead and induce fatigue faster than a single cognitive task [31]. The letter/number task was implemented using the PsychoPy framework [32] for experiment design and was administered on a laptop while participants were seated. During $S3$, participants were presented a 2 × 2 square grid on a grey background. On each trial, a combination of two characters – a letter followed by a number – appeared in one of the squares (see Fig. 2). If the characters appear in one of the *top* two squares, participants had to respond to the *letter* and ignore the number. In this case, they were asked to press the 'c' key on their keyboard if the letter was a consonant and the 'm' key if it was a vowel. On the other

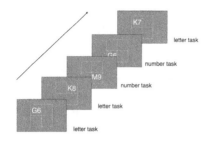

Fig. 2. Dual task to induce mental fatigue.

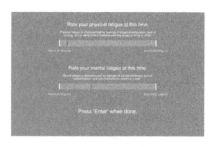

Fig. 3. Fatigue visual analog scales.

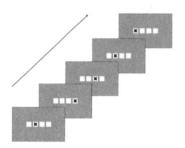

Fig. 4. Choice reaction time task.

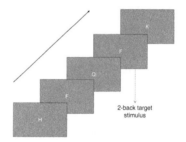

Fig. 5. N-back task.

hand, if the characters appeared in one of the *bottom* two squares, participants were required to respond to the *number* and ignore the letter. Based on whether the number was even or odd, participants had to respond by pressing 'c' or 'm' respectively. The task consisted of 200 trials and lasted approximately 15 min, which has been shown to be enough to induce mental fatigue [31]. Performance on the dual task was not analyzed, since the objective was only to induce mental fatigue by virtue of time on task.

3.4   Fatigue and Fatigability Measurements

To measure the impact of physical activity on mental fatigue and fatigability, we obtained self-reported fatigue scores and performance on two distinct cognitive tasks three times during each session - before physical activity ($M1$), between physical activity and mental fatigue induction ($M2$), and after the induction of mental fatigue ($M3$).

Measurement of Fatigue: Participants were asked to report their physical and mental fatigue on two computerized VAS scales ranging from "Not at all fatigued" to "Maximally fatigued" (see Fig. 3). Prior work has validated the use of simple VAS scales to measure fatigue, suggesting their utility over more complex multi-dimensional scales [11]. Participants were instructed to rate their levels of fatigue *at this time* by clicking or dragging the mouse along the scale, and were provided the following definitions of physical and mental fatigue in an attempt to ensure a similar understanding of the terms across participants:

Physical fatigue is characterized by feelings of physical exhaustion, lack of energy, and a disinclination towards exerting physical force or effort. Mental fatigue is characterized by feelings of mental tiredness, lack of concentration, and low motivation to continue a task.

Physical and mental fatigue ratings were converted to integers between 0–100 based on the distance from the "Not at all fatigued" end of the scale.

Measurement of Mental Fatigability: Participants were asked to perform two short cognitive tasks, and their performance was measured in terms of reaction times and errors committed. The difference in performance as compared to the baseline measurement $M1$ was used as an indicator of fatigability.

The first task was the Deary-Liewald Choice Reaction Time (CRT) task [10], which requires participants to select and make the appropriate response to each of several stimuli. The CRT task has been used as an indicator of processing speed, and reaction times have been shown to be affected by physical exertion [22]. In our study, participants were presented with four white squares stacked horizontally on a grey background (see Fig. 4). The squares were each mapped to a different key on the keyboard – 'z', 'x', ',' (comma), and '.' (period) respectively from left to right. During each trial, a black cross appeared in one of the squares and participants had to press the corresponding key as soon as possible after the appearance of the cross. The stimulus stayed on the screen until a key was pressed. Once responded, the stimulus disappeared and the next one appeared after a random inter-stimulus interval of 1 to 3 s. Each performance measurement consisted of 36 trials of the CRT task, with the stimulus appearing in each of the 4 boxes an equal number of times (Fig. 4).

In addition to the CRT task, participants were also asked to complete a 2-back task to assess their working memory [17]. In this task, a sequence of

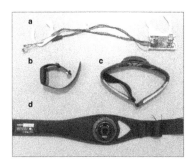

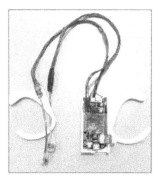

Fig. 6. Wearables for data collection: (a) our earable prototype, (b) E4 wristband, (c) Muse S headband, (d) BioHarness ECG chest band.

Fig. 7. The eSense earable prototype contains IMU and PPG sensors in each earbud.

letters appeared briefly at the center of the screen for 0.5 s, with a 2-s gap
between letters (see Fig. 5). Participants were asked to respond with the 'm' key
on their keyboard if the current letter was the same as the one that appeared
two letters before it. If not, they were asked to withhold their response and not
press any key. Each round of fatigability measurement consisted of 20 trials of
the 2-back task, lasting approximately 50 s with target trials (which required a
response) occurring four times.

3.5 Physiological Measurements

A range of physiological signals were recorded throughout the experiment sessions using four different wearable devices (see Fig. 6): (i) our earable prototype
with inertial measurement units and photoplethysmographic sensors in each earbud, developed based on Nokia eSense [2,18], (ii) a Muse S EEG headband [3],
(iii) a Zephyr BioHarness 3.0 chestband [4], and (iv) an Empatica E4 wristband [1]. Table 1 has a detailed description of the sensors on each device.

Table 1. Sensor data collected from each wearable device.

Sensor	Units/Range	Sampling rate
Earable prototype		
Accelerometer	g {−2:+2}	100 Hz
Gyroscope	°/s {−500:+500}	100 Hz
PPG - green, infrared, and red channels	−	100 Hz
Muse S EEG headband		
Accelerometer	g {−2:+2}	52 Hz
Gyroscope	°/s {−245:+245}	52 Hz
EEG raw waveform	uV {0.0:1682.815}	256 Hz
EEG absolute band power (alpha, beta, delta, gamma, theta bands)	Bels	10 Hz
Zephyr BioHarness 3.0 chest band		
Accelerometer	bits {0–4094}	100 Hz
Breathing sensor raw output	bits {1:16777215}	25 Hz
Breathing rate	breaths per minute {4:70}	1 Hz
Breath-to-breath interval	ms	−
ECG raw waveform	bits {0:4095}	250 Hz
Heart rate	beats per minute {25:240}	1 Hz
Heart rate variability	ms {0:65534}	1 Hz
RR interval	ms {0:32767}	−
Posture	degrees from vertical {−180:180}	1 Hz
Empatica E4 wristband		
Accelerometer	g {−2:+2}	32 Hz
Blood volume pulse	−	64Hz
Average heart rate	1 Hz	
Inter-beat interval	ms	−
Electrodermal activity	microsiemens	4 Hz
Skin temperature	C	4 Hz

4   Preliminary Results

The collected dataset consisted of 36 sessions – twelve sessions each of low, medium, and high physical activity – with a total duration of almost 13 h of physiological and behavioral recordings. The average duration of each recording was 21.24 min (SD: 3.23 min). No significant difference in session length was observed across the physical activity conditions ($F = 1.57$, $p = 0.24$).

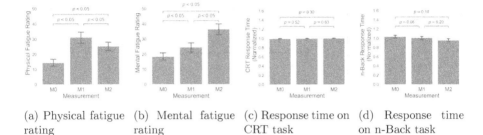

(a) Physical fatigue rating   (b) Mental fatigue rating   (c) Response time on CRT task   (d) Response time on n-Back task

Fig. 8. Fatigue and fatigability measures at baseline ($M1$), after physical activity ($M2$), and after cognitive task ($M3$).

4.1   Fatigue and Fatigability Measurements

We first investigated the overall difference between fatigue and fatigability measurements at different stages – at baseline ($M0$), after physical activity ($M1$), and after cognitive task ($M2$) – pooling all experimental conditions together. As shown in Fig. 8a, physical fatigue ratings increased significantly following the treadmill activity and decreased following the cognitive task. This is expected since the cognitive task was completed while participants were seated, allowing them to use this extended period of seating to recover from the physical activity session. Mental fatigue ratings showed a small increase following physical activity, and a larger increase after the cognitive task (see Fig. 8b). We failed to observe a significant difference in response times measured at different points during the experimental session for either the CRT or the n-back task (see Figs. 8c and 8d). The above analysis shows that the study design was able to successfully induce physical and mental fatigue, but significant mental fatigability was not observed when not accounting for physical activity conditions.

We also found no significant correlation ($p > 0.05$) between fatigue scores and response times on either the CRT or n-back tasks, indicating that participants' perception of fatigue did not correspond to their objective cognitive performance.

4.2   Effect of Physical Activity on Fatigue and Fatigability

Next, we explore the effect of the level of physical activity on mental fatigue and fatigability. To this end, we first look into mental fatigue and fatigability

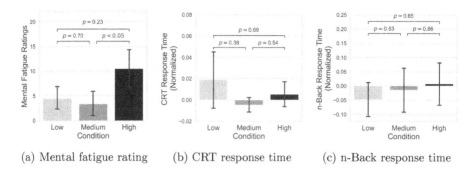

(a) Mental fatigue rating   (b) CRT response time   (c) n-Back response time

Fig. 9. Mental fatigue and fatigability after physical activity ($M2 - M1$).

after participants completed physical activity on the treadmill by calculating the difference between $M2$ and the baseline measurement $M1$ for each activity condition. As shown in Fig. 9a, there was a positive trend in mental fatigue ratings across all conditions, but the increase in self-reported fatigue was significantly higher during the "High" physical activity condition compared to the "Medium" condition. In terms of fatigability, average response times on the CRT task increased during "Low" and "High" intensity activity and decreased during the "Medium" condition, but differences across conditions were not significant (see Fig. 9b). For the n-back task, response times decreased during "Low" and "Medium" conditions and increased slightly during "High" activity, though no significant differences were observed across conditions (see Fig. 9c). "Medium"-level activity was associated with both the least increase in subjective fatigue and slight improvements in performance on both cognitive tasks following physical activity.

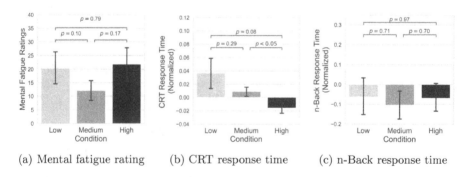

(a) Mental fatigue rating   (b) CRT response time   (c) n-Back response time

Fig. 10. Mental fatigue and fatigability after cognitive activity ($M3 - M1$).

We also investigated mental fatigue and fatigability following the subsequent cognitive task (difference between $M3$ and $M1$). We found that all physical activity conditions were associated with an increase in fatigue ratings after the dual cognitive task, though the difference between conditions was not found to be significant (Fig. 10a). In terms of fatigability, "High" physical activity exhibited a significant decline in CRT response times compared to the other two conditions (see Fig. 10b). No significant differences between conditions were found on the more cognitively-demanding n-back task (Fig. 10c), where participants may have overcome performance declines by expending more effort.

5   Conclusion

In this work, we present FatigueSet, a multi-modal dataset for understanding the impact of physical and cognitive activity on the development of mental fatigue and fatigability. Based on a preliminary analysis of experimental data recorded from twelve participants over 36 sessions, we show that cognitive performance and fatigability are poorly associated with individuals' perception of fatigue. This demonstrates the need to independently consider experiential and behavioral dimensions of fatigue while developing fatigue-aware applications. Our analysis also reveals a difference in mental fatigue and fatigability across different physical activity conditions, illustrating the importance of accounting for the interplay between physical and mental fatigue. We hypothesize that these goals can be achieved by taking into account physiological correlates of fatigue and fatigability. Our publicly available dataset is an effort in this direction, and contains EEG, ECG, PPG, EDA, skin temperature, accelerometer, and gyroscope data from four devices at different on-body locations to facilitate a deeper understanding of mental fatigue and fatigability in daily life.

References

1. E4 Wristband. https://www.empatica.com/research/e4/
2. eSense overview. https://www.esense.io/
3. Introducing Muse S. https://choosemuse.com/muse-s/
4. Zephyr^{TM} performance systems. https://www.zephyranywhere.com/
5. Fatigue, July 2021. https://www.ccohs.ca/oshanswers/psychosocial/fatigue.html
6. Ahlstrom, C., et al.: Fit-for-duty test for estimation of drivers' sleepiness level: eye movements improve the sleep/wake predictor. Transp. Res. Part C: Emerg. Technol. **26**, 20–32 (2013)
7. Borg, G.: Perceived exertion as an indicator of somatic stress. Scand. J. Rehabil. Med. **2**(2), 92–98 (1970)
8. Chmura, J., Nazar, K., Kaciuba-Uścilko, H.: Choice reaction time during graded exercise in relation to blood lactate and plasma catecholamine thresholds. Int. J. Sports Med. **15**(04), 172–176 (1994)
9. Craig, A., Tran, Y., Wijesuriya, N., Nguyen, H.: Regional brain wave activity changes associated with fatigue. Psychophysiology **49**(4), 574–582 (2012)
10. Deary, I.J., Liewald, D., Nissan, J.: A free, easy-to-use, computer-based simple and four-choice reaction time programme: the deary-liewald reaction time task. Behav. Res. Methods **43**(1), 258–268 (2011)
11. Dittner, A.J., Wessely, S.C., Brown, R.G.: The assessment of fatigue: a practical guide for clinicians and researchers. J. Psychosom. Res. **56**(2), 157–170 (2004)

12. Elshafei, M., Shihab, E.: Towards detecting biceps muscle fatigue in gym activity using wearables. Sensors **21**(3), 759 (2021)
13. Gjoreski, M., et al.: Datasets for cognitive load inference using wearable sensors and psychological traits. Appl. Sci. **10**(11), 3843 (2020)
14. Häkkinen, K.: Neuromuscular fatigue and recovery in male and female athletes during heavy resistance exercise. Int. J. Sports Med. **14**(02), 53–59 (1993)
15. Janveja, I., Nambi, A., Bannur, S., Gupta, S., Padmanabhan, V.: Insight: monitoring the state of the driver in low-light using smartphones. Proc. ACM Interact. Mob. Wearable Ubiquit. Technol. **4**(3), 1–29 (2020)
16. Jetté, M., Sidney, K., Blümchen, G.: Metabolic equivalents (METS) in exercise testing, exercise prescription, and evaluation of functional capacity. Clin. Cardiol. **13**(8), 555–565 (1990)
17. Kane, M.J., Conway, A.R., Miura, T.K., Colflesh, G.J.: Working memory, attention control, and the n-back task: a question of construct validity. J. Exp. Psychol. Learn. Mem. Cogn. **33**(3), 615 (2007)
18. Kawsar, F., Min, C., Mathur, A., Montanari, A.: Earables for personal-scale behavior analytics. IEEE Pervasive Comput. **17**(3), 83–89 (2018)
19. Kluger, B.M., Krupp, L.B., Enoka, R.M.: Fatigue and fatigability in neurologic illnesses: proposal for a unified taxonomy. Neurology **80**(4), 409–416 (2013)
20. Krausman, A.S., Crowell III, H.P., Wilson, R.M.: The effects of physical exertion on cognitive performance. Technical report, Army Research Lab Aberdeen Proving Ground MD (2002)
21. Krupp, L.B., LaRocca, N.G., Muir-Nash, J., Steinberg, A.D.: The fatigue severity scale: application to patients with multiple sclerosis and systemic lupus erythematosus. Arch. Neurol. **46**(10), 1121–1123 (1989)
22. Levitt, S., Gutin, B.: Multiple choice reaction time and movement time during physical exertion. Res. Q. Am. Assoc. Health Phys. Educ. Recreation **42**(4), 405–410 (1971)
23. Li, F., Chen, C.H., Xu, G., Khoo, L.P., Liu, Y.: Proactive mental fatigue detection of traffic control operators using bagged trees and gaze-bin analysis. Adv. Eng. Inform. **42**, 100987 (2019)
24. Lorist, M.M., Klein, M., Nieuwenhuis, S., De Jong, R., Mulder, G., Meijman, T.F.: Mental fatigue and task control: planning and preparation. Psychophysiology **37**(5), 614–625 (2000)
25. Luo, H., Lee, P.A., Clay, I., Jaggi, M., De Luca, V.: Assessment of fatigue using wearable sensors: a pilot study. Digit. Biomarkers **4**(1), 59–72 (2020)
26. Maman, Z.S., Yazdi, M.A.A., Cavuoto, L.A., Megahed, F.M.: A data-driven approach to modeling physical fatigue in the workplace using wearable sensors. Appl. Ergon. **65**, 515–529 (2017)
27. Marcora, S.M., Staiano, W., Manning, V.: Mental fatigue impairs physical performance in humans. J. Appl. Physiol. **106**(3), 857–864 (2009)
28. Monk, T.H.: A visual analogue scale technique to measure global vigor and affect. Psychiatry Res. **27**(1), 89–99 (1989)
29. Norton, K., Norton, L., Sadgrove, D.: Position statement on physical activity and exercise intensity terminology. J. Sci. Med. Sport **13**(5), 496–502 (2010)
30. Ortega, F.B., et al.: The international fitness scale (IFIS): usefulness of self-reported fitness in youth. Int. J. Epidemiol. **40**(3), 701–711 (2011)
31. O'Keeffe, K., Hodder, S., Lloyd, A.: A comparison of methods used for inducing mental fatigue in performance research: individualised, dual-task and short duration cognitive tests are most effective. Ergonomics **63**(1), 1–12 (2020)

32. Peirce, J., et al.: Psychopy2: experiments in behavior made easy. Behav. Res. Methods **51**(1), 195–203 (2019)
33. Phillips, R.O.: A review of definitions of fatigue-and a step towards a whole definition. Transport. Res. F: Traffic Psychol. Behav. **29**, 48–56 (2015)
34. Rammstedt, B., John, O.P.: Measuring personality in one minute or less: a 10-item short version of the big five inventory in English and German. J. Res. Pers. **41**(1), 203–212 (2007)
35. Roenneberg, T., Wirz-Justice, A., Merrow, M.: Life between clocks: daily temporal patterns of human chronotypes. J. Biol. Rhythms **18**(1), 80–90 (2003)
36. Rogers, R.D., Monsell, S.: Costs of a predictible switch between simple cognitive tasks. J. Exp. Psychol. Gen. **124**(2), 207 (1995)
37. Shahid, A., Wilkinson, K., Marcu, S., Shapiro, C.M.: Stanford sleepiness scale (SSS). In: Shahid, A., Wilkinson, K., Marcu, S., Shapiro, C.M. (eds.) STOP, THAT and One Hundred Other Sleep Scales, pp. 369–370. Springer, Heidelberg (2011). https://doi.org/10.1007/978-1-4419-9893-4_91
38. Shen, K.Q., Li, X.P., Ong, C.J., Shao, S.Y., Wilder-Smith, E.P.: EEG-based mental fatigue measurement using multi-class support vector machines with confidence estimate. Clin. Neurophysiol. **119**(7), 1524–1533 (2008)
39. Silverman, M.N., Heim, C.M., Nater, U.M., Marques, A.H., Sternberg, E.M.: Neuroendocrine and immune contributors to fatigue. PM&R **2**(5), 338–346 (2010)
40. Smith, M.R., Chai, R., Nguyen, H.T., Marcora, S.M., Coutts, A.J.: Comparing the effects of three cognitive tasks on indicators of mental fatigue. J. Psychol. **153**(8), 759–783 (2019)
41. Van Cutsem, J., Marcora, S., De Pauw, K., Bailey, S., Meeusen, R., Roelands, B.: The effects of mental fatigue on physical performance: a systematic review. Sports Med. **47**(8), 1569–1588 (2017)
42. Van Dongen, H., Belenky, G., Krueger, J.M.: Investigating the temporal dynamics and underlying mechanisms of cognitive fatigue (2011)
43. Wan, J., Qin, Z., Wang, P., Sun, Y., Liu, X.: Muscle fatigue: general understanding and treatment. Exp. Mol. Med. **49**(10), e384–e384 (2017)

Exploring Unique App Signature
of the Depressed and Non-depressed Through
Their Fingerprints on Apps

Md. Sabbir Ahmed$^{(\boxtimes)}$ (iD) and Nova Ahmed (iD)

Design Inclusion and Access Lab, North South University, Dhaka, Bangladesh
sabbir.eu.bd@gmail.com, nova.ahmed@northsouth.edu

Abstract. Growing research on re-identification through app usage behavior reveals the privacy threat in having smartphone usage data to third parties. However, re-identifiability of a vulnerable group like the depressed is unexplored. We fill this knowledge gap through an in the wild study on 100 students' PHQ-9 scale's data and 7 days' logged app usage data. We quantify the uniqueness and re-identifiability through exploration of minimum hamming distance in terms of the set of used apps. Our findings show that using app usage data, each of the depressed and non-depressed students is re-identifiable. In fact, using only 7 h' data of a week, on average, 91% of the depressed and 88% of the non-depressed are re-identifiable. Moreover, data of a single app category (i.e., Tools) can also be used to re-identify each depressed student. Furthermore, we find that the rate of uniqueness among the depressed students is significantly higher in some app categories. For instance, in the Social Media category, the rate of uniqueness is 9% higher (P = .02, Cohen's d = 1.31) and in the Health & Fitness category, this rate is 8% higher (P = .005, Cohen's d = 1.47) than the non-depressed group. Our findings suggest that each of the depressed students has a unique app signature which makes them re-identifiable. Therefore, during the design of the privacy protecting systems, designers need to consider the uniqueness of them to ensure better privacy for this vulnerable group.

Keywords: Depressed · Non-depressed · Re-identification · Privacy · Unique app signature · Social media · Health & fitness · Smartphone

1 Introduction

Third party apps and websites can collect sensitive information from the users in different ways. Without users' awareness, apps can collect sensitive data such as SMS [4, 5], location [19], phone number [5, 19], even the collection of installed apps from the smartphone [5]. It is possible to uniquely re-identify the users through their data of music preferences [18], app usage [3, 6, 8–11, 23, 32], and mobility [2, 7] which increases the risk of privacy leakage. Moreover, attacks can be designed through the use of leaked data [14]. In fact, study [4] found that malware detects and matches with the users' installed

H. Lewy and R. Barkan (Eds.): PH 2021, LNICST 431, pp. 218–239, 2022.
https://doi.org/10.1007/978-3-030-99194-4_15

apps to perform pre-determined tasks. Due to attacks like cyber-attacks, victims can suffer from various mental illness (e.g., frustration [15]). Therefore, in the case of the people who are already depressed, the situation can worsen. Given the significance of better privacy for vulnerable groups, we explore the unique app signature of the depressed group by which they can be re-identified only from the app usage data.

Scholarly studies [20–22, 29, 33, 41–44, 47] have been conducted regarding depression and technology. A substantial amount of studies [6, 7, 10, 11, 14, 30, 32, 35, 40] also presented the approach to re-identify. Depressed people may have identifiable unique app signatures as previous studies show different preferences of the depressed. For instance, people with major depressive disorder are more likely to prefer sad and low energy music [44]. However, none of these studies have explored the unique app signature of the depressed students by which they can be re-identified from a dataset where any direct identity (e.g., name, email) is not available. If the depressed students are more unique in some app categories, then they are more likely to be vulnerable in having data of those app categories to the third parties which can be a privacy threat. This motivated us to explore the following research questions.

- Can the depressed be uniquely re-identified only from a set of used apps?
- Is there any statistically significant difference between the depressed and non-depressed, in terms of re-identifiability?

To answer the research questions, using our developed app, we collected 7 days' actual app usage data and response of the PHQ-9 scale [12] from 100 Bangladeshi students. Then, following scholarly studies [13, 28, 29], we divided the participants based on their PHQ-9 score. Participants having scores of less than 10 were grouped as the non-depressed and others as the depressed. To understand the re-identifiability, we calculated the hamming distance. Our analysis of regardless app category shows that all of the depressed and non-depressed students are re-identifiable. We also find that students of both groups are more unique on weekdays. However, still, on weekends, about 25 apps are needed to make them anonymous. Our findings also show that using data of the app categories, it is possible to re-identify a significant number of depressed and non-depressed students. In fact, analysis of the Tools category shows that with 12 h data of each day of a week all of the students can be re-identified. It was also interesting to see that depressed students' uniqueness rate is significantly higher in some app categories. For instance, the uniqueness rate among the depressed is 9% higher (p = .02) in the Social Media and 8% higher (p = .005) in the Health & Fitness category.

Our research has several contributions. Firstly, we explored the depressed students' uniqueness in app signatures which is the first study (to our best knowledge) regarding any group suffering from mental health problems where possibility of re-identification is presented. Secondly, we have presented the differences of this group from the non-depressed in terms of re-identifiability. Thirdly, we have presented that depressed and non-depressed students can be uniquely re-identified through the data of app categories which was not explored previously even in terms of general people. Lastly, through higher uniqueness of the depressed students, we have discussed about their support seeking behavior which can be insightful in designing apps to overcome depression.

2 Related Work

2.1 Difference in Smartphone Usage Among Various Groups of People

Smartphone usage behavior varies between different groups of people, from teens [16] to older [17]. The substantial diversity of smartphone usage behavior is presented by some previous studies [3, 48]. Researchers presented that the number of interactions, number of apps [48], diurnal usage pattern [8, 48], frequency of using apps [3] varies between the users. The usage behavior can vary by place [49] and day of the week [3, 49] also. Bentley et al. found that teens' smartphone usage behavior is different from the general population [16] and Gordon et al. [17] found that smartphone usage of the older adults is different from the younger adults. Indeed, smartphone usage behavior varies by platform. For instance, iPhone users have a higher number of apps per session [40] than the Android users. App usage behavior differ between the risk and non-risk smartphone users also [8]. However, none of the studies explored the behavioral difference between the depressed and non-depressed in terms of re-identifiability.

2.2 Smartphone Usage and Mental Health

Smartphones have been widely used in assessing different types of mental health problems such as depression [13, 29, 33, 41, 42, 53, 54] and loneliness [52, 55]. Noë et al. [22] found that smartphone addiction does not correlate with interaction regarding every app category. Rozgonjuk et al. [20] found a negative relation of depression and anxiety with the frequency of unlocking phone screens. However, there are several studies who did not find a negative relation. For instance, a previous study found that addiction to smartphone usage has a significant positive correlation with depression [21]. In another study [29], researchers found that though the depressed and non-depressed students do not differ by total smartphone usage data, they differ significantly in terms of app categories usage data. Using smartphone sensed data, researchers [33, 42] found that students having symptoms of depression and non-depression can be classified accurately. In our study, we discuss the support seeking nature of the depressed students through their unique characteristics of app usage.

2.3 Re-identification of the Users and Privacy Leakage

Most of the ad (advertisement) libraries of the apps collect personal information [5]. Installed apps in users' phones can expose location information to the servers of advertisers without implicit or explicit consent of the users [19]. This is a threat to the privacy of the users as based on location data they can be re-identified [7, 11], and also their demographic attributes can be inferred [14]. The ad libraries [5], popular social media apps like Twitter [36, 37] collect the information regarding installed apps from the users' phone. Moreover, a study [38] showed that 42.55% of the apps share data with Facebook. This data is shared even when the people do not use Facebook [39]. Information collected through different ways can later be used for identification purposes [5]. In fact, combining data that is shared with Facebook can reveal personal information related to activities, interests, health etc. [39]. With the available data, previous studies presented several ways by which people can be re-identified. Tu et al. [11] investigated the risk of re-identification and privacy leakage through the use of spatial and temporal information. Welke et al. [6] found that 99.67% of the users can be uniquely identified under consideration of 500 most frequent apps. Moreover, they found that even after restricting to 60 most frequent apps, it is still possible to uniquely find out 99.4% users. Surprisingly, few other studies [10, 11, 35] showed that even with 4 random apps, most users can be uniquely re-identified which is a threat to privacy. However, this re-identification varies by season, country [10], mobility, activity in social networks, and gender [11]. Therefore, distinct characteristics regarding fingerprints on apps need to be considered to protect privacy of the users. However, the re-identification of the depressed is unexplored which could be useful in designing technology having better privacy of the depressed.

Apart from the usage of apps' data, previous studies [18, 30] demonstrated some other ways of re-identification. By doing four experiments, Hirschprung and Leshman [18] showed that users can be re-identified by their music selection. Gulyás et al. [32] found that using a combination of font and screen size, users can be re-identified. Their findings also showed that by 100 cameras for 40 lac people, it is possible to re-identify a number of users from the Call Detail Record (CDR) dataset [32]. On the other hand, using data regarding transactions, Montjoye et al. [30] showed that with four spatiotemporal points, 90% credit card users can be uniquely re-identified. Their findings also presented that uniqueness varies by gender, income level. For instance, they found that women can be more easily identified than the men. However, Tu et al. [11] found that men are more distinguishable in terms of app usage data. However, the difference between the depressed and non-depressed is unexplored in terms of re-identification through the app usage data which could be insightful to understand the depressed better and to come up with a better technology ensuring the privacy of this vulnerable group.

3   Methodology

Using our developed automatic logger app (Sect. 3.1), we collected 7 days' actual app usage data (Sect. 3.2). After pre-processing and categorization of the apps (Sect. 3.3), to understand the re-identifiability, we calculated the hamming distance (Sect. 3.3). Apart from this, we did statistical analysis (Sect. 3.3) to explore the difference statistically in uniqueness between the depressed and non-depressed.

3.1   Data Collection Tool

App Usage Data. We developed an Android app to collect actual smartphone usage data and self-reported psychological data. With the proper consent of the user, this app retrieves past 7 days' app usage data very accurately. To get the foreground and background events of the used apps, we used *UsageStatsManager* class of Java and to save the data, we used Google Firebase. Except for the metadata, our app does not collect or store any sensitive data like photo, message etc. We released the app in Google Play store as this app store is known to the Android users (Fig. 1).

Testing the Data Collection Tool. We tested the app in different ways. First of all, we compared the retrieved app usage data of our tool with the manually calculated app usage

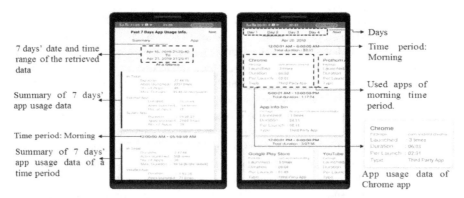

Fig. 1. Screenshots of our developed Android app which was used to collect data.

data. Secondly, we compared the retrieved app usage data of our tool with such apps [57, 58] of Google Play store. Finally, we tested the tool on 9 different smartphones. We find that in each of the mentioned approaches, our data collection tool can calculate 7 days' app usage data (e.g., duration) very accurately.

Scale to Detect Depression. In the data collection tool, to measure the depression, we include the PHQ-9 scale [12]. In our app, the scale was available in English as well as in native language Bengali. Amid the pandemic, depression increased among the young. In fact, a previous study [34] conducted before COVID found a 69.5% depression rate among the first-year university students of Bangladesh. As a word like dead may worsen the mental health of a depressed student while responding to the questions, we have consulted with three lecturers (one is from the department of CSE and two is from Sociology), and a program coordinator of a university who have good connections with the students. Due to various concerns, all of them suggested removing the word dead. For instance, the program coordinator was concerned about the mental health of the depressed students after being asked a question regarding death. In addition, we talked with 3 more doctors who served the COVID patients. They remarked that the word hurting in the ninth item may present the suicide intention of the depressed one. Moreover, we found that the word dead is not preferable in all cultural contexts. For example, religious participants may not feel comfortable in responding to this item [56]. Therefore, we removed the bold word dead to make the 9th item comfortable for the participants. Finally, we translated the questionnaire in Bengali where three researchers, 2 final year students, and 4 other undergraduate students were involved.

3.2   Data Collection Procedure and Participants

Data Collection Procedure. Using the snowball sampling method [24], the data were collected from 100 students of 12 different higher institutions of Bangladesh and they were from department of BBA (Bachelor of Business Administration), CSE (Computer Science & Engineering), EEE (Electrical & Electronic Engineering), LLM (Master of Laws), MBBS (Bachelor of Medicine, Bachelor of Surgery), Sociology, and Textile

Engineering. But the majority of them were studying in the CSE department. We collected data during COVID period and due to COVID, it was not possible for us to collect all participants' data through a face to face meeting. From most of the participants, we collected data by arranging group meetings and one to one meetings through a virtual platform like Google Meet, Messenger depending participants' availability and their preferences. During data collection, at first we briefly described our research and then asked the participants to read the consent form, download the app from Google Play store. As exams may have an impact on students' mental health, we did not collect data from the students who had mid-term or semester final exams during the data collection time.

Categorization of the Participants. Following previous studies [13, 28, 29], we divide the participants into depressed and non-depressed on the basis of their self-reported response to the PHQ-9 scale. The participants whose score was at least 10 were categorized as depressed and the participants whose score were less than 10 were categorized as non-depressed. For major depression detection, both the sensitivity and specificity of PHQ-9 score 10 was 88% [12].

Depression of the Participants. In the PHQ-9 questionnaire [12], there are 9 symptoms and participants had the option to select the days (not at all, several days, more than half the days, and nearly every day) they bothered each of those symptoms in the past 14 days. In the case of the depressed students, 36.4% responses were nearly every day and 82.6% responses were at least several days (Fig. 2 (a)). On the other hand, in case of non-depressed students more than 50% responses were not at all (56.5%) and only 10.7% responses were more than half the days and nearly every day. (Fig. 2(b)) This presents that in the depressed group, the symptoms appeared at a much higher number of days in comparison to the non-depressed group.

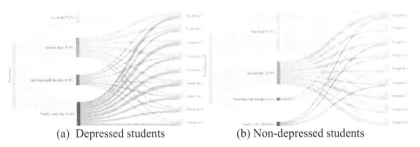

(a) Depressed students   (b) Non-depressed students

Fig. 2. The frequency (not at all, several days, more than half the days, nearly everyday) of appearance of different depressive symptoms, in (a) depressed and (b) non-depressed group.

Demographic Characteristics. We explored whether there is any difference between the depressed and non-depressed group in terms of gender, age, and social circumstances such as monthly income as these can be confounders. In the depressed group, there were 13.7% female which is close to the female participants' percentage (12.2%) of the non-depressed group (Fig. 3(a)). There were also almost similar percentages of male participants (86.3% and 87.8%) in both of the groups. Our statistical analysis also shows that there is no significant difference of age between these two groups of students (Fig. 3(b)). Mean age of the depressed was 23.25 years (SD = 2.33) and non-depressed was 22.86 years (SD = 1.62) which are statistically not different (t(89) = 0.99, P = .32). We also find that there is no statistically significant difference (depressed: BDT 62,488.9 vs non-depressed: BDT 51,541.7, U = 1160.5, P = .54) of monthly income (Fig. 3(c)).

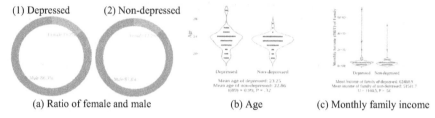

(a) Ratio of female and male   (b) Age   (c) Monthly family income

Fig. 3. Difference between the depressed and non-depressed group in terms of (a) ratio o female and male participants, (b) age, and (c) monthly family income (in BDT: Bangladeshi Taka).

3.3 Data Analysis

App Categorization. In 7 days, participants used 1129 unique apps in total. To understand their uniqueness regarding app categories, we grouped those apps into 26 categories. During categorization, we considered the features of the apps, volunteers' opinion, developers' referred category in different apps stores, and app categorization of the previous studies (e.g., [1, 40]). For some apps, we did not use the developers' referred category. For instance, though Zoom and Google Meet were categorized as Business apps in the Google Play store, we categorized those as Education apps since participants of our study were students and amid COVID-19, their classes were held virtually using these apps. There were some apps for which detailed information was not available. We kept those in unknown app category like Böhmer et al. [1]. Moreover, in Art & Design category (e.g., Autodesk SketchBook app), there was only 1 participant. Thus, we excluded that app category also keeping 24 categories for statistical analysis.

Analysis to Find the Uniqueness. Finding the uniqueness of a smartphone user, one can be identified easily by an attacker which is a direct privacy leakage [11]. To identify the uniqueness of the both depressed and non-depressed students, we calculate the minimum hamming distance [25] of a user as used by previous studies in case of other groups of people [6, 11, 40]. Let's say, there are two participants named participant 1 and participant 2. The set of apps used by participant 1 is {*WorldGK, Wikipedia*} and the set of apps used by participant 2 is {*Dictionary, Wikipedia, EnglishGrammarFull*}. In terms of app usage, the hamming distance (*D*) between these two participants can be calculated using the following formula:

$$D = (S_1 \cup S_2) - (S_1 \cap S_2)$$

Here, $S_1 \cup S_2$ presents the set of all the apps used by the participant 1 and participant 2. $S_1 \cap S_2$ presents the common set of apps used by both of these two participants. D represents the distance between participant 1 and participant 2. In the case of the given set of apps, the distance will be 3 ({*WorldGK*, *Dictionary*, *Wikipedia*, *English GrammarFu*ll} − {*Wikipedia*}). In this way, we calculate the hamming distance of a participant from all other participants. After that, to find the uniqueness of a participant (U_i), we find out the user with whom the hamming distance is minimum.

$$U_i = min\{D_1, D_2, D_3, D_4, ..., D_n\}$$

Here, U_i represents the uniqueness of the ith participant. This value will represent the minimum number of apps that will be required to use for the ith participant to be anonymous as described by a previous study [6].

Statistical Analysis. After calculating the minimum hamming distance, we explore whether the uniqueness of depressed and non-depressed students is different. As most of our data were not normally distributed, we did mostly non-parametric Mann-Whitney U Test using scipy library [26]. However, in those cases where data were normally distributed and had equal variance among the groups of students, we did Standard T-Test. In some categories where both groups did not have equal variance, we did the Welch T-Test. As multiple comparisons can produce false positive results, we controlled

Table 1. Brief description about the used phrases in this study.

Phrase	Brief description
App usage fingerprint	The fingerprint on the used set of apps [10, 11]. Here, we used the word fingerprint to denote the touch on the screen of smartphones while using an app
App signature	App signature is defined as the set of mobile apps which were used at least for one time in the participant's phone [6]
Uniqueness	The uniqueness is measured by calculating hamming distance [25] from one participant to another. The higher the hamming distance, the more unique a participant is (for more, please see subsection named "Analysis to Find the Uniqueness") of Methods
Rate of uniqueness	The percentage of participants (e.g., depressed) who used at least one different app from the other participants
Uniqueness through app categories	The uniqueness in terms of the participants' used apps of a particular app category (e.g., Social Media)
Re-identification	Possibility to re-identify [10, 11] a participant. For example, in this study, we used app usage data to present the re-identification of the depressed and non-depressed students, without having any other information (e.g., demographic characteristics)

the type I error using False Discovery Rate (FDR) method [27]. We considered each app category as a separate family as depending on app category, depressed and non-depressed students' smartphone usage behavior varies [29] (Table 1).

3.4 Research Ethics

This study is a part of a research project which was approved by the Center of Research & Development of a university. We collected data with all of the participants' informed consent where we mentioned explicitly details of the study like data we are collecting, data security which we will provide. During the data donation, one had to give two permissions (to access the IMEI number and to access app usage data) which was also mentioned in the consent form.

4 Results

After analysing the response of the PHQ-9 scale [12], we find that among 100 students, 51 participants had depression scores of at least 10. Therefore, based on the classification criteria [13, 28, 29], 51% participants were depressed and 49% participants were non-depressed. We also find that all of the depressed students and non-depressed students can be uniquely re-identified without considering any app category (Sect. 4.1). However, analysis of Tools app category shows that with app usage data of only a single category, it is possible to re-identify each of the depressed and non-depressed students (Sect. 4.2). Moreover, we find that with 24 h data of 7 days, a significant number of participants can be re-identified by the popular app categories such as Communication, Photo & Video, Productivity (Sect. 4.2). After exploring the uniqueness difference between these two groups of students, we find that depressed students are significantly more unique in some app categories (Sect. 4.3). For example, in Social Media, the rate of uniqueness among the depressed students was 9% higher and it was statistically significant ($P = .02$, Cohen's $d = 1.31$).

4.1 Uniqueness While Considering Apps of All Categories

About 37 Apps are Needed to Make the Depressed and Non-depressed Anonymous. To understand how unique the depressed and non-depressed students are, we calculated the minimum hamming distance to the nearest participant. Here, during finding the nearest participant, we did not consider that participant's group (e.g., depressed) since we wanted to understand their uniqueness among all participants. From Table 2, we see that under consideration of a week's app usage data only, both in case of depressed and non-depressed students, on average, about 37 apps will be required to be anonymous.

Both of the Depressed and Non-depressed are More Unique on Weekdays. We present the uniqueness of each student on 7 days, weekdays, and on weekends. We find that both the depressed and non-depressed students are more unique on weekdays in comparison to weekends. On weekdays, the average distance to the nearest user is about 34 whereas on weekends, this distance is about 25 (Table 2).

Table 2. Depressed and non-depressed students' hamming distance. SD: Standard Deviation.

Days	Depressed students' Hamming distance				Non-depressed students' Hamming distance			
	Minimum	Maximum	Mean	SD	Minimum	Maximum	Mean	SD
7 days	16.0	137.0	37.73	17.84	16.0	122.0	36.7755	14.995
Weekdays	4.0	76.0	33.53	11.98	4.0	101.0	34.20	12.94
Weekends	7.0	79.0	24.61	9.898	7.0	94.0	24.61	12.055

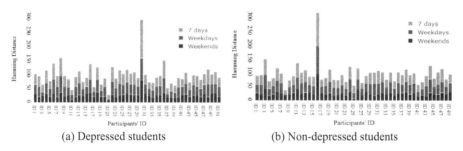

(a) Depressed students   (b) Non-depressed students

Fig. 4. Hamming distance to the nearest user for each of the depressed and non-depressed.

In Each Hour, Depressed and Non-depressed Can Be Uniquely Re-identified.
Supporting the findings of each individual student's uniqueness as presented in Fig. 4,
Fig. 5 also shows that in each hour of the day, on weekdays, their uniqueness level is
higher. The difference in uniqueness between weekdays and weekends becomes higher
from mid day. In addition, Fig. 5 shows that as we move from morning (6 AM) to
afternoon both the depressed and non-depressed students use more unique apps. However, from 10 PM, their uniqueness begins to move downwards and in case of the non-
depressed students (Fig. 5(b)), this decrease is approximately linear on weekdays. On
the other hand, in case of depressed students (Fig. 5(a)), from 7 AM on weekdays, their
average uniqueness increment is almost linear.

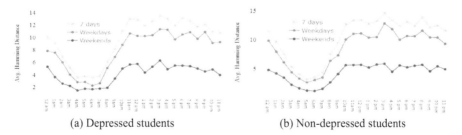

(a) Depressed students   (b) Non-depressed students

Fig. 5. Average hamming distance of the depressed and non-depressed students in each hour of
weekdays, weekends, and 7 days (weekdays + weekends).

4.2 Uniqueness Through App Categories

To understand how many students can be uniquely re-identified if adversaries have only an app category's data of particular hours of 7 days, we calculate the average percentage of unique students in terms of 8 different hour intervals (1 h, 2 h, 3 h, 4 h, 6 h, 8 h, 12 h, 24 h). To do this analysis, at first, we calculate the percentage of students that are unique in terms of each time range (e.g., 12 AM–2 AM, 2 AM–4 AM) of 7 days under consideration of a particular interval (e.g., 2 h interval). After that, we calculate the average percentage of students that are unique, in terms of the corresponding interval.

Tools Category's Data Can Re-identify Each of the Depressed and Non-depressed. Our findings show that regardless of the app category, all of the participants can be uniquely re-identified using 12 h' data of each day of a week (Fig. 6(a)). In fact, considering 1 h's data of each day of a week, our findings show that on average 91% depressed and 88% non-depressed students are unique (Fig. 6(a)). This motivated us to explore how uniquely both the depressed and non-depressed students can be re-identified with app categories usage data. Analysis of the Tools app category shows that like the findings of regardless app category, each of the students of both groups can be re-identified when we consider the 12 h interval's data of this app category. Our findings also show that if an attacker gets just 1 h's data of each day of a week (i.e., 7 h data of a week), about 70% of students can be re-identified through the Tools category (Fig. 6(b)).

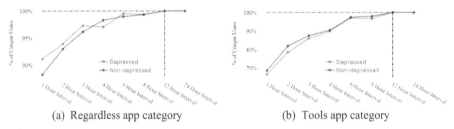

(a) Regardless app category   (b) Tools app category

Fig. 6. Percentage of the users that can be re-identified while considering (a) Without consideration of app category and (b) Tools app category.

Through Data of Popular App Categories Also, Depressed Can Be Uniquely Re-identified. As the popular app categories are used more by the students, we explored how the popular app categories can be used to uniquely re-identify the depressed and non-depressed students. Here, we visualize the app categories which can be used for re-identification of at least 50% users. Our findings show that in the case of Communication (Fig. 7(a)), Photo & Video (Fig. 7(b)), and Productivity (Fig. 7(c)) app categories, more than 75% users can be uniquely re-identified with usage data of only a single app category. In fact, in the Communication category, with 7 h data of a week (1 h interval), it is possible to re-identify more than 50% depressed and non-depressed students (Fig. 7(a)). We also find in terms of Games category, more than 50% depressed students are unique (Fig. 7(d)).

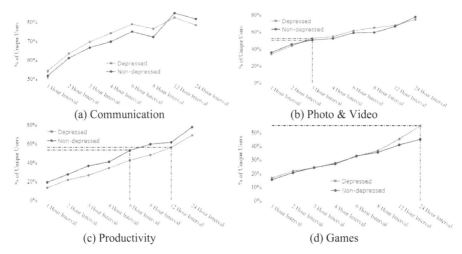

Fig. 7. Percentage of users that can be re-identified while considering (a) Communication (b) Photo & Video (c) Productivity (d) Games app categories. The dashed line indicates the interval using which one can uniquely re-identify at least 50% of students of a group (e.g., depressed).

4.3 Difference in Uniqueness Between the Depressed and Non-depressed Students

Depressed are Significantly more Unique in 7 App Categories. To understand whether there is any difference in uniqueness between the depressed and non-depressed students, we did a comparative study (for methodology, please see Sect. 3.3). After analyzing the data of 26 app categories, we find that in the Finance ($P = .01$, $d = 1.7$), Food & Drink ($P = .004$, $d = 1.69$), Health & Fitness ($P = .005$, $d = 1.47$), Launcher Like App ($P = .003$, $d = 3.4$), Lifestyle ($P = .005$, $d = 1.77$), Social Media ($P = .02$, $d = 1.31$), and Sports ($P = .0004$, $d = 3.13$) app categories, there is a significant difference in percentage of uniquely identifiable students between the depressed and non-depressed group (Table 3). In each of these app categories, more depressed students can be re-identified. As these percentages are based on hamming distance, higher uniqueness represents that the depressed students use a diverse set of apps than the non-depressed students. For instance, in the Health & Fitness category, we find that a student of the depressed group uses an app (Quit Tracker: Stop Smoking) to quit her/his smoking habit. Few others of that group use apps to create and communicate with replica friends (by an app, Replika: My AI Friend), to concentrate more, to reduce body weight etc. However, these types of apps were not used by the the non-depressed students.

Depressed are 9% More Unique in Social Media and 8% More Unique in the Health & Fitness Category. Our findings also show that in terms of Social Media category, after considering all of the 8 different hour intervals' percentage, on average 21% students can be uniquely re-identified (Table 3). However, analysis of the same app category shows that on average 13% students can be uniquely re-identified in case of non-depressed students which is 9% less ($P = .02$). Moreover, we find that in the Health & Fitness

Table 3. App categories which show significant differences between the depressed and non-depressed groups in percentage of re-identifiable students. Here, mean represents the average percentage of uniqueness after considering the percentages of 8 different hour intervals.

App Category	Example Apps	% of Depressed		% of Non-depressed		Statistics Value	P Value	Cohen's d
		Mean	Max.	Mean	Max.			
Finance	ALLEX, bKash	6	12	2	3	t(51) = 3.41	0.01	1.7
Food & Drink	eFood, CoSRe	2	4	0.9	2	t(98) = 3.38	0.004	1.69
Health & Fitness	Replika: My AI Friend	10	24	2	6	U= 59	0.005	1.47
Launcher Like App	System UI, Launcher3	9	10	4	8	U = 61	0.003	3.4
Lifestyle	SmartThings, Athan	5	10	1	4	U = 59	0.005	1.77
Social Media	Instagram, Facebook	21	31	13	22	t(98) = 2.62	0.02	1.31
Sports	Goal News, CricBall	6	10	0.6	1	t(52) = 6.26	0.0004	3.13

app category, 8% more (P = .005) students of the depressed group can be re-identified. Though in some other app categories (e.g., Food & Drink), we find that depressed students are significantly (P < .05) more unique (Table 3), in this section and the following sections of this paper, we will talk about Social Media and Health & Fitness app categories as using other app categories (which show significant difference) very less number (less than 10%) of students can be re-identified.

Supporting the findings mentioned in Table 3, Fig. 8 also shows that in the case of Social Media and Health & Fitness app categories, depressed students are more unique in both of these app categories. In fact, considering 24 h data of 7 days, in the Health & Fitness category, 6% non-depressed students are unique whereas in the depressed group, 24% are unique (Fig. 8(b)).

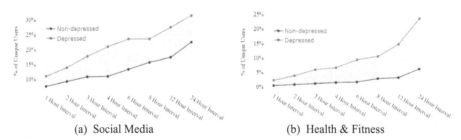

(a) Social Media   (b) Health & Fitness

Fig. 8. Difference between depressed and non-depressed students in percentage of users that can be re-identified while considering (a) Social Media (b) Health & Fitness app categories.

As using Social Media category, a significantly higher percentage of depressed students can be re-identified, we were motivated to explore this app category more. To understand whether in this app category, two groups of students have different diurnal usage patterns or not, following previous studies [3, 8], we divide a day into four equal periods taking 6 h as an interval: Night: 12:01 AM to 6:00 AM; Morning: 6:01 AM to 12:00 PM; Afternoon: 12:01 PM to 6:00 PM; Evening: 6:01 PM to 12:00 AM.

Depressed are More Unique in the Afternoon and Evening Time Period. Table 4 shows that considering Social Media usage of the night and morning time, there is no significant

Table 4. Difference of hamming distance between the depressed and non-depressed students, in terms of their Social Media app category usage data of different time ranges.

Time Range	Distance of Depressed		Distance of Non-depressed		Statistics Value	P	Cohen's d
	Mean	Maximum	Mean	Maximum			
Night	0.24	3	0.16	2	U=1250.5	0.995	0.15
Morning	0.18	1	0.1	1	U=1342.5	0.385	0.27
Afternoon	0.41	5	0.1	1	U=1475	0.046	0.47
Evening	0.35	3	0.1	2	U=1490	0.046	0.47

difference in hamming distance between the depressed and non-depressed students. However, in the afternoon time, the hamming distance of the depressed students to the nearest user is much higher than the non-depressed students and the difference is statistically significant (dep. 0.41 vs non-dep. 0.1, P = .046). Cohen's d of 0.47 also shows that the effect is not smaller. After analysing data of evening time range also, we find that depressed students can be more uniquely re-identified than the other group (dep. 0.35 vs non-dep 0.1, P = .046, Cohen's d = 0.47) using Social Media category usage data. Higher hamming distance of the depressed students in the afternoon and evening time ranges reveal that they use a more diverse set of apps in these time periods. Moreover, this analysis also presents that in terms of unique signature on apps of Social Media, depressed students have significantly different diurnal usage patterns than the non-depressed students.

In Several App Categories, Though Both the Depressed and Non-depressed are Unique, There is No Significant Difference. Several app categories do not show any significant difference between the depressed and nondepressed students' groups. Though using data of Tools app category, a large number (more than 90%) of students of each group can be uniquely re-identified, there is no significant difference (dep. 89% vs non-dep 90%, P = .84, Cohen's d = −0.1) in percentage of uniqueness between these two groups of students (Table 5). We also find similar insignificant (P > .05) differences in the case of several other app categories (Table 5). For instance, from analysis (Table 5 and Fig. 7(c)) of the Productivity category, it seems that a higher number of non-depressed students can be uniquely re-identified. However, the difference is not statistically significant (dep. 39% vs non-dep. 47%, P = .41, Cohen's d = −0.42). This says that in terms of percentage of uniquely re-identifiable students, the depressed group is more likely to be similar to the non-depressed group, in case of the app categories as presented in Table 5.

Table 5. App categories which do not show statistically significant differences between the depressed and non-depressed in percentage of uniquely re-identifiable students. Here, mean is the average percentage of uniqueness after considering the percentages of 8 different intervals.

App category	Example apps	% of Depressed		% of Non-depressed		Statistics value	P	Cohen's d
		Mean	Max.	Mean	Max.			
Books & Reference	World GK, Translate	16	24	18	29	$t(98) = -0.73$	0.48	−0.36
Browser & Search	Browser, Search	27	35	32	47	$t(98) = -1.03$	0.32	−0.51
Business	Pymetrics, TallyKhata	5	10	8	16	$t(98) = -1.27$	0.22	−0.64
Communication	TalkSign, Messenger	72	82	70	85	$t(98) = 0.38$	0.71	0.19
Education	ZOOM, Learn PHP	6	14	10	18	$t(98) = -1.62$	0.13	−0.81
Entertainment	Football TV, Adere	13	27	10	16	$t(98) = 0.97$	0.35	0.49
Games	Among Us, Archero	32	55	30	45	$t(98) = 0.39$	0.7	0.19
Medical	Daktarbhai, Patient Aid	2	2	0.8	2	$U = 47$	0.12	1.04
Music & Audio	Harmonium, i Music	15	25	16	35	$t(98) = -0.3$	0.77	−0.15
News & Magazines	Reddit, Job Circular	5	8	3	6	$t(98) = 1.97$	0.07	0.98
Personalization	Theme Store, Themes	7	10	5	9	$t(98) = 1.51$	0.15	0.75
Photo & Video	Camera, Collage Maker	57	75	56	78	$t(98) = 0.14$	0.89	0.07
Productivity	Scanner, Calendar	39	69	47	78	$t(98) = -0.84$	0.41	−0.42
Shopping	Pickaboo, AliExpress	6	14	6	7	$t(60) = 0.27$	0.79	0.14
Tools	Settings, Download Mp3	89	100	90	100	$t(98) = -0.2$	0.84	−0.1

(*continued*)

Table 5. (*continued*)

App category	Example apps	% of Depressed		% of Non-depressed		Statistics value	P	Cohen's d
		Mean	Max.	Mean	Max.			
Travel & Local	NOVOAIR, Rail Sheba	6	10	5	12	t(98) = 0.44	0.67	0.22
Weather	Weather	2	6	3	4	U = 16	0.1	−0.43
Regardless App Category	Browser, Weather	97	100	97	100	t(98) = 0.29	0.78	0.14

5 Discussion

Our findings show that 51% of the students (N = 100) are depressed which is close to the depression rate found in the previous studies [50, 51]. Our analysis on re-identification shows that using only 7 h of data a week, 91% of the depressed and 88% of the non-depressed students can be re-identified. Moreover, in comparison to the non-depressed, depressed students' rate of uniqueness is 9% (P = .02) and 8% (P = .005) higher in the Social Media and Health & Fitness app categories respectively. Our findings are novel and to our best knowledge, this is the first study which explored the re-identification of a group suffering from mental disease. We believe that our findings will be worthwhile to bring better privacy to the depressed one.

5.1 Depressed and Non-depressed Students Can Be Uniquely Re-identified

Based on only 7 days' data, on average, both the depressed and non-depressed students' minimum hamming distance to the nearest user is about 37 apps which represents that a higher number of apps will be needed to make them anonymous. This finding showing the uniqueness of the depressed extend the previous studies [6, 10, 11] which were conducted on the general people. Going beyond the previous studies, we also explore the app categories and find that using data of a single app category named Tools, it is possible to uniquely re-identify all of the depressed and non-depressed students. This highlights the possible threat to privacy, if the adversaries get data even of a single app category. Thus, to ensure better privacy, instead of focusing only on total set of used apps, researchers and designers need to utilize the data of app categories also.

It was interesting to see that depressed students have more uniqueness on weekdays than the weekends. Previous studies found that app usage behavior varies by days of a week [3, 49] and on weekdays people are more unique [11]. Researchers [11] also remark that this difference can be due to variation in profession. However, our findings suggest that despite being in the same group and having similar characteristics (student, no significant difference in age, monthly family income) of the depressed participants, they can be more uniquely re-identified on weekdays than the weekends. This indicates that during designing systems to protect privacy of the depressed, their uniqueness on weekdays should get more weight in differential privacy [60].

5.2 Depressed Students Are More Unique in Some App Categories

Through statistical analysis, we find that the depressed students are significantly more unique in some app categories, notably in the Social Media category. This finding contrast with the previous study [29] which did not find any significant difference in terms of total usage duration, frequency of launcing Social Media apps. We speculate about depressed students' less energy to do real world interaction [43] which may encourage them to use a more diverse set of Social Media apps to communicate with others. In fact, we find that a depressed student having a PHQ-9 score of 17 uses an AI based app (Replika: My AI Friend) which is used to create and communicate with a replica friend. Meanwhile, we find that depressed students use significantly more diverse set of Social Media apps in the afternoon (12 PM–6PM] and evening (6 PM–12AM] time period of weekdays which are peak time for class and self-study respectively in Bangladesh. Supporting our findings, previous study also shows that depressed have peak usage Social Media during the working hour [43]. A plausible reason for having peak during the class time can be due to having online classes instead of on-campus class amid the pandemic. Moreover, negative emtions can cause higher apps use to find distraction [62]. Going beyond our study's focus of re-identification, these findings demonstrate the support seeking nature of the depressed students which opens up opportunities for the researchers to explore further.

Our findings show that in the Health & Fitness category also, more depressed students can be uniquely re-identified and it is significantly more than the non-depressed. Wang et al. [33] show that physical activity has a negative relation with depression score. However, findings of another previous study [47] shows that the relation of physical activity with a patient's state can vary by person as well as time period of a day. Different app usage behavior of the depressed students of our study regarding Health & Fitness category represents that they may want to improve their situation since we find that depressed students use such apps of this category which are usually used to improve health. For example, a depressed student uses an app which has a feature to stop smoking and another student uses an app which is used to concentrate more. Therefore, our findings suggest to integrate the the physical and mental health professionals in the Health & Fitness apps, as having proper guidance (e.g., through counselling [61]) based on medical sciences can help the depressed to overcome their depression.

Since our findings demonstrate that the depressed students use statistically significantly more unique apps in some categories, specially, in the Health & Fitness and Social Media categories, more noises [59] can be added to the data of these app categories to make the depressed anonymous. Moreover, our findings present that the depressed are significantly more unique in the afternoon and evening usage of Social Media. Therefore, a higher weight to the noise can be added for those time periods to preserve depressed students' privacy.

6 Limitations

Though we have several novel contributions as mentioned in the introduction section, we have some limitations also. Since mental health is a taboo topic in Bangladesh [45, 46], it was difficult to collect such data from a large number of participants. In addition, we used the snowball sampling method [24] and thus, a research through random sampling is required to inspect the generalizability of the findings. Beside these, though we removed the dead word from the 9th item of the PHQ-9 scale [12] through an approach (Sect. 3.1), having a clinical validation will increase the reliability. However, without the 9th item of the PHQ-9 scale, still all of the depressed participants remain depressed in PHQ-8 scale [31] and this may present the efficacy of our findings.

7 Conclusion

In our in the wild study, using the 100 students' actual smartphone usage data, we present how uniquely the depressed and non-depressed students can be re-identified. We find that using fingerprints of 7 days' usage data regardless of app category, it is possible to re-identify each of the depressed and non-depressed students. Moreover, we find that using data of a single category named Tools, we can get the same (100%) percentage of re-identification. Our findings also show that depressed students are significantly more unique in case of some app categories. The reason behind their uniqueness is the use of a diverse set of apps as presented by the value of hamming distance. These reveal that during designing the privacy protection system, designers should consider the high uniqueness of the vulnerable group like the depressed students.

References

1. Böhmer, M., Hecht, B., Schöning, J., Krüger, A., Bauer, G.: Falling asleep with Angry Birds, Facebook and Kindle. In: Proceedings of the 13th International Conference on Human Computer Interaction with Mobile Devices and Services - MobileHCI 2011. ACM Press (2011). https://doi.org/10.1145/2037373.2037383
2. Zang, H., Bolot, J.: Anonymization of location data does not work. In: Proceedings of the 17th Annual International Conference on Mobile Computing and Networking - MobiCom 2011. ACM Press (2011). https://doi.org/10.1145/2030613.2030630
3. Zhao, Š., Ramos, J., Tao, J., et al.: Discovering different kinds of smartphone users through their application usage behaviors. In: Proceedings of the 2016 ACM International Joint Conference on Pervasive and Ubiquitous Computing. ACM (2016). https://doi.org/10.1145/2971648.2971696
4. Zhou, Y., Jiang, X.: Dissecting Android malware: characterization and evolution. In: 2012 IEEE Symposium on Security and Privacy. IEEE (2012). https://doi.org/10.1109/sp.2012.16
5. Grace, M.C., Zhou, W., Jiang, X., Sadeghi, A.-R.: Unsafe exposure analysis of mobile in-app advertisements. In: Proceedings of the Fifth ACM Conference on Security and Privacy in Wireless and Mobile Networks - WISEC 2012. ACM Press (2012). https://doi.org/10.1145/2185448.2185464
6. Welke, P., Andone, I., Blaszkiewicz, K., Markowetz, A.: Differentiating smartphone users by app usage. In: Proceedings of the 2016 ACM International Joint Conference on Pervasive and Ubiquitous Computing. ACM (2016). https://doi.org/10.1145/2971648.2971707
7. de Montjoye, Y.-A., Hidalgo, C.A., Verleysen, M., Blondel, V.D.: Unique in the crowd: the privacy bounds of human mobility. Sci. Rep. 3(1) (2013). https://doi.org/10.1038/srep01376
8. Lee, U., Lee, J., Ko, M., et al.: Hooked on smartphones. In: Proceedings of the SIGCHI Conference on Human Factors in Computing Systems. ACM (2014). https://doi.org/10.1145/2556288.2557366

9. Shin, C., Dey, A.K.: Automatically detecting problematic use of smartphones. In: Proceedings of the 2013 ACM International Joint Conference on Pervasive and Ubiquitous Computing. ACM (2013). https://doi.org/10.1145/2493432.2493443

10. Sekara, V., Alessandretti, L., Mones, E., Jonsson, H.: Temporal and cultural limits of privacy in smartphone app usage. Sci. Rep. **11**(1) (2021). https://doi.org/10.1038/s41598-021-822 94-1

11. Tu, Z., Li, R., Li, Y., et al.: Your apps give you away: distinguishing mobile users by their appusage fingerprints. Proc. ACM Interact. Mob. Wearable Ubiquitous Technol. **2**(3), 1–23 (2018). https://doi.org/10.1145/3264948

12. Kroenke, K., Spitzer, R.L., Williams, J.B.W.: The PHQ-9: validity of a brief depression severity measure. J. Gen. Intern. Med. **16**(9), 606–613 (2001). https://doi.org/10.1046/j.1525-1497.2001.016009606.x

13. Sarda, A., Munuswamy, S., Sarda, S., Subramanian, V.: Using passive smartphone sensing for improved risk stratification of patients with depression and diabetes: cross-sectional observational study. JMIR Mhealth Uhealth **7**(1), e11041 (2019). https://doi.org/10.2196/11041

14. Li, H., Zhu, H., Du, S., Liang, X., Shen, X.: Privacy leakage of location sharing in mobile social networks: attacks and defense. IEEE Trans. Dependable Secure Comput. **15**(4), 646–660 (2018). https://doi.org/10.1109/tdsc.2016.2604383

15. Guynn, J.: Anxiety, depression and PTSD: The hidden epidemic of data breaches and cyber crimes. USA Today. https://www.usatoday.com/story/tech/conferences/2020/02/21/data-breach-tips-mental-health-toll-depression-anxiety/4763823002/. Accessed 23 Feb 2021

16. Bentley, F., Church, K., Harrison, B., Lyons, K., Rafalow, M.: Three Hours a Day: Understanding Current Teen Practices of Smartphone Application Use (2015)

17. Gordon, M.L., Gatys, L., Guestrin, C., Bigham, J.P., Trister, A., Patel, K.: App usage predicts cognitive ability in older adults. In: Proceedings of the 2019 CHI Conference on Human Factors in Computing Systems. ACM (2019). https://doi.org/10.1145/3290605.3300398

18. Hirschprung, R.S., Leshman, O.: Privacy disclosure by de-anonymization using music preferences and selections. Telematics Inform. **59**, 101564 (2021). https://doi.org/10.1016/j.tele.2021.101564

19. Enck, W., Gilbert, P., Han, S., et al.: TaintDroid: an information-flow tracking system for realtime privacy monitoring on smartphones. ACM Trans. Comput. Syst. **32**(2), 1–29 (2014). https://doi.org/10.1145/2619091

20. Rozgonjuk, D., Levine, J.C., Hall, B.J., Elhai, J.D.: The association between problematic smartphone use, depression and anxiety symptom severity, and objectively measured smartphone use over one week. Comput. Hum. Behav. **87**, 10–17 (2018). https://doi.org/10.1016/j.chb.2018.05.019

21. Mohamed, S.M., Mostafa, M.H.: Impact of smartphone addiction on depression and self-esteem among nursing students. Nurs Open **7**(5), 1346–1353 (2020). https://doi.org/10.1002/nop2.506

22. Noë, B., Turner, L.D., Linden, D.E.J., Allen, S.M., Winkens, B., Whitaker, R.M.: Identifying indicators of smartphone addiction through user-app interaction. Comput. Hum. Behav. **99**, 56–65 (2019). https://doi.org/10.1016/j.chb.2019.04.023

23. Seneviratne, S., Seneviratne, A., Mohapatra, P., Mahanti, A.: Your installed apps reveal your gender and more! In: Proceedings of the ACM MobiCom Workshop on Security and Privacy in Mobile Environments. ACM (2014). https://doi.org/10.1145/2646584.2646587

24. Wikipedia contributors. Snowball sampling. Wikipedia, The Free Encyclopedia (2020). https://en.wikipedia.org/w/index.php?title=Snowball_sampling&oldid=993212057. Accessed 25 Feb 2021

25. Wikipedia contributors. Hamming distance. Wikipedia, The Free Encyclopedia (2021). https://en.wikipedia.org/w/index.php?title=Hamming_distance&oldid=1007490112. Accessed 25 Feb 2021
26. Virtanen, P., Gommers, R., et al.: SciPy 1.0: fundamental algorithms for scientific computing in Python. Nat. Methods **17**(3), 261–272 (2020). https://doi.org/10.1038/s41592-019-0686-2
27. Benjamini, Y., Hochberg, Y.: Controlling the false discovery rate: a practical and powerful approach to multiple testing. J. Roy. Stat. Soc.: Ser. B (Methodol.) **57**(1), 289–300 (1995). https://doi.org/10.1111/j.2517-6161.1995.tb02031.x
28. Manea, L., Gilbody, S., McMillan, D.: A diagnostic meta-analysis of the Patient Health Questionnaire-9 (PHQ-9) algorithm scoring method as a screen for depression. Gen. Hosp. Psychiatry **37**(1), 67–75 (2015). https://doi.org/10.1016/j.genhosppsych.2014.09.009
29. Ahmed, Md.S., Rony, R.J., Hasan, T., Ahmed, N.: Smartphone usage behavior between depressed and non-depressed students. In: Adjunct Proceedings of the 2020 ACM International Joint Conference on Pervasive and Ubiquitous Computing and Proceedings of the 2020 ACM International Symposium on Wearable Computers. ACM (2020). https://doi.org/10.1145/3410530.3414441
30. de Montjoye, Y.-A., Radaelli, L., Singh, V.K., Pentland, A.S.: Unique in the shopping mall: on the reidentifiability of credit card metadata. Science **347**(6221), 536–539 (2015). https://doi.org/10.1126/science.1256297
31. Kroenke, K., Strine, T.W., Spitzer, R.L., Williams, J.B.W., Berry, J.T., Mokdad, A.H.: The PHQ-8 as a measure of current depression in the general population. J. Affect. Disord. **114**(1–3), 163–173 (2009). https://doi.org/10.1016/j.jad.2008.06.026
32. Gulyás, G.G., Acs, G., Castelluccia, C.: Near-optimal fingerprinting with constraints. Proc. Priv. Enhancing Technol. **2016**(4), 470–487 (2016). https://doi.org/10.1515/popets-2016-0051
33. Wang, R., Wang, W., daSilva, A., et al.: Tracking depression dynamics in college students using mobile phone and wearable sensing. Proc. ACM Interact. Mob. Wearable Ubiquitous Technol. **2**(1), 1–26 (2018). https://doi.org/10.1145/3191775
34. Islam, S., Akter, R., Sikder, T., Griffiths, M.D.: Prevalence and factors associated with depression and anxiety among first-year university students in bangladesh: a cross-sectional study. Int. J. Ment. Heal. Addict. 1–14 (2020). https://doi.org/10.1007/s11469-020-00242-y
35. Achara, J.P., Acs, G., Castelluccia, C.: On the unicity of smartphone applications. In: Proceedings of the 14th ACM Workshop on Privacy in the Electronic Society. ACM (2015). https://doi.org/10.1145/2808138.2808146
36. Marshall, J.: Twitter is tracking users' installed apps for ad targeting. Wall Street J. (2014). https://www.wsj.com/articles/BL-269B-2167. Accessed 9 Mar 2021
37. Dredge, S.: Twitter scanning users' other apps to help deliver 'tailored content'. The Guardian (2014). https://www.theguardian.com/technology/2014/nov/27/twitter-scanning-other-apps-tailored-content. Accessed 9 Mar 2021
38. Binns, R., Lyngs, U., Van Kleek, M., Zhao, J., Libert, T., Shadbolt, N.: Third party tracking in the mobile ecosystem. In: Proceedings of the 10th ACM Conference on Web Science. ACM (2018). https://doi.org/10.1145/3201064.3201089
39. Privacy International. How Apps on Android Share Data with Facebook. Privacy International (2018). https://privacyinternational.org/sites/default/files/2018-12/How%20Apps%20on%20Android%20Share%20Data%20with%20Facebook%20-%20Privacy%20International%202018.pdf. Accessed 10 Mar 2021
40. Morrison, A., Xiong, X., Higgs, M., Bell, M., Chalmers, M.: A large-scale study of iphone app launch behaviour. In: Proceedings of the 2018 CHI Conference on Human Factors in Computing Systems. ACM (2018). https://doi.org/10.1145/3173574.3173918

41. Doherty, K., Marcano-Belisario, J., Cohn, M., et al.: Engagement with mental health screening on mobile devices. In: Proceedings of the 2019 CHI Conference on Human Factors in Computing Systems. ACM (2019). https://doi.org/10.1145/3290605.3300416
42. Xu, X., Chikersal, P., Doryab, A., et al.: Leveraging routine behavior and contextually-filtered features for depression detection among college students. Proc. ACM Interact. Mob. Wearable Ubiquitous Technol. **3**(3), 1–33 (2019). https://doi.org/10.1145/3351274
43. Park, S., Kim, I., Lee, S.W., Yoo, J., Jeong, B., Cha, M.: Manifestation of depression and loneliness on social networks. In: Proceedings of the 18th ACM Conference on Computer Supported Cooperative Work & Social Computing. ACM (2015). https://doi.org/10.1145/2675133.2675139
44. Yoon, S., Verona, E., Schlauch, R., Schneider, S., Rottenberg, J.: Why do depressed people prefer sad music? Emotion **20**(4), 613–624 (2020). https://doi.org/10.1037/emo0000573
45. Rahman, M.: 16.8% Bangladeshi adults suffer from mental health issues. Dhaka Tribune (2019). https://www.dhakatribune.com/bangladesh/dhaka/2019/11/07/survey-nearly-17-of-bangladeshi-adults-suffer-from-mental-health-issues. Accessed 16 Mar 2021
46. Deshwara, M., Eagle, A.: Taking on taboos. The Daily Star (2017). https://www.thedailystar.net/backpage/taking-taboos-1486447. Accessed 16 Mar 2021
47. Osmani, V., Maxhuni, A., Grünerbl, A., Lukowicz, P., Haring, C., Mayora, O.: Monitoring activity of patients with bipolar disorder using smart phones. In: Proceedings of International Conference on Advances in Mobile Computing & Multimedia - MoMM 2013. ACM Press (2013). https://doi.org/10.1145/2536853.2536882
48. Falaki, H., Mahajan, R., Kandula, S., Lymberopoulos, D., Govindan, R., Estrin, D.: Diversity in smartphone usage. In: Proceedings of the 8th International Conference on Mobile Systems, Applications, and Services - MobiSys 2010. ACM Press (2010). https://doi.org/10.1145/1814433.1814453
49. Do, T.M.T., Blom, J., Gatica-Perez, D.: Smartphone usage in the wild: a large-scale analysis of applications and context. In: Proceedings of the 13th International Conference on Multimodal Interfaces - ICMI 2011. ACM Press (2011). https://doi.org/10.1145/2070481.2070550
50. Islam, Md.A., Barna, S.D., Raihan, H., Khan, Md.N.A., Hossain, Md.T.: Depression and anxiety among university students during the COVID-19 pandemic in Bangladesh: a web-based cross-sectional survey. PLoS ONE **15**(8), e0238162 (2020). https://doi.org/10.1371/journal.pone.0238162. Pakpour, A.H. (ed.)
51. Koly, K.N., Sultana, S., Iqbal, A., Dunn, J.A., Ryan, G., Chowdhury, A.B.: Prevalence of depression and its correlates among public university students in Bangladesh. J. Affect. Disord. **282**, 689–694 (2021). https://doi.org/10.1016/j.jad.2020.12.137
52. Doryab, A., Villalba, D.K., Chikersal, P., et al.: Identifying behavioral phenotypes of loneliness and social isolation with passive sensing: statistical analysis, data mining and machine learning of smartphone and fitbit data. JMIR Mhealth Uhealth **7**(7), e13209 (2019). https://doi.org/10.2196/13209
53. Saeb, S., Zhang, M., Karr, C.J., et al.: Mobile phone sensor correlates of depressive symptom severity in daily-life behavior: an exploratory study. J. Med. Internet Res. **17**(7), e175 (2015). https://doi.org/10.2196/jmir.4273
54. Ben-Zeev, D., Buck, B., Chu, P.V., Razzano, L., Pashka, N., Hallgren, K.A.: Transdiagnostic mobile health: smartphone intervention reduces depressive symptoms in people with mood and psychotic disorders. JMIR Ment. Health **6**(4), e13202 (2019). https://doi.org/10.2196/13202
55. Li, Z., Shi, D., Wang, F., Liu, F.: Loneliness recognition based on mobile phone data. In: Proceedings of the 2016 International Symposium on Advances in Electrical, Electronics and Computer Engineering (2016). https://doi.org/10.2991/isaece-16.2016.3

56. Velloza, J., Njoroge, J., Ngure, K., et al.: Cognitive testing of the PHQ-9 for depression screening among pregnant and postpartum women in Kenya. BMC Psychiatry **20**(1) (2020). https://doi.org/10.1186/s12888-020-2435-6

57. Lu, S.: App Usage - Manage/Track Usage. https://play.google.com/store/apps/details?id=com.a0soft.gphone.uninstaller. Accessed 28 Mar 2021

58. Labs, M.: YourHour - Phone Addiction Tracker & Controller. https://play.google.com/store/apps/details?id=com.mindefy.phoneaddiction.mobilepe. Accessed 28 Mar 2021

59. Dwork, C., McSherry, F., Nissim, K., Smith, A.: Calibrating noise to sensitivity in private data analysis. In: Halevi, S., Rabin, T. (eds.) TCC 2006. LNCS, vol. 3876, pp. 265–284. Springer, Heidelberg (2006). https://doi.org/10.1007/11681878_14

60. Yang, Y., Zhang, Z., Miklau, G., Winslett, M., Xiao, X.: Differential privacy in data publication and analysis. In: Proceedings of the 2012 International Conference on Management of Data - SIGMOD 2012. ACM Press (2012). https://doi.org/10.1145/2213836.2213910

61. Holden, J.M., Sagovsky, R., Cox, J.L.: Counselling in a general practice setting: controlled study of health visitor intervention in treatment of postnatal depression. BMJ **298**(6668), 223–226 (1989). https://doi.org/10.1136/bmj.298.6668.223

62. Sarsenbayeva, Z., Marini, G., van Berkel, N., et al.: Does smartphone use drive our emotions or vice versa? A causal analysis. In: Proceedings of the 2020 CHI Conference on Human Factors in Computing Systems. ACM (2020). https://doi.org/10.1145/3313831.3376163

A Serious Game for Nutritional Education of Children and Adolescents with Neurodevelopmental Disorders

Francesca Santini[1]([envelope]), Giovanni Tauro[1], Maddalena Mazzali[1], Silvia Grazioli[2], Maddalena Mauri[2,3], Eleonora Rosi[2], Marco Pozzi[4], Arianna Tarabelloni[2], Federica Tizzoni[2], Filippo Maria Villa[2], Massimo Molteni[2], Maria Nobile[2], Marco Sacco[1], Sara Arlati[1], and Vera Colombo[1,5]

[1] Institute of Intelligent Industrial Technologies and Systems for Advanced Manufacturing, Italian National Research Council, Via Previati 1/E, 23900 Lecco, Italy
{francesca.santini,giovanni.tauro,maddalena.mazzali,marco.sacco, vera.colombo}@stiima.cnr.it
[2] Child Psychopathology Unit, Scientific Institute, IRCCS E. Medea, via Don Luigi Monza 20, 23842 Bosisio Parini, Lecco, Italy
{silvia.grazioli,maddalena.mauri,eleonora.rosi, arianna.tarabelloni,federica.tizzoni,filippo.villa, massimo.molteni,maria.nobile}@lanostrafamiglia.it
[3] School of Medicine and Surgery, University of Milano-Bicocca, Milan, Italy
[4] Scientific Institute, IRCCS Eugenio Medea, 23842 Bosisio Parini, Italy
marco.pozzi@lanostrafamiglia.it
[5] Department of Electronics, Information and Bioengineering, Politecnico di Milano, via Ponzio 34, 20133 Milan, Italy

Abstract. Children and young people with neurodevelopmental disorders seem to be more susceptible to developing obesity and eating disorders. To prevent this, therapeutic programs including nutritional education are, therefore, needed. Serious games (SGs) represent a promising solution to improve adherence to the treatment in different populations, including children/adolescents with Attention-Deficit/Hyperactivity Disorder (ADHD) and Autism Spectrum Disorder (ASD). The present paper describes the design and development of a SG to promote a healthy diet and lifestyle. To the best of our knowledge, this is the first SG specifically focused on nutritional education developed for young individuals with ADHD or ASD. The SG is made of four mini-games contextualized within a single narrative frame. Through his/her avatar, the player has to challenge four opponents, one for each educational topic, with the help of a wise character that educates him/her throughout the story. The SG can be experienced with a tablet or a PC, and with the supervision of an adult. A pilot study will be carried out to evaluate the feasibility, engagement, and usability of the SG, involving children with ADHD, ASD, and a group of typically developing peers. Based on the results, some adaptations will be implemented to improve the SG before conducting a larger trial to evaluate the effectiveness of the SG in promoting a healthy diet and lifestyle.

Keywords: ADHD · ASD · Serious game · Nutritional education · Healthy diet

1 Introduction

1.1 Background and Significance

Attention-Deficit/Hyperactivity Disorder (ADHD) and Autism Spectrum Disorder (ASD) are among the most common neurodevelopmental disorders in childhood, affecting 8.4% of children (in the case of ADHD) [1] and 1.8% of children in the case of ASD [2]. ADHD is characterized by impairing symptoms of inattention and/or hyperactivity and impulsive behavior, hampering the child's development. ASD presents a constellation of early-appearing social communication deficits and repetitive sensory-motor behaviors and it is associated with a strong genetic component (and other causes).

Literature suggests a significant association between both ADHD and ASD and obesity [3, 4] and an increased risk of developing eating disorders [5] due to abnormal eating patterns, sedentary lifestyle, and possible common genetic alteration. Diet plays a crucial role in physical and mental health, especially for growing children, and some studies suggest a healthy diet can help in ameliorating symptoms of ADHD and ASD [6, 7].

Serious games (SGs), based on technologies of video-gaming, have been proposed for the assessment and treatment of ADHD and/or ASD [8, 9]. It could be expected that children with ADHD and ASD present difficulties engaging with video games due to their shorter attention span; however, children with ADHD and ASD can focus for long periods of time on activities they enjoy, a phenomenon referred to as hyperfocus [10]. SGs are therefore a promising tool to enhance engagement and motivation and promote adherence to therapeutic interventions.

According to these premises, the goal of the SG described in this paper is to educate and encourage healthy eating in children with neurodevelopmental disorders in an engaging way, consequently promoting symptoms amelioration and overall health. The SG is designed considering the needs of the specific target population, such as short attention span and need of positive-feedback to increase motivation.

1.2 Related Works

Two recent reviews of SG interventions for children with neurodevelopmental disorders [8, 9] reported that the main type of intervention for ADHD children was cognitive training, i.e. a series of tasks aimed at improving executive functioning, such as attention, working memory and reaction time. Most studies used a PC as a platform, with a minority using a tablet or Xbox Kinect. SGs for children with ASD are aimed at assisting them in acquiring emotional competencies [11] or promoting reading skills [12]. Therapeutic interventions based on SGs were well accepted and generally effective in improving cognitive functions and ameliorating ADHD/ASD symptoms. This appears to be due to the mechanism of *gamification*, which enhances children's engagement and possibly promotes neuroplasticity. Despite this, Peñuelas-Calvo et al. [8] identified some limitations of currently available applications and suggested strengthening the collaboration between developers and healthcare professionals to further improve the potential of this technology.

In the field of nutritional education, many mobile applications and games have been developed for typically developing (TD) children and adolescents: to increase vegetable consumption [13], to teach about digestive health [14], to encourage healthy eating [15, 16], to improve the measurement of their food consumption [15]. SGs were generally well accepted and effective in increasing children's knowledge about healthy diet and lifestyle, however, the limitation of these studies is that only short-term effects are assessed, which means it is not known whether the positive effects will be maintained in the longer term.

To the authors' knowledge, no SG for nutritional education of children or adolescents with ADHD/ASD has been previously developed.

2   The Serious Game "Captain Chomp and the Great FoodAdventure"

2.1   Design

The design process was carried on throughout a collaboration between biomedical engineers, neuropsychiatrists, psychologists, nutritional experts, and designers. All these professionals collaborated to define the characteristics of the SGs to develop, in terms of graphics, educational content, and interaction. The definition of requirements took place through brainstorming sessions during which collaborative design tools, in particular Figma[1] and Miro[2], were used to support the creative process. Indeed, the process of developing a serious game for a fragile category of users takes seriously the focus on the usability concept, i.e., how easy a System Interface (SI) is to use. Factors to consider in order to achieve usability are Effectiveness, Efficiency, Satisfaction, Learnability, Memorability, Low Error Rate and Cognitive Load; the category of final users, their characteristics, their need, and their preferences; what type of goal needs to be achieved while using the app, and finally the context of use [18–20].

The target users are 6–16-year-old children and adolescents with ADHD or ASD, as well as their parents, who are the primary gatekeepers to children's food intake. The SG is designed for the parent and child to use jointly, either in the clinics or at home, according to the therapeutic path defined by the clinical personnel. The SG has been developed in Unity and deployed for Windows OS personal computer and Android OS tablet, to accommodate the devices already available in children's homes.

The SG "Captain Chomp and the Great FoodAdventure" consists of four different mini-games, which have been framed in the same narrative. The child chooses an avatar and follows the adventures of "Captain Chomp", a positive leading character, defeating four enemies and learning lessons about food and healthy diet along the way. The player starts from the first mini-game, and as the levels are completed, the following mini-games are unlocked. A schematic wireframe of the SG structure is presented in Fig. 1. Each mini-game covers a different topic: food categories, the food pyramid, the

---

[1] Figma: the collaborative interface design tool. https://www.figma.com.
[2] https://miro.com.

importance of physical activity, and the Healthy Eating Plate, recommended by Harvard University [21]. A more detailed description of the content of each mini-game is provided in Sect. 2.2.

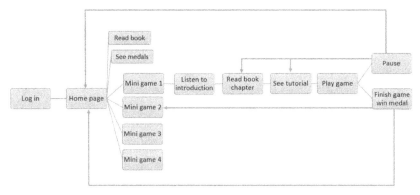

Fig. 1. Wireframe of the Serious Game structure. After the log-in, the user is directed to the home page, where he/she can read the educational content, or see the medals he/she has won, or go to one of the mini-games. Before playing each mini-game, the user listens to an introductory explanation, reads the educational content related to the nutritional topic and sees the tutorial. During the game, the user can pause the game to go back to the home page, or review the book or the tutorial. When the user finishes the mini-game, he/she wins a medal, and can either play the following mini-game, or go back to the home page.

The graphics of the SG have been developed focusing on the needs of the target audience. The graphics are 2D, simplified, with flat colors following the wide list of characters liked by children analyzed during the research phase, such as *Peppa Pig*, *La Pimpa*, etc. The leading character, the four enemies, and the avatars are drawn with the same style and technique (see Fig. 2), with four available options for the avatar (male/female, white/dark skin), to help player identification of the child [22].

On the other hand, to display the food, we chose 3D realistic images to promote the transfer of the knowledge acquired during the use of the SG to the real world. We selected more than 200 food images, from different countries and cultures.

In order to simplify the learning process, each mini-game provides a tutorial where gestures and tasks are shortly introduced. We expect this feature to maximize the Learnability and Memorability process, consequently reducing the possibility to commit errors (Low Error Rate). By adding a recorded audio clip to each written message, we aimed to keep the attention level high and increase Efficiency (resources expended to achieve the goal).

To further promote Learnability, we collected all the diet-related information in a unique and easily-findable place. A dedicated section of the app, "The Book of Captain Chomp", gathers educational content about each of the four topics, with short sentences and images. The child needs to read the corresponding pages of the diary before playing a game; such pages are available throughout the whole game as well. During each mini-game, educational information is delivered through short messages. As reinforcement improves cognitive performance, especially in children with ADHD/ASD [23,

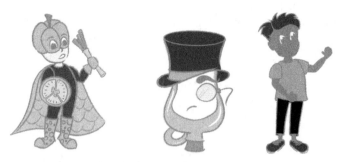

Fig. 2. The leading character, "Captain Chomp", the enemies and the player avatar are designed with 2D, simplified graphics.

24], we focused on positive, encouraging messages throughout the mini-games, instead of penalties. If the player makes a mistake, a different message is displayed based on the gravity of the error: a "yellow light" if it's a minor error, a "red light" if it's more serious. Moreover, after completing each game, the players win a medal, and they are encouraged to complete the four mini-games to collect all the medals: this is expected to increase Effectiveness and Satisfaction. In order to reduce the Cognitive Load, children are expected to use the app in a focused environment, sitting in front of the PC or with a tablet, with the supervision of an adult, who is supposed to help them with the educational content, and at the same time learn with them.

Importantly, the SG communicates a *flexible* food culture underlining the importance of varying diet, i.e. there are no strict rules or banned food, but food that should be eaten more or less often. This first version of the SG does not include specific diets for each individual, e.g. vegetarian or vegan diets or allergies have not been considered. Instead, the content has been selected to adapt to the most widespread diet in Italy, i.e. the Mediterranean diet.

2.2 Development

As previously mentioned, the SG is composed of four mini-games: "Food in the Cart", "Playing with Pyramid Blocks", "Fit and Healthy", "The Food Puzzle, the Fuzzle" (Fig. 3). For each game, the application generates a report file (XML format) including information on the child performance. In particular, information about the player (age, sex, traditional cuisine), total playing and reading time, and the performances of each mini-game (completion time, number and type of errors) are included.

Food in the Cart. The goal of the first mini-game, "Food in the Cart", is to learn to recognize which nutritional category the foods belong to. In the first level there are 10 carts, each labeled with a category: fruit and vegetables, meat and fish, legumes, tubers, oils and fats, cereals and derivatives, milk and derivatives, eggs, sweets and packaged foods, and water (see Fig. 4). In the second level, the two categories of carbohydrates and proteins are introduced. One food at a time is shown, and the child needs to drag and drop it into the correct cart. Twenty foods need to be correctly placed in their corresponding cart to complete the level. Such foods are picked from a pool of over 200

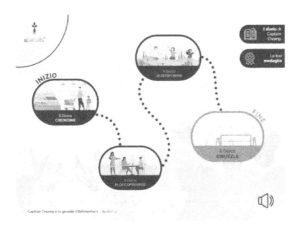

Fig. 3. Screenshot of the Home Page of the Serious Game, when the player has unlocked the third mini-game by completing the first two. The fourth is still locked. Each mini-game has a different color and graphic. On the upper left, the logo of the project, on the upper right, the player can visualize the medals he/she has won already and read the educational content.

elements, in a pseudo-random way (e.g. there are always 3 items belonging to the "fruit and vegetables" category, 2 items of the "legumes" category, etc.). When one food is correctly or incorrectly placed, a message is displayed, congratulating or encouraging the child to retry, and giving further information about "tricky" food (e.g. "*Potatoes are not vegetables, as you might think, but belong to the tubers family. They provide carbohydrates and must be eaten after cooking.*").

Playing with Pyramid Blocks. The goal of the second mini-game, "Playing with Pyramid Blocks", is to learn about the Food Pyramid and how often we should eat some foods. The Food Pyramid is a visual representation of how different foods contribute towards a healthy balanced diet. The Food Pyramid organizes foods into 5 blocks, starting from water and physical activity at the base of the pyramid, and decreased advised frequency of consumption in the upper blocks ("every meal", "every day", "twice a week or more", "twice a week max", "the least possible") [25]. The game has 3 levels of increasing difficulty. In the first level, the pyramid is full of food, and the child has to choose the correct food item between three options, and insert it in the highlighted pyramid block. In the second level, one block of the pyramid is empty, and the child has to select the food item belonging to the empty block. In the third level, the pyramid is empty, and the child has to drag and drop the food items on the correct blocks (see Fig. 4). Every time a food is placed, a congratulating or encouraging message is displayed, suggesting to the child if that food should be eaten more or less frequently.

Fit and Healthy. The goal of the third mini-game, "Fit and Healthy", is to take a break from the educational content while conveying the information that physical activity is important for our health. The child's avatar is running in a field, and the child has to make it jump – by tapping on the screen or clicking the mouse – to avoid the enemy, "Chef Atica", a chubby and lazy chef (see Fig. 5).

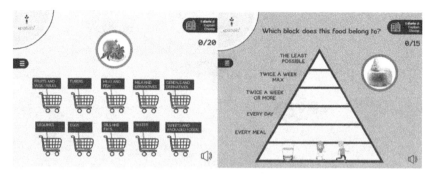

Fig. 4. On the left: Screenshot of the first mini-game, "Food in the Cart". An image of a food, e.g. a pomegranate, is displayed, and the child has to drag and drop it in the cart labeled with the category the food belongs to, e.g. "Fruit and Vegetables". On the right: Screenshot of the third level of the second mini-game, "Playing with Pyramid Blocks". The child has to drag and drop the food, i.e. parmesan cheese, in the correct pyramid block, i.e. twice a week max.

The Food Puzzle, the Fuzzle. The goal of the fourth mini-game, "The Food Puzzle, the Fuzzle", is to recognize and learn how to compose a Healthy Eating Plate. The Healthy Eating Plate is a guide for creating healthy, balanced meals: ½ of your plate should be vegetables and fruits, ¼ whole grains and ¼ protein [26]. In the first level, the child can choose the healthy plate from three options. While one of the incorrect options is "almost correct", with 2 food items out of 4 belonging to the same category, the other one is unbalanced, with 3 food items of the same category. The plates represent balanced main meals, as well as breakfasts and snacks. In the second level, an empty plate (accompanied by a glass of water and a bottle of oil) and 12 random foods are displayed: the child needs to compose a healthy plate with 4 food items (see Fig. 5). If the child chooses a plate with 2 food items of the same category, a "yellow light" message is displayed, while with 3 food items of the same category a "red light" is displayed, explaining the error and encouraging the child to try again.

3   Protocol of the Pilot Study

At first, in order to evaluate the feasibility and the engagement related to the SG "Captain Chomp and the Great FoodAdventure", the research group will present it to a small number of children and adolescents.

Participants with a diagnosis of ADHD and/or ASD, according to DSM-5 criteria [27], will be recruited from the Child Psychopathology Unit of IRCCS E. Medea Scientific Institute. The participation will be proposed to a group of TD peers. We estimate to recruit 10 children with ADHD, 10 children with ASD and 10 TD peers between 6 and 16 years of age. The exclusion criteria will include the presence of intellectual disability, neurological diseases, epilepsy, genetic syndromes, and treatment with psychotropic drugs. A diagnosis of other psychiatric disorders (e.g., anxiety, specific learning disorders) will not be an exclusion criterion.

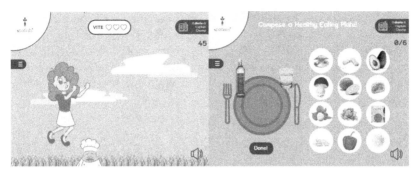

Fig. 5. On the left: Screenshot of the third mini-game, "Fit and Healthy". The player taps on the screen to make the avatar jump and avoid the enemy, Chef Atica. On the upper part of the screen, the number of remaining lives are displayed (three hearts), and the seconds left to finish the game. On the right: Screenshot of the second level of the fourth mini-game, "The Food Puzzle, the Fuzzle!". The child is asked to build a Healthy Eating Plate, by dragging 4 of the food items on the right inside the plate, accompanied by olive oil and water, on the left.

The primary aim of this first study is to collect preliminary observations about the feasibility of the proposed intervention both in the clinic and at home, the degree of satisfaction linked to the digital tool, and the SG effectiveness. Our secondary aim is to compare the degree of feasibility and of effectiveness between the recruited samples. To achieve these aims, the SG will be proposed to children and their parents.

Our pilot study has been approved by our institute's ethics committee, "Comitato Etico IRCCS E. Medea—Sezione Scientifica Associazione La Nostra Famiglia", in accordance with the Declaration of Helsinki (1989) as part of the sPatials3 study, which aims to develop instruments for food intake evaluation. Written informed consent and assent will be obtained from all caregivers and participants.

The SG "Captain Chomp and the Great FoodAdventure" will be administered during the first evaluation at IRCCS E. Medea Scientific Institute and will be installed on personal devices to also train at home for 1 week. After 1 week of home-fruition, each participant will be asked to return to the Institute. Researchers will hence save the output files that are generated during each game session, to evaluate each child's adherence and performances. Through the pilot study we will collect qualitative information regarding possible partial modifications to the SG that the participants' family would suggest. Finally, participants and their parents will fill in self-report questionnaires or tests to assess socio-economic status, behavioral and neuropsychological traits, the SG usability, the degree of satisfaction and involvement of the SG, and the learned knowledge about healthy eating. Specifically, we will use "System Usability Scale (SUS)" to assess the SG usability, which consists of a 10-item questionnaire with five response options for respondents from "strongly agree" to "strongly disagree" [28]. It allows the evaluation of a wide variety of products and services, and will be adapted for the SG application. It will be filled out by parents or adolescents. In addition, we will use an observation grid to qualitatively assess execution time, errors, questions and spontaneous comments of children or adolescents during the use of the SG. Furthermore, we will use questionnaires to assess involvement of the SG through "Game Engagement Questionnaire" [29]. We expect the intervention to be feasible, usable and engaging for all children groups. We also expect to find significant differences in background knowledge and motivation about healthy eating between ADHD, ASD and TD groups, especially in ADHD and ASD groups with relative peculiarities. Finally, we expect to find significant improvements regarding the knowledge about healthy eating in all groups, possibly with inter-group differences.

4 Conclusions

This work offers an approach to improve knowledge of children and adolescents with ADHD or ASD about a healthy diet by developing a cross-platform SG. Therapeutic interventions for children and adolescents with ADHD or ASD based on SGs have been proved to be well accepted and effective, however, no SG aimed at nutritional education of this target population has been previously developed.

We expect that children who will be engaged in our study could improve their knowledge about healthy eating, and consequently improve their eating habits thus ameliorating their overall health. We also expect a high degree of satisfaction linked to the digital tool. Inter-age and pathology-dependent differences may arise.

Based on the results of the pilot study and on the suggestions of the children and their parents, the SG will possibly be adjusted to better respond to the target population's needs. For example, ASD children may respond abnormally to rewards and error-feedback during learning [24]. After the implementation of these modifications, the SG will be tested in a larger trial in order to assess its effectiveness in improving nutritional habits in children with ADHD or ASD.

Acknowledgments. This research was funded by Regione Lombardia under the POR FESR 2014–2020 Asse Prioritario I-Call Hub Ricerca e Innovazione, project "sPATIALS3-Miglioramento delle produzioni agroalimentari e tecnologie innovative per un'alimentazione più sana, sicura e sostenibile" ID 1176485.

References

1. Danielson, M.L., Bitsko, R.H., Ghandour, R.M., Holbrook, J.R., Kogan, M.D., Blumberg, S.J.: Prevalence of parent-reported ADHD diagnosis and associated treatment among U.S. children and adolescents, 2016. J. Clin. Child Adolesc. Psychol. 47(2), 199–212 (2018)
2. Maenner, M.J., Shaw, K.A., Baio, J., et al.: Prevalence of autism spectrum disorder among children aged 8 years—autism and developmental disabilities monitoring network, 11 sites, United States, 2016. MMWR Surveill. Summ. 69(SS-4), 1–12 (2020)
3. Cortese, S., Tessari, L.: Attention-deficit/hyperactivity disorder (ADHD) and obesity: update 2016. Curr. Psychiatry Rep. 19(1), 1–15 (2017). https://doi.org/10.1007/s11920-017-0754-1
4. Liu, T., Kelly, J., Davis, L., Zamora, K.: Nutrition, BMI and motor competence in children with autism spectrum disorder. Medicina (Kaunas) 55(5), 135 (2019)
5. Nazar, B.P., Bernardes, C., Peachey, G., Sergeant, J., Mattos, P., Treasure, J.: The risk of eating disorders comorbid with attention-deficit/hyperactivity disorder: a systematic review and meta-analysis. Int. J. Eat. Disord. 49(12), 1045–1057 (2016)

6. Heilskov Rytter, M.J., et al.: Diet in the treatment of ADHD in children - a systematic review of the literature. Nord J. Psychiatry **69**(1), 1–18 (2015)
7. Peretti, S., et al.: Diet: the keystone of autism spectrum disorder? Nutr. Neurosci. **22**(12), 825–839 (2019)
8. Peñuelas-Calvo, I., Jiang-Lin, L.K., Girela-Serrano, B., et al.: Video games for the assessment and treatment of attention-deficit/hyperactivity disorder: a systematic review [published online ahead of print, 18 May 2020. Eur Child Adolesc Psychiatry (2020)
9. Kokol, P., Vošner, H.B., Završnik, J., Vermeulen, J., Shohieb, S., Peinemann, F.: Serious game-based intervention for children with developmental disabilities. Curr. Pediatr. Rev. **16**(1), 26–32 (2020)
10. Ashinoff, B.K., Abu-Akel, A.: Hyperfocus: the forgotten frontier of attention. Psychol. Res. **85**(1), 1–19 (2019). https://doi.org/10.1007/s00426-019-01245-8
11. Cunha, P., Brandão, J., Vasconcelos, J., Soares, F., Carvalho, V.: Augmented reality for cognitive and social skills improvement in children with ASD. In: Proceedings of the 13th International Conference on Remote Engineering and Virtual Instrumentation, Madrid, Spain, pp. 334–335. Institute of Electrical and Electronics Engineers, Piscataway (2016)
12. Gomez, J., Jaccheri, L., Torrado, J.C., Montoro, G.: Leo con lula, introducing global reading methods to children with ASD. In: Proceedings of the 17th ACM Conference on Interaction Design and Children, Trondheim, Norway, pp. 420–6. Association for Computing Machinery, New York (2018)
13. Farrow, C., et al.: Using repeated visual exposure, rewards and modelling in a mobile application to increase vegetable acceptance in children. Appetite **141** (2019)
14. Putri, R.C.R.W.: NomNom, mobile app about digestive health for children. In: 2015 3rd International Conference on New Media (CONMEDIA). IEEE (2015)
15. Fuentes, E.M., Varela-Aldás, J., Palacios-Navarro, G., García-Magariño, I.: Immersive virtual reality app to promote healthy eating in children. In: Stephanidis, C., Antona, M. (eds.) HCII 2020. CCIS, vol. 1225, pp. 9–15. Springer, Cham (2020). https://doi.org/10.1007/978-3-030-50729-9_2
16. Putnam, M.M., et al.: Influence of a character-based app on children's learning of nutritional information: should apps be served with a side of media characters? Games Health J. **7**(2), 121–126 (2018)
17. Bissell, K., Conlin, L.T., Zhang, X., Bie, B., McLemore, D.: Let Go of My iPad: Testing the Effectiveness of New Media Technologies to Measure Children's Food Intake and Health Behaviors, Mass Communication and Society (2016)
18. Nielsen, J.: Usability Engineering. Morgan Kaufmann Publication (1994)
19. ISO 9241: Ergonomics Requirements for Office Work with Visual Display Terminals (VDTs) International Standards Organisation, Geneva (1997)
20. Adams, R.: Applying advanced concepts of cognitive overload and augmentation in practice; the future of overload. In: Schmorrow, D., Stanney, K.M., Reeves, L.M. (eds.) Foundations of Augmented Cognition, 2nd edn., pp. 223–229. Springer, Heidelberg (2006)
21. The Nutrition Source. https://www.hsph.harvard.edu/nutritionsource/healthy-eating-plate/. Accessed 10 Sept 2021
22. Turkay, S., Kinzer, C.K.: The effects of avatar-based customization on player identification. IJGCMS **6**(1), 1–25 (2014)
23. Fosco, W.D., Hawk, L.W., Rosch, K.S., et al.: Evaluating cognitive and motivational accounts of greater reinforcement effects among children with attention-deficit/hyperactivity disorder. Behav. Brain Funct. **11**, 20 (2015)
24. Schuetze, M., et al.: Reinforcement learning in autism spectrum disorder. Front. Psychol. **8**, 2035 (2017)
25. The Food Pyramid from Healthy Ireland; Department of Health. https://www.gov.ie/en/publication/70a2e4-the-food-pyramid/. Accessed 20 Sept 2021

26. The Nutrition Source. Healthy Eating Plate. https://www.hsph.harvard.edu/nutritionsource/healthy-eating-plate/. Accessed 23 Sept 2021
27. American Psychiatric Association. Diagnostic and Statistical Manual of Mental Disorders (DSM-5®); AmericanPsychiatric Publication, Washington (2013)
28. Brooke, J.: SUS: A "quick and dirty" usability scale. In: Jordan, P.W., Thomas, B., Weerdmeester, B.A., McClelland, A.L. (eds.) Usability Evaluation in Industry. Taylor and Francis, London (1996)
29. Brockmyer, J.H., Fox, C.M., Curtiss, K.A., McBroom, E., Burkhart, K.M., Pidruzny, J.N.: The development of the game engagement questionnaire: a measure of engagement in video game-playing. J. Exp. Soc. Psychol. **45**(4), 624–634 (2009)

Elderly Care and Technologies

Designing Conversational Assistants to Support Older Adults' Personal Health Record Access

Pegah Karimi[✉], Kallista Ballard, Pooja Vazirani,
Ravi Teja Narasimha Jorigay, and Aqueasha Martin-Hammond

Indiana University Purdue University Indianapolis, Indianapolis, IN, USA
{pkarimi,kadeball,pvaziran,rjorigay,aqumarti}@iu.edu

Abstract. Older adults often rely on information provided during doctors' visits or online to manage their health but can experience challenges accessing this information at home. Recently, conversational assistants are being explored to aid navigation of health information included in online portals, but we still know little about users' perceptions of using these tools for managing personal health information. In this paper, we conducted a wizard-of-oz study to better understand older adults' perceptions of a conversational assistant, MIHA, to help with navigating personal health information. Participants saw value in using a tool such as MIHA to help facilitate access to their personal health information and to help them become more engaged in their health. Participants believed MIHA's features helped build confidence in the responses returned, but made suggestions for improving the interactions. We share insights of potential uses and design implications for conversational assistants that help older adults navigate personal health information.

Keywords: Older adults · Conversational assistants · Online health portals · Wizard of Oz

1 Introduction

Formal caregivers including doctors and nurses play an important role in helping older adults manage their health care [1]. Older patients often regard formal caregivers as a preferred and trusted resource to provide answers to health-related questions [2,3]. However, older adults also rely on patient e-health portals [4] to access and remember health-care providers' advice. E-health portals linked to electronic health records (EHRs) can be useful for older adults to access information associated with a visit. Patients can use these portals to review lab results, medications, or doctors' advice provided during visits [5]. E-health portals, however, can pose challenges for older adults with low digital literacy skills or access

This research is based on work supported by the National Science Foundation under Grant #2130583.

H. Lewy and R. Barkan (Eds.): PH 2021, LNICST 431, pp. 253–271, 2022.
https://doi.org/10.1007/978-3-030-99194-4_17

barriers, which in turn makes it harder for them to access the personal health information they need [6,7]. In parallel, online information can often supplement older adults understanding the content provided by their doctors or through e-health portals [8], but older adults can still face difficulties searching for health information due to negative perceptions about online sources [9] making it difficult for them to trust the information [10].

More recently, with advances in artificial intelligence (AI) and speech recognition, there has been an emerging interest in using conversational assistants (CAs) such as voice assistants and chatbots to assist users with their health-care needs [11–16]. However, there are still gaps in understanding of how CAs can best support individuals' health care needs and promote transparent, trustworthy interactions with users. To uncover older adults' perceptions of CAs for navigating personal health information, we developed a conversational assistant called MIHA (Multimodal Intelligent Health Assistant). MIHA supports older adults with searching and navigating information provided by their doctor and provides tailored answers to users' questions. It also includes several features to support users' understanding of information. Through a within-subjects wizard-of-oz (WOZ) study with ten older adults, we explored perceptions of MIHA and its potential usefulness for supporting access to information stored in e-health portals. We found that participants saw value in using an interface such as MIHA to improve their access to information shared by their physician once outside the doctor's office, but also the ability to stay informed about their health and empower them to better participate as patients. We also found that participants felt that MIHA's features including retrieving responses from verified sources and providing options to understand how responses were derived were useful to improve confidence in responses. However, despite enthusiasm participants also felt that MIHA needed improvements particularly for gauging and responding to user intent in question-answering interactions as well as a broader set of features for summarizing and simplifying medical content. We discuss the potential for CAs such as MIHA to support older adults' access to personal health information and how we might facilitate transparent interactions with CAs for health.

2   Related Work

With aging, self-care and managing personal health and wellness becomes important to acquire better health outcomes [18,19]. To improve health outcomes, it is essential for individuals to maintain their health by making informed decisions [17]. Studies have shown older patients often rely on various sources, including personal notes, information communication technologies (e.g., phone calls, emails), and informal caregivers to manage their health and make decisions at home [3,20]. Personal notes can include information, such as recently prescribed medications, medications schedules, or dietary or treatment plans [4]. However, it can be challenging to organize notes from different doctors [4] and finding relevant information across multiple notes can be time-consuming [21]. Some, therefore, make use of phone calls or emails to connect to their healthcare providers and follow up with questions [21]; however, this method may take more time as the doctor may not be available to address a concern immediately. Finally, older adults may rely on informal caregivers (i.e., family caregivers), who often seek collaboration with formal caregivers (i.e., doctors, nurses) to provide care by helping them gather and manage information to facilitate care at home [22]. However, family caregivers may not always be available [23].

Online patient portals (i.e., personal health records, e-health portals) are another common tool to help patients access medical records and information shared by doctors during visits. Patient portals often allow individuals to access lab results, treatment plans, and medications discussed during doctor's appointments. However, portals also pose three main challenges for older adults: (1) accessing and navigating portals can be difficult [24], (2) they lack personalization [25], and (3) they have limited support for older patients with low health literacy [27]. Studies have shown that older adults often do not use patient portals for their intended purposes - managing health information [7] - and instead, use them only as a communication channel, diminishing the portal's usefulness. In addition, some older adults have found it challenging to manage multiple portal accounts between different providers [7], which in turn leads to non-use of portals and increases preference for talking directly to a healthcare provider [28]. Some patient portals also do not include doctors' notes which can be valuable to help patients recall information from their visits [56].

Researchers have found that providing patients with access to doctors' notes can positively impact patients' participation in their health [29–31]. For instance, in their study of retrospective use of OpenNotes, an effort that allows patients access to doctors' notes directly, researchers found that groups of patients, including older adults, found significant benefits from reading doctors' notes directly [31]. Karimi and Martin-Hammond, for example, found potential for AI-assisted tools that enable older adults' access to doctors' notes to aid in their recall of information shared during visits [4]. In parallel, researchers have also introduced AI-assisted note-taking tools that automatically generate encounter notes based on patient-physician conversations during a visit. These tools have also been useful for physicians. For example, a study of EmpowerMD [32], demonstrates the potential of AI-based features to document patients' health data for doctors. However, there are still open questions of the value of providing similar access to patients through their personal health records.

To overcome some of the usability issues associated with navigating online portals [26, 33–36], conversational assistants (CAs) have gained attraction in health and research has found that these systems can support patients with mental health issues, chronic illnesses, and breast cancer among others [11–16, 37]. CAs are a class of technologies, including chatbots and voice-based systems that use conversational interactions to engage users in dialog [38]. A systematic review of using voice interactions to navigate online portals suggests that users perceive CAs as an efficient way to navigate information provided in online portals [39]. In particular, for people with certain disabilities such as motor impairments that prevent them from typing with keyboards, conversational interactions through voice-based input is seen as a way to make online portals more accessible [40]. CAs are also being explored to support adherence to treatments and medications for different user populations [41,42]. Researchers have found that older adults view CAs that provide medical instructions included in EHR systems as useful [12]. Others noted that some see CAs as potentially useful for navigating electronic health records if challenges can be addressed [39]. This paper builds on this prior work to investigate older adults' perceptions of a CA for navigating patient information included in doctors' notes provided in an EHR system.

3 MIHA: A Health-Related Question Answering Prototype

To enable older patients retrieve and navigate their personal health information, we developed a conversational assistant prototype, called MIHA (Fig. 1). There are three main design principles for MIHA. First, it provides answers to the user's health-related questions from a verified source (e.g., doctor's notes). Trust and transparency are top concerns for patients when interacting with health related intelligent assistants [43]. Therefore, we envision MIHA as being able to support access to existing patient information provided from a trusted source. Second, MIHA aims to provide transparency by enabling users to verify answers provided in the conversational interaction. Prior work suggests that conversational interactions for health search can be less transparent posing potential risk to patients [44]. In an effort to address these concerns, we provide a mechanism for "explainability" by allowing users to view the text used to answer the questions. Third, MIHA attempts to simplify health information search tasks by providing additional support for specific questions about an illness or medication using a trusted consumer health source (Medlineplus [45] and WebMD [46]).

MIHA includes several features to support users' understanding of the responses provided (see Fig. 1). After posing a question (1), MIHA returns a response and additionally (2) asks the user if they would like to view how the response was derived using the doctor's note. A preview of the note including the highlighted portion of text that was used to generate the response is provided. If the user wants to view the entire note, (3) MIHA provides a preview of the file that includes the entire note. (4) To help users with medical terminologies (e.g., prescribed medications), the system asks the user if they want additional information. (5) If the user selects "yes", the system provides the user with a summary of the medication generated from a valid source. Users can enter questions using an open text field or preselected questions recommended by MIHA.

3.1 AI Model for Question and Answering

Recently, transfer learning has been used as an efficient learning method in natural language processing. In this case, a pre-trained model is trained on a large corpus of texts that can solve various tasks, such as question answering, sentence

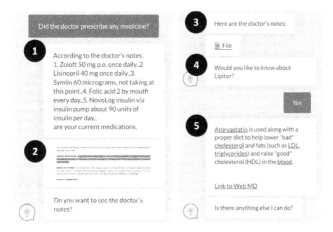

Fig. 1. Once users receive a response, (1) they can preview (2) or view the full doctor's note (3) and ask follow-up questions (4–5).

completion, and summarization [47]. We used the Text-to-Text Transfer Transformer model (T5) [48] to return answers to questions posed to MIHA using the transcription of the doctor's note. T5 is a large Transformer [49] model that is pre-trained on the large Colossal Clean Crawled Corpus (C4). The model is able to differentiate between similar questions (e.g., asking about past vs. current medications) and it supports conditional information extraction (e.g., asking about the patient's history or the doctor's recommendations). The answers returned are a paraphrased version of the corresponding note content.

To test the effectiveness of the T5 model, we used a public benchmark called *Medical Transcriptions* [50] that contains a dataset of 5000 anonymized doctors' note samples. Notes contained four different fields: description, medical specialty, sample name, transcription, and keywords. To prepare the dataset of notes, we first removed duplicates by merging their specialties and keywords, because the same text could appear under different specialties. We then split the different sections and assigned a topic based on the prefix. Due to a large number of different prefixes, we merged labels belonging to the same topic. Finally, we separated each section in the constituent sentences, inheriting the section topic, to obtain the cleaned dataset. For the purpose of our study, we only used two fields: medical specialty and transcription. Figure 2 shows an example of a cardiovascular medical note along with questions and answers returned. We set the minimum and maximum number of words for the returned answer to 10 and 150, respectively. This range allowed the AI model to provide an answer of appropriate length for our application. Initial testing showed that the model was able to handle various types of questions, such as conditional or yes/no questions.

4 Method

We conducted a user study with older adults to evaluate their perceptions of CAs for navigating personal health information (i.e., doctor's notes about visits)

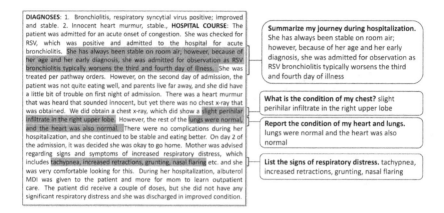

Fig. 2. An example of medical transcript of cardiovascular note highlighted to show answers returned by the T5 model.

and their perceptions of the answers MIHA returned. For the purpose of our study, we used the *Medical transcriptions* [42] dataset that includes doctors' notes available in EHRs. The dataset includes wide range of medical terms that are focused on patients' care. Therefore, while we asked about MIHA's features, we also ask participants how they thought a tool like MIHA might impact access to personal health information more broadly.

4.1 Participants

We recruited 10 older adults, age 60 years and older by reaching out to senior centers that provide services such as wellness and health programs, transportation services and public benefit counseling. Six participants self-identified as female and four participants as male. Participants' ages ranged from 61 to 83 (avg = 66.5, std = 7.38). The number of formal caregivers (e.g., doctors or nurses) involved in participants' health care teams ranged from one to three, whereas the number of informal caregivers ranged from zero to more than five. Moreover, seven participants reported they always use computers, one sometimes, and two rarely. All participants reported they always use smartphones except for one who often uses smartphones. Five participants described themselves as very familiar with computers, two familiar, and three somewhat familiar. Five participants described themselves as very familiar with smartphones, four familiar, and one somewhat familiar. More demographic data is shown in Table 1.

4.2 Wizard-of-Oz Study and Procedure

To test older adults' perceptions of CAs for navigating personal health information and the answers returned, we conducted a within-subjects, wizard-of-oz study (WOZ) followed by semi-structured interview questions. We defined four

Table 1. Demographic data

ID	Age	Doctors' visits in the last 12 months	Chronic illnesses	Num of years managing illnesses	Level of difficulty navigating online portals
P1-M	62	1–2 times	Hypercholesterolemia	1–2 years	Somewhat difficult
P2-F	60	3–5 times	No chronic illness	NA	Somewhat difficult
P3-M	64	3–5 times	Blood pressure, Hypercholesterolemia	>10 years	Somewhat easy
P4-F	61	3–5 times	No chronic illness	NA	No usage
P5-F	62	0 times	Ulcers, Asthmalittle Arthritis	4–10 years	Somewhat difficult
P6-M	69	3–5 times	Blood pressure, Hypercholesterolemia	>10 years	Moderately difficult
P7-M	67	3–5 times	No chronic illness	>10 years	Moderately easy
P8-F	75	3–5 times	Diabetes, Hypertension	>10 years	Moderately easy
P9-F	62	3–5 times	Not reported	>10 years	Somewhat difficult
P10-F	83	3–5 times	Blood pressure	>10 years	Moderately easy

different scenarios to capture situations in which users pose questions to MIHA about a recent doctor's visit: (1) asking the type of medication their doctor prescribed for type I diabetes, (2) asking the test result following a visit for high blood pressure, (3) asking the results following a visit for chest pain, and (4) asking the treatment plan for various aches and pains after a follow up visit. Within each scenario we asked participants to complete four tasks. The first task required participants to ask a question pertaining to the scenario and type it into the system. Unlike the other tasks, the question was not pre-generated, and participants could type any question of their interest. The purpose of the first task was two-fold: to better understand what types of questions the user might pose and to see if there might be differences in participants' ratings of answers returned by MIHA compared to the answers given to our pre-selected questions. The second task required participants to select a pre-selected question (e.g., "what was my diagnosis?"). The objective of this task was to give users options to select from instead of requiring them to type. The third task gave users the option to select the returned response from MIHA and view the response in the transcript. The purpose of this task was to understand whether providing an explanation of how the answer was derived altered users' perceptions of the system's answer. The fourth task asked participants to select a follow-up question to learn more about a prescribed medication or treatment. Similar to the third task, the goal for this task was to see how transparency pertaining to the information derived contributed to users' perception of the information. The order of the four scenarios were counterbalanced to account for any ordering effect.

For the study, MIHA was implemented using landbot (https://landbot.io/) an interactive interface for prototyping chatbot applications. Landbot was chosen because it included functionality that allowed researchers to return answers from the T5 model in real-time through the chatbot interface as well as send other responses to the user as needed. Therefore, we could mimic a working intelligent chatbot prototype. Participants were first introduced to the purpose of the study, our chatbot (MIHA), and its features. Studies were conducted remotely via Zoom or phone depending on the participants' preferences. At the beginning of the study, we read aloud the study information sheet. We then asked participants a set of demographic and background questions. After completing the questionnaire, we asked participants to start the first task in the first scenario. Each task was followed by two questions asking participants their perceptions of the systems' response and if they felt it was accurate. A third question included a Likert-scale question that asked users to rate the response on a scale of not relevant to very relevant. After the participant completed the last task, we asked them interview questions focusing on their experience completing the tasks and opinions about the usefulness of the MIHA for assisting them with navigating their own personal health information. All interviews were audio recorded. Our study was reviewed and approved by the institutional review board at Indiana University before any data collection began. Each session took approximately 60–90 min. We provided participants a $20 gift card for their involvement.

4.3 Data Analysis

We analyzed the post task data using descriptive statistics. Additionally, we performed thematic analysis using transcripts of participants' responses to interview questions. In doing so, we first used closed coding based on the interview questions to understand participants overall experiences. We then performed open coding to explore potential themes that might emerge about the design of MIHA and participants' experiences using similar technologies.

5 Results

5.1 Users Initial Thoughts of MIHA

Participants shared that they had a positive experience using MIHA. They were able to recognize without explanation that MIHA provides answers to medical questions. P1 stated: "*We can have multiple medical questions and the system answers my questions regarding the treatment plan, the lab result and future plan.*" Participants also recognized MIHA's ability to remind patients about instructions provided by their doctor and access their medical information after the visit. P6 stated:"*if you forgot to ask something [during doctors' visits]...you can use the system to find out and refresh your memory.*" Therefore, our findings confirm that users' mental models of the system matched our conceptual model of MIHA's design. However, participants also shared other envisioned uses of MIHA and how it compared with their experiences using patient portals.

Envisioned Uses of MIHA. Participants described different scenarios, in which MIHA could be useful to them. This included providing them with the option to verify answers to medical questions after a visit, manage information from multiple doctors, organize personal notes, alleviate health anxiety, and providing an alternative when not being able to see the doctor. Users mentioned situations in which they felt a system such as MIHA could be used to obtain an answer to their questions at their convenience. For instance, P5 commented: *"sometimes I've noticed some of my friends that are older, they're afraid to ask the doctor questions...So, when you are able to go home and actually look at this in the privacy of your own home, it would help you because you could be able to look at it and process it a little bit easier."* Another situation was to reference conversations with doctors to track health over time. P9 stated: *"I see the same doctor every six months, so it also gives a reference as to what we talked about last time. And how has things gone with my health."* Therefore, participants felt that MIHA could provide an alternative way of allowing patients to access and track health information shared during doctors' visits.

Other participants specified that the system could be useful to confirm answers to medical questions while at home. For instance, when asking about examples of situations in which the tool could be useful, P7 commented: *"To verify the definition of a diagnosis...the treatment plan that has already been established...[and] how I should take medication if it's not already on the bottle."* Some users specified that when they need to have answers to a medical question due to an immediate health concern, the tool can relieve some of the anxiety. For example, P2 commented: *"When you have some symptoms, or you know something [is] going on with [you], you want to know as soon as possible."* Thus, participants felt that MIHA could supplement following-up with their doctors to also help them become more empowered and informed patients.

Additionally, participants suggested that the tool could help creating personal notes from doctors' records. P5 suggested that MIHA could be helpful for them to organize and track personal notes. They discussed, *"If I would like to have a personal message area..., it [MIHA] would help me to go back from previous visits to see what the doctor had prescribed for me."* P2 and P9 suggested similar uses of MIHA. P2 stated, *"I can create a history in my notes, because every time I can go to the tool, access it, and use it pretty easily for any questions and add it to my notes."* Thus, participants saw MIHA as an opportunity to better organize their personal note inventories to manage their health.

Several participants discussed that the system would also give them the opportunity to be more involved in their health. P7 shared, *"It [having access to the doctor's note] would also help to answer questions that I may not have thought about during the visit. It also helped me to read information that the doctor perhaps said during the office visit, but I as the patient didn't hear it."* P5 made a similar observation, they stated, *"If I go to the doctor...I would appreciate being able to see the doctor's notes and also a verification of what they said."* Therefore participants felt that MIHA could improve their ability and willingness to engage with information shared in conversations with their doctors.

MIHA's Comparison to Online Patient Portal Experiences. Given that MIHA answers questions using notes generated from an electronic health record system, we asked participants to compare their interactions with the system to online portals. Participants felt that MIHA could improve their ability to find information. Some participants mentioned that doctor's notes are not always included in the portal, but if they were, the system could allow them to save time in getting an answer to their health questions by using the chat feature. For instance, P9 commented: *"My current portal...they do not have doctor's notes...You can see your test results...but the doctor may [or may not] put his notes in the body of an answer (report)."* P9 also shared, *"I believe this is a good tool for the medical community to have, it would lighten their load as far as me calling into the office...It's actually better than the portal...because it gives you more information."* Another participant, P1, provided similar feedback stating: *"One of the most useful advantage of using MIHA system is saving time. Because I can see the right answer to my question as soon as possible, whereas with online portals I have to go over all the note to find my answer."* This implies that the tool has the potential to enhance search by directing users to information which might be more difficult to find when reading through an entire note. Participants also expressed that when the system provides more detailed information about a medical term, it enhances their ability to find information faster. For instance, P5 commented: *"It's [MIHA] just a lot easier to use and it gives you more straightforward answers. Some of the ones [portals] that I had been on have been very confusing. You have to switch back and forth between two to three different screens. And this [MIHA] is a lot more user-friendly."* Therefore, participants felt that MIHA offered features that could make it easier and faster to navigate information such as non-structured doctors' notes compared to online portals.

5.2   Perceptions for Answering Personal Health Questions

To understand users' perceptions of engaging in dialog with MIHA to answer questions, we examined the conversational interactions supported by MIHA.

Types of Questions Users Posed to MIHA. We collected the open-ended questions submitted to our prototype and examined how participants might engage conversationally with the system to find answers to a question. Out of the 40 open-ended questions posted, we found that nearly 78% (31/40) were interrogatives that asked the system to do something. Interrogative sentences follow the traditional question format of a question word (Who, What, Where, When, Why, or How) followed by an auxiliary, subject, main verb, and optionally extra information. Examples include "What is the result of my chest pain?" and "What type of medication do I need?" The other 22% (9/4) of questions were imperative sentences or commands that tell the system to do something. Examples include "Tell me more about the medication you prescribed" and "I want to know about my results." Half of the participants (N = 5) posed interrogative questions only, and the other half (N = 5) posed a mix of questions and commands. The details provided by participants when posing their questions varied. The majority (67%) of questions (27/40) were basic questions that did not include any additional information to clarify intent. Approximately 33% of questions posed included an auxiliary, subject, main verb, and additional information such as the name of the illness or symptoms.

Users Perceptions of MIHA's Responses and Explanations. We also asked users to provide feedback on the answers to the questions that the T5 model returned. We were particularly interested in whether or not, based on their perspective, the responses returned were relevant and accurate. We did not provide participants with formal definitions unless they asked us to clarify. Our goal was to therefore distinguish between responses viewed by participants as pertinent or related in some way based on their expectations.

Overall, participants felt that the system returned relevant responses. Open-ended questions were majority positive, with 63% of responses (25/40) rated as relevant or very relevant and 37% (15/40) rated as not relevant or somewhat relevant. We saw a similar trend for closed-ended questions with 80% of responses (32/40) rated as relevant or very relevant and 20% of responses (8/40) rated as somewhat relevant or not relevant. While participants viewed most answers to open and closed-ended questions as relevant, they were more positive about closed-ended responses compared to open-ended. Participants' perceptions of the accuracy of responses were also majority positive. For open-ended questions, participants rated 87% of responses (25/40) as accurate compared to 13% (5/40) as not accurate. Closed-ended questions also received more positive responses. Participants rated 95% of responses (38/40) as accurate compared to 5% (2/40) as not accurate. We believe that the significant positive change found between open and closed-ended questions may have been due to limitations with the T5 model and its sensitivity to question phrasing and also that participants perceptions of responses and explanations were influenced by factors other than relevance and accuracy.

Participants rated 90% of responses as relevant or very relevant after viewing the note compared to 80% before viewing the note. Participants rated 10% of responses as somewhat relevant or not relevant after viewing the "explainability" note compared to 20% before viewing the note. Some participants also changed their views about accuracy after viewing the note, however the majority (34/40) remained positive before and after viewing. Four participants' ratings changed from not accurate to accurate after viewing the note and one participant changed from accurate to not accurate. However, several themes emerged from interviews suggesting that participants' perceptions of the responses returned by MIHA (i.e., the T5 model) were influenced by other factors.

Participants discussed knowing that the responses were coming from validated sources (i.e., doctors' notes, validated online sources, and patients' records) increased their confidence in the information MIHA provided. P2 commented: *"In the beginning for some questions, I didn't receive an accurate answer but after reviewing doctors' notes [I felt] the answer was relevant."* In a similar vein, P5 said: *"Because you can see responses correlates back and forth with the doctor's notes."* These statements imply that participants felt that the ability to go back and forth between the answer and note improved their confidence in the answers.

Similar comments were made about being able to view follow-up information that was provided by WebMD, an online source participants trusted. Therefore, participants discussed that having trusted information available increased their confidence in the system. Participants also shared it was helpful when the responses either aligned with their prior knowledge or helped to facilitate learning. When the systems' responses matched their prior knowledge, participants noted that it improved their confidence in the answers. P8 shared that they felt the response to questions were generally relevant because, *"I take diabetes medication. I take hypertension medication, but I knew that Lipitor was cholesterol medication."* Additionally, participants liked that the system supported learning of how answers were derived within the tool through showing the note. When asked if users could better trust the answer after seeing where the answer was located in the doctor's notes, P8 commented: *"Yes, it did...because it was explained more."* Including mechanisms to help users understand how answers were derived were viewed as helpful to build confidence in the tool.

5.3   Improving MIHA

Participants also provided suggestions on how MIHA could better serve their needs. These recommendations include simplifying interaction with medical terms, supporting better conversational interactions, and integrating new design features. For example, when asking about how the tool might improve to meet their needs, P4 commented: *"Changing the terminology for the responses, making them simpler, reader friendly. Because if I'm not a doctor or I don't know anything about the medication, I need the medication information to be simplified."* P8 shared that the systems' inability to simplify information led to some lower ratings. They shared, *"because at one time, it [MIHA] named another medication, it didn't say it was a generic name, it should have explained it."* Therefore in addition to simplifying navigation, participants also felt more needed to be done to facilitate understanding of medical terminologies.

Participants shared that improvements in MIHA's ability to gauge the intent of the question would further build their confidence in the system. They mentioned while answers were relevant, they were not always what they were expecting. P7 shared, *"The majority of the answers were relevant, but there was one where I as a patient was asking a very broad question - Tell me more about the medications that I was prescribed? - and the system just answers what would be on the bottle. That's not more information."* P4 shared a similar experience, they stated that in one instance, *"Yeah it [MIHA] didn't answer my question accurately. I asked what side effects and it just gave me the prescribed medicine. So I guess I am just supposed to go look that up."* Participants also mentioned that they preferred when the system provided them with different options to choose from instead of requiring them to type in questions. For instance, P5 commented: *"I liked the idea of just having the choices to click on...rather than typing it out myself."* Participants discussed that this would remove the challenges they might have while typing but also help with reducing cognitive burden of formulating a query. Some users also suggested using voice as an alternative option to interact with the system. P5 also commented: *"That sounds excellent [using voice]. Especially for older folks that have problems with typing or with clicking buttons or whatever, it's a lot easier to just talk-to-text."* Participants made other suggestions for improving conversational interactions such as restating questions and providing features to show that MIHA is thinking.

Finally, users pointed to potential interface design features that could improve the usefulness of MIHA. Features included adding a calendar that shows doctors' visits with notes organized all in one place. Some participants discussed making MIHA more personable such as including a photo of the doctor. P6 shared, *"I miss the old days ... we used to have doctors...they knew your family, the kid's ages, what they are doing now. Now you go and there are just numbers...a lot of times you don't see your own doctor."* Participants also suggested including an option to chat with the doctor directly in case the system could not find an appropriate answer. For example, P4 and P6 noted that sometimes people are not able to go to the doctor in person. Both participants shared that it would be useful if they could connect with the doctor using MIHA as well.

6   Discussion

Our findings suggest that participants perceived a conversational assistant such as MIHA that supports navigating and improving interactions with personal health data as useful. Participants also felt that the features to support understanding and transparency of information were helpful for building their confidence in the responses. We discuss design implications for designing conversational interactions that support older adults' access to health information and for facilitating user confidence in conversational tools for health information search.

6.1   Using CAs to Support Older Adults' Access to Health Information

Several researchers have found that older adults prefer talking directly with a healthcare provider to ask questions about their health [3,8], though individuals' experiences can vary [3]. Some older patients are not comfortable following-up with their doctor during or after visits [3,8], or may sometimes miss information due to anxiety, stress, or accessibility challenges [51]. At the same time, tools such as online portals which allow patients to revisit instructions from their doctor can be challenging for older adults to navigate [7,25,27]. For these reasons, our participants envisioned that having a tool like MIHA that was connected to a verified source could alleviate some of the challenges they experience accessing their personal health information. Participants felt that a tool similar to MIHA could empower them to become more knowledgeable and involved in their health.

Aligned with prior findings [52,53], participants suggested that drawing information from a verified source would be ideal for a CA. While providing patients with access to doctors' notes is not yet widely available [30,31], the concept of using conversational interactions through online portals is being actively explored. Azevedo and colleagues found that older adults saw conversational interactions useful for explaining medical instructions included in EHR systems [12]. Kumah-Crystal and colleagues, have also explored using voice technologies to navigate electronic health-records. They note many benefits but also the open challenges such as improving contextual awareness of understanding what information users may want to communicate [39]. Building on this work, our findings highlight older adults' beliefs that conversational interactions would be useful to access and navigate personal health information shared on EHR systems. Several participants discussed that sometimes they are not able to understand, hear, or focus on what the doctor discussed during visits. Thus, they felt having access to a tool similar to MIHA could improve their engagement by allowing them to search and ask questions at their leisure at home. Some users discussed that they currently do not have access to their doctors' notes outside of the visit even within the online patient portal. While providing patients with access to doctors' notes is still controversial [29,30], there has been a move to provide patients with this information which suggests we may see more access in the future. However, doctors have long provided notes [54] to support patients' recall of information, which might be alternative sources of data to support patients.

Participants also discussed potential improvements that they believed would enhance their experiences during conversational interactions including improving query experiences by reducing typing (i.e., pre-selected questions) or introducing voice. These findings suggest that a multimodal approach should be considered due to the variations in preferences among participants. Similarly, we found that participants engaged with MIHA mostly with questions opposed to the commands which are often used to execute voice-based queries on devices such as Alexa and Google Home. This suggests a need to further understand expected interactions with CAs for health. For example, some participants noted that while providing pre-selected questions reduces cognitive burden of generating a query and mobility challenges, it reduces the question set. While voice interaction reduces the above challenges, it also introduces concerns related to speech recognition accuracy that might outweigh ease of use. Therefore, we would need to explore the best way of reducing challenges related to open-ended questions. Participants noted that while MIHA often returned something relevant or accurate, it did not always consider intent highlighting the limitations of the AI model. Thus, in addition to conversational design, improving AI models to support intelligent Q&A will be needed.

6.2   Building Confidence in Conversational Tools for Health Search

While conversational assistants have been used quite often for supporting health tasks [11–16], recent findings have raised concerns about participants' abilities to gauge information from certain types of conversational agents such as voice assistants in consumer health environments [44]. As such, we explored different ways of integrating user confidence into the interaction. Reflecting on [55] and methods for improving transparency in intelligent systems through design, we summarized what needed better explanation to build users' confidence in MIHA's responses. Participants agreed that connecting MIHA to a verified source would improve their confidence in the responses. In addition, providing an understanding of how the response was derived helped build confidence as they could compare and contrast the two. Participants appreciated the inclusion of some sort of "explainability" feature which allowed them to verify responses if they wish. However, some participants also discussed the need to balance between providing information and assisting understanding. Exploring how to explain features beyond showing the source can be further investigated in the future.

We also found that confidence in the responses differed, which we believe occurred due to the AI model's sensitivity to question wording. One approach could be to include post processing steps to aid users in query generation. However, participants' feedback suggests the need for a broader exploration of methods to reduce challenges related to query generation (e.g., cognitive load) and to provide responses that better match users' intent. Because some responses were related but did not match what participants expected, they questioned MIHA's abilities. In the future, it would be useful to explore approaches to increase the likelihood that responses match users' intent. It might also be helpful to consider whether personalization could support better reasoning. The majority of participants omitted specific details about medical conditions or medications from their questions suggesting an expectation that the system would "know" about prior health history.

Finally, we found that apart from improving characteristics of the responses, participants suggested that MIHA needed additional ways to improve their understanding of medical terminologies. Both simplifying medical terminologies and summarizing medical texts [4,12,52] have been noted as concerns among older adults when interacting with intelligent health tools and we found similar concerns among our participants. Participants mentioned that it was not enough to provide an answer and therefore suggested including features to help simplify and facilitate understanding of content. Other efforts have also highlighted that for older adults, providing content may not be sufficient without also increasing comprehension and presentation of medical content [12,52]. Therefore, future efforts would need to consider factors beyond navigation and access that can help older adults better interact with their personal health information.

7   Conclusion

In this paper, we explore older adults' perceptions of a conversational assistant, MIHA, that aids with navigation and access of health information at home. We conduct a within-subjects WOZ study followed by semi-structured interviews to understand participants' perceptions of the tool. Our findings suggest that MIHA facilitates access and helps older adults to become more engaged in their health. Participants envisioned MIHA as a supplement to doctors' visits and a way to help them manage information about their health. Participants also felt that MIHA's connection to a verified health source and ability to explain how responses were derived were useful for supporting trusting interactions with the

CA. However, they also felt that MIHA could do more to support understanding of complex medical terminology, simplify language, and understand about question intent.

References

1. Li, J., Song, Y.: Formal and informal care. In: Gu, D., Dupre, M.E. (eds.) Encyclopedia of Gerontology and Population Aging, pp. 1–8. Springer, Cham (2019)
2. Chaudhuri, S., Le, T., White, C., Thompson, H., Demiris, G.: Examining health information-seeking behaviors of older adults. Comput. Inform. Nurs. **31**(11), 547–553 (2013)
3. Hall, A.K., Bernhardt, J.M., Dodd, V.: Older adults' use of online and offline sources of health information and constructs of reliance and self-efficacy for medical decision making. J. Health Commun. **20**(7), 751–758 (2015)
4. Karimi, P., Martin-Hammond, A.: Understanding barriers to medical instruction access for older adults: implications for AI-assisted tools. In: Adjunct Proceedings of the 2020 ACM International Joint Conference on Pervasive and Ubiquitous Computing and Proceedings of the 2020 ACM International Symposium on Wearable Computers, pp. 42–45 (2020)
5. Portz, J.D., et al.: Using the technology acceptance model to explore user experience, intent to use, and use behavior of a patient portal among older adults with multiple chronic conditions: descriptive qualitative study. J. Med. Internet Res. **21**(4), e11604 (2019)
6. Sakaguchi-Tang, D.K., Bosold, A.L., Choi, Y.K., Turner, A.M.: Patient portal use and experience among older adults: systematic review. JMIR Med. Inform. **5**(4), e38 (2017)
7. Son, H., Nahm, E.-S.: Older adults' experience using patient portals in communities: challenges and opportunities. Comput. Inform. Nurs. **37**(1), 4–10 (2019)
8. Medlock, S., et al.: Health information- seeking behavior of seniors who use the internet: a survey. J. Med. Internet Res. **17**(1), e3749 (2015)
9. Waterworth, S., Honey, M.: On-line health seeking activity of older adults: an integrative review of the literature. Geriatr. Nurs. **39**(3), 310–317 (2018)
10. Miller, L.M.S., Bell, R.A.: Online health information seeking: the influence of age, information trustworthiness, and search challenges. J. Aging Health **24**(3), 525–541 (2012)
11. Alagha, E.C., Helbing, R.R.: Evaluating the quality of voice assistants' responses to consumer health questions about vaccines: an exploratory comparison of Alexa, Google Assistant and Siri. BMJ Health Care Inform. **26**(1), e100075 (2019)
12. Azevedo, R.F.L., et al.: Using conversational agents to explain medication instructions to older adults. In: AMIA Annual Symposium Proceedings 2018, pp. 185–194 (2018)
13. Dojchinovski, D., Ilievski, A., Gusev, M.: Interactive home healthcare system with integrated voice assistant. In: 2019 42nd International Convention on Information and Communication Technology, Electronics and Microelectronics (MIPRO), pp. 284–288 (2019)
14. Keller, R., et al.: Are conversational agents used at scale by companies offering digital health services for the management and prevention of diabetes? (2021). http://alexandria.unisg.ch/

15. Laranjo, L., et al.: Conversational agents in healthcare: a systematic review. J. Am. Med. Inform. Assoc. **25**(9), 1248–1258 (2018)
16. Nallam, P., Bhandari, S., Sanders, J., Martin-Hammond, A.: A question of access: exploring the perceived benefits and barriers of intelligent voice assistants for improving access to consumer health resources among low-income older adults. Gerontol. Geriatr. Med. **6**, 2333721420985975 (2020)
17. Terris, M.: Concepts of health promotion: dualities in public health theory. J. Public Health Policy **13**(3), 267–276 (1992)
18. McDonald-Miszczak, L., Wister, A.V., Gutman, G.M.: Self-care among older adults: an analysis of the objective and subjective illness contexts. J. Aging Health **13**(1), 120–145 (2001)
19. Morrongiello, B.A., Gottlieb, B.H.: Self-care among older adults. Can. J. Aging/La Revue canadienne du vieillissement **19**(S1), 32–57 (2000)
20. Family Caregiver Alliance: Caregiver assessment: principles, guidelines and strategies for change: report from a National Consensus Development Conference. Family Caregiver Alliance (2006)
21. Harris, M., Bayer, A., Tadd, W.: Addressing the information needs of older patients. Rev. Clin. Gerontol. **12**(1), 5–11 (2002)
22. Keating, N., Fast, J., Dosman, D., Eales, J.: Services provided by informal and formal caregivers to seniors in residential continuing care. Can. J. Aging/La Revue canadienne du vieillissement **20**(1), 23–46 (2001)
23. Glasser, M., Prohaska, T., Gravdal, J.: Elderly patients and their accompanying caregivers on medical visits. Res. Aging **23**(3), 326–348 (2001)
24. Wildenbos, G.A., Maasri, K., Jaspers, M., Peute, L.: Older adults using a patient portal: registration and experiences, one year after implementation. Digit. Health **4**(2018), 2055207618797883 (2018)
25. Price-Haywood, E.G., Harden-Barrios, J., Ulep, R., Luo, Q.: eHealth literacy: patient engagement in identifying strategies to encourage use of patient portals among older adults. Popul. Health Manag. **20**(6), 486–494 (2017)
26. Irizarry, T., Shoemake, J., Nilsen, M.L., Czaja, S., Beach, S., Dabbs, A.D.: Patient portals as a tool for health care engagement: a mixed-method study of older adults with varying levels of health literacy and prior patient portal use. J. Med. Internet Res. **19**(3), e99 (2017)
27. Kim, S., Fadem, S.: Communication matters: exploring older adults' current use of patient portals. Int. J. Med. Inform. **120**, 126–136 (2018)
28. Anthony, D.L., Campos-Castillo, C., Lim, P.S.: Who isn't using patient portals and why? Evidence and implications from a national sample of US adults. Health Aff. **37**(12), 1948–1954 (2018)
29. Wolff, J.L., et al.: Inviting patients and care partners to read doctors' notes: Open-Notes and shared access to electronic medical records. J. Am. Med. Inform. Assoc. **24**(e1), e166–e172 (2017)
30. Bell, S.K., et al.: When doctors share visit notes with patients: a study of patient and doctor perceptions of documentation errors, safety opportunities and the patient-doctor relationship. BMJ Qual. Saf. **26**(4), 262–270 (2017)
31. Walker, J., et al.: OpenNotes after 7 years: patient experiences with ongoing access to their clinicians' outpatient visit notes. J. Med. Internet Res. **21**(5), e13876 (2019)
32. Microsoft. Project EmpowerMD: Medical conversations to medical intelligence (2018). https://www.steelcase.com/research/articles/topics/healthcare/exam-rooms-that-empower-people/

33. Friedberg, M.W., et al.: Factors affecting physician professional satisfaction and their implications for patient care, health systems, and health policy. Rand Health Q. **3**(4) (2014)
34. King, J., Patel, V., Jamoom, E.W., Furukawa, M.F.: Clinical benefits of electronic health record use: national findings. Health Serv. Res. **49**(1pt2), 392–404 (2014)
35. Middleton, B., et al.: Enhancing patient safety and quality of care by improving the usability of electronic health record systems: recommendations from AMIA. J. Am. Med. Inf. Assoc. **20**(e1), e2–e8 (2013)
36. Turner, A.M., et al.: Use of patient portals for personal health information management: the older adult perspective. In: AMIA Annual Symposium Proceedings, vol. 2015, p. 1234. American Medical Informatics Association (2015)
37. Chen, C., et al.: Understanding barriers and design opportunities to improve healthcare and QOL for older adults through voice assistants. In: The 23rd International ACM SIGACCESS Conference on Computers and Accessibility (Virtual Event, USA) (ASSETS 2021). Association for Computing Machinery, Virtual Event (2021). https://doi.org/10.1145/3441852.3471218
38. Moore, R.J., Arar, R.: Conversational UXDesign: A Practitioner's Guide to the Natural Conversation Framework. Morgan & Claypool (2019)
39. Kumah-Crystal, Y.A., Pirtle, C.J., Whyte, H.M., Goode, E.S., Anders, S.H., Lehmann, C.U.: Electronic health record interactions through voice: a review. Appl. Clin. Inform. **9**(3), 541 (2018)
40. Garrett, J.T., Heller, K.W., Fowler, L.P., Alberto, P.A., Fredrick, L.D., O'Rourke, C.M.: Using speech recognition software to increase writing fluency for individuals with physical disabilities. J. Spec. Educ. Technol. **26**(1), 25–41 (2011)
41. Bauermeister, J., et al.: Interactive voice response system: data considerations and lessons learned during a rectal microbicide placebo adherence trial for young men who have sex with men. J. Med. Internet Res. **19**(6), e207 (2017)
42. Reidel, K., Tamblyn, R., Patel, V., Huang, A.: Pilot study of an interactive voice response system to improve medication refill compliance. BMC Med. Inform. Decis. Making **8**(1), 1–8 (2008)
43. Martin-Hammond, A., Vemireddy, S., Rao, K.: Exploring older adults' beliefs about the use of intelligent assistants for consumer health information management: a participatory design study. JMIR Aging **2**(2), e15381 (2019)
44. Bickmore, T.W., et al.: Patient and consumer safety risks when using conversational assistants for medical information: an observational study of Siri, Alexa, and Google Assistant. J. Med. Internet Res. **20**(9), e11510 (2018)
45. MedlinePlus - Health Information from the National Library of Medicine. https://medlineplus.gov/. Accessed 13 May 2021
46. WebMD - Better information. Better health. https://www.webmd.com/. Accessed 13 May 2021
47. Wolf, T., et al.: Transformers: state-of-the-art natural language processing. In: Proceedings of the 2020 Conference on Empirical Methods in Natural Language Processing: System Demonstrations, pp. 38–45 (2020)
48. Raffel, C., et al.: Exploring the Limits of Transfer Learning with a Unified Text-to-Text Transformer (2019). arXiv:1910.10683 [cs.LG]
49. Vaswani, A., et al.: Attention Is All You Need (2017). arXiv:1706.03762 [cs.CL]
50. Boyle, T.: Medical Transcriptions. Kaggle (2018). https://www.kaggle.com/tboyle10/medicaltranscriptions
51. Cohen, J.M., et al.: Studies of physician-patient communication with older patients: how often is hearing loss considered? A systematic literature review. J. Am. Geriatr. Soc. **65**(8), 1642–1649 (2017)

52. Martin-Hammond, A., Gilbert, J.E.: Examining the effect of automated health explanations on older adults' attitudes toward medication information. In: Proceedings of the 10th EAI International Conference on Pervasive Computing Technologies for Healthcare (Cancun, Mexico) (PervasiveHealth 2016). ICST (Institute for Computer Sciences, Social-Informatics and Telecommunications Engineering), Brussels, BEL, pp. 186–193 (2016)

53. Sanders, J., Martin-Hammond, A.: Exploring autonomy in the design of an intelligent health assistant for older adults. In: Proceedings of the 24th International Conference on Intelligent User Interfaces: Companion (IUI 2019), pp. 95–96. ACM, New York (2019)

54. Brown, T.F., Massoud, E., Bance, M.: Informed consent in otologic surgery: prospective study of risk recall by patients and impact of written summaries of risk. J. Otolaryngol. **32**(6), 368–372 (2003)

55. Eiband, M., Schneider, H., Bilandzic, M., Fazekas-Con, J., Haug, M., Hussmann, H.: Bringing transparency design into practice. In: 23rd International Conference on Intelligent User Interfaces (IUI 2018), pp. 211–223. ACM, New York (2018)

56. Karimi, P., Bora, P., Martin-Hammond, A.: Scribe: improving older adults' access to medical instructions from patient-physician conversations. In: Proceedings of the 18th International Web for All Conference, April 2021, pp. 1–11 (2021)

Helping People to Control Their Everyday Data for Care: A Scenario-Based Study

Pei-Yao Hung$^{(\boxtimes)}$ and Mark S. Ackerman

University of Michigan, Ann Arbor, MI 48109, USA
{peiyaoh,ackerm}@umich.edu

Abstract. With the advent of pervasive sensing devices, data captured about one's everyday life (e.g., heart rate, sleep quality, emotion, or social activity) offers enormous possibilities for promoting in-home health care for severe chronic care, such as can be found in Spinal Cord Injury or Disorders or the like. Sharing these Everyday Data for Care (EDC) allows care team personnel (e.g., caregivers and clinicians) to assist with health monitoring and decision-making, but will also create tension and concerns (e.g., privacy) for people with health conditions due to the detailed nature of the data. Resolving these tensions and concerns is critical for the adoption and use of a pervasive healthcare environment.

We examine data sharing of EDC to determine how we can better manage the tradeoffs between privacy on one hand and the pro-active sharing of data that one needs for better care. In this paper, we target one critical aspect of using EDC, the problem of sharing an overwhelming number of sensor outputs with numerous care team recipients. We report the results of a scenario-based study that examined ways to reduce the burden of setting policies or rules to manage both the pro-active data sharing and the privacy aspects of care with EDC. In summary, we found that our participants were able to use self-generated groupings of EDC data, and more importantly, largely kept those groupings when creating to share data with potential recipients and when dealing with changes in their health trajectory. These findings offer hope that we can reduce the burden of authoring and maintaining data sharing and privacy policies through semi-automatic mechanisms, where the system suggests policies that are consistent with the users' preferences - especially as health changes.

Keywords: Data sharing · Patient-generated health data · Chronic care · Privacy · Control · Self-care · Care team · Care network

1 Introduction

Support for people with chronic diseases is becoming more important in the US and around the world [68]. In the US, it is estimated that 6 out of 10 adults

© ICST Institute for Computer Sciences, Social Informatics and Telecommunications Engineering 2022
Published by Springer Nature Switzerland AG 2022. All Rights Reserved
H. Lewy and R. Barkan (Eds.): PH 2021, LNICST 431, pp. 272–301, 2022.
https://doi.org/10.1007/978-3-030-99194-4_18

have a chronic condition [26]. Because of this, there has been extensive interest in supporting people with chronic conditions in the Computer-Supported Collaborative Work and Social Computing (CSCW) community [9,20,41,63,76,80].

Recently, using data captured during one's everyday life for supporting care, or Everyday Data for Care (EDC), has received significant attention from the research community (e.g., including Observations of Daily Living (ODLs) [70] or Patient-Generated Health Data [30]) as well. EDC are defined as data captured about the everyday life of people with health conditions that could be useful for care, including data such as heart rate, fluid intake, sleep quality, and loneliness. These data could be generated automatically through sensors in a pervasive healthcare environment, wearable devices, or captured by care team members of people with health conditions. The use of EDC could provide benefits by bridging the hospital and home care environments by extending the monitoring of people' health outside of a traditional medical setting.

To unlock the full potential of EDC technologies while protecting the concerns of people with health conditions[1], we are examining how we might support people in their use and dissemination of EDC. Based on the prior literature:

- We want to achieve appropriate *data sharing* for *care*. Data sharing not only includes the protective aspects of privacy, but it also has a pro-active component. For care, it is critical to consider disseminating the necessary health data to actors who can help. In general privacy research, some authors consider both aspects of data sharing, but others do not. Following Kariotis et al.'s call [44], we use the term "data sharing" to foreground both the protective and pro-active aspects of dealing with EDC data.
- Data sharing must be done in the context of care teams. People with severe chronic conditions often need to rely on teams of people who help with daily life, including self-care [4,19,20,80]. Care teams are critical in supporting the health of people with health conditions. These care teams consist of the person with a health condition and caregivers (family members and/or paid/volunteer staff), who provide immediate day-to-day care, as well as clinicians [35]. Care teams are often dynamic, adding and losing members as health conditions change and as members turn over [20]. For illustration here, we consider spinal cord injury and disorder (SCI/D) [61], where the condition is life-time and where care teams of 10–20 people are not unusual.

To do this, we are exploring the designs that promote the following goals:

- Data sharing should be under the control of the people with health conditions or their surrogates to allow them take an active role in conducting care [8,9,

---

[1] We use the term "person with a health condition" interchangeably with "patient" in this paper, to emphasize her identity as a human being. We recognize the unfortunate connotations of "patient" in that it privileges the medicalization of care and the clinical participants in care. However, we use "patient" in some parts of the paper, such as in the related work, to avoid confusion and to maintain consistency with some existing literature.

35, 63]. We want to find ways to allow people to control their own data sharing, instead of putting it under the purview of large corporations or healthcare systems [44].

- If data sharing is to be under the purview of individuals, we have to keep the control from being overwhelming. With severe chronic care, a person with a health condition is likely to need to change sharing settings as their health deteriorates, a time in which they may not be able to focus or find the energy to do so. Moreover, this will become an increasingly difficult problem for users as healthcare sensors become cheaper and proliferate.

In this paper, we report a card sorting study to investigate whether EDC could be shared in groupings (i.e., grouping EDC types together as units to be shared) to simplify configuration. In short, we found our study participants were able to create groupings based on sorting Everyday Data for Care (EDC) into 5 bins based on their levels of comfort about sharing the EDC. More importantly, these groupings demonstrate their utility as high-level units that allow participants to discuss how to share EDC with care team members conveniently, as opposed to describing sharing settings for each EDC type. The use of these user-generated groupings allows us to observe people's inclination to share more EDC when a person's health deteriorates.

We view these results as preliminary but provocative. The findings suggest possibilities for creating new technical mechanisms that can help patients and caregivers in severe chronic care, and they also may resolve some of the difficulties of setting privacy policies overall.

Our contributions, then, from these results include:

- Showing that users can create groupings of EDC data that are meaningful to themselves and can be used to create EDC data sharing settings. Users can easily create these groupings.
- Demonstrating that our participants could reuse these user-defined groupings as high-level units to specify sharing settings in study tasks, implying that it may be possible to create stable groupings for each user that would simplify creating and potentially maintaining data sharing and privacy settings.

In the following sections, we first review related work on care team collaboration, everyday data for care, and support for data sharing and privacy. We then describe our study design, data collection, and analysis. We next present our findings. We conclude with implications for designing interactive systems to facilitate the creation and maintenance of sharing and privacy settings, as well as discuss the limitations of our study and future work.

2   Related Work

2.1   Chronic Care

With the prevalence of chronic conditions [26, 68], how to support chronic care becomes an important challenge to tackle. Chronic care refers to the tasks and steps that are necessary to do on a daily basis to maintain and improve health for the long term [5]. This includes adjusting routines (e.g., taking medicine), making conscious lifestyle choices (e.g., diet), and monitoring one's health at home (e.g., monitoring urination) [33,61]. As mentioned, managing a severe health condition (e.g., SCI/D) at home will often require the participation of a care team that consists of family members (e.g., as caregivers), other personnel (e.g., hired caregivers), and occasionally medical professionals (e.g., occupational therapists) so as to effectively manage different aspects of care and everyday life [4,14,19,20,80].

While early studies focused more on design to support patient-clinician [59] or patient-caregiver [14,94] interaction, recent work, including Consolvo et al. [25], has called for a design to support the care team as a whole [65], with particular attention to diverse roles, the communication structure, and the importance of sharing information [25]. Designing systems to support the entire care team requires careful consideration of the diverse expertise of team members [25], relationships among them [20], how team members with different time commitments collaborate in a loosely coupled manner (e.g., with non-overlapped shifts) [14], and how the team membership changes constantly [25]. Team members need to collaboratively monitor changes in a patient's health [19], and adapt to the patient's priorities in life [69]. This paper builds on this previous literature about care teams and examines how users' control over data sharing within care teams can be facilitated.

We next review literature on the use of data captured about people's everyday life to support collaboration for chronic care.

2.2   Everyday Data for Care

Everyday data for care (EDC) hold great potential for supporting chronic care. EDC are defined as data captured about the everyday life of people with health conditions that could be useful for care. These data could be generated through different mechanisms (e.g., including sensors in a futuristic pervasive environment or captured by care team members of people with health conditions). These data could include those that are commonly collected during clinic visits (e.g., heart rate or blood pressure), data that characterize a patient's behavior (e.g., sleep pattern) or emotional wellbeing (e.g., mood), and even contextual factors that could be influential on the patient's life (e.g., weather).

The definition of EDC is very similar to Patient-Generated Health Data (PGHD), which is defined as health-related data captured by patients or their care team members (e.g., caregivers) outside of medical environments [30]. Another term that is closely related to EDC is Observations of Daily Living (ODLs), for ODLs contain patterns and observations about patients' lives that were not traditionally included in the medical record [70]. In this paper, we use EDC to include PGHD and ODLs in order to focus on potential data sources generated from a pervasive environment (e.g., a person's home) full of different sensors that could be used to support care.

EDC's definition also overlaps with Quantified Self (QS) [77] and Personal Informatics (PI) [53]. The prominent difference is that EDC specifically focus on using data for health, while QS and PI can include anything of personal interest. In this section, we will briefly review the literature on the benefits and concerns of using EDC. For more comprehensive review (especially patient-generated health data), please refer to Figueiredo and Chen [30].

EDC could be used to support all kinds of health decision-making. However, the range of data included in EDC and the context of data capture (e.g., at home) make EDC especially applicable to severe, long-term chronic conditions such as irritable bowel syndrome (IBS) [23], and spinal cord injury/disorders [19]. As chronic care requires consistent monitoring of how the lifestyle of person with a health condition affects the person's health and life, care team members could use EDC to investigate how different factors (e.g., diet) trigger changes in the patient's health (e.g., symptoms) and quality of life (e.g., sleep quality) [45]. EDC provide an excellent opportunity for people to get involved and take an active role in understanding their health as well as decision-making. Indeed, existing work has shown multiple benefits of using EDC for them, including allowing them to understand their conditions [8], increasing their sense of control [8,35], supporting the planning of chronic care [29], empowering them to have a voice in the discussion of their health [9,63], and supporting interaction with clinicians [23,76].

While EDC provide a great number of benefits, existing research has also highlighted multiple challenges. First, tracking a wide range of data (e.g., including context [8]) could be overwhelming. Moreover, every person with a health condition might have a unique perspective on what is important to track [75]. Second, people with health conditions might have difficulty making sense of EDC [22]. Third, while care team members could help to make sense of EDC, care team members might have different expectations of what to track, the purpose of tracking, and consequently how to properly interpret the data [9,41,55].

Lastly, people with health conditions need to share EDC to support collaborative monitoring while maintaining a sense of control [63] and independence [20]. Our work follows this line of research to investigate how people think about sharing a variety of EDC to support care while respecting their sense of control and the need for privacy (i.e., avoiding surveillance). Maintaining the appropriate balance will be crucial for the success of a pervasive healthcare environment. We next review existing work on supporting sharing control and identify gaps for further investigation.

2.3   Privacy and Data Sharing

While sharing data can support our professional [16,17] and daily lives [81], people might naturally want to perform impression management [21,87,89] and avoid negative consequences such as undesirable inferences about oneself [48,81, 84] or data being leaked unexpectedly [51,66,87].

Concerns about the negative effects from sharing data have engendered research centered on privacy. Privacy has been generally defined as the ability to decide "when, how, and to what extent, information about them is communicated to others [93]."

One approach to helping people with their privacy concerns consists of technical research that augments or facilitates user control.

Considerable research has been devoted to creating and editing privacy policies (and by extension data sharing policies). Privacy policies consist of computational statements [15] in first-order predicate calculus, specialized computer languages, and the like [32,73]. Despite this considerable research, end-users cannot or will not write and edit policy statements, finding them too complex and difficult [49,58,95].

Instead, practice swung to another approach to allow users to create privacy settings through easier-to-use interfaces that used toggle buttons, elaborate tables, and other user interface widgets to manually manipulate privacy settings (e.g., Google's privacy settings). Again studies have been largely technical. This research includes designing user interfaces that allow people to control the audience [40,50,60,71,72] and data presentation [28,74,88,91], as well as interfaces that provide feedback (e.g., visualization or notifications) to help people understand the effects of privacy settings [2,3,36,46,85,86,92]. Despite the considerable evidence that users have trouble with these privacy interfaces [42,56], these interfaces persist.

A third approach consists of studies that attempt to understand and model people's privacy and data sharing preferences so as to ease the burden of configuration for different contexts, including social media [78], mobile application permission [67,79], and Internet of Things (IoT) [6,10,11,21,27,37,52]. For example, Choe et al. [21], through a survey, found that self-appearance, intimacy, cooking and eating, media use, oral expression, personal hygiene, physical activity, and sleep are among the most frequently mentioned categories people would not want to be recorded at home. Emami-Naeini et al. [27], Barbosa et al. [11], and Apthorpe et al. [6] found that safety and security (e.g., an emergency situation) was a prominent reason, on the other hand, that people generally would approve data collection and sharing. Similarly, Lee and Kobsa [52] and Bahirat et al. [10] have found that people would be more willing to disclose information for a health-related reason.

Additionally, there are numerous studies that attempt to create one taxonomy or classification scheme that will be appropriate for all users. For example, Li et al. [54] used Mechanical Turk to create a taxonomy of "sensitive" photo features that classifiers could use to suggest photos that every user would not want to share. Others have developed ontologies of IoT sensors or healthcare devices (e.g., [7,43,57,90]) to support privacy protection in larger IoT environments (e.g., hospitals or offices).

Finally, there are a handful of studies that examine user-generated groupings for privacy, such as using groups of locations to create privacy settings for mobile applications (Toch et al. [82]) and a set of privacy profiles for social media and marketing use (Knijnenburg [47]). These studies attempt to create groupings that work for all individuals. As far as we know, there are no studies that examine whether having users group the types of data for themselves might help users, especially in healthcare settings. In this paper, we examine the possibility of using user-generated groupings of EDC to simplify sharing in a pervasive health care environment.

3   Methods

3.1   Participants and Recruitment

The goal of our study was to understand whether groupings of everyday data for care (EDC) could be created by users for simplifying data sharing with care team members in a chronic care setting. To obtain an initial understanding of whether such groupings were possible and potentially useful, we invited participants with different backgrounds to participate in our study. Anyone can potentially have a severe chronic condition later in their lives. However, we specifically encouraged people with caregiving experience or people with a close family member who has a chronic condition to participate so that their understanding of care and navigating health challenges for a range of chronic conditions could be properly brought into the discussion on EDC sharing.

Participants were recruited in the U.S. through university mailing lists and personal networks. We recruited 25 participants, all of whom had college degrees (or above) or were currently enrolled in a college program. There were 21 females and 4 males, with ages between 18 to 63 (22 as the median). Among the participants, 24 (out of 25) participants had either caregiving experience or at least one close family member with a chronic condition (see Table 2 in the Appendix for more details, including background). We excluded the data from P20 as P20 only provided partial data for this study. Participants with caregiving experience had provided care for people with a range of conditions, including epilepsy, autism, auto-immune disease, severe motor impairment, traumatic brain injury, and stroke.

3.2   Study Design

The study used card sorting followed by semi-structured interviews to investigate the possibility of using user-generated groupings for managing the sharing of EDC. As participants might not have had experience sharing a diverse list of EDC, using the card sorting allowed participants to engage in the process of comparing different EDC types before creating sharing settings. The semi-structured interviews allowed the research investigator to follow up with participants to understand the process of grouping and sharing EDC. All the study activities were done remotely through video conferencing software (i.e., Zoom [96]) and an online whiteboard platform (i.e., Miro [62]).

To properly help participants consider sharing data in a specific chronic care context, we presented each participant with a scenario that described a person with spinal cord injury and disorder (SCI/D). The scenario was designed to introduce the setting of a particular kind of severe chronic care that requires a care team to assist the person. Many people with SCI/D utilize moderately sized care teams (8–25 people), whose members have different roles and expertise. Furthermore, monitoring ongoing health concerns would be beneficial for many people with SCI/D [19,61]. The scenario was realistic for our purposes: As sensors become more and more available in a pervasive health care environment, people and caregivers will have to make data sharing and privacy decisions.

In this scenario, the person was injured severely as the result of a car accident. The person then required assistance from caregivers and health professionals to manage her health and everyday life throughout her lifetime (chronic care). The participants were asked to put themselves in the role of this person during the study to consider how they would group data about different aspects of their lives for sharing with a list of care team members. This list includes primary care-givers (e.g., family members such as a parent or a spouse), secondary caregivers (e.g., family members who occasionally help), hired caregivers, primary care physicians, psychotherapists, physical therapists, healthcare system/hospital IT workers, a nurse (e.g., from a spinal cord clinic), and an Emergency Room doctor.

A list of EDC was presented as everyday data for care that could be useful to share with care team members to support monitoring and diagnosis. Participants were first asked to review the list of EDC types and to understand the details captured in EDC. Inspired by prior work on people's attitudes toward sharing data [18,21,64] and common care activities for people with SCI/D and their care teams [1,19,20,61], 32 types of data were selected, which covered a range of aspects of a person's life and her health condition (see Table 1).

Participants were asked to sort the data types into 5 bins based on how comfortable they were in sharing data with their care teams, from bin 1 (most comfortable) to bin 5 (least comfortable). We did not define "comfort", but let participants supply their own definition. This ambiguity has been found to be useful in many card sorting studies (e.g., [13, p. 269] and [12, p. 249]).

Table 1. Selection of data types

Computer game	Exercise	Fluid intake	Flatulence
Food/diet	Hanging out	Heart rate	Internet history
Intimate behavior	Location	Loneliness	Medication
Messages	Mobile app usage	Mood	Conversational dialogs
Pain	Phone calls	Stool	Recreational drug use
Relaxation	Religious behavior	Romantic dates	Skin condition
Sleep	Smoking	Social media status	Stress
Urine	Video use	Weight	Work activity

This list of EDC types was entered into Miro [62] as digital cards for sorting (See Fig. 1 in the Appendix). In this paper, we will use "bins" to denote the pre-determined number of containers given to every participant in the Miro-based card sort, and use "groupings" to denote the resulting collections of data types, which may be different for every participant, in the various bins.

Prior work on design for chronic care has suggested how changes in a person's health requires the care team to revise care routines (e.g., maintain proper fluid intake) and hence the use of data (e.g., monitoring) [19,38]. We used three situations (see below) in our study to examine whether EDC groupings could be used to support sharing when there were changes in health, and whether there were patterns that could be useful for simplifying EDC sharing.

- New normal: a regular day living with the chronic condition.
- Something going on: exhibiting new symptoms with the causes unknown.
- Emergency: feeling ill and being rushed to the emergency room.

After observing participants' sorting with a think-aloud protocol, we then conducted semi-structured interviews to understand how easy or difficult it was to group the EDC, and how these groupings could be useful for expressing sharing settings with different care team members under different care situations.

The guiding questions for the interviews were, for the presented scenario:

- How would you describe the data in this grouping?
- Were there data that were tricky to assign to a grouping? What were they (walking through each grouping)?
- When you stated how you would share data with this care team member (walking through each potential recipient), what went through your mind?
- When you stated how you would share data in this care situation (walking through each potential recipient), how was it different than the other situations?

3.3   Data Analysis

We used Clarke's Situational Analysis [24], an updated version of Grounded Theory, to analyze the interview transcripts and think-aloud data. Open coding was applied to interview notes and transcripts using Atlas.ti [34] to generate initial themes. The authors discussed themes and categories through weekly meetings to identify emerging themes. Analytic memos were written summarizing the emerging themes, and themes that emerged were used to re-code all the transcripts to maintain consistency. This process was repeated iteratively.

Participants who successfully finished the study were compensated with a $20 e-gift card for their time and effort. This study was reviewed by our university's Institutional Review Board. Any data presented here have been anonymized; we have lightly edited some of the data presented here for presentation clarity.

4   Findings

In this section, we describe our participants' sharing preferences for EDC generated in a pervasive healthcare environment. We provide a description of whether our participants were able to group the set of EDC types, as well as how any groupings were used to express sharing settings both with different care team members and in varying care situations. We start with a description of how our participants grouped data types and whether they found these groupings useful and usable.

4.1   Grouping EDC is Usable and Useful

In our study, we asked our participants to perform a card sorting activity to put a list of EDC types into 5 bins, telling them to sort the types by their "comfort" of sharing that data with care team members (1: most comfortable, 5: least comfortable).

The participants were able to utilize the bins to group the EDC types. Figure 2 in the Appendix visualizes how participants grouped the data types. Three things leap out. First, all 5 bins were used by nearly all participants. In fact, only P01 excluded bin 5, while all other participants distributed the EDC to all 5 bins. Participants were at ease in doing so, as their think-aloud data indicated.

Second, there was some agreement among participants about the contents of each bin, but overall the contents could differ widely. Participants put largely physiological data in bin 1, as can be seen in Fig. 2, and all participants felt most comfortable sharing that data. (Remember this was in a scenario about health care.) Bin 5 tended to include deeply personal data, such data about sexual activity or drug use, and was not shared frequently:

> Um, religious behavior, I don't really see the health relationship with my health, but I guess I would worry about how people perceive me based on religious practice. (P19)

and

> These data [phone calls, social media messages, and recreational drug use] are the most personal. We don't share that with people that often. (P08)

However, the contents in bins 2–4 varied widely. There was some consistency. For example, phone calls were commonly assigned to bins 4 and 5 but also to other bins. If we look at how often participants used the same bin, one can see the variation: One data type (i.e., heart rate) was assigned to adjacent bins (i.e., within one bin of one another); 4 data types are assigned to one of consecutive three bins, but the rest of the 27 data types were assigned to more than three. For example, participants differed on their comfort level with sharing data such as smoking and location, where they could be placed by different participants in bins 1 through 5:

> Mostly like loneliness, relaxation, stress, work, and mood, I was mostly considering whether it was important for them [the care team members] to know that... and whether I would want to share that. (P24)

It follows that some EDC types were likely to be collocated within a grouping. For instance, heart rate and pain as well as stool and urine were pairs of data types that typically were put into the same grouping. On the other hand, heart rate and intimate behavior were less likely to be put into the same grouping, as people typically considered sharing data about intimate behavior to be uncomfortable.

Admittedly, some participants did signal that they found some EDC types to be challenging to assign to a specific grouping, resulting in ambivalence about the correct grouping. Note this ambivalence was not about what was uncomfortable to share per se – they could assign a data type that was uncomfortable to share to bin 5 (the most uncomfortable). Debating what grouping to which to assign a type was relatively uncommon, and what types were challenging was idiosyncratic to the individual.

Some participants who were found themselves ambivalent about a grouping indicated that their ambivalence resulted when a EDC type's potential connection to health and the benefits of sharing were unclear to them:

> I think maybe weight and work, that are the ones I am debating,... because it's not like... the most embarrassing thing and it is for your health... but I am still hesitant. [P21]

This ambivalence, however, only adds to the difficulty of finding *one* set of groupings that will hold across all users. The differences in individuals' binning could be significant; our participants did not agree on what EDC data types should go in a specific bin (i.e., a comfort level). Figure 2 in the Appendix shows the variance in the groupings. Because of this variance, it is unlikely that any *one* taxonomy or classification scheme will suit all users.

Regardless, individuals were able to group the data types for themselves, suggesting that groupings could be potentially usable. While some participants needed to deliberate slightly more about a relatively small set of data, they were able to settle quickly. In other words, sorting EDC into groupings based on comfort level was a rather doable process for our participants.

Somewhat to our surprise, while our participants did not always agree on the types that went into each comfort grouping, these groupings seemed useful for themselves to allocate data to care team members. (To make it clear that we are talking about the individuals' set of groupings, we will call these "user-groupings".) *That is, once participants grouped the data types, they were able to use those user-groupings to describe their sharing preferences for different care-team members and care situations efficiently*, finding the grouping they did useful and usable for themselves. This strongly suggests their own groupings could be used to reduce the number of data sharing or privacy policies that users might need to construct and maintain.

In summary, participants were able to put EDC into groupings based on how comfortable they were in sharing these EDC with care team members. These groupings were idiosyncratic enough to each individual that one classification scheme for all users is impossible or unlikely. While the exact data types in each grouping varied from individual to individual, the user-groupings appeared to be useful, since each individual participant was able to use her groupings consistently as units in expressing sharing settings.

Below we will discuss how participants used the groupings to deal with the subtleties of who might receive the data, namely by varying the groupings specific recipients could see. We will then deal with how participants also used the user-groupings to share data when the patient's health situation changed.

4.2 Utility of Groupings for Sharing Within a Care Team

Many patients with SCI/D, as discussed above, rely on care teams. For a condition such as SCI/D, patients might experience different degrees of neurological impairment, and for those with more severe conditions, they often require a care team to assist with different tasks in everyday life. Sharing EDC within the care team would allow team members to collaboratively monitor the patient's health and handle changes that might arise.

The care team for a patient with SCI/D is not homogeneous. Primary care givers, who are likely to be parents or spouses, are generally trusted more than paid or volunteer caregivers. Secondary care givers, such as siblings or other relatives, may lie between primary care givers and paid caregivers. Care teams may also involve a range of clinicians including different kinds of doctors, nurses, physical and occupational therapists, and the like. In this section, we described how the user-created groupings (user-groupings) were useful for sharing data with different care team roles.

In the process of determining what EDC to share with different care team members, the user-groupings provided guidance for our participants to quickly identify what to share with a particular care team member. Instead of considering every single EDC type, the user-groupings served as units for our participants in their evaluations of what to share. Indeed, participants often considered multiple groupings at the same time for inclusion or exclusion. For instance, P02 commented on how she decided what to share with the primary caregiver and paid caregivers; she excluded three groupings at once and decided to share the other two groupings:

> I think [groupings] 3 to 5 is like more personal... The first group... everyone in my team should know. The second group ... I spend most of time with primary caregivers and hired caregivers, so I would like to share [data about] my life [in group 2 for this participant] with them. [P02]

Similarly, P03 explained how she would share EDC with her primary care doctor by including and excluding the groupings she created.

> For my primary care doctor, this one is more like... they [have to] kind of know my condition overall. That is why I share [up to] group 3, so that they would have a basic idea of how I feel and how my physical body works [groupings 1 and 2 for this participant], but they don't necessarily need to know my personal activities [groupings 4 and 5 for this participant]. (P03)

As shown in the comments above, our participants found their EDC user-groupings, created based on comfort level, were useful units for determining sharing with specific care team members. In the study tasks, our participants went through each role and decided what groupings to share. (See Table 3 in the Appendix for the set of roles given to participants in the study tasks.) Only two participants deviated from using their initial user-created groupings, and they did so only once each.

That is, with the exception of P06 and P07, participants did not feel the need to restart the grouping process in order to specify sharing preferences for each role.

These user-generated groupings are by no means perfect, as some groupings might contain data that were not as relevant for a given care team personnel. Participants might decide to share the whole group when (1) there were data that were relevant or even critical to share, and (2) they don't feel strong discomfort for sharing those less relevant data.

> Data such as loneliness, religious behavior, social media [, some data types from those groupings I share)... I would be more comfortable sharing these data with psychotherapists because they are more socially and mentally oriented. They probably wouldn't need to know my skin conditions [a data type from those groupings I share), but I would be comfortable with them knowing more. [P10]

Again, we stress that the exact groupings for any given individual are not what is interesting here – it is, instead, that individually participants were able to reuse these user-groupings to create sharing settings without major challenges or re-grouping.

While our participants were able to use their groupings for assigning sharing to care team roles, we acknowledge that a role is quite abstract. Sharing may differ from abstract roles (e.g., paid caregiver) to specific individuals (e.g., Sally, a specific person who has been with the patient for a decade). Changes to the groupings might be required, for example, to allow different sharing settings for different individuals in the same role. Changes might also be required as patients or caregivers better understand their sharing and privacy needs; this could be seen with P06 and P07, who changed their groupings in specific study tasks. However, we must note that the groupings would still be useful in jump-starting a process of customization. We will return to this point in the Discussion.

In summary, our participants found the user-created groupings of EDC useful for deciding how to share EDC with a specific care team roles. One major benefit for participants was to use the groupings to quickly assess the sharing threshold for a given recipient. Participants were able to consider multiple EDC at the same time, without the need to examine every single EDC type for each recipient, which for this number or slightly more care team members or sensors would have been an overwhelming task.

4.3   Utility of Groupings for Sharing with Changes in Health Condition

Chronic care involves working with a care team to address any health changes over time. To design support for people to control EDC sharing for severe chronic care contexts, for example SCI/D, it is critical to understand how sharing preferences might change across care situations. We prompted participants to express their preferences about sharing EDC in three care situations: a regular day (the baseline condition), a situation where something may be starting to affect the patient's health, and an emergency. We found that these user-groupings created based on comfort level for sharing, again, provides a good framework for participants to decide what EDC data to share in different care situations. We also found that the care situation did affect the threshold for sharing (i.e., sharing up to grouping X), generally in a positive direction as the patient's health condition deteriorated. In other words, people are inclined to share either the same or additional groupings of EDC when their health situations escalate in severity.

Table 4 in the Appendix shows how sharing increased as the health needs were perceived to have become greater. We show the sharing threshold (i.e., the highest grouping that will be shared) for primary and paid caregivers, as well as two doctors, the primary care physician and an Emergency Room doctor.

For departures from a regular day (i.e., when there is a change in the patient's health), the necessity of sharing increases. Such an increase is motivated by the need to have more people monitoring a patient and help with care and treatment, including both medical professionals and non-medical care team members. As seen in Table 4 in the Appendix, participants tended to keep or raise the threshold for each care team member in order to share more with each of them so as to allow EDC to flow smoothly to care team members. On average, 30% of the care team members were given access to all data (group 1 to group 5) in when there were changes in health (i.e., the something going on situation), a 5% increase from the normal situation.

> The data is important for them [primary care doctors] to make medical decisions. Hopefully, they are working in my best interest. ...so a proper decision is made for my health. (P19)

> Even if they [hired caregivers] are college kids without medical training, they might be like the next best option [when there is a health change and other caregivers are not around]. (P13)

Participants wanted to share the most data in emergency situations. On average, 56% of the care team members were given access to all data (group 1 to group 5).

There were only two exceptions to the general trend, sharing the same or more data when the situation worsened. P25 preferred sharing rather limited data with primary caregivers, secondary caregivers, and psychotherapists when her health deteriorated (in the something going on condition). P16 preferred to maintain a sense of control when there was a non-threatening change (i.e., something going on), but would let go of the control and entrust recipients with more data in an emergency when her life was at stake. Both P16 and P25 explained that a lack of medical expertise and the situation (e.g., health deterioration) were the main factors for such adjustments. For instance, primary caregivers, who were highly involved in care but were considered to have less medical expertise, were given even fewer EDC groupings in an emergency compared to a regular day.

Again, our results showed that the user-generated EDC groupings appear to be a useful way for people to express sharing preferences – this time across care situations. As people's health changed, the inclination to share more EDC was observed at the grouping level: participants either share the same groupings or share more groupings of EDC, as the people's health condition escalates.

5   Discussion

Repeatedly in our study, we saw evidence that our participants could bin EDC data types into groupings based on a criteria of "comfort". *We also observed them reusing those user-generated groupings. The groupings differed from individual to individual, but one's groupings appeared to be valuable for the individual participant.* These groupings were not perfect, but seemed to be robust enough to support EDC sharing configuration. Few participants changed their groupings when setting up privacy and data sharing, and more importantly, they constructed a number of nuanced settings using them in a number of study tasks. Our participants were able to use these user-groupings to select what EDC to share with different care team members and in changing health conditions.

As far as we know, these findings have not been studied or observed before. These findings need to be confirmed, but they suggest that these user-groupings could be a valuable tool in easing the burden of dealing with the increasing amount of sensors and EDC data in a pervasive healthcare environment. Our study substantially extends the ideas of Toch et al. [82], Knijnenburg [47], and Li et al. [54]. Toch et al., Knijnenburg, and Li et al. merely examined user-generated taxonomies that were supposed to fit everyone; we found that such taxonomies are not likely to do as well as individualizing groupings. We, on the other hand, showed that user-groupings (i.e., individualized groupings) could be useful for configuring data sharing (e.g., of EDC).

In the next subsections, we consider the possibilities we believe our study uncovered – namely, the semi-automatic configuration of data sharing – as well as the potential limitations of this study and future work.

5.1   Creating Semi-automatic Assistance

The findings above strongly suggest that allowing people with health conditions or their caregivers the ability to bin EDC data types creates valuable shortcuts and forms of assistance to people and caregivers in creating and potentially maintaining privacy and data sharing settings. A wizard-like mechanism would allow the simple binning of EDC data types and then the creation of straight-forward sharing rules.

Future work could also apply the methodologies proposed by Knijnenburg [47] and Li et al. [54] to investigate semi-automated approaches for EDC shar-ing configuration, where sharing profiles could be extracted from some user-generated groupings and applied to new types of data. The individual differences we observed, however, indicate that some user involvement will be necessary. For users, allowing them to further customize automatically generated settings would still be easier than creating settings from scratch.

In addition to the possibility of using user-generated groupings for data shar-ing configuration [47,83], our findings further suggest that such groupings could be reused across different care situations, which is important in severe chronic care as care team members need to collaboratively monitor and adapt to changes in health and care [19,69]. Reusing groupings in different health situations would reduce the user burden of configuration, again reiterating the utility of such user-generated groupings for the chronic care context.

Finally, extending the findings of prior work that suggest safety and health could be reasons for people to share data [6,10,11,27,52], our findings further demonstrate that in the context of chronic care, people have the general tendency to share more at the grouping level when health problems escalate. Architec-tures or frameworks designed to support EDC data management should consider explicitly supporting the interaction between care situations and the threshold of comfort for sharing. For instance, having a system that made suggestions of sharing settings, potentially with customization, would ease the burden of people with health conditions or their caregivers. This would avoid the burden of cre-ating separate settings for different health situations. Future work may uncover similar tendencies for roles. For example, the sharing with a secondary caregiver (e.g., a family member) will likely be a superset of the sharing with a hired caregiver. Such tendencies based on user-generated groupings of recipients (e.g., roles) could provide further simplification of EDC sharing to empower patients in directing their care [9,20,23,29,63,76].

5.2 Limitations and Future Work

There are several potential limitations to this work.

Our exploratory study used non-probability sampling, but we believe our study has theoretical generalizability [24]: The use of user-generated groupings without requesting major changes was prevalent in this study. Yet, while we were careful when prompting participants to double-check that they were satisfied with their groupings, it is admittedly an unknown and surprising result. We do recognize that to gain widespread acceptance in health informatics or in medicine, additional studies, especially empiricist studies, will be required.

Additionally, we provide a pre-determined number of bins to guide the EDC grouping process. While the number seems to provide a good scaffolding for par-ticipants in our study, future studies could consider systematically examining other numbers to structure the grouping process. One direction worth exploring could be to identify whether there exists an ideal range where the resultant number of groupings is still manageable (under a certain threshold) while providing enough distinction (above a certain threshold) that supports the necessary differential treatment for different care team members and under different situations.

In this study, we asked participants, who understand the care context (i.e., through caregiving or having a close family member with a chronic condition) but were not people with health conditions (except one), to role-play a person with a health condition. This allowed us to obtain initial results about whether EDC could be shared in groups to simplify sharing configurations and to understand considerations participants have when sharing EDC in groups. However, we acknowledge that people with health conditions might have additional perspectives on the utility of user-groupings. Future studies should examine using people with health conditions as well to develop a more thorough understanding.

Moreover, as we noted earlier in this paper, we asked about sharing with abstract roles, but real sharing occurs with specific people in specific contexts. This issue remains for future studies to reaffirm the usefulness of user-groupings.

As well, we examined only the ambiguously-defined criteria of "comfort" in this study, and participants were clear that "comfort" included understanding how the data might be used in a care context. Future work should examine these and additional factors related to the care context to guide user-grouping creation.

Finally, our findings were generated through a one-time engagement with participants. In reality, supporting chronic care, by definition, will engender a different style of engagement across a longer period of time. Future studies should examine how stable these user-generated groupings are and factors that necessitate changes in these groupings. It is also possible that the attitudes toward sharing these EDC data types might change for people with health conditions as they encounter different events in their health journeys and develop a better understanding of the benefits and risks of sharing. Future research could consider exploring machine-initiated intervention (e.g., using intelligent agents [31]) that will periodically examine EDC groupings and call for attention (e.g., check-in after a new development in one's health). This method could be integrated with other methods that provide an estimate of a person's understanding and expertise in EDC (e.g., using expertise estimation based on user behavior logs [39]). The integrated approach will allow adjustments based on people's educational backgrounds or experiences to allow interactive systems to reassess whether and what aspects of the EDC groupings need to be modified to reflect people's preferences and expertise.

6   Conclusion

Our work aims to support patients and their caregivers in a pervasive healthcare environment through controlling their sharing of Everyday Data for Care (EDC), specifically in the context of severe chronic conditions that require a care team and healthcare over time. This paper presented findings that examine how to help users set sharing and privacy preferences for EDC. Through a scenario-based study with think-aloud card sorting and semi-structured interviews, we found that our participants were able to use self-generated groupings of EDC data, and more importantly, kept those groupings, with only minor exceptions, when creating sharing settings for potential recipients and when dealing with changes in the health trajectory. The major contribution from this work was the surprising and speculative finding that users could garner assistance from their user-generated groupings of EDC data. This work offers hope that we can reduce the burden of authoring and maintaining data sharing and privacy policies through semi-automatic mechanisms, where the system suggests policies that are consistent with the users' preferences - especially as health changes and especially in difficult chronic care.

A   Appendix

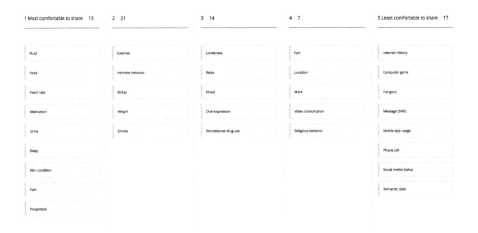

Fig. 1. Participants created groupings of EDC by the level of comfort from the most comfortable (bin 1 on the left) to the least comfortable (bin 5 on the right).

Table 2. Participant description: "Caregiver" (C) refers to a participant who has caregiving experience (including as a nursing professional), "person"(P) refers to "a person with a chronic condition and/or a disability", and "PFC" refers to "a person with a close family member who has a chronic condition".

	Age	Gender	Background	Occupation	Experience
P01	26–30	F	Fashion	Student	PFC
P02	26–30	F	Counseling	Research assistant	C
P03	26–30	F	Linguistic	Student	PFC
P04	31–35	F	Education	Instructional designer	PFC
P05	26–30	M	Computer Science	Software engineer	PFC
P06	31–35	M	Computer Science	UX designer	PFC
P07	36–40	M	Social Work	Social worker	C
P08	31–35	F	Linguistic	Student	No
P09	31–35	M	Computer Science	Student	PFC
P10	18–25	F	Nursing	Student	C
P11	18–25	F	Nursing	Patient Care Technician	C
P12	18–25	F	Nursing	Student	C
P13	18–25	F	Nursing	Patient Care Technician	C
P14	18–25	F	Nursing	Student	C
P15	18–25	F	Nursing	Nurse aide	C
P16	18–25	F	Nursing	Nursing assistant	C
P17	18–25	F	Nursing	Student	C
P18	18–25	F	Nursing	Student	C
P19	18–25	F	Nursing	Student	C
P20	61–65	F	Nursing	Clinical nurse educator	C
P21	18–25	F	Nursing	Student	C
P22	26–30	F	Psychology	Care navigator	P & C
P23	18–25	F	Nursing	Student	C
P24	18–25	F	Nursing	Student	C
P25	18–25	F	Nursing	Student	C

Table 3. EDC groupings shared with different care team roles: primary caregiver (primary), secondary caregiver (secondary), hired or paid caregiver (hired), primary care physician (PCP), psychotherapist (psych), physical therapist (PT), and healthcare system IT specialist (IT). The value represents the highest grouping shared. The last column shows whether a participant adjusted groupings in the process of creating sharing settings. (P20 was omitted since their data was partial.)

	Primary	Second	Hired	PCP	Psych	PT	IT	Grouping changes
P01	3	4	2	2	3	2	0	No
P02	2	3	2	1	2	1	1	No
P03	5	5	3	3	3	1	2	No
P04	5	2	1	3	3	2	2	No
P05	5	3	2	4	5	2	1	No
P06	4	4	4	3	1	1	0	Yes
P07	5	4	3	3	5	3	2	Yes
P08	2	2	2	2	2	2	2	No
P09	4	4	1	5	4	3	3	No
P10	3	1	3	3	4	2	0	No
P11	5	5	5	5	5	5	5	No
P12	2	2	2	5	5	5	1	No
P13	3	4	4	4	5	2	1	No
P14	4	3	2	3	5	2	1	No
P15	2	2	2	5	5	5	0	No
P16	5	2	2	3	5	2	1	No
P17	3	3	3	5	4	3	2	No
P18	2	2	4	3	5	3	1	No
P19	3	0	0	2	2	1	1	No
P21	5	2	3	5	5	2	0	No
P22	3	3	3	4	5	2	2	No
P23	2	2	2	5	4	3	5	No
P24	5	5	1	4	4	1	0	No
P25	3	3	0	2	3	2	0	No

Table 4. EDC groupings shared with care team roles increase when health situation deteriorates. Roles include: primary caregiver (PC), hired caregiver (HC), primary care physician (PCP), and emergency room doctor (ERD). The health situations included a regular day (Normal), when symptoms begin to emerge (Symptom), and an emergency requiring a trip to the ER (Emergency). We did not include the hired caregiver role in the emergency situation in our study; we omit participants for which we have only partial data.

Participant	Normal			Symptoms			Emergency		
	PC	HC	PCP	PC	HC	PCP	PC	HC	ERD
P06	4	4	3	4	4	4	4		4
P07	5	3	3	5	4	5	5		5
P08	2	2	2	2	2	3	2		3
P09	4	1	5	4	2	5	4		4
P10	3	3	3	3	3	3	4		4
P11	5	5	5	5	5	5	5		5
P12	2	2	5	2	2	5	5		5
P13	3	4	4	3	5	5	3		5
P14	4	2	3	5	3	5	5		5
P15	2	2	5	2	2	5	2		5
P16	5	2	3	3	2	5	3		5
P17	3	3	5	4	4	5	5		5
P18	2	4	3	2	4	3	2		3
P19	3	0	2	3	0	2	4		4
P21	5	3	5	5	3	5	5		5
P22	3	3	4	4	3	4	5		5
P23	2	2	5	3	3	5	4		5
P24	5	1	4	5	1	4	5		4
P25	3	0	2	2	0	2	2		2

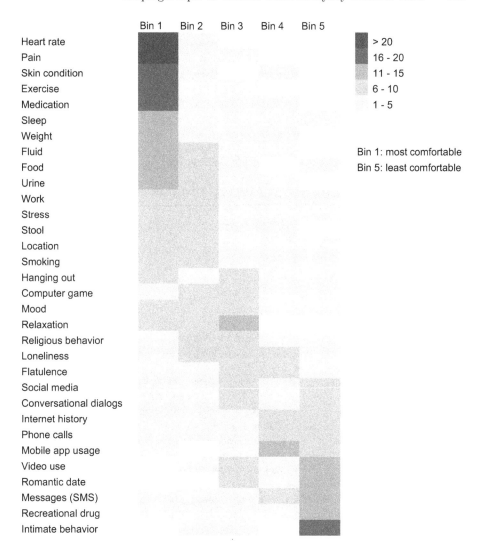

Fig. 2. Heatmap showing how frequently participants assigned an EDC type to each bin. Very light pink 1–5, light pink 6–10, medium pink 5–10, dark pink 11–15, red 16–20, dark red >20 (n = 24). Some participants omitted because of partial data. (Color figure online)

References

1. Ackerman, M.S., Büyüktür, A.G., Hung, P.-Y., Meade, M.A., Newman, M.W.: Socio-technical design for the care of people with spinal cord injuries. In: Designing Healthcare That Works, pp. 1–18. Elsevier (2018)
2. Ackerman, M.S., et al.: Simplifying user-controlled privacy policies. IEEE Pervasive Comput. **8**, 28–32 (2009)

3. Almuhimedi, H., et al.: Your location has been shared 5,398 times!: a field study on mobile app privacy nudging. In: Proceedings of the 33rd Annual ACM Conference on Human Factors in Computing Systems, CHI 2015, pp. 787–796. ACM, New York (2015). https://doi.org/10.1145/2702123.2702210. http://doi.acm.org/10.1145/2702123.2702210

4. Amir, O., Grosz, B.J., Gajos, K.Z., Swenson, S.M., Sanders, L.M.: From care plans to care coordination: opportunities for computer support of teamwork in complex healthcare. In: Proceedings of the 33rd Annual ACM Conference on Human Factors in Computing Systems, CHI 2015, pp. 1419–1428. ACM, New York (2015). https://doi.org/10.1145/2702123.2702320. http://doi.acm.org/10.1145/2702123.2702320

5. Anderson, G.: Chronic care: making the case for ongoing care (2010)

6. Apthorpe, N., Shvartzshnaider, Y., Mathur, A., Reisman, D., Feamster, N.: Discovering smart home internet of things privacy norms using contextual integrity. Proc. ACM Interact. Mob. Wearable Ubiquitous Technol. **2**(2), 59:1–59:23 (2018). https://doi.org/10.1145/3214262

7. Arruda, M.F., Bulcão-Neto, R.F.: Toward a lightweight ontology for privacy protection in IoT. In: Proceedings of the 34th ACM/SIGAPP Symposium on Applied Computing, SAC 2019, pp. 880–888. Association for Computing Machinery, New York, April 2019. https://doi.org/10.1145/3297280.3297367

8. Ayobi, A., Marshall, P., Cox, A.L., Chen, Y.: Quantifying the body and caring for the mind: self-tracking in multiple sclerosis. In: Proceedings of the 2017 CHI Conference on Human Factors in Computing Systems, CHI 2017, Denver, Colorado, USA, pp. 6889–6901. Association for Computing Machinery, May 2017. https://doi.org/10.1145/3025453.3025869

9. Bagalkot, N., Sokoler, T.: MagicMirror: towards enhancing collaborative rehabilitation practices. In: Proceedings of the ACM 2011 Conference on Computer Supported Cooperative Work, CSCW 2011, pp. 593–596. ACM, New York (2011). https://doi.org/10.1145/1958824.1958922. http://doi.acm.org/10.1145/1958824.1958922

10. Bahirat, P., He, Y., Menon, A., Knijnenburg, B.: A data-driven approach to developing IoT privacy-setting interfaces. In: 23rd International Conference on Intelligent User Interfaces, IUI 2018, pp. 165–176. ACM, New York (2018). https://doi.org/10.1145/3172944.3172982. http://doi.acm.org/10.1145/3172944.3172982

11. Barbosa, N.M., Park, J.S., Yao, Y., Wang, Y.: "What if?" predicting individual users' smart home privacy preferences and their changes. Proc. Priv. Enhancing Technol. **2019**(4), 211–231 (2019). https://doi.org/10.2478/popets-2019-0066

12. Bernard, H.R.: Research Methods in Anthropology: Qualitative and Quantitative Approaches. Rowman & Littlefield (2017). Google-Books-ID: 2Fk7DwAAQBAJ

13. Bernard, H.R.: Social Research Methods: Qualitative and Quantitative Approaches. SAGE (2000). Google-Books-ID: VDPftmVO5lYC

14. Birnholtz, J., Jones-Rounds, M.: Independence and interaction: understanding seniors' privacy and awareness needs for aging in place. In: Proceedings of the SIGCHI Conference on Human Factors in Computing Systems, CHI 2010, pp. 143–152. ACM, New York (2010). https://doi.org/10.1145/1753326.1753349. http://doi.acm.org/10.1145/1753326.1753349

15. Borders, K., Zhao, X., Prakash, A.: CPOL: high-performance policy evaluation. In: Proceedings of the 12th ACM conference on Computer and communications security, CCS 2005, pp. 147–157. Association for Computing Machinery, New York, November 2005. https://doi.org/10.1145/1102120.1102142

16. Bowser, A., Shilton, K., Preece, J., Warrick, E.: Accounting for privacy in citizen science: ethical research in a context of openness. In: Proceedings of the 2017 ACM Conference on Computer Supported Cooperative Work and Social Computing, CSCW 2017, Portland, Oregon, USA, pp. 2124–2136. Association for Computing Machinery, February 2017. https://doi.org/10.1145/2998181.2998305

17. Bowyer, A., Montague, K., Wheater, S., McGovern, R., Lingam, R., Balaam, M.: Understanding the family perspective on the storage, sharing and handling of family civic data. In: Proceedings of the 2018 CHI Conference on Human Factors in Computing Systems, CHI 2018, pp. 136:1–136:13. ACM, New York (2018). https://doi.org/10.1145/3173574.3173710. http://doi.acm.org/10.1145/3173574.3173710

18. Bélanger, F., Crossler, R.E., Hiller, J.S., Park, J.M., Hsiao, M.S.: POCKET: a tool for protecting children's privacy online. Decis. Support Syst. **54**(2), 1161–1173 (2013). https://doi.org/10.1016/j.dss.2012.11.010. http://www.sciencedirect.com/science/article/pii/S0167923612003429

19. Büyüktür, A.G., Ackerman, M.S., Newman, M.W., Hung, P.-Y.: Design considerations for semi-automated tracking: self-care plans in spinal cord injury. In: Proceedings of the 11th EAI International Conference on Pervasive Computing Technologies for Healthcare, PervasiveHealth 2017, pp. 183–192. ACM, New York (2017). https://doi.org/10.1145/3154862.3154870. http://doi.acm.org/10.1145/3154862.3154870

20. Büyüktür, A.G., Hung, P.-Y., Newman, M.W., Ackerman, M.S.: Supporting collaboratively constructed independence: a study of spinal cord injury. Proc. ACM Hum.-Comput. Interact. **2**(CSCW), 26:1–26:25 (2018). https://doi.org/10.1145/3274295. http://doi.acm.org/10.1145/3274295

21. Choe, E.K., Consolvo, S., Jung, J., Harrison, B., Kientz, J.A.: Living in a glass house: a survey of private moments in the home. In: Proceedings of the 13th International Conference on Ubiquitous Computing, UbiComp 2011, Beijing, China, pp. 41–44. Association for Computing Machinery, September 2011. https://doi.org/10.1145/2030112.2030118

22. Choe, E.K., Lee, N.B., Lee, B., Pratt, W., Kientz, J.A.: Understanding quantified-selfers' practices in collecting and exploring personal data. In: Proceedings of the SIGCHI Conference on Human Factors in Computing Systems, CHI 2014, pp. 1143–1152. ACM, New York (2014). https://doi.org/10.1145/2556288.2557372. http://doi.acm.org.proxy.lib.umich.edu/10.1145/2556288.2557372

23. Chung, C.F., et al.: Identifying and planning for individualized change: patient-provider collaboration using lightweight food diaries in healthy eating and irritable bowel syndrome. Proc. ACM Interact. Mob. Wearable Ubiquitous Technol. **3**(1), 7:1–7:27 (2019). https://doi.org/10.1145/3314394

24. Clarke, A.: Situational Analysis: Grounded Theory After the Postmodern Turn. SAGE Publications, Thousand Oaks (2005)

25. Consolvo, S., Roessler, P., Shelton, B.E., LaMarca, A., Schilit, B., Bly, S.: Technology for care networks of elders. IEEE Pervasive Comput. **3**(2), 22–29 (2004). https://doi.org/10.1109/MPRV.2004.1316814

26. Centers for Disease Control and Prevention: About Chronic Diseases—CDC (2020). https://www.cdc.gov/chronicdisease/about/index.htm

27. Emami-Naeini, P., et al.: Privacy expectations and preferences in an IoT world. In: Thirteenth Symposium on Usable Privacy and Security (SOUPS 2017), pp. 399–412. USENIX Association, Santa Clara (2017). https://www.usenix.org/conference/soups2017/technical-sessions/presentation/naeini

28. Epstein, D.A., Borning, A., Fogarty, J.: Fine-grained sharing of sensed physical activity: a value sensitive approach. In: Proceedings of the 2013 ACM International Joint Conference on Pervasive and Ubiquitous Computing, UbiComp 2013, pp. 489–498. ACM, New York (2013). https://doi.org/10.1145/2493432.2493433. http://doi.acm.org/10.1145/2493432.2493433

29. Felipe, S., Singh, A., Bradley, C., Williams, A.C., Bianchi-Berthouze, N.: Roles for personal informatics in chronic pain. In: 2015 9th International Conference on Pervasive Computing Technologies for Healthcare (PervasiveHealth), pp. 161–168, May 2015. https://doi.org/10.4108/icst.pervasivehealth.2015.259501

30. Figueiredo, M.C., Chen, Y.: Patient-generated health data: dimensions, challenges, and open questions. Found. Trends® Hum.-Comput. Interact. **13**(3), 165–297 (2020). https://doi.org/10.1561/1100000080

31. Fischer, G., Lemke, A.C., Mastaglio, T., Morch, A.I.: Using critics to empower users. In: Proceedings of the SIGCHI Conference on Human Factors in Computing Systems, CHI 1990, pp. 337–347. ACM, New York (1990). https://doi.org/10.1145/97243.97305. http://doi.acm.org/10.1145/97243.97305

32. Fong, P.W.: Relationship-based access control: protection model and policy language. In: Proceedings of the First ACM Conference on Data and Application Security and Privacy, CODASPY 2011, San Antonio, TX, USA, pp. 191–202. ACM, New York (2011). https://doi.org/10.1145/1943513.1943539. http://doi.acm.org/10.1145/1943513.1943539

33. Glasgow, R.E., Anderson, R.M.: In diabetes care, moving from compliance to adherence is not enough. Diab. Care **22**(12), 2090–2092 (1999)

34. Scientific Software Development GmbH: ATLAS.ti: The Qualitative Data Analysis & Research Software (2020). https://atlasti.com/

35. Grönvall, E., Verdezoto, N.: Beyond self-monitoring: understanding non-functional aspects of home-based healthcare technology. In: Proceedings of the 2013 ACM International Joint Conference on Pervasive and Ubiquitous Computing, UbiComp 2013, pp. 587–596. ACM, New York (2013). https://doi.org/10.1145/2493432.2493495

36. Harbach, M., Hettig, M., Weber, S., Smith, M.: Using personal examples to improve risk communication for security & privacy decisions. In: Proceedings of the SIGCHI Conference on Human Factors in Computing Systems, CHI 2014, pp. 2647–2656. ACM, New York (2014). https://doi.org/10.1145/2556288.2556978. http://doi.acm.org/10.1145/2556288.2556978

37. He, Y., Bahirat, P., Knijnenburg, B.P., Menon, A.: A data-driven approach to designing for privacy in household IoT. ACM Trans. Interact. Intell. Syst. (TiiS) **10**(1), 10:1–10:47 (2019). https://doi.org/10.1145/3241378

38. Hong, M.K., Wilcox, L., Machado, D., Olson, T.A., Simoneaux, S.F.: Care partnerships: toward technology to support teens' participation in their health care. In: Proceedings of the 2016 CHI Conference on Human Factors in Computing Systems, CHI 2016, pp. 5337–5349. ACM, New York (2016). https://doi.org/10.1145/2858036.2858508. http://doi.acm.org/10.1145/2858036.2858508

39. Hung, P.-Y., Ackerman, M.S.: Discount expertise metrics for augmenting community interaction. In: Proceedings of the Work-In-Progress Track of the 7th International Conference on Communities and Technologies, vol. 12, pp. 43–52 (2015)

40. Iachello, G., et al.: Control, deception, and communication: evaluating the deployment of a location-enhanced messaging service. In: Beigl, M., Intille, S., Rekimoto, J., Tokuda, H. (eds.) UbiComp 2005. LNCS, vol. 3660, pp. 213–231. Springer, Heidelberg (2005). https://doi.org/10.1007/11551201_13

41. Jacobs, M.L., Clawson, J., Mynatt, E.D.: Comparing health information sharing preferences of cancer patients, doctors, and navigators. In: Proceedings of the 18th ACM Conference on Computer Supported Cooperative Work & Social Computing, CSCW 2015, pp. 808–818. ACM, New York (2015). https://doi.org/10.1145/2675133.2675252. http://doi.acm.org/10.1145/2675133.2675252

42. Junior, M.P., Xavier, S.I.D.R., Prates, R.O.: Investigating the use of a simulator to support users in anticipating impact of privacy settings in Facebook. In: Proceedings of the 18th International Conference on Supporting Group Work, GROUP 2014, pp. 63–72. ACM, New York (2014). https://doi.org/10.1145/2660398.2660419. http://doi.acm.org/10.1145/2660398.2660419

43. Kanaan, H., Mahmood, K., Sathyan, V.: An ontological model for privacy in emerging decentralized healthcare systems. In: 2017 IEEE 13th International Symposium on Autonomous Decentralized System (ISADS), pp. 107–113, March 2017. https://doi.org/10.1109/ISADS.2017.37

44. Kariotis, T., et al.: Emerging health data platforms: from individual control to collective data governance. Data Policy **2** (2020). https://doi.org/10.1017/dap.2020.14

45. Karkar, R., et al.: TummyTrials: a feasibility study of using self-experimentation to detect individualized food triggers. In: Proceedings of the 2017 CHI Conference on Human Factors in Computing Systems, CHI 2017, pp. 6850–6863. ACM, New York (2017). https://doi.org/10.1145/3025453.3025480. http://doi.acm.org/10.1145/3025453.3025480

46. Kelley, P.G., Cranor, L.F., Sadeh, N.: Privacy as part of the app decision-making process. In: Proceedings of the SIGCHI Conference on Human Factors in Computing Systems, CHI 2013, pp. 3393–3402. ACM, New York (2013). https://doi.org/10.1145/2470654.2466466. http://doi.acm.org/10.1145/2470654.2466466

47. Knijnenburg, B.P.: Information disclosure profiles for segmentation and recommendation. In: SOUPS2014 Workshop on Privacy Personas and Segmentation (2014)

48. Kumar, P., Schoenebeck, S.: The modern day baby book: enacting good mothering and stewarding privacy on Facebook. In: Proceedings of the 18th ACM Conference on Computer Supported Cooperative Work & Social Computing, CSCW 2015, Vancouver, BC, Canada, pp. 1302–1312. Association for Computing Machinery, February 2015. https://doi.org/10.1145/2675133.2675149

49. Kumaraguru, P., Cranor, L., Lobo, J., Calo, S.: A survey of privacy policy languages. In: Workshop on Usable IT Security Management (USM 2007): Proceedings of the 3rd Symposium on Usable Privacy and Security. ACM (2007)

50. Könings, B.: User-centered awareness and control of privacy in Ubiquitous Computing. Dissertation, Universität Ulm, July 2015. https://doi.org/10.18725/OPARU-3240. https://oparu.uni-ulm.de/xmlui/handle/123456789/3267

51. Langheinrich, M.: Privacy by design—principles of privacy-aware ubiquitous systems. In: Abowd, G.D., Brumitt, B., Shafer, S. (eds.) UbiComp 2001. LNCS, vol. 2201, pp. 273–291. Springer, Heidelberg (2001). https://doi.org/10.1007/3-540-45427-6_23

52. Lee, H., Kobsa, A.: Privacy preference modeling and prediction in a simulated campuswide IoT environment. In: 2017 IEEE International Conference on Pervasive Computing and Communications (PerCom), pp. 276–285, March 2017. https://doi.org/10.1109/PERCOM.2017.7917874. ISSN 2474-249X

53. Li, I., Dey, A., Forlizzi, J.: A stage-based model of personal informatics systems. In: Proceedings of the SIGCHI Conference on Human Factors in Computing Systems, Atlanta, Georgia, USA, 10–15 April 2010, CHI 2010, pp. 557–566. ACM, New

York (2010). https://doi.org/10.1145/1753326.1753409. http://doi.acm.org.proxy. lib.umich.edu/10.1145/1753326.1753409

54. Li, Y., Vishwamitra, N., Hu, H., Caine, K.: Towards a taxonomy of content sensitivity and sharing preferences for photos. In: Proceedings of the 2020 CHI Conference on Human Factors in Computing Systems, CHI 2020, pp. 1–14. Association for Computing Machinery, New York, April 2020. https://doi.org/10.1145/3313831. 3376498

55. Liu, L.S., et al.: Improving communication and social support for caregivers of high-risk infants through mobile technologies. In: Proceedings of the ACM 2011 Conference on Computer Supported Cooperative Work, CSCW 2011, pp. 475–484. ACM, New York (2011). https://doi.org/10.1145/1958824.1958897. http:// doi.acm.org/10.1145/1958824.1958897

56. Liu, Y., Gummadi, K.P., Krishnamurthy, B., Mislove, A.: Analyzing Facebook privacy settings: user expectations vs. reality. In: Proceedings of the 2011 ACM SIGCOMM Conference on Internet Measurement Conference, pp. 61–70 (2011)

57. Loukil, F., Ghedira-Guegan, C., Boukadi, K., Benharkat, A.N.: LIoPY: a legal compliant ontology to preserve privacy for the Internet of Things. In: 2018 IEEE 42nd Annual Computer Software and Applications Conference (COMPSAC), vol. 02, pp. 701–706, July 2018. https://doi.org/10.1109/COMPSAC.2018.10322. ISSN 0730-3157

58. Luca, A.D., Zezschwitz, E.V.: Usable privacy and security. IT - Inf. Technol. **58**(5), 215–216 (2016). https://doi.org/10.1515/itit-2016-0034. https://www.degruyter. com/document/doi/10.1515/itit-2016-0034/html

59. Mamykina, L., Mynatt, E., Davidson, P., Greenblatt, D.: MAHI: investigation of social scaffolding for reflective thinking in diabetes management. In: Proceedings of the SIGCHI Conference on Human Factors in Computing Systems, CHI 2008, pp. 477–486. ACM, New York (2008). https://doi.org/10.1145/1357054.1357131. http://doi.acm.org/10.1145/1357054.1357131

60. Mazzia, A., LeFevre, K., Adar, E.: The PViz comprehension tool for social network privacy settings. In: Proceedings of the Eighth Symposium on Usable Privacy and Security, SOUPS 2012, pp. 13:1–13:12. ACM, New York (2012). https://doi.org/ 10.1145/2335356.2335374. http://doi.acm.org/10.1145/2335356.2335374

61. Meade, M.A.: Health Mechanics: Tools for the Self-Management of Spinal Cord Injury and Disease. University of Michigan, Ann Arbor (2009)

62. Miro: Miro—Free Online Collaborative Whiteboard Platform (2020). https://miro. com/

63. Murnane, E.L., Walker, T.G., Tench, B., Voida, S., Snyder, J.: Personal informatics in interpersonal contexts: towards the design of technology that supports the social ecologies of long-term mental health management. Proc. ACM Hum.-Comput. Interact. **2**(CSCW), 127:1–127:27 (2018). https://doi.org/10.1145/3274396

64. Nissen, B., et al.: Should I Agree?: delegating consent decisions beyond the individual. In: Proceedings of the 2019 CHI Conference on Human Factors in Computing Systems, CHI 2019, Glasgow, Scotland UK, pp. 515:1–515:13. ACM, New York (2019). https://doi.org/10.1145/3290605.3300745. http://doi.acm.org/ 10.1145/3290605.3300745

65. Nunes, F., Fitzpatrick, G.: Self-care technologies and collaboration. Int. J. Hum.-Comput. Interact. **31**(12), 869–881 (2015). https://doi.org/10.1080/10447318. 2015.1067498

66. Odom, W., Sellen, A., Harper, R., Thereska, E.: Lost in translation: understanding the possession of digital things in the cloud. In: Proceedings of the SIGCHI

Conference on Human Factors in Computing Systems, CHI 2012, Austin, Texas, USA, pp. 781–790. Association for Computing Machinery, May 2012. https://doi. org/10.1145/2207676.2207789

67. Olejnik, K., Dacosta, I., Machado, J.S., Huguenin, K., Khan, M.E., Hubaux, J.P.: SmarPer: context-aware and automatic runtime-permissions for mobile devices. In: 2017 IEEE Symposium on Security and Privacy (SP), pp. 1058–1076, May 2017. https://doi.org/10.1109/SP.2017.25. ISSN 2375-1207

68. World Health Organization: WHO—Integrated chronic disease prevention and control (2020). https://www.who.int/chp/about/integrated_cd/en/

69. Pina, L.R., et al.: From personal informatics to family informatics: understanding family practices around health monitoring. In: Proceedings of the 2017 ACM Conference on Computer Supported Cooperative Work and Social Computing, CSCW 2017, pp. 2300–2315. ACM, New York (2017). https://doi.org/10.1145/2998181. 2998362. http://doi.acm.org/10.1145/2998181.2998362

70. Piras, E.M.: Beyond self-tracking: exploring and unpacking four emerging labels of patient data work. Health Inform. J. **25**(3), 598–607 (2019). https://doi.org/10. 1177/1460458219833121

71. Raber, F., Luca, A.D., Graus, M.: Privacy wedges: area-based audience selection for social network posts. In: Twelfth Symposium on Usable Privacy and Security (SOUPS 2016). USENIX Association, Denver (2016). https://www.usenix.org/ conference/soups2016/workshop-program/wpi/presentation/raber

72. Reeder, R.W., et al.: Expandable grids for visualizing and authoring computer security policies. In: Proceedings of the SIGCHI Conference on Human Factors in Computing Systems, CHI 2008, pp. 1473–1482. ACM, New York (2008). https:// doi.org/10.1145/1357054.1357285. http://doi.acm.org/10.1145/1357054.1357285

73. Sandhu, R.S., Coyne, E.J., Feinstein, H.L., Youman, C.E.: Role-based access control models. Computer **29**(2), 38–47 (1996). https://doi.org/10.1109/2.485845

74. Schaub, F., Könings, B., Lang, P., Wiedersheim, B., Winkler, C., Weber, M.: Pri-Cal: context-adaptive privacy in ambient calendar displays. In: Proceedings of the 2014 ACM International Joint Conference on Pervasive and Ubiquitous Computing, UbiComp 2014, pp. 499–510. ACM, New York (2014). https://doi.org/10. 1145/2632048.2632087. http://doi.acm.org/10.1145/2632048.2632087

75. Schroeder, J., et al.: Examining self-tracking by people with migraine: goals, needs, and opportunities in a chronic health condition. In: Proceedings of the 2018 Designing Interactive Systems Conference, DIS 2018, Hong Kong, China, pp. 135–148. Association for Computing Machinery, June 2018. https://doi.org/10.1145/ 3196709.3196738

76. Schroeder, J., Hoffswell, J., Chung, C.F., Fogarty, J., Munson, S., Zia, J.: Supporting patient-provider collaboration to identify individual triggers using food and symptom journals. In: Proceedings of the 2017 ACM Conference on Computer Supported Cooperative Work and Social Computing, CSCW 2017, pp. 1726–1739. ACM, New York (2017). https://doi.org/10.1145/2998181.2998276. http:// doi.acm.org/10.1145/2998181.2998276

77. Quantified Self: Quantified Self - Self Knowledge Through Numbers. https:// quantifiedself.com/, library Catalog: quantifiedself.com

78. Sharma, A., Cosley, D.: Studying and modeling the connection between people's preferences and content sharing. In: Proceedings of the 18th ACM Conference on Computer Supported Cooperative Work & Social Computing, CSCW 2015, Vancouver, BC, Canada, pp. 1246–1257. Association for Computing Machinery, February 2015. https://doi.org/10.1145/2675133.2675151

79. Smullen, D., Feng, Y., Zhang, S.A., Sadeh, N.: The best of both worlds: mitigating trade-offs between accuracy and user burden in capturing mobile app privacy preferences. Proc. Priv. Enhancing Technol. **2020**(1), 195–215 (2020). https://doi.org/10.2478/popets-2020-0011. https://content.sciendo.com/view/journals/popets/2020/1/article-p195.xml

80. Suh, J., Williams, S., Fann, J.R., Fogarty, J., Bauer, A.M., Hsieh, G.: Parallel journeys of patients with cancer and depression: challenges and opportunities for technology-enabled collaborative care. Proc. ACM Hum.-Comput. Interact. 4(CSCW1), 038:1–038:36 (2020). https://doi.org/10.1145/3392843

81. Thayer, A., Bietz, M.J., Derthick, K., Lee, C.P.: I love you, let's share calendars: calendar sharing as relationship work. In: Proceedings of the ACM 2012 conference on Computer Supported Cooperative Work, CSCW 2012, Seattle, Washington, USA, pp. 749–758. Association for Computing Machinery, February 2012. https://doi.org/10.1145/2145204.2145317. https://doi.org/10.1145/2145204.2145317

82. Toch, E., et al.: Empirical models of privacy in location sharing. In: Proceedings of the 12th ACM International Conference on Ubiquitous Computing, UbiComp 2010, pp. 129–138. Association for Computing Machinery, New York, September 2010. https://doi.org/10.1145/1864349.1864364

83. Toch, E., et al.: Locaccino: a privacy-centric location sharing application. In: Proceedings of the 12th ACM International Conference Adjunct Papers on Ubiquitous Computing - Adjunct, UbiComp 2010, pp. 381–382. Adjunct, ACM, New York (2010). https://doi.org/10.1145/1864431.1864446. http://doi.acm.org/10.1145/1864431.1864446

84. Tolmie, P., Crabtree, A., Rodden, T., Colley, J., Luger, E.: "This has to be the cats": personal data legibility in networked sensing systems. In: Proceedings of the 19th ACM Conference on Computer-Supported Cooperative Work & Social Computing, CSCW 2016, pp. 491–502. ACM, New York (2016). https://doi.org/10.1145/2818048.2819992. http://doi.acm.org/10.1145/2818048.2819992

85. Tsai, L., et al.: Turtle guard: helping android users apply contextual privacy preferences. In: Thirteenth Symposium on Usable Privacy and Security (SOUPS 2017), pp. 145–162. USENIX Association, Santa Clara (2017). https://www.usenix.org/conference/soups2017/technical-sessions/presentation/tsai

86. Van Kleek, M., Liccardi, I., Binns, R., Zhao, J., Weitzner, D.J., Shadbolt, N.: Better the devil you know: exposing the data sharing practices of smartphone apps. In: Proceedings of the 2017 CHI Conference on Human Factors in Computing Systems, CHI 2017, pp. 5208–5220. ACM, New York (2017). https://doi.org/10.1145/3025453.3025556. http://doi.acm.org/10.1145/3025453.3025556

87. Vertesi, J., Kaye, J., Jarosewski, S.N., Khovanskaya, V.D., Song, J.: Data narratives: uncovering tensions in personal data management. In: Proceedings of the 19th ACM Conference on Computer-Supported Cooperative Work & Social Computing, CSCW 2016, pp. 478–490. ACM, New York (2016). https://doi.org/10.1145/2818048.2820017. http://doi.acm.org/10.1145/2818048.2820017

88. Vescovi, M., Perentis, C., Leonardi, C., Lepri, B., Moiso, C.: My data store: toward user awareness and control on personal data. In: Proceedings of the 2014 ACM International Joint Conference on Pervasive and Ubiquitous Computing: Adjunct Publication, UbiComp 2014, pp. 179–182. Adjunct, ACM, New York (2014). https://doi.org/10.1145/2638728.2638745. http://doi.acm.org/10.1145/2638728.2638745

89. Voida, A., Grinter, R.E., Ducheneaut, N., Edwards, W.K., Newman, M.W.: Listening in: practices surrounding iTunes music sharing. In: Proceedings of the SIGCHI

Conference on Human Factors in Computing Systems, CHI 2005, Portland, Oregon, USA, pp. 191–200. Association for Computing Machinery, April 2005. https://doi.org/10.1145/1054972.1054999

90. Wang, S., Hou, Y., Gao, F., Ma, S.: Ontology-based resource description model for Internet of Things. In: 2016 International Conference on Cyber-Enabled Distributed Computing and Knowledge Discovery (CyberC), pp. 105–108, October 2016. https://doi.org/10.1109/CyberC.2016.29

91. Wang, Y., Gou, L., Xu, A., Zhou, M.X., Yang, H., Badenes, H.: VeilMe: an interactive visualization tool for privacy configuration of using personality traits. In: Proceedings of the 33rd Annual ACM Conference on Human Factors in Computing Systems, pp. 817–826. ACM (2015)

92. Wang, Y., Leon, P.G., Acquisti, A., Cranor, L.F., Forget, A., Sadeh, N.: A field trial of privacy nudges for Facebook. In: Proceedings of the SIGCHI Conference on Human Factors in Computing Systems, CHI 2014, pp. 2367–2376. ACM, New York (2014). https://doi.org/10.1145/2556288.2557413. http://doi.acm.org/10.1145/2556288.2557413

93. Westin, A.F.: Privacy and Freedom (1968). Google-Books-ID: EqGAfBTQreMC

94. Yu, S.H., et al.: A mobile mediation tool for improving interaction between depressed individuals and caregivers. Pers. Ubiquitous Comput. **15**(7), 695–706 (2011). https://doi.org/10.1007/s00779-010-0347-z

95. Zhao, J., Binns, R., Van Kleek, M., Shadbolt, N.: Privacy languages: are we there yet to enable user controls? In: Proceedings of the 25th International Conference Companion on World Wide Web, WWW 2016, pp. 799–806. Companion, International World Wide Web Conferences Steering Committee, Republic and Canton of Geneva, CHE, April 2016. https://doi.org/10.1145/2872518.2890590

96. Zoom: Video Conferencing, Web Conferencing, Webinars, Screen Sharing (2020). https://zoom.us/

The Peer Support for Elderly Breast Cancer Patients' Continuing Care at Home Through Smart Service System

Bo Gao[1,2(✉)] and Siying Chen[2]

[1] The Joint NTU-UBC Research Centre of Excellence in Active Living for the Elderly (LILY),
Nanyang Technological University, Singapore, Singapore
bo.gao@ntu.edu.sg
[2] Tongji University, Shanghai, China

Abstract. Breast cancer is the first most frequent cancer and cancer with the highest incidence and the most frequent cancer among women globally. Elderly female patients with breast cancer need peer support to maintain their physiological and psychological health. Strengthening peer support in the continuing care at home requires maintaining the continuation of information between home and hospital, strengthening the relationship between the stakeholders, helping elderly patients recover physically and mentally through enhancing the user experience. We present the progress and results from the research adopted a series of UCD (user-center design) methods since 2018. We did the co-creation workshops with four breast cancer hospitals, 68 breast cancer patients, and eight families to clarify the needs and capture the experience of the patients and family caregivers. We designed the "Bcare," the smart service system for peer support in daily routine care at home based on these research. Through the testing, "Bcare" has been proved to improve the satisfaction of patients and family caregivers' experience and reduce the burden of care for family caregivers.

Keywords: Breast cancer · Continuing care · Peer support · UCD (user-center design) · User experience

1 Introduction

The number of breast cancer patients had reached 2.26 million, becoming the "world's largest cancer" [1]. It is a cancer with the highest incidence and the most frequent cancer among women in the world, with an incidence of 24.2% [2]. After breast cancer surgery, patients need to receive regular long-term physical examinations, once every 3 months within 2 years, every six months for 3–5 years, and once a year after 5 years [3]. The risk of recurrence is two peak periods in the second and fifth years after surgery, and the peak of the former is higher than the latter [4]. The long-term and periodic breast cancer treatment will experience life-long treatment. Many patients began to take it lightly after the 5-year peak of recurrence, which lead to recurrence [6]. Continuing care

H. Lewy and R. Barkan (Eds.): PH 2021, LNICST 431, pp. 302–317, 2022.
https://doi.org/10.1007/978-3-030-99194-4_19

after breast cancer surgery is closely related to the recurrence rate. Elder patients need to switch between the different scenarios, such as hospital, community, and family after breast cancer surgery. Continuing care is to ensure that when patients transfer between different scenarios, the health services they receive are coordinated and continuous, and prevent or reduce the deterioration of the patient's health [5].

The existing medical system in Shanghai mainly deals with acute and sudden medical services, lacks sufficient medical resources to take care of patients after surgery. Breast cancer as the cancer with the reproductive organs, the treatment is affected by social ethics, social relations and self-awareness during rehabilitation [3]. After tracked the data of the breast cancer patients after their recovery for three years in Yangpu Central Hospital Shanghai, China. We found that the hospitals only remind patients of regular physical examinations and medication guidance, but psychological communication needs to be strengthened, especially for targeted counseling based on elderly patients' psychological characteristics. Elderly breast cancer patients often have strong negative psychology and a sense of uncertainty about the disease. The depression rate of elderly patients accounts for 32.76%, which is much higher than that of younger patients [8]. At the same time, elder patients experience a reduction of their social support structure due to life events, such as widowhood and retirement. This may lead to isolation and loneliness, which may exacerbate their emotional response to cancer [9]. Elderly patients have a strong sense of psychological anxiety and need to obtain close and lasting interpersonal relationships [18].

Peer support, which is underpinned by components of social cognitive theory [19] and the theory of planned behavior [20], uses trained individuals who have shared experiences and who provide knowledge, emotional, social and/or practical help to support others. Peer support is mostly used for the management of chronic diseases. In recent years, peer support has been effectively applied to breast cancer continuing care with the trend of "treat cancer as a chronic disease". Peer support creates the necessary emotional communication scenarios to control disease and maintain health, provide social and rehabilitation assistance, and supple other health-care services [10]. Peer support therapy combined with social support can reduce patients' loneliness, assists in the implementation of medical care programs more fully, and improves the quality of patient self-management [12].

The previous research on peer support in China used in the hospital, mainly in offline face-to-face communication with the breast cancer patients, medical staff and volunteers [11]. The face-to-face offline peer support has difficulty continuing for elderly patients or during the isolation in Covid-19 [26]. And previous research on peer support online is mostly conducted in hospitals [13, 14], lacks the research on homecare.

The purpose of this research and the design of "Bcare" are to enhance the peer support for elder breast cancer patients in continuing care service at home. Breast cancer continuing care at home in Shanghai needs to focus on three continuations [7]:

1) The continuation of information refers to patients to ensuring the accuracy of patient information during the referral process in different medical scenarios.
2) The continuation of medical services refers to patients to ensure patients always receive continuous health care throughout the health service system.

3) The continuation of relationship between doctors and nurses, patients and families refer to patients receive services from different health caregivers while maintaining a good relationship between stakeholders.

This paper is divided into the following parts: Sect. 1 introduces some background of peer support in continuing care of breast cancer; Sect. 2 analyzes related works. Section 3 presents the design process of the smart service system, named "Bcare"; Sect. 4 introduces the development and the results of the testing of the design prototype. Section 5 introduces the conclusion and future work.

This paper highlights two key contributions to the field of HCI and UCD for home-care: 1) combined the method of UCD (user-center design) to gain insight into the physical and psychological needs of elder breast cancer patients and their families in homecare, and transfer the insight into the practice design 2) Focus on the special patient groups of elderly breast cancer patients, and explore the use of ICT technology to establish a hospital-community-family peer-supported service system in the informal family care that may inform similar or future research.

2   Related Works

There are four core functions of peer-support in continuing care of breast cancer in the previous research [11]:

1) assist in daily management.
2) provide social and emotional support.
3) establish connections with hospital care and community resources.
4) provide active, flexible, and continuous long-term follow-up service.

At present, in Europe and the United States, peer support combined with the local primary medical systems. Most of the companion support therapy in China used in the hospital, mainly in offline communication with the breast cancer patients, medical staff, and volunteers.

2.1   Peer Support in Offline Communities

Peer support programs which consist of cancer survivors as mentors furnish cancer patients with unique emotional and educational benefits [21, 27]. The research from Japan examining the sources of supportive care in breast cancer illustrated a high need for peer support in addressing medical-psychological, social-spiritual, and sexual needs [22]. The Corsi di Cucina cooking class on healthy diets for cancer patients' families in in Milan. Peer support is mainly the teaching and answering of experts and the sharing and communication between patients and family caregivers. The highlight of peer support is the table sharing the link of cooking teaching results sharing. All stakeholders can easily find topics from the cooking teaching content and the patient's recovery experience and effectively communicate with high emotional concentration.

2.2 Peer Support in Online Communities

The research from Japan explored the differences in peer support received by lurkers and posters in online breast cancer communities. The posters felt they received more benefits from online communities than lurkers did, including emotional support, helping other patients, and expressing their emotions. And the lurkers were found to gain a certain amount of peer support through online communities, especially about advice and insight/universality [13]. In 2017, a study on the discovery of peer support to improve the benefits of breast cancer patients at the Chinese Academy of Medical Sciences and Peking Union Medical College Hospital. It has been proved that most of the positive psychological indicators of the experimental group patients have improved [14].

2.3 Peer Support in Online + offline Communities

The characteristics of China's urban and rural development and the one-child policy have affected the composition of families and communities, making the offline implementation of peer support face greater resistance. At the same time, China's smart medical development and internet penetration quickly, the peer support via online and offline communities can break geographical boundaries, communicate more efficiently and instantly, connect various scenario of patients' lives to ensure the continuity and effectiveness of health services. The Shanghai Cancer Center built the "Yankang e-follow-up" online community in wechat platform, patients and their families can complete preliminary screening, diagnosis, and establish communication with experts through this platform, which is convenient for postoperative chemotherapy, endocrine therapy, medication dispensing, follow-up, etc. [15]. The online community also provides a channel for patients to talk to each other, which relieves patients' psychological anxiety and pressure. Yankang e-follow-up also organizes various offline communities' activities to provide patients with psychological counseling or professional lectures, play a role in alleviating psychological anxiety.

2.4 UCD (User-Center Design) Adopted in Breast Cancer Continuing Care

More medical research results on patients' diseases and treatment experience show that medical services provided from this biomedical perspective alone cannot produce satisfactory results, and interventions from a perspective beyond treatment are required [25]. Users have begun to participate in the process of design and innovation as an indispensable factor, their involvement lead to more effective, efficient and safer products and contributed to the acceptance and success of products [14, 24]. User-centered design (UCD) is a general term for a philosophy and methods which focus on designing for and involving users in the design of computerized systems [23]. The user-centered rule in the medical-related design process has gradually shifted to center on the user experience. UCD (user-center design) has been used in health care, the methods of UCD such as "empathy design", "service design", and "collaborative design", "design thinking" have been developed to integrate the patient's status, experience, and psychological feelings, etc. into the scope of design considerations [15, 16, 28].

The existing projects have helped to establish "peer support" in continuing care, such as the "HOPE" series of continuing care services by the National Breast Cancer Foundation USA. The "HOPE" service helping more stakeholders to support patients build confidence in defeating cancer. The Moira course for breast cancer in Italy follows the EBCD (Experience-based co-design) principles and provides breast cancer patients with opportunities for peer communication to promote the patients' full physical and mental recovery. The "Staying the Course" project designed by the Royal College of Art in 2017, produced a smartphone application to help patients conduct cognitive education, build a bridge between patients and caregivers, and provide relevant information about their specific treatment. In 2018, Northeast Illinois University launched "My Guide", a community-supported method of building applications to help patients with community-based peer support. The Breast Cancer Integrated Care Collaborative (ICC) at North York General Hospital (NYGH) have more than 40 experts, including patients and families, through extensive consultation co-designed the new care model. Using an innovative approach to link medical and support services together, with evidenced-based practice as a lever for change, the ICC was developed to provide a seamless, integrated patient-and family-centred care approach from diagnosis to survivorship.

3 Methods

3.1 UCD (User-Center Design) Adopted in Breast Cancer Continuing Care

Since 2018, we did the multi-discipline research by using UCD (user-center design) in three phases, worked with four breast cancer hospitals, 68 breast cancer patients (the age from 65–80, $\geq$1-month post-treatment), eight families, 18 family caregivers (the age of from 22–46, 9 female and 9 male). The age ranged from 22 to 80 years. Then, we summarized the direction of design from the perspective of patients and family caregivers.

In the investigation phase, we investigated and observed the situation of peer support in the continuing care by the patients, family caregivers, medical staff, and online and offline community organization workers. Then, we conducted structured interviews and semi-structured interviews with selected users, recorded and analyzed the different psychological feelings of patients during the transition of different continuous service scenarios, then gained insights and sum up the needs of patients.

In the design phase: the research team held two co-creation workshops using tool A, B, C, D to develop the patient's journey map of continuing care, patients' information chart and peer support experience chart, and service scenario.

In the evaluation phase, the patients, family caregivers and doctors evaluated the "Bcare" service system prototype.

3.2 UCD (User-Center Design) Tools

We organized two co-creation workshops in discussed the five questions raised by investigation research:

1) The basic information of the patients and the status of peer support in the breast cancer continuing care.
2) The method of the patients do the self-management after the surgery and the role of the family caregiver in this process.
3) The medium for patients to use for recording data in continuing care.
4) The method for family caregivers to obtain patients' information in daily routine care.
5) The patient's experience of participating in the online and offline peer support community in homecare.

There are three participants in the first co-creation workshop, including two patients recovering at home after the operation, one is 54 years old and the other is 72 years old. The 72 years patient's daughter also participated in the workshop as a family caregiver. The workshop lasted two hours. We used tool A, B, C to collect reviews of the pains in body and the comments of the service and activities in the treatment, developed the patient's postoperative treatment journey map, patients' information chart and patient's experience. Based on the first cocreation workshop, we designed tool D and used it in the second co-creation workshop to develop the service scenario. There are nineteen participants, including eight patients recovering at home after the operation (the age from 65–80, ≥1-month post-treatment), and 4 fully-registered, practicing medical staffs (2 doctors and 2 nurses), seven patient's families also participated in the workshop as a family caregiver (the age from 22–46, 4 female and 3 male). Informed consent was obtained from each participant before the workshop. Shopping vouchers worth 100 RMB were received by each participant after the experiment as compensation. Then, we summarized the direction of design from the perspective of patients and family caregivers.

Tool A: To Develop the Patients' Information Chart
Tool A including the panda dolls and rehabilitation record is used to develop patients' information chart. We use panda dolls wearing postoperative lymphatic massage patterns to guide patients and family members to recall their memory of the mental journey after surgery. It worked well as an ice-breaking tool in opening the topic and enlivening the atmosphere. The rehabilitation record lists the questions including patients' habit of making recovery records, the way of patients to record rehabilitation data. From outcome of the patients' information chart, we find that the most important information points need to be recorded are medication, exercise, diet, doctor's advice, recovery time management, and family caregivers should provide supervision and rewards during the continuing care period. The information channels are mainly paper-based newspapers and wechat in mobile phone, a small amount of TV and related reports on health websites (Fig. 1).

Tool B: To Develop the Patient's Continuing Care Journey Map
We used Tool B to develop the patient's continuing care journey map. At first, we used Tool B to guide the participants to share their experience of peer support in continuing care and fill the information into the map. The horizontal headings of Tool A are five

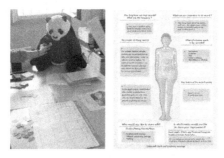

Fig. 1. Tool A including the panda dolls and rehabilitation record to develop the patients' information chart.

phases of the continuous care to be defined by the patient from left to right, and the vertical headings from top to bottom are the specific experiences of peer support, including the patient's actions, ideas, and suggestions. We learned from the conversations between patients and family caregivers that family caregiver learned that the mother was in a state of depression and extreme lack of self-confidence for a long time after surgery. From the patient's continuing care journey map, we found that the patient needs are the assistance of rehabilitation exercise and the sense of companionship throughout the whole continuing care process. The patient's adherence to postoperative self-management stems from the internal drive to reintegrate into the social circle, family caregivers should act in it as the role of encourager and supervisor in homecare (Fig. 2).

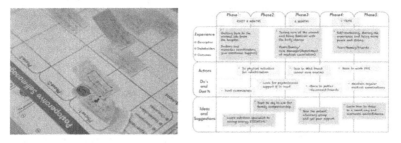

Fig. 2. Tool B is to develop patient's continuing care journey map.

Tool C: To Develop the Peer Support Experience Chart

Tool C is designed to understand the patient's experience of participating in peer support online and offline communities' activities, the relevance of activity types and personal hobbies, and the help that family caregivers can provide during the activities. We selected 12 kinds of activities usually acted in the continuing care, including dance, yoga, online course, sing, massage, art creating, online game, jogging, gardening, storytelling, recipe sharing and book club. We drew these 12 kinds of activities cards for patients to choose 4 of them and set a blank area next to the selection area for patients to fill in freely. Participants can share experiences and thoughts while doing physical exercises (Fig. 3).

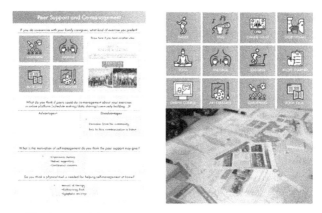

Fig. 3. Tool C is to develop peer support experience chart.

Tool D: To Develop the Service Scenarios

Based on the outcome of the first co-creation workshop, we put forward the design hypotheses and designed tool D and used it in the second co-creation workshop. Tool D includes seven visualized service scenarios, including: access to services, daily records, one meeting a week, good moments, social activities, monthly summaries, and harvest memories. Then we showed the seven service scenario with the explanation of the service story to six patients, four fully-registered, practicing medical staffs (2 doctors and 2 nurses) and seven patient's families. Then, the participations expressed their opinions and used the different colored notes we provided to fill in their opinions. The green notes are from middle-aged postoperative patients, the red notes are from elderly postoperative patients, the orange notes are from family caregivers, and the purple notes are from medical staffs. Based on the perspectives of different stakeholders, we have a deeper understanding of the key points of the adaptability of the adjustment plan, and after adjustments we developed the new service scenario (Fig. 4).

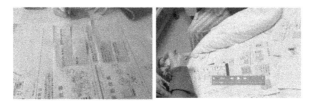

Fig. 4. Tool D is to develop the service scenarios.

3.3   The Direction of the Design

Based on the results of the co-creation workshop, we put forward a framework of the peer support of homecare in continuing care, and use this framework to guide the direction of design. The framework is divided into three steps, peer support norms, peer support cooperation and peer support target. Three steps promote each other, and will continue to update with the social environment changes and technological applications, forming one recycled service. We believe that the concept of "patient-centered" needs to be transformed into "family center", it is important to treat patients and their families as a whole and focus on the cooperation relationship in the family care. The experience of family caregiver will affect the patient's experience and physical and mental recovery. The "family center" is the center of this service system.

Peer support norms is the first step. Patients, family caregivers, and medical staff are aware of the importance of incentive, communication, and accessibility tools, and agree that they are the prerequisites for promoting innovation in peer support services. Peer support cooperation is the second step. Optimizing the interactive experience of patients to families, doctors to patients, and patients to platforms in the service system can promote the completion of the third step. The third step is the peer support target. The peer support target not only requires individual improvement, optimal usage, but also treat the physical and mental health, the individuals and groups patients' health as the holistic health (Fig. 5).

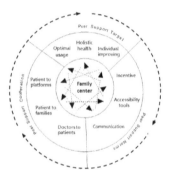

Fig. 5. The framework of the peer support of homecare in continuing care

We summarized the design direction from the framework. There are three design direction, including the psychological rehabilitation support, physical rehabilitation support, and the form of the information communication platform.

1) The design focus on the psychological rehabilitation support is to allow patients to experience the sense of companionship brought by family caregivers and to encourage patients to get rehabilitation achievements in different phase.
2) The design focus on the physical rehabilitation support is for family caregivers to supervise the patients' medication, diet, etc. Implementation of exercises, physical examinations, etc., and participation in offline peer support activities with patients.
3) The design focus on the information communication platform that assist patients in completing rehabilitation data records efficiently and help family caregivers and medical teams can track the data and give feedback in time.

4 "Bcare" Design

The research team designed the "Bcare", a smart service system of peer supported for elderly breast cancer patients' continuing care, is mainly composed of four parts, the Bcare service platform for patients, the Bcare App for family caregivers, "Bcare WeChat Mini Program" for patients and "Bcare" hospital continuing service management linking with the hospital.

4.1 "Bcare" Service Platform for Patient

"Bcare" service platform for patients, help patients to continuously record rehabilitation data, and trigger discussion and information exchange between family caregivers and patients. Patients learn about the knowledge of post-operative rehabilitation both through the "Bcare" App for the family caregiver and paper based "Bcare" rehabilitation manuals, images and video guidelines for post-operative exercises, guidelines for healthy eating, etc.

The elderly patients who are inconvenient to use mobile phones and prefer to use traditional paper materials, can mark in the record page with three items (medication/diet/exercise) in the patient's paper rehabilitation manual, and write down the memo (physical examination schedule/doctor's advice). Paper-based "Bcare" rehabilitation manuals are suitable for elderly patients to identify and learn, and record quickly, the daily recording time is within 5 min.

When family caregivers communicate with patients every weekend, they can check paper based "Bcare" rehabilitation manuals and continuously upload the patient's data into the "Bcare" App for the family caregiver.

4.2 "Bcare" App for the Family Caregiver

The main functional interfaces of the "Bcare" App for family caregivers include the welcome page, registration page, home page, data entry page, activity page, appointment page, and communication page, etc. The four major functions of the navigation bar are "Homepage", "Supervision", "Moments ", and "Community". The "Homepage" section provides rehabilitation guidelines and peer support information to family caregivers; family caregivers can browse the patient's past rehabilitation records and the information of phased curve changes on the "Supervision" section; In "Moments" section, the family caregivers can upload the pictures of memorable moments in the patient's recovery process; "Community" section includes the connection of the online and offline peer support community activities. Family caregivers can share the latest information and discussing with the patients to make an appointment. In the "appointment" section, family caregivers can make appointments to hospitals, and online offline community activities. It also can make online modifications according to the needs of patients. Patients will be encouraged to develop personal hobbies and expand social interactions through these peer support activities. It is synchronized with the information on the "Bcare WeChat Mini Program" used by the patients, and family caregivers can send messages to remind the patient to have a face-to-face consultation on time.

Family caregivers can connect with the hospital's continuation service on the "communication" page, to keep in touch with the medical team from hospital, obtain timely recommendations, as well as the continuation service made by the hospital based on the patient's recovery. At the end of each month, the family caregivers will receive the patient's overall recovery data and targeted suggestions from the "Bcare" App system. The system will also encourage and reminders based on the input and data of patients and family caregivers. The system will also send reference questions for family caregivers to stimulate discussion and communication with patients (Fig. 6).

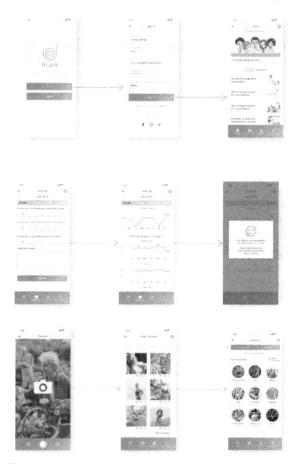

Fig. 6. The interface of "Bcare" App for the family caregiver.

4.3 "Bcare WeChat Mini Program" for Patients

According to the different digital literacy of patients, Bcare also set up in WeChat Mini Program, which is convenient for elderly patients who can use mobile phones. WeChat

Mini Programs are "sub-applications" within the WeChat ecosystem. They enable to provide advanced features to users such as e-commerce, task management, coupons, etc. in China [17]. Patients who can log in to the "Bcare" WeChat Mini Program on their own mobile phone, they can quickly check in the medication, diet, and exercise in the daily check-in section. Patients can write down their memos by converting voice to text. The patient also can share the check-in list results to the WeChat patient peer support group, and invite other patients to join the "Bcare" WeChat Mini Program.

The patient's "Bcare" WeChat Mini Program set up an associated account with the family cares' App terminal. The family caregiver can view and remind the patient's appointments, such as physical examination in real-time, and also can get the information about the patient's daily check-in status in the "supervision" function.

4.4 "Bcare" Hospital Continuing Service Management

"Bcare" hospital continuing service management is mainly a computer web page, consider that main usage scenarios and interaction habits of medical staff from the hospital. "Bcare" hospital's continuing service management port mainly has two sections: (1) Doctors can quickly manage related patients, review the patient's treatment status and recent physical reports, and deal with them promptly. At the same time, the service system will automatically match the relevant knowledge and send it to the patients and caregivers, according to the keywords of the doctor's order; (2) Doctors can communicate with patients and caregivers in time and can also communicate with another stakeholder (such as they can make connections between different hospitals, introduce the online and offline peer support community), to achieve the continuation of information, relationships, and care for patients.

5 Preliminary Results

In the user testing session, the research team invited 25 users, including ten elder patients (the age from 65–80, $\geq$1-month post-treatment), 10 family caregivers, and 5 fully-registered, practicing medical staffs (3 doctors and 2 nurses) to test the design prototypes and give the scoring. The specific process of the testing was: 1) We treated 10 elder patients and 10 family caregivers as the "Bcare" main users, they were asked to rate the satisfaction of the existing continuous care services by using Table 1, a seven-point Likert scale (1 = Strongly disagree, 2 = Disagree, 3 = Slightly disagree, 4 = Neutral, 5 = Slightly agree, 6 = Agree, 7 = Strongly agree) 2) through the introduction of the research team, users tried and experienced the "Bcare" step by step. The users communicated with the research team and gave comments and suggestions. 3) the users completed the Table 1 again after testing the prototype of "Bcare" to do the comparison.

The scoring focus on the evaluation of the user's experience about service scenario: 1) The experience in the switchover between medical institutions and continuing care service scenarios, such as home and offline community. 2) The experience in the participation of online and offline communities' activities. 3) The experience of communication and interaction within the family members.

The scoring items are the acquisition of rehabilitation and health care information, communication and interaction with peers, and peer support in physical rehabilitation and peer support in psychological rehabilitation. A total of 13 questions about physical examination, peer support activities and peer support at home to evaluate the user's experience. The instrument is shown in Table 1.

Table 1. The satisfaction score of user's experiences

Physical examination	Score
1: Satisfied with the rehabilitation health information provided by physical examination in continuing care	1 2 3 4 5 6 7
2: Satisfied with the communication with the doctor or other stakeholders support physical examination in continuing care	1 2 3 4 5 6 7
3: Physical rehabilitation status in the medical examination is good	1 2 3 4 5 6 7
4: Emotional state is good in the physical examination of the continuing care	1 2 3 4 5 6 7
Peer support activities	Score
5: Satisfied with the rehabilitation information obtained during the offline peer support community activity	1 2 3 4 5 6 7
6: Satisfied with the communication with the doctor or other stakeholders during the offline peer support community activity	1 2 3 4 5 6 7
7: physical rehabilitation status during attending the offline peer support community activity is good	1 2 3 4 5 6 7
8: Emotional state is good during attending the offline peer support community activity	1 2 3 4 5 6 7
Peer support at home	Score
9: Satisfied with the information of continuing care at home	1 2 3 4 5 6 7
10: The support received from a doctor in continuing care at home	1 2 3 4 5 6 7
11: I had the support received from a family caregiver at home is good	1 2 3 4 5 6 7
12: Physical rehabilitation while receiving support from a family caregiver is good	1 2 3 4 5 6 7
13: Emotions while receiving support from a family caregiver in the continuing care at home is good	1 2 3 4 5 6 7

1: Strongly disagree; 2: Disagree; 3: Slightly disagree; 4: Neutral; 5: Slightly agree; 6: Agree; 7: Strongly agree.

The average score of the existing continuous care services by 10 elder patients is 2.9. The average score is 5.4 after they tested the prototype of "Bcare". The test results show that the satisfied rated by elder patients has improved by average score 2.5 points. Among them, the largest improvement was about the physical rehabilitation while receiving support from a family caregiver in the twelfth question, reaching 3.8 points. The improvement of physical examination is 2.625 points, the average score for the improvement of peer support activities is 2 points, and the total score for the improvement of peer support at home is 2.88 points.

The average score of the existing continuous care services by ten family caregivers is 2.8. The average score is 5.4 after they tested the prototype of "Bcare". The test results show that the satisfied rated by family caregivers has improved by average score 2.6 points. Among them, the largest improvement was about the satisfaction of the information about continuing nursing at home in the ninth question, reaching 3.2 points. The improvement of physical examination is 2.475 points, the average score for the improvement of peer support activities is 2.4 points, and the total score for the improvement of peer support at home is 2.9 points.

The scores had reflected that "Bcare" has indeed improved the satisfaction of users' experience. And it is prominently manifested in the scenarios of taking physical examinations after surgery and the communication and interaction scenarios within the family, especially the acquisition of rehabilitation and health care information in the scenarios and the communication and interaction with peers.

Five fully registered, practicing medical staffs (three doctors and two nurses) were involved in the feedback exercise. A nurse believes that the interactive form of the patient's check-in can be combined with the patient's social sharing habits, and a doctor suggested that the content of the communication with the doctor and patients can be incorporated into the electronic medical record as a reference.

Some experience design needs to be updated:

1) Patients and family caregivers thought doctor-patient communication is very important in the whole continuing care process. They hope to obtain online Q&A from medical staff in a timely and efficient manner, and patients can get promptly remind of appointment information, such as physical examinations.
2) Patients and stakeholders had a higher demand for a healthy diet and knowledge guidance on rehabilitation exercises for patients.
3) Patients believed that the companionship of relatives and friends is an important form of psychological rehabilitation support.
4) Patients believed that the participation of offline peer support community activities should be selectively based on the patient's interests and hobbies.
5) Patients are more inclined to use online platforms to complete daily records, and especially hope to build the platform on a communication platform that is frequently used daily, such as WeChat. At the same time, they worried about the privacy of personal information.
6) Patients believed that it is the patient's responsibility to complete the daily rehabilitation record and companionship by family caregivers is already the best form of family support.

6   Conclusion

Breast cancer rehabilitation after surgery is a long and tortuous process, elderly breast cancer patients and their family caregivers need the help to maintain comprehensive and effective chronic disease management of the patient's physiology, psychology, and quality of life in homecare. In this paper, we present the design process of "Bcare", we used the UCD (user-center design) to gain insight into the physical and psychological needs from elder patients and family caregivers and put forward a framework of the peer support of homecare in continuing care. We designed the "Bcare" to make the effective media channel for elder patients and family caregivers to get the rehabilitation and health care information and increase the communication and interaction between the family caregivers and hospital. To evaluate the developed design prototype, we have conducted 25 users including 10 elder patients, 10 family caregivers, and 5 fully registered, practicing medical staff to test the prototypes. The great majority of them gave overall good score on "Bcare", they also believe the developed system will be useful for elderly breast cancer patients in terms of getting peer support in continuing care at home.

When applicability of these results to other cultural populations, we need to notice that peer support has different manifestations in different social. The peer support activities need to focus on local patients' real needs, integrate into the local social resources, medical resources, and maximize peer support activities' benefits.

In future, we would like to 1) Based on user feedback, iterate plans to improve elder user experience and to protect users' privacy. 2) Strengthen the research of peer support in emotional to deal with the psychological problems that plague female patients in the continuing care. 3) Increasing technical to matches the hospital medical system, cooperate with more stakeholders, and considering the adaptability to be used in post-epidemic era.

Acknowledgments. Specials thanks to the all the participations in this research. This research is supported, in part, by the National Research Foundation, Prime Minister's Office, Singapore under its IDM Futures Funding Initiative; AISG-RP-2019-050.

References

1. The International Agency for Research on Cancer (IARC): Latest global cancer data: cancer burden rises to 19.3 million new cases and 10.0 million cancer deaths in 2020
2. Lancet, T.: GLOBOCAN 2018: Counting the toll of cancer. Lancet **392**(10152), 985 (2018)
3. Aizpurua-Perez, I., Perez-Tejada, J.: Resilience in women with breast cancer: a systematic review. Eur. J. Oncol. Nurs. **49**, 101854 (2020). https://doi.org/10.1016/j.ejon.2020.101854
4. Demicheli, R., Abbattista, A., Miceli, R., Valagussa, P., Bonadonna, G.: Time distribution of the recurrence risk for breast cancer patients undergoing mastectomy: further support about the concept of tumor dormancy. Breast Cancer Res. Treat. **41**(2), 177–185 (1996). https://doi.org/10.1007/BF01807163
5. Coleman, E.A.: Falling through the cracks: challenges and opportunities for improving transitional care for persons with continuous complex care needs. J. Am. Geriatr. Soc. **51**(4), 549–555 (2003)
6. Dowsett, M., et al.: Integration of clinical variables for the prediction of late distant recurrence in patients with estrogen receptor-positive breast cancer treated with 5 years of endocrine therapy: CTS5. J. Clin. Oncol. **36**(19), 1941–1948 (2018)
7. Haggerty, J.L., Reid, R.J., Freeman, G.K., et al.: Continuity of care a multidisciplinary review. BMJ **327**(7425), 1220–1223 (2003)

8. Diao, L.H., Niu, Y.H., Li, Y.L.: Nursing and investigation of correlation between depression and social support of elderly patients with cancer. Chin. J. Nurs. **37**(05), 16–18 (2002)
9. Hu, Y., Huang, Y.L.: To Be with You and Support with You. Shanghai Scientific and Technical Publishers (2008)
10. Solomon, P.: Peer support/peer provided services underlying processes, benefits, and critical ingredients. Psychiatr. Rehabil. J. **27**(4), 392–401 (2004)
11. Mead, S., Hilton, D., Curtis, L.: Peer support: a theoretical perspective. Psychiatr. Rehabil. J. **25**(2), 134–141 (2001)
12. Setoyama, Y., Yamazaki, Y., Namayama, K.: Benefits of peer support in online Japanese breast cancer communities: differences between lurkers and posters. J. Med. Internet Res. **13**(4), e122 (2011)
13. Zhao, H.Y., Zhang, Y.B., Ma, Y.F.: The experience of peer support to improve the discovery of benefits for patients after breast cancer surgery. J. Nurs. **24**(14), 76–78 (2017)
14. Dong, F.: Breast cancer patients: please leave it to WeChat to take care of it. Comfort Life (12), 10–11 (2015)
15. Mannonen, P., Kaipio, J., Nieminen, M.P.: Patient-centred design of healthcare services: meaningful events as basis for patient experiences of families. Stud. Health Technol. Inform. **234**, 206–210 (2017)
16. Yu, E., Sangiorgi, D.: Service design as an approach to new service development: reflections and futures studies. In: ServDes 2014. Fourth Service Design and Innovation Conference, Lancaster, United Kingdom (2014)
17. ECOVIS R&G Consulting Ltd. (Beijing) and Advantage Austria. E-commerce in China, Industry report (2015)
18. Kadambi, S., et al.: Social support for older adults with cancer: Young International Society of Geriatric Oncology review paper. J. Geriatr. Oncol. **11**(2), 217–224 (2020)
19. Ajzen, I.: The theory of planned behaviour is alive and well, and not ready to retire: a commentary on Sniehotta, Presseau, and Araujo-Soares. Health Psychol Rev. **9**(2), 131–137 (2015)
20. Mirrielees, J.A., et al.: Breast cancer survivor advocacy at a university hospital: development of a peer support program with evaluation by patients, advocates, and clinicians. J. Cancer Educ. **32**(1), 97–104 (2017)
21. Umezawa, S., Fujisawa, D., Fujimori, M., Ogawa, A., Matsushima, E., Miyashita, M.: Prevalence, associated factors and source of support concerning supportive care needs among Japanese cancer survivors. Psychooncology **24**(6), 635–642 (2015)
22. Abras, C., Maloney-Krichmar, D., Preece, J.: User-centered design. In: Bainbridge, W. (ed.) Encyclopedia of Human-Computer Interaction. Sage Publications, Thousand Oaks (2004)
23. Preece, J., Rogers, Y., Sharp, H.: Interaction Design: Beyond Human-Computer Interaction. Wiley, New York (2002)
24. Qiu, J., et al.: Quality of life and psychological state in Chinese breast cancer patients who received BRCA1/2 genetic testing. PLoS ONE **11**(7), e0158531 (2016). https://doi.org/10.1371/journal.pone.0158531
25. Epstein, R.M., Street, R.L.: The values and value of patient-centered care. Ann. Fam. Med. **9**(2), 100–103 (2011). https://doi.org/10.1370/afm.1239
26. Satish, T., et al.: Care delivery impact of the COVID-19 pandemic on breast cancer care. JCO Oncol. Pract. **17**(8), e1215–e1224 (2021). https://doi.org/10.1200/OP.20.01062
27. Hu, J., et al.: Peer support interventions for breast cancer patients: a systematic review. Breast Cancer Res. Treat. **174**(2), 325–341 (2019). https://doi.org/10.1007/s10549-018-5033-2
28. Hou, I.-C., et al.: The development of a mobile health app for breast cancer self-management support in Taiwan: design thinking approach. JMIR MHealth UHealth **8**(4), e15780 (2020). https://doi.org/10.2196/15780

RITA: A Privacy-Aware Toileting Assistance Designed for People with Dementia

Irene Ballester[1]([⊠]) ⓘ, Tamar Mujirishvili[2] ⓘ, and Martin Kampel[1] ⓘ

[1] Computer Vision Lab, TU Wien, Vienna, Austria
{irene.ballester,martin.kampel}@tuwien.ac.at
[2] Department of Nursing, University of Alicante, Alicante, Spain
tamar@ua.es

Abstract. Dementia is one of the leading causes of disability and dependence among older people, currently affecting more than 55 million people and estimated to increase to 139 million by 2050. A growing number of technologies are being developed to assist people with dementia in their daily lives, but assistance with toileting remains a neglected area.

In this work, we present RITA, a system to automatically guide people with mild dementia in the toilet. The system detects activities that the user performs and compares them to a predefined model that maps out the correct toilet procedure. If problems are detected, such as wandering around the toilet or sitting on the bowl for longer than a certain time, instructions are given on what to do next. As only depth images are used, the privacy of the users is guaranteed at all times, a crucial factor in such an intimate context as toilet-going.

For an automated assistance system to be effective, the adequate design of its interaction with the user is essential. For this reason, our design is not only based on the available technological solutions, but also on the conclusions derived from focus groups with healthcare professionals. We report these findings with the aim of contributing to reducing the information gap in interaction design for people with dementia.

Keywords: AAL · Dementia · Privacy-aware technology

We gratefully acknowledge the participation in this study of the healthcare professionals of the Rey Ardid Rosales Residence. This work is partially funded by JP-AAL under grant number AAL-2019-6-150-C for the DIANA project and by the European Union's Horizon 2020 research and innovation programme under the Marie Skłodowska-Curie grant agreement No. 861091 for the visuAAL project.

1 Introduction

Dementia is defined by the WHO[1] as a syndrome in which there is a deterioration in cognitive functioning beyond what might be expected from normal ageing.

In recent years, the international community has recognised the urgent need for action on dementia [15] and the Global action plan on the public health response to dementia 2017–2025 [16] includes among its key actions the development of support and services for dementia caregivers as well as the promotion of research and innovative technologies as a way to significantly improve the lives of people with dementia, their families and caregivers.

The severity of dementia progresses from the mildest stage, when the person's functionality is just beginning to be affected, to the most severe stage, when the person becomes completely dependent on others in order to complete activities of daily living (ADL)[2], which makes it one of the major causes of disability and dependence among older people globally [15].

With the aim of promoting the independence of people with dementia by supporting ADL, we present RITA (Respect for Intimacy in Toilet Assistance), which, by targeting users with mild cognitive impairment, is intended to provide step-by-step guidance to the person using the toilet in such a way that they do not need any assistance from a second person.

Applications to support people with dementia in the usage of toilet could benefit both caregivers and patients themselves [3]. However, assistance in the toilet seems to have been overlooked in the development of assistive technologies, which may be due to the high privacy requirements in this intimate context. RITA addresses these high privacy requirements through the use of a 3D sensor and edge computing, which eliminates the need to transmit images, ensuring that user privacy is respected at all times.

Moreover, given that dementia affects individuals differently (See footnotes 1 and 2), identifying the optimal approach to design interactions with people with dementia is a non-trivial task and there is currently not enough information to determine which is the best option. As this is a key determinant of the overall effectiveness of the system, considerable effort has been made to assess the range of interaction possibilities and our findings on this topic are also presented in this paper.

2 Related Work

An increasing number of technologies are being developed to support the autonomy of the older population. Yet, despite toileting being the third main ADL with which older people have difficulty [5], very little progress has been made in this area compared to other assistance applications.

---

[1] World Health Organization. https://www.who.int/news-room/fact-sheets/detail/dementia (accessed September 25, 2021).

[2] National Institute on Aging's ADEAR Center. https://www.nia.nih.gov/health/what-dementia-symptoms-types-and-diagnosis (accessed September 18, 2021).

An exception is, for example [1], which describes a public smart toilet developed for the older and disabled population. This is a continuation of work done at [13] and [18], to develop a modular toileting system for older adults.

In terms of the technologies designed for people with dementia, the systematic review presented in [4] provides an overview and emphasises the need to employ user-centred designs to successfully develop assistive technologies for this range of users. However, there is not much information available on how to design interaction with users with dementia and most of the studies on this topic are limited to providing general design guidelines without addressing specific aspects of design choices. An example is [17], where the authors present a series of recommendations for the design of smart homes for people with dementia, focusing on user interface aspects.

Lumetzberger et al. [12] developed a vision-based solution to assist users with cognitive impairment in the toilet. An avatar and simple visual and textual instructions are the proposed forms of interaction, but the adequacy of the selected interaction methods for people with dementia is not specifically addressed.

In general terms, many of the studies (e.g. [6,8,11]) place particular emphasis on the importance of designing a system that can be tailored to the individual in order to ensure the effectiveness of the indications. Smith et al. [19] and Fried et al. [6] mention the effectiveness of using multi-modal inputs for dementia patients and conclude that communication strategies should be based on multiple modalities to build on the patient's strengths.

Mihailidis et al. [14] test the performance of a system to assist people with severe dementia during hand-washing through verbal prompting, but no comparison with other prompting modes is provided. In fact, they note that more research should be done on the types of interactions and the effectiveness of prompts for people with dementia, suggesting the incorporation of video-based prompting strategies.

Of particular relevance is the work done in [10], where the authors compared verbal and audio-visual prompts to guide patients with moderate to severe cognitive impairment in the task of hand-washing. The results reveal little differences between the efficiency achieved with the two modes of automated assistance, with audio-visual assistance resulting in statistically fewer caregiver interventions. However, the authors conclude that the efficacy depends on many factors, such as the physical environment or the nature of prompts as well as their speed and timing. Therefore, further research is needed, possibly including other modalities in the comparison too.

The study conducted in [8], as part of the ACT@HOME project, presents a qualitative evaluation of an intelligent virtual assistant to assist Alzheimer's sufferers during hand-washing. The authors provide guidelines for the design of prompting methods and, in general, the design of virtual assistants for people with cognitive impairment. Despite the relevance of this study to our application, the results are limited to qualitative interviews with people with dementia and their caregivers about the virtual agent's physical appearance and acceptance, without delving into alternative modalities of prompting.

Virtual agents as personal assistants were also proposed in [20] framed in the Living Well project[3], which seeks to adapt a virtual ICT assistant for users with dementia or other age-related cognitive problems.

Lighting signals are used in the PETAL project[4], aimed to develop a platform for personalising remote assistance for adults with mild cognitive impairment (MCI) to support their spatio-temporal orientation. However, no concrete data is provided to validate the hypothesis that communication using light signals is effective for patients with MCI, nor is this interaction modality compared with alternative solutions.

Only the works described in [8,10,14] provide a comparison between modalities or a validation of the effectiveness of the modalities investigated. Thus, when it comes to making specific design choices, not enough information is available for selecting the most appropriate interaction modality for people with dementia. This work aims at reducing this information gap as well as using these findings to provide a privacy-aware solution than can successfully guide people with dementia in the toilet.

3   Interaction with People with Dementia: Methodology and Results

The effectiveness of an automatic assistance system critically depends on how it interacts with the user. Dementia causes communication difficulties, even for skilled caregivers[5]. So, it is clear that the interaction strategies need to be carefully designed to successfully convey the messages issued by automatic systems. In the lack of well-established methods, this work has devoted special attention to this aspect. It takes into consideration not only available technological solutions, but also the knowledge and recommendations from experienced carers as the most valuable input to define effective communication strategies.

3.1   Methodology

As a first step, we conduct a thorough review of possible solutions. This, in addition to saving resources, is particularly important when the users are people with dementia, as exposing users to early-stage devices as faulty prototypes can lead to anxiety and future rejection [17]. Orpwood et al. [17] advocate involving users in the design process, but propose collaborating in the first instance with caregivers and then, when relatively mature prototypes become available, conducting specific tests with the patients themselves.

Apart from ethical issues, caregivers seem to be the best placed to estimate the needs of dementia patients, to provide an overview of specific challenges and

---

[3] Living Well with Anne. https://livingwellwithanne.eu/ (accessed September 18, 2021).

[4] PETAL - PErsonalizable assisTive Ambient monitoring and Lighting. http://www.aal-petal.eu/ (accessed September 18, 2021).

[5] Alzheimer's Association. https://www.alz.org/ (accessed April 26, 2021).

to assess the effectiveness of possible solutions [17]. For this reason, two focus group sessions are held with care home professionals.

3.2 Communication in Dementia

Communication difficulties tend to become more pronounced as the disease progresses (See footnote 5). However, dementia affects each person very differently, meaning that in addition to the stage of the disease, symptoms may vary depending on other factors, such as the specific type of dementia, the impact of the disease or the person's personality before becoming ill (See footnotes 1 and 2).

Due to the heterogeneity of the particular abilities and constantly changing needs of people with dementia, studies such as [6,22] claim that communication strategies should be adapted to the specific needs and abilities of each person, evolving throughout the course of the disease. Moreover, consideration should also be given to the patient's socioeconomic status when opting for a specific communication strategy [22]. For example, in the case of considering text as a prompting modality, it should be borne in mind that written communication will be more effective for a person with a higher education level, than for someone who had difficulties in reading even before their dementia.

Multi-modal approaches can be effective ways to bridge the difficulty imposed by the inter-variability of dementia patients when communication cannot be tailored to each specific patient [6,8,19]. The use of multiple modalities provides more channels for the delivery of the message, giving more opportunities for the message to be received effectively by the target person. Finally, the challenge of the multi-modal approach lies in selecting complementary modalities with the highest cost-benefit ratio.

3.3 Review of Possible Solutions

The following is a brief description of the possible interaction solutions:

- **Verbal prompts.** Verbal guidance consists of using spoken language to give instructions to the user. Factors that play an important role in the effectiveness of messages in this modality may include, but are not limited to, tone of voice, speed of speech, choice of vocabulary, sentence structure, or whether the voice is familiar to the user.
- **Text.** Textual messages are displayed on a screen for the user to read.
- **Audiovisual prompts.** The use of audio-visual technologies falls, by definition, within multi-modal approaches, as it uses images or videos as a visual support and, generally, verbal language to transmit the information using the sense of hearing.
- **Agents.** A special sub-type of audio-visual approaches is involving the use of virtual or real agents. Virtual agents refer to embodied entities displayed on a screen designed in a way that encourages natural interaction with the user, while real agents involve the recording of a real person.

- **Light- or sound-based solutions.** Lights or audio sources are placed next to the objects involved in the toileting process, which will be switched on and off to guide the patient's attention as he or she moves through the process, offering a less intrusive form of guidance.

3.4   Focus Groups

To complement the information extracted from the literature review, two focus groups are organised with health professionals from a nursing home.

Participants. Focus groups are conducted with health professionals of a specialised facility for residents with Alzheimer's and other types of dementia in Zaragoza (Spain). Two sessions are held with two different groups of healthcare providers (n = 4 and n = 9, respectively), with a total of 13 participants:

- Group 1: Higher level health professionals, including a psychologist, a nurse, an occupational therapist and a physiotherapist.
- Group 2: Professional caregivers composed of 9 nursing assistants.

All participants were female, aged between 23 and 58 years (mean: 40, standard deviation: 11.5) and had different lengths of work experience (minimum: less than 1 year, maximum: 20 years, mean: 7.4, standard deviation: 6).

Procedure. Each focus group session lasted about 1 h and 15 min and started with an explanation of the research project. Participants were told that the sessions would be voice-recorded and they agreed by signing a consent form.

The focus group guide was structured in two parts: the first part included a brief description of the proposed technology and the possible interaction modalities and questions on the interaction design while the second part was dedicated to perceived usefulness and barriers such as privacy and trust issues. Figure 1 presents three of the videos shown as example to the participants. The methodology used for the preparation of the sessions is described in [2] and [9].

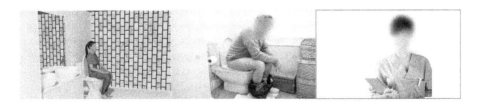

Fig. 1. Samples of the videos presented to the participants. Left: Virtual avatar showing the action to perform. This option was preferred by all the participants in Group 1. Centre: Real person showing the action to perform. Right: Caregiver addressing the patient. The latter two were the options supported by participants in Group 2.

Focus Groups Results. The results presented here are a brief summary of a qualitative content analysis from the audio recordings and the notes collected during the focus group sessions. Conclusions about the interaction design and perceived usefulness and barriers are discussed.

Interaction Design

- **Separate systems for patients with mild and with moderate dementia.** Participants from both groups highlighted the need to create two different systems for users with mild and moderate dementia, as there is a significant difference in the symptomatology of these patients. Consequently, our target group has been reduced to people with mild dementia.
- **Overall preferred modalities: video and verbal messages.** In general, the combination of video and verbal messages was preferred over these modalities used separately. In addition, the use of text was perceived to be distracting rather than supportive if used in combination with these modalities. Participants of both groups concurred that a familiar voice would play a crucial role in the effectiveness of the instructions and that using the voice of a caregiver from the care facility where the system will be deployed is the best option. In line with this, video instructions were undoubtedly preferred to be recorded in the familiar physical setting too, such as the very same bathroom that patients are using. And if synthetic imagery is preferred, the design of facility's bathrooms should be reproduced. There was no consensus on which would be more effective: having the agent perform the action or only addressing the user. As for the appearance of the agent, participants in Group 1 opted for a virtual agent with a realistic appearance, while those in Group 2 preferred a real person (see Fig. 1).
  Both groups discouraged the use of sounds, as they may frighten users, and lights were only considered useful for people with moderate dementia.
- **Structure of verbal messages: clear and short.** Both groups agreed that verbal messages should be clear and as short as possible. However, there were different opinions regarding the appropriate level of imperiousness of the prompts. Group 1 (higher level health professionals) indicated that instructions should always be imperative to convey clearly the message. Conversely, all the participants in Group 2 (professional caregivers) pointed out that although imperative instructions are sometimes necessary, their usual preferred way of proceeding is to first kindly ask to perform a certain action. Two participants pointed out that when residents are asked in a polite way, using a kind tone, "they even listen more".
- **Initiate interaction only after a problem is detected** for people with mild dementia. Participants of both groups expressed that, in the case of mild dementia, the system should delay interaction with the patient until a problem is detected, otherwise it could be upsetting or frightening to patients. For patients with moderate dementia, conversely, interaction should be initiated as soon as the patient enters the room.

Perceived Usefulness and Barriers. Participants of both groups have positively evaluated the proposed system, stating that "it can be a great alleviation for patients as well as caregivers' work". Increasing patient's autonomy and thus reinforcing their self-esteem and sense of dignity was named among the main benefits, especially for people with mild dementia in need for support. Caregivers pointed out that this technology could greatly lighten their workload (Caregiver: "The most time-consuming task is accompanying them (the patients) to the toilet"), which would also be reflected in the reduction of their stress level. Furthermore, participants of both groups expressed their special interest and usefulness of the system's ability to detect falls.

As for barriers, both groups said that a period of adaptation would be necessary, but they were also confident that the residents would eventually accept the system. Higher level professionals also commented that caregivers might be initially reluctant, as the implementation process might be perceived as additional work. However, this claim was not supported by the caregivers themselves, who indicated the system could be a positive relief, although many residents would still need to be supervised. Practical aspects were mentioned, such as the use of diapers, which would prevent the system from being accessible to all users.

Regarding privacy issues, it is worth noting that no such concerns were raised by the participants themselves and that, only after specifically drawing their attention to the potential threats, they voiced some possible issues. Most of the participants were not concerned about being filmed, 8 out of 13 clearly stated that they would not mind it "at all". Two of the participants in Group 1 stated that they did not consider depth images as "images", "videos" or "recordings", as people cannot be identified and the images are not saved, thus it is not a threat to privacy. In contrast, all participants gave a categorical negative response when asked about the feasibility of using RGB instead of depth images. Caregivers were not concerned about appearing in such images either, even if a fall of a patient was captured while they were supervising them, stating that such falls are often inevitable even in their presence. However, when one participant expressed a worry that such images could be exploited by relatives as evidence against them (if the images were saved) in the case of a serious accident, several participants echoed this concern. Another participant noted that the use of "fuzzy images" could lead to different interpretations of their actions. Despite health professionals' general openness towards the suggested system, they also noted that patients relatives might be quite sensitive about privacy concerns. They strongly emphasised the importance of using the right language when explaining the technology as the use of terms such as "recording" or "video" could lead to misunderstanding and rejection of the system from the patients' families.

4   Implementation of the System

RITA has been implemented as a prototype, including both hardware and software components.

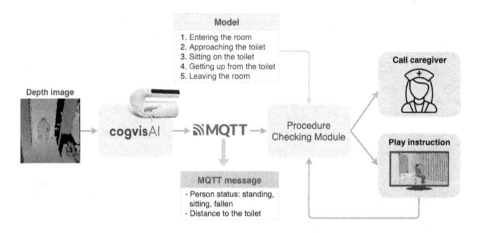

Fig. 2. Block diagram of RITA.

4.1   Overview of the System

Figure 2 is a block diagram of RITA. First, a modified version of the cogvisAI sensor[6] processes the depth image and publishes an MQTT message with the following information: status of the person (standing, sitting or fallen) and distance of the person from the toilet. The Procedure Checking Module then verifies whether the person's action conforms to the predefined model of the toilet procedure and, if not, it plays a message with the corresponding instruction. The instruction is repeated up to 3 times, with a time interval between repetitions, and in case the corresponding action is not completed after these 3 repetitions, a call is sent to the caregiver and a message informing that a caregiver is arriving to help is played. In the event of a fall, the system acts in the same way: an alert is sent to the caregiver and a reassuring message is displayed to the user.

4.2   Procedure Checking Module

Based on the inputs from the cogvisAI sensor, the model for the Procedure Checking Module features the following actions: entering the room, approaching the toilet, sitting on the toilet, getting up from the toilet and leaving the room.

The Procedure Checking Module determines what action the user is currently performing and waits for the user to perform the next action within a specified time. If the user does not perform the action, RITA plays the message giving the instruction. For development purposes, the time thresholds have been set heuristically and should be investigated further in the future. Furthermore, for the user's performance to be considered correct, the actions listed in the model must be performed in a specific order and any deviation from this sequence would cause the system to initiate interaction with the user.

---

[6] Cogvis. https://cogvis.ai/cogvis-en/ (accessed September 18, 2021).

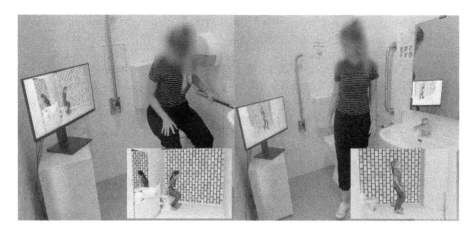

Fig. 3. Photos of the demonstration of the system. Left: "Stand up" action. Right: "Leave the room" action.

The Procedure Checking Module identifies the current action of the person following a rule-based logic that takes as input the last message received from the cogvisAI sensor and previous actions identified by the module. For instance, for the action to be set as "approaching the toilet", the conditions to be met are: distance from the toilet below a distance threshold, not sitting on the toilet, and the previous action being "entering the room".

4.3   Interaction Module

The conclusions drawn from the focus group sessions helped to narrow down the design options and, together with some insights gained from literature surveys, largely determined the design of interaction procedures. We decided to select people with mild dementia as target users and adopt a multi-modal approach to overcome the challenge posed by the inter-variability of communication impairments in people with dementia. The modalities selected are a video showing an avatar performing the action and an audio recording giving the instruction verbally, and no text was included in the visual support. Figure 3 shows photos taken during the demonstration of the system in the lab. The design decisions can be summarised as follows:

- **Audio messages recorded by a caregiver.** In addition to being a voice familiar to the residents as recommended by [17] and the participants of the focus groups, this allows the vocabulary and local accent to be matched to improve the effectiveness of the instruction as well as to harness the experience of caregivers in communicating with people with dementia.
- **Verbal messages: short, clear and polite.** Given that, as stated in [17], assistive technologies should be designed to emulate the behaviour of the caregiver, we followed the guidelines on communication strategies for health

professionals[7] [7] to design verbal messages as clear and brief as possible. In addition, instructions start with the word "please" to reduce the level of imperiousness as recommended by [8] and by the Group 2 participants.

- **Virtual agent with a realistic appearance.** A virtual agent was selected over a real agent, as respondents in Group 1 stated that a real agent would not have a positive impact on the effectiveness of the modality, but instead could cause discomfort to users. As for the appearance of the agent, we opted for realistic appearance and avoided a cartoon-like design, as it is also proposed, for example, in [21].
- **Interaction only after a problem has been detected** in order to minimise the risk that the system will be perceived as unduly intrusive by users, as recommended by participants of the focus groups.

4.4   Prototype Implementation

For the prototype, an MQTT broker has been installed on a Raspberry PI where both the cogvisAI sensor and the computer in charge of the Procedure Checking Module are connected. In this way, the cogvisAI sensor publishes messages in topics to which the computer subscribes. The monitor and speakers used to play the instructions are wired to this computer. A wireless router acting as a mobile Wi-Fi access point ensures that all devices have Internet connection.

5   Conclusions

RITA has been implemented as a prototype to guide people with mild dementia in the toilet. Preliminary tests in the lab confirm RITA's ability to detect actions performed by the user and to identify whether he/she is following the correct sequence and, if not, issuing suitable instructions to the user or to a caregiver.

Since interaction is a critical factor for the effectiveness of an automatic assistant, significant effort has been put into determining the best communication strategy. To this end, focus groups were conducted with healthcare professionals from a care home specialising in dementia. Findings from these sessions are presented, as they have been crucial for the design process and they may be of value to future researchers too.

Furthermore, although the focus group sample is insufficient to draw statistical conclusions, participants in both groups positively rated the potential of RITA to increase patient independence and self-esteem, and to reduce workload for caregivers. These preliminary results also suggest the feasibility of using depth images to protect personal privacy and ensure greater user acceptance.

The directions in which RITA is planned to be further developed include the incorporation of the detection of hand-washing actions, the implementation of an action acknowledgment message when the user performs the action after being guided by the system and the definition and evaluation of test cases. The latter

---

[7] National Health Service (NHS) - UK. https://www.nhs.uk/conditions/dementia/communication-and-dementia/ (accessed April 27, 2021).

may include seeking additional feedback from healthcare professionals as part of the collaborative design process, conducting simplified testing in controlled environments, and investigating end-user reactions to the prototype.

References

1. Balaceanu, C., Marcu, I., Suciu, G., Dantas, C., Mayer, P.: Developing a smart toilet system for ageing people and persons with disabilities. In: Proceedings of the 6th Conference on the Engineering of Computer Based Systems, pp. 1–4 (2019)
2. Blandford, A.E.: Semi-structured qualitative studies. Interaction Design Foundation (2013)
3. Drennan, V.M., Cole, L., Iliffe, S.: A taboo within a stigma? A qualitative study of managing incontinence with people with dementia living at home. BMC Geriatr. **11**(1), 1–7 (2011). https://doi.org/10.1186/1471-2318-11-75
4. Evans, J., Brown, M., Coughlan, T., Lawson, G., Craven, M.P.: A systematic review of dementia focused assistive technology. In: Kurosu, M. (ed.) HCI 2015. LNCS, vol. 9170, pp. 406–417. Springer, Cham (2015). https://doi.org/10.1007/978-3-319-20916-6_38
5. Fänge, A., Iwarsson, S.: Changes in accessibility and usability in housing: an exploration of the housing adaptation process. Occup. Ther. Int. **12**(1), 44–59 (2005)
6. Fried-Oken, M., Mooney, A., Peters, B.: Supporting communication for patients with neurodegenerative disease. NeuroRehabilitation **37**(1), 69–87 (2015)
7. Jootun, D., McGhee, G.: Effective communication with people who have dementia. Nurs. Stand. **25**(25), 40–46 (2011)
8. König, A., Malhotra, A., Hoey, J., Francis, L.E.: Designing personalized prompts for a virtual assistant to support elderly care home residents. In: PervasiveHealth, pp. 278–282 (2016)
9. Krueger, R.A., Casey, M.A.: Designing and conducting focus group interviews (2002)
10. Labelle, K.L., Mihailidis, A.: The use of automated prompting to facilitate handwashing in persons with dementia. Am. J. Occup. Ther. **60**(4), 442–450 (2006)
11. Lapointe, J., Bouchard, B., Bouchard, J., Potvin, A., Bouzouane, A.: Smart homes for people with Alzheimer's disease: adapting prompting strategies to the patient's cognitive profile. In: Proceedings of the 5th International Conference on Pervasive Technologies Related to Assistive Environments, pp. 1–8 (2012)
12. Lumetzberger, J., Ginzinger, F., Kampel, M.: Sensor-based toilet instructions for people with dementia. In: Nunes, I.L. (ed.) AHFE 2021. LNNS, vol. 265, pp. 101–108. Springer, Cham (2021). https://doi.org/10.1007/978-3-030-79816-1_13
13. Mayer, P., Panek, P.: Involving older and vulnerable persons in the design process of an enhanced toilet system. In: Proceedings of the 2017 CHI Conference Extended Abstracts on Human Factors in Computing Systems, pp. 2774–2780 (2017)
14. Mihailidis, A., Boger, J., Canido, M., Hoey, J.: The use of an intelligent prompting system for people with dementia. Interactions **14**(4), 34–37 (2007)
15. World Health Organization: Global status report on the public health response to dementia. World Health Organization (2021)
16. World Health Organization, et al.: Global action plan on the public health response to dementia 2017–2025 (2017)
17. Orpwood, R., Gibbs, C., Adlam, T., Faulkner, R., Meegahawatte, D.: The design of smart homes for people with dementia-user-interface aspects. Univ. Access Inf. Soc. **4**(2), 156–164 (2005). https://doi.org/10.1007/s10209-005-0120-7

18. Panek, P., et al.: On the prototyping of an ICT-enhanced toilet system for assisting older persons living independently and safely at home. In: eHealth, pp. 176–183 (2017)
19. Smith, E.R., et al.: Memory and communication support in dementia: research-based strategies for caregivers. Int. Psychogeriatr. **23**(2), 256 (2011)
20. Stara, V., et al.: The design adaptation of the Virtual Assistant Anne for moderate dementia patients and their formal caregivers in protected environment tests. In: Lightner, N.J., Kalra, J. (eds.) AHFE 2019. AISC, vol. 957, pp. 270–279. Springer, Cham (2020). https://doi.org/10.1007/978-3-030-20451-8_27
21. Straßmann, C., Krämer, N.C.: A categorization of virtual agent appearances and a qualitative study on age-related user preferences. In: Beskow, J., Peters, C., Castellano, G., O'Sullivan, C., Leite, I., Kopp, S. (eds.) IVA 2017. LNCS (LNAI), vol. 10498, pp. 413–422. Springer, Cham (2017). https://doi.org/10.1007/978-3-319-67401-8_51
22. Suijkerbuijk, S., Nap, H.H., Cornelisse, L., IJsselsteijn, W.A., De Kort, Y.A., Minkman, M.: Active involvement of people with dementia: a systematic review of studies developing supportive technologies. J. Alzheimer's Dis. **69**(4), 1041–1065 (2019)

Design of a Rule-Based and ADL Analysis System to Support Care of the Elderly

Naomi Irvine[1]([⊠]), Catherine Saunders[1], Matias Garcia-Constantino[1],
Paul Moorhead[2], David Branagh[3], and Chris Nugent[1]

[1] School of Computing, Ulster University, Jordanstown, UK
{n.irvine,ce.saunders,m.garcia-constantino,
cd.nugent}@ulster.ac.uk
[2] Kraydel, Belfast, UK
paul.moorhead@feature-creep.com
[3] Connected Health Innovation Centre (CHIC), Ulster University, Jordanstown, UK
d.branagh@ulster.ac.uk

Abstract. Medical advances have allowed people to live longer and this has presented different challenges to support them to keep living independently at home. The COVID-19 pandemic has affected the situation with less care staff and resources available for the elderly, which have also been spending more time at their homes without external contact. Elderly people are typically looked after by formal (professional carers) and informal (relatives and friends) carers. The work of carers has been increasingly supported using technologies for communication and wellbeing monitoring of Activities of Daily Living (ADLs) that elderly people perform in order to detect abnormal events that could negatively affect their wellbeing. This paper presents the design of a rule-based and ADL analysis system that takes data from different sensors as input and presents a number of visualisations in a dashboard as output. The dashboard is as user friendly as possible for both formal and informal carers of elderly people. It is intended that the proposed system can identify both immediate problems, but also trends and deviations from the individual's norm, or that of a comparable cohort, which indicate the opportunity for pro-active care. This research has been done in collaboration with the Kraydel company, whose staff supported with ideas and with the commercial needs to be considered in the solution design presented in this paper.

Keywords: Activity recognition · Activities of Daily Living · Sensors

1 Introduction

Enabling elderly people to live independent lives safe and well in their own homes is a key challenge of our age. This need has been amplified by the COVID-19 pandemic and the need for the elderly (and other vulnerable) people to shield themselves from external contacts. The gradual affordability and widespread use of technologies for communication and for wellbeing monitoring have supported the work of formal (professional

H. Lewy and R. Barkan (Eds.): PH 2021, LNICST 431, pp. 331–345, 2022.
https://doi.org/10.1007/978-3-030-99194-4_21

carers) and informal (relatives and friends) carers of elderly people. It is of particular interest to monitor the Activities of Daily Living (ADLs) that elderly people perform to detect abnormal events that could negatively affect their wellbeing and send notifications to their carers to act promptly. In addition, care is slowly pivoting towards a model of preventive rather than reactive action, and that is only possible if we have reliable information on people's physical and mental well-being and any trends which suggest an intervention is required.

This paper presents the design of a rule-based and ADL analysis system that takes data from different sensors as input and presents a number of visualisations in a dashboard as output. The dashboard is intended to be as user friendly as possible for both formal and informal carers of elderly people. It is intended that the proposed system can identify both immediate problems, but also trends and deviations from the individual's norm, or that of a comparable cohort, which indicate the opportunity for pro-active care. The solution design presented is the output of a project collaboration with the Kraydel company, whose staff supported with ideas and with the commercial needs to consider for this solution. Kraydel has developed a hub with onboard sensors to be deployed within the home. Kraydel's hub has integration with third party sensors such as motion, smart plugs, and room temperature, and also biomedical devices such as blood-pressure cuffs, pulse-oximeters, clinical thermometers and weighing scales. Kraydel have also developed a proof-of-concept event processing engine that demonstrates some of the principles necessary for identifying ADLs and which was used as foundation of the event processing engine presented in this paper.

The remainder of the paper is organised as follows. Section 2 presents the related work on the motivation for the use of Smart Homes and different types of approaches. Section 3 describes the type of data and the dataset considered. Section 4 introduces the rule syntax approach used. Section 5 explains an event processing engine that uses rules to detect that an ADL has occurred. Section 6 presents a dashboard user interface in which the inferred ADLs are visualised. Finally, Sect. 7 presents conclusions and future work.

2 Related Work

This section presents the related work in two areas: (i) the motivation for the use of Smart Homes, and (ii) different types of Smart Home approaches (knowledge-driven, data-driven, and hybrid).

2.1 Motivation for Smart Home Research

The World Health Organisation (WHO) have recently stated concerns regarding the ageing population, expressing that "In 2019, the number of people aged 60 years and older was 1 billion, and this number will increase to 2.1 billion by 2050" [1]. Health decline of the ageing population through disability and the development of chronic illnesses has had an adverse impact upon the continually increasing healthcare costs, in addition to increasing the strain upon healthcare providers due to staff deficiencies [2]. Thus, an alternative cost-effective care provision is required.

The concept of "ageing in place" has emerged due to the concerns outlined, which aims to support the ageing population through enabling them to live independently for longer within their own homes, thus increasing their quality of life [2]. According to [3], a large majority of the ageing population are reluctant to reside in dedicated care facilities, therefore the progression of supportive measures are required to maintain independent living within their own homes.

Smart home research involving ambient intelligence and the development of assistive technologies has emerged to tackle the specified concerns, with Ambient Assisted Living (AAL) transpiring as one technology-focused approach to support independent living amongst the ageing population. For example, these technologies may monitor an inhabitant's movements within the home and may detect health decline or abnormal behaviours through activity tracking, which may indicate a health or behavioural problem that requires intervention. ADLs are often monitored in smart homes to ascertain the status of health and wellbeing of inhabitants [4]. During an assessment, an inhabitant's independence is observed and evaluated to ensure they have adequate cognitive and physical capabilities to perform basic activities, such as maintaining personal hygiene, dressing, preparing meals and taking medication. An inhabitant must be capable of performing ADLs independently to ensure they can safely live and function in their home environment [5, 6].

Several technologies exist and can be deployed within smart homes to track the movements of inhabitants and automatically recognise activities performed. These are commonly categorised as either vision-based or sensor-based activity recognition approaches [7]. Vision-based approaches, such as the deployment of video cameras, often raise privacy concerns which restrict their adoption. For example, according to [8], a large majority of the ageing population express privacy concerns with vision-based approaches and therefore are reluctant to their installation. Instead, sensor-based approaches are often preferred to eliminate privacy issues within health and wellbeing application areas. These can be body-worn sensors such as smart watches, or environmentally deployed sensors such as Passive Infrared (PIR) sensors, contact switches, vibration, pressure, temperature/light/humidity or Radio-Frequency Identification (RFID) sensors, which can unobtrusively monitor smart home inhabitants [8].

2.2 Knowledge-Driven vs Data-Driven Approach

Sensor-based activity recognition is generally categorised as either knowledge-driven or data-driven [9]. Data-driven approaches require large-scale datasets and the application of data mining and machine learning methods to learn activity models [10], whereas knowledge-driven approaches build activity models through exploiting rich prior knowledge within the focused domain [11]. Data-driven approaches are able to handle temporal information and uncertainty, and this may be deemed beneficial, however their successful implementation relies upon the use of large-scale datasets and reusability concerns have emerged as the learnt models may underperform when applied to a range of users [10]. Another concern that continues to challenge the successful implementation of data-driven approaches is the widely-acknowledged shortage in publicly available, accurately annotated and high-quality datasets [12]. In a study conducted by [13], a data-driven approach was designed and implemented to monitor the health and wellbeing of an elderly smart home inhabitant through detecting both normal and abnormal behaviours whilst performing ADLs. The proposed framework was able to analyse and process environmental sensor data, which were subsequently classified as either normal or abnormal ADLs using the k-Nearest Neighbour (kNN) algorithm. Considering instances of abnormal ADLs, the system generated alerts to notify care providers, in addition to generating a detailed report of the detected behaviour sent via email. The proposed system appeared promising, with the researchers indicating that experiments with real-time data streams were required to further evaluate the effectiveness of the proposed system.

The acknowledged concerns pertaining to data-driven techniques are overcome through the alternative application of knowledge-driven approaches, for example, they eliminate reusability concerns as knowledge-driven approaches generate generic models which can apply to a range of users. Nevertheless, these models are weaker at handling temporal information and uncertainty [11], and they are often weaker in dealing with complex activities due to providing insufficient human knowledge to capture their fine-grained components. Instead, human knowledge is commonly provided upon simplistic activities involving only the fundamental steps required to complete each activity. In a recently conducted study [14], a knowledge-driven solution to activity recognition was developed which combined elements of both static and recurrent models. A smart home inhabitant's behaviour was monitored through implementing a rule-based method which resembled a Finite State Machine (FSM). The developed method involved defining both "signature" sensors, i.e. those that only activated during one particular activity, and "descriptive" sensors, i.e. those that were consistently activated within multiple activities. ADL recognition was performed through detecting activity sequences within binary sensor event streams using the developed FSM-based method, followed by manually adjusting the designed rules based on the training data. Results demonstrated the effectiveness of the developed method; however, researchers stated the general applicability of their method was poor. Another recent study [15], proposed a knowledge-driven activity profiling technique based on training data. The defined activity profiles were used to induce additional features, i.e. fingerprinting, to help distinguish activities performed by smart home residents. A fingerprint vector was defined per activity which held distinguishing sensor events. The windowed training data was then augmented by incorporating the profiled features, for example if a particular window contained two distinguishing sensor events defined within an activity profile, the activity associated with those sensor events was chosen. Experimental results demonstrated the success of the proposed method in comparison to benchmarked techniques.

Recently, hybrid approaches have emerged which integrate both knowledge-driven and data-driven techniques to overcome the acknowledged limitations of each technique. For example, hybrid approaches are able to adjust and learn user preferences continuously, rather than generating static models. A promising hybrid method developed in [16] produced an Intelligent Decision Support System for dementia care. The proposed system involved two levels of decision making i.e. short-term and long-term. Short-Term Decision Making (STDM) was performed to raise alerts for abnormally detected ADLs, whereas Long-Term Decision Making (LTDM) supported decisions upon the rate of progression in the occupant's developmental stage of dementia. The STDM framework integrated data-driven decision making to learn abnormal behaviours and their associated alerts (low, high or emergency), and knowledge-driven rule-based decision making. Experimental results demonstrated the success of the proposed system in terms of classification accuracies obtained in comparison to the benchmarked methods.

Although hybrid methods have appeared promising recently, it was decided to develop a knowledge-driven, rule-based approach within this project due to the acknowledged limitations of data-driven methods. Particularly, the identified shortage of large-scale, accurately annotated datasets. The availability of domain knowledge provided by project partners has further motivated the exploration of a knowledge-driven approach.

3 ADL Dataset Considered

Given that changes in circumstances resulted in an inability to generate specific data for this study, external smart home data was used to evaluate the system. The data comprised of similar sensors and ADLs that were originally considered.

3.1 UCAmI

The chosen dataset was generated by researchers within the UJAmI smart lab over a period of 10 days. The smart lab, presented in Fig. 1, comprised five areas: an entrance, a kitchen, a living room and a bedroom merged with a bathroom. A single male inhabitant performed 24 ADLs whilst manually annotating the dataset during typical morning, afternoon and evening time routines. The recorded activities included: take medication, prepare breakfast, prepare lunch, prepare dinner, breakfast, lunch, dinner, eat a snack, watch tv, enter smart lab, leave smart lab, play a videogame, relax on the sofa, leave smart lab, visitor to smart lab, put waste in the bin, wash hands, brush teeth, use the toilet, wash dishes, put washing in the machine, work at the table, dressing, go to bed, and finally, wake up. A range of binary sensors were deployed throughout the smart lab comprising 4 PIR motion sensors, 24 contact switches and 2 pressure sensors. Pressure sensors were located within the sofa and the bed, contact switches were attached to, or integrated within, various objects and doors, and the PIR motion sensors were located within the main areas of the smart lab i.e., the kitchen, bedroom, bathroom and living area to detect movement.

It was decided to focus initially upon a small subset of ADLs as some were deemed relatively less integral and Kraydel currently had no available sensors to distinguish the following ADLs: wash dishes, laundry, washing hands and housekeeping/cleaning. Consequently, those ADLs were removed. The enter/leave home ADLs were also removed as the only available sensor, i.e., the motion sensor located in the hallway, currently provided insufficient information in distinguishing whether an inhabitant had entered or left the home. Finally, the resting/relax ADL was removed as the motion sensor within the Kraydel hub or the infra-red sensor in the living room could only determine that an inhabitant was in the living area, which was deemed insufficient in distinguishing this ADL. It was discussed that an additional sensor, for example a pressure sensor in the sofa, would provide more detailed information to distinguish the relaxing/resting ADL. Consequently, the ADL subset chosen for this project included the get up, go to bed, prepare meal, visitor, watch TV and use toilet activities.

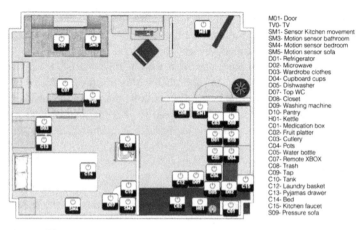

M01- Door
TV0- TV
SM1- Sensor Kitchen movement
SM3- Motion sensor bathroom
SM4- Motion sensor bedroom
SM5- Motion sensor sofa
D01- Refrigerator
D02- Microwave
D03- Wardrobe clothes
D04- Cupboard cups
D05- Dishwasher
D07- Top WC
D08- Closet
D09- Washing machine
D10- Pantry
H01- Kettle
C01- Medication box
C02- Fruit platter
C03- Cutlery
C04- Pots
C05- Water bottle
C07- Remote XBOX
C08- Trash
C09- Tap
C10- Tank
C12- Laundry basket
C13- Pyjamas drawer
C14- Bed
C15- Kitchen faucet
S09- Pressure sofa

Fig. 1. Location of binary sensors in the UJAmI smart lab

3.2 Dataset Preparation

All activity instances and sensor activations pertaining to the following ADLs were removed from the UCAmI dataset: wash dishes, laundry and washing hands, which involved sensors C09, D03, C13. As for the enter/leave home and resting/relax ADLs, the data for these activities was retained by merging them with others. For example, instances of enter/leave home were relabelled as visitor to efficiently use the available data, in addition to also including synthetic data to represent a binary doorbell activation. The pressure sensor located on the sofa (S09) was also retained within the dataset to provide additional information in distinguishing the watching TV ADL.

The data was then further reduced to remove any additional sensors that the UCAmI dataset contained which did not emulate the Kraydel environment. For example, to recognise the prepare meal ADL, both Kraydel and UCAmI have microwave (D02) and kettle (H01) sensors available, however the UCAmI dataset has an additional 15 kitchen sensors which were removed, including a trash sensor (C08), kitchen motion (SM1), cutlery (C03), closet (D08), refrigerator (D01), pantry (D10), water bottle (C05), cups cupboard (D04), pots (C04), washing machine (D09), laundry basket (C12), dishwasher (D05), kitchen faucet (C15), medication box (C01) and fruit platter (C02). The remaining redundant sensors chosen for removal included the Xbox remote (C07) and a motion sensor at the sofa (SM5) as these were not required to distinguish the chosen subset of ADLs. Finally, the UCAmI dataset was collected over 10 non-consecutive days in 2017, therefore the timestamps were updated and gaps in the data were removed to simulate data collection over 10 consecutive days.

Note that over time additional sensors will become available and it is intended for the approach presented in this paper to be extensible and handle both signature sensors and ADLs detectable through correlation of information from multiple sensors.

4 Rules Syntax

ADLs are used to monitor inhabitants within a smart home. They can be useful in assessing the wellbeing of the inhabitant and their ability to live independently in their own home. The project identified 6 core ADLs that an individual needs to be able to carry out in order for the person to be deemed capable of living independently. 6 ADLs were created based on the sensor data from the UCAmI dataset: Sleep, Get Up, Prepare Meal, Watching TV, Visitor, and Use Toilet.

The UCAmI sensor dataset was modified so that it contained only sensor events that are needed to trigger one of these 6 ADLs. To trigger an ADL, each rule requires a combination of more than one type of sensor event to occur within a specified time window. The rules are stored in the format shown in Fig. 2, each rule lists a number of key-values that are used by the code to determine if an ADL has occurred. Each of the 6 rules requires a minimum of 2 sensor events to happen within a specified time. This section explains each JSON key-value pair as well as describing how daily time routines are used to detect abnormal behaviour on the part of the inhabitant.

The rules specify the conditions that must be met for an ADL to trigger. An example of the rule for the Sleep ADL is shown in Fig. 2, this ADL is used in conjunction with the 'Get Up' ADL to calculate sleep duration. It is expected that this ADL will be triggered at 'Night', if it occurs during one of the other 3 routines (Morning, Afternoon, Evening) then the 'Identified Time Routine' column on the Dashboard UI will give one of these values this instead of 'Night'. Caregivers that are monitoring the Dashboard can determine that the inhabitant is not sleeping during the expected time routine, this could indicate physical illness or degradation of their mental state.

```
{
  "name": "Sleep",
  "type": "Sequence",
  "rearm_time": 480,
  "time_window": 600,
  "events": ["EM1_On", "L1_Off"],
  "expected_routine": ["Morning", "Afternoon", "Evening", "Night"],
  "min_values": [0,0,0,1],
  "max_values": [0,0,0,1]
},
```

Fig. 2. JSON format for the Sleep ADL

There are two *'types'* of rules that can be specified in the JSON rules file, these are Combination and Sequence. If the rule states that it is a 'Sequence' rule then the sensor events that it requires must happen in a specific order. The order is determined by the "events" section, in Fig. 2 the EM1_On sensor must occur before the L1_Off sensor otherwise the rule will not be triggered.

The *"rearm_time"* is the amount of time in seconds that must have elapsed before the ADL can be triggered again. If the Sleep ADL is detected, it can only be detected again after 480 s or 8 min. The UCAmI dataset initially had multiple sensor events going Off and On at the same Date and Time, this generated multiple ADLs of the same type when in fact only 1 ADL had occurred. The re-arm time feature was created to mitigate this, the dataset was eventually modified to remove all duplicate instances. However, this feature could be useful when using real-time sensors especially pressure sensors as they may give erroneous data.

The *"time_window"* value is used in conjunction with the current sensor event's date and time to find other sensor events. When a sensor event is read in, an initial check is performed against the rules file to see if this event matches the final sensor event in any of the rules *"events"* section. If any of the 6 rules' final *"event"* match the current sensor event then that rule is flagged for a further check. That rule's time window value is subtracted from the current sensor event's time to create a historic time window, the first event is then searched for within this window. In Fig. 2 the final sensor event that the Sleep Rule requires is L1_Off (Light turned off), if this L1_Off event is read in from the sensor events file, the code then searches for the first event EM1_On (Mattress pressure sensor on) in the sensor data.

The *"events"* section consists of 2 or more sensor events, all must occur within the stated time window. If the rule is a Sequence rule then the events must occur in the order listed, a Combination rule only requires all specified events to occur.

The expected routine lists all 4 times of day (Morning, Afternoon, Evening, Night), the number of times the ADL is expected to occur for each is listed in Min Values and Max Values. In Fig. 2, the Min and Max Values for sleep is 1 for the Night routine, it is not expected to occur more than once or during the other 3 routines.

It is important to be able to detect what is considered to be normal and abnormal behaviour as this can indicate a decline in physical health or a cognitive decline. The *"expected_routine"* is used to keep track of when the ADLs are activated and whether this is in keeping with the individual's normal routine or if it is an abnormal behaviour and perhaps a cause for concern and further investigation. The Dashboard UI was designed so that the routine time frames are customizable for an individual, this helps to ensure that the detection of abnormal behaviour is more accurate for each individual user.

5   Event Processing Engine

In this part, the main objective was to develop an event processing engine that could receive sensor events and recognize ADLs by using a rule-based system. The event processing engine was developed using Python, the web application was created using Flask. This section explains how the event processing engine uses the rules to detect that an ADL has occurred.

The UCAmI dataset is evaluated against a set of rules to check if an activity has taken place. When each line of the dataset is read in, the code performs a preliminary check to determine if the current sensor event matches any of the rule's events. All rules that require that particular sensor event are then added to a dataframe for potential matches. The code iterates through each rule and calculates the historic time window by subtracting the rule's *'time_window'* value from the current sensor event's time. The events that occurred within this window are compared to each of the potential rules' other required events. If a match occurs, then the ADL is added to a list of Detected ADLs and displayed on the web application Dashboard.

The two Rule 'types' are Combination and Sequence rules, the event checking code differs for each, with the sequence check code being more complex. A Sequence rule can only be activated if the sensor events occur in the order stated in the rule's events list. A Combination rule does not require the events to happen in a specific order, only that they both occur within the time window. The rationale behind the Sequence rule is that logically certain sensor events should take place before other events. In the case of the Get Up ADL, the bedside lamp (L1_On) must be in the On state before the mattress (EM1_Off) sensor is in the Off state. Note that this is just an example of a sequence rule and some conditions might change based on the individual's habits and routines. The Sequence check only performs the time window check if the current sensor event matches the final event in the rule's event list. This ensures that if the other rule event(s) are discovered within the time window they will have happened before the current event.

A broken or missing event ADL check was created to keep track of ADLs that are partially activated but not completed. This could give a Caregiver or Clinician some insight into the inhabitant's behaviour, if key ADLs such as 'Prepare Meal' are started but not finished then this is flagged on the Dashboard. When either the Combination or Sequence check methods are called, both methods perform a further check to look for broken Combination/Sequence events. A Broken Combi/Sequence ADL is when a sensor event matches a rule but the other events the rule requires do not occur. To detect that a broken ADL has occurred, the Combination and Sequence check methods add any sensor events to a list of potential broken ADLs. The list is also checked when the methods are called, and any event that has since been used to trigger an ADL is removed from the broken ADL list.

Other health metrics that are included in the analysis are Sleep Duration and Bathroom Frequency, both are displayed on the Dashboard. If the sleep duration is less than 6 h or more than 10 h an alert is created, this is shown in a DataTable on the Dashboard UI. The code requires both a Sleep and Get Up ADL to calculate duration, if Get Up doesn't occur then the sleep duration is not calculated. Future work would include a feature to notify if a Sleep ADL was not followed by a Get Up ADL within a certain amount of time. Another important health indicator is bathroom frequency, excessive visits that deviate from the inhabitant's norm may indicate illness. A daily upper limit is set within the code, when this value is exceeded this is flagged on the dashboard.

6 ADL Dashboard UI

The Dashboard User Interface (UI) was developed using the Python web application framework Flask. This section describes the analysis output presented on the Dashboard. The original UCAmI dataset is from 2017, the dates were changed to 2021 to reduce the amount of scroll back when using the date dropdowns.

6.1 Daily Summaries

The Daily Summaries stacked bar chart in Fig. 3 shows the number of ADLs that were triggered for a given day. The dates are shown on the Y axis, and an ADL frequency count (1, 2, 3…10) is on the X axis. Each day's bar consists of different colours representing different ADLs, the size of each section of the bar visually depicts how many times the ADL occurred that day (X axis count). A dropdown Date Picker allows the user to choose a date range, the bar chart updates according to the range chosen. The legend lists the ADLs, it is clickable and allows the user to remove ADLs from the chart, this is useful as it allows the user to simplify the chart, especially when comparing the same ADL over multiple days.

The stacked bar chart can be further customized with the Routines radio buttons underneath the chart. In Fig. 4, the 'Night' routine is selected, the chart then updates to only show the ADLs that took place during that time range. This feature is a good way of visually comparing the frequency of ADLs for several days, e.g., how many bathroom visits occurred during the night. The chart also includes a hover menu that appears when the mouse hovers over a bar, this lists the ADLs and the count for that day.

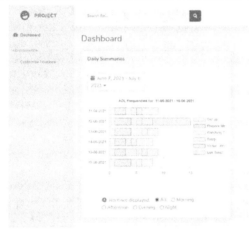

Fig. 3. Stacked Bar chart showing the frequency of all ADLs per day.

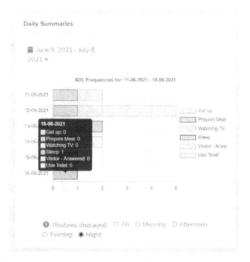

Fig. 4. Stacked Bar chart with Night routine selected.

6.2 Detected ADLs

The Detected ADL DataTable is shown in Fig. 5, it displays all of the ADLs for the entire dataset. The table includes the following columns – Date, Time, ADL, Identified Time Routine. The number of entries shown can be modified using the dropdown menu in the top right, the default is 10 entries. An ADL search function is included that enables the user to search for and display only the entries for that ADL. The Identified Time Routine gives the general time of day (Morning, Afternoon, Evening, Night) when the ADL occurred, this may be different to when an ADL is expected to occur. When an ADL occurs during a 'Time Routine' other than the one in which it is expected to occur, this could indicate a new illness or worsening of an existing condition.

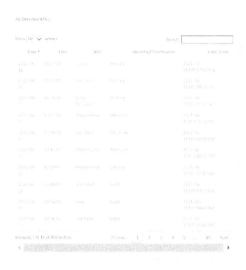

Fig. 5. Detected ADLs DataTable.

6.3 Daily Summary

The Daily Summary bar chart in Fig. 6 shows all ADLs that occurred on one day, the date can be changed using a dropdown menu. The Y Axis shows frequency count, this is the number of times that the ADL occurred, e.g., Sleep = 1, Prepare Meal = 2 times. The X axis lists the 6 ADLs (Sleep, Get Up, Prepare Meal, Watch TV, Visitor, Use Toilet). This chart is useful if the user wants to quick visual update on the current day as opposed to comparing multiple days and trends.

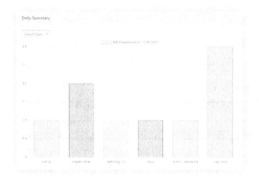

Fig. 6. Daily Summary Bar chart for one day.

6.4 Notification Alerts

This table is an amalgamation of the bathroom frequency and sleep duration alerts. The table is shown in Fig. 7, the columns are – Alert Type, Date, Alert, Information. Alert Type can be either 'Bathroom Alert' or 'Sleep Alert'. The Alert column gives the number of bathroom visits e.g., *"7 bathroom visits today"*, for Sleep it will state the sleep duration e.g. *"You slept for 12:13:00 h"*. The Information column then gives more detail as to why this activity has been flagged as an alert. For the sleep alert, it simply states "Overslept", the rule uses less than 6 and more than 10 h as the cut off values for sleeping too little or too much. The dataset does not include any instances of sleep duration being less than 6 h, so only the overslept alert is displayed. The information section for the bathroom alerts gives the upper limit of expected daily bathroom visits. This upper limit

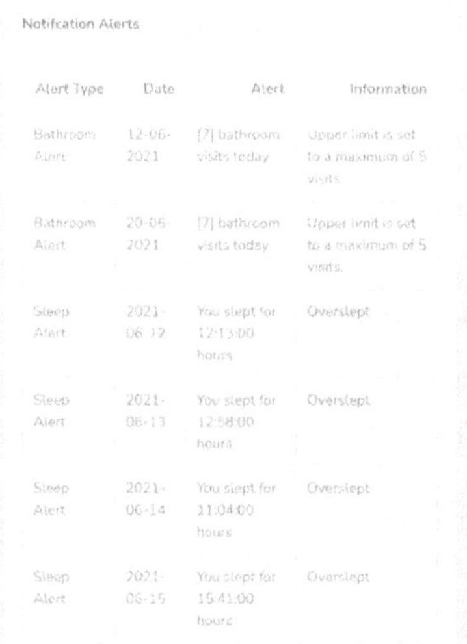

Alert Type	Date	Alert	Information
Bathroom Alert	12-06-2021	[7] bathroom visits today	Upper limit is set to a maximum of 5 visits
Bathroom Alert	20-06-2021	[7] bathroom visits today	Upper limit is set to a maximum of 5 visits
Sleep Alert	2021-06-12	You slept for 12:13:00 hours	Overslept
Sleep Alert	2021-06-13	You slept for 12:58:00 hours	Overslept
Sleep Alert	2021-06-14	You slept for 11:04:00 hours	Overslept
Sleep Alert	2021-06-15	You slept for 15:41:00 hours	Overslept

Fig. 7. Notification alerts table, this includes sleep and bathroom frequency alerts.

value can be customized for the inhabitant to give a more tailored experience. The actual number of daily visits is displayed in the Alert column.

6.5 Broken ADLs

The tables shown in Fig. 8 display all sensor events that were a partial match for a rule but did not result in an ADL activating, due to the other events needed not occurring in the time window. The tables include the sensor type (L1 is a lamp sensor), the value column indicates whether the sensor was on or off, the status, timestamp data, and the name of the partially triggered ADL rule. The Sequence rules table in Fig. 8(a) lists all ADL rules that require the sensor events to occur in a particular order. The Broken Combination table in Fig. 8(b) displays the sensor events and rule's that do not have to occur in any specific order.

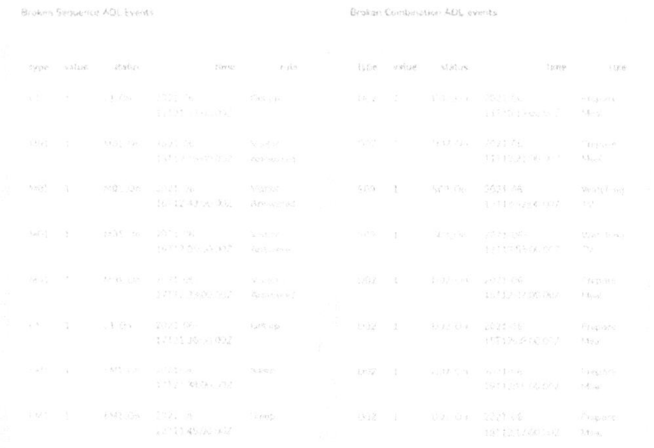

Fig. 8. (a) Broken sequence ADL table; (b) Broken combination ADL table.

7   Conclusions and Future Work

This paper presented the design of a rule-based and ADL analysis system that takes data from different sensors as input and presents a number of visualisations in a dashboard as output. The main parts of the system are: (i) a syntax to represent ADL rules, (ii) an event processing engine to process the ADL rules, and (iii) a dashboard user interface that includes a number of visualisations. The solution design presented is the output of a project collaboration with the Kraydel company, whose staff supported with ideas and with the commercial needs to consider for this solution. The project identified 6 core ADLs that an individual needs to be able to carry out for the person to be deemed capable of living independently: sleep, get up, prepare a meal, watch TV, have a visitor, and use toilet. Alternative forms of entertainment can be accommodated.

It was not possible to use real data collected from Kraydel because there was not enough at the time of the development of the system. As an alternative, the UCAmI dataset was used because the types of sensors considered (motion sensors, contact switches and pressure sensors) were the same as those used by Kraydel. Using a dataset collected at a smart lab instead of a dataset from Kraydel comprised by data from real situations did not affect the design presented in this paper. In terms of further data analysis and improvements, using a larger amount of real data collected from Kraydel will help in the development of the event processing engine and its ADL detection accuracy. While the number of sensors considered was determined by the sensors used by Kraydel, the modular design of the system allows adding or removing sensor data as required. Future work will consider the use of data collected from Kraydel and from other datasets to keep testing and improving the system. The use of more data from different sources to improve the functioning of the system and the accuracy in detecting abnormal behaviour will be investigated.

Acknowledgements. Invest Northern Ireland is acknowledged for supporting this project under the Competence Centre Programs Grant RD0513853 – Connected Health Innovation Centre.

References

1. WHO: Ageing. World Health Organisation (2020). https://www.who.int/health-topics/ageing. Accessed 18 Nov 2020
2. World Health Organisation: Global Strategy and Action Plan on Ageing and Health (2017)
3. Schomakers, E.-M., Heek, J.-V., Ziefle, M.: Attitudes towards aging and the acceptance of ICT for aging in place. In: Zhou, J., Salvendy, G. (eds.) Human Aspects of IT for the Aged Population. Acceptance, Communication and Participation. LNCS, vol. 10926, pp. 149–169. Springer, Cham (2018). https://doi.org/10.1007/978-3-319-92034-4_12
4. Krishnan, N.C., Cook, D.J.: Activity recognition on streaming sensor data. Pervasive Mob. Comput. **10**(Part B), 138–154 (2014)
5. Mlinac, M.E., Feng, M.C.: Assessment of activities of daily living, self-care, and independence. Arch. Clin. Neuropsychol. **31**(6), 506–516 (2016)
6. Yan, S., Liao, Y., Feng, X., Liu, Y.: Real time activity recognition on streaming sensor data for smart environments. In: IEEE International Conference on Progress in Informatics and Computing, pp. 51–55 (2016)
7. Ahmed, N., Rafiq, J.I., Islam, M.R.: Enhanced human activity recognition based on smartphone sensor data using hybrid feature selection model. Sensors **20**(1), 1–18 (2020)
8. Chen, L., Nugent, C.D.: Sensor-based activity recognition review. In: Chen, L., Nugent, C.D. (eds.) Human Activity Recognition and Behaviour Analysis, pp. 23–47. Springer, Cham (2019). https://doi.org/10.1007/978-3-030-19408-6_2
9. Lago, P., Inoue, S.: A hybrid model using hidden Markov chain and logic model for daily living activity recognition. In: Multidisciplinary Digital Publishing Institute Proceedings, vol. 2, no. 19, p. 1266 (2018)
10. Chen, L., Hoey, J., Nugent, C.D., Cook, D.J., Yu, Z.: Sensor-based activity recognition. IEEE Trans. Syst. Man Cybern. Part C (Appl. Rev.) **42**(6), 790–808 (2012)
11. Azkune, G., Almeida, A., López-De-Ipiña, D., Chen, L.: Extending knowledge-driven activity models through data-driven learning techniques. Expert Syst. Appl. **42**(6), 3115–3128 (2015)

12. Cleland, I., Donnelly, M.P., Nugent, C.D., Hallberg, J., Espinilla, M.: Collection of a diverse, naturalistic and annotated dataset for wearable activity recognition. In: PerCom (2018)
13. Pirzada, P., White, N., Wilde, A.: Sensors in smart homes for independent living of the elderly. In: 5th International Multi-Topic ICT Conference Technologies for Future Generations, IMTIC 2018 - Proceedings, pp. 1–8 (2018)
14. Karvonen, N., Kleyko, D.: A domain knowledge-based solution for human activity recognition: the UJA dataset analysis. In: MDPI Proceedings UCAmI 2018, pp. 1–8 (2018)
15. Rawashdeh, M., Al Zamil, M.G., Samarah, S., Hossain, M.S., Muhammad, G.: A knowledge-driven approach for activity recognition in smart homes based on activity profiling. Future Gener. Comput. Syst. **107**, 924–941 (2020)
16. Gayathri, K.S., Elias, S., Easwarakumar, K.S.: Assistive dementia care system through smart home. In: Somani, A.K., Srivastava, S., Mundra, A., Rawat, S. (eds.) Proceedings of First International Conference on Smart System, Innovations and Computing. SIST, vol. 79, pp. 455–467. Springer, Singapore (2018). https://doi.org/10.1007/978-981-10-5828-8_43
17. Tkinter. https://docs.python.org/3/library/tkinter.html. Accessed 8 July 2021
18. Dash. https://plotly.com/dash/. Accessed 8 July 2021
19. Chart.js. https://www.chartjs.org/. Accessed 8 July 2021

Design for Discordant Chronic Comorbidities (DCCs): A DC³ Model

Tom Ongwere[1]([⊠]), Erik Stolterman[2], Patrick C. Shih[2], Clawson James[2], and Kay Connelly[2]

[1] University of Dayton, Dayton, USA
tongwere1@udayton.edu
[2] Indiana University Bloomington, Bloomington, USA
{estolter,patshih,clawson,connelly}@indiana.edu

Abstract. Patients with complex conditions and treatment plans often find it challenging to communicate with multiple providers and to prioritize various management tasks. The challenge is even greater for patients with discordant chronic comorbidities (DCCs), a situation where a patient has conditions that have unrelated and/or conflicting treatment plans. We present results that highlight these challenges from two studies. The first is a photo-elicitation study with patients with DCCs (n = 16), and the second is an interview study of health providers (n = 8). In an attempt to address these challenges, we introduce a model that captures the different stages of synthesizing information about symptoms and suggested medical treatments, decision making around possible treatment plans including prioritizing different portions of the plan, and implementing their plan. This model is iterative, such that changes in a plan can impact symptoms and necessitate revisiting the plan. We call this model the Discordant Chronic Condition Care (DC³) model.

Keywords: Contextual model · Care and treatment · Type-2 diabetes · Discordant chronic conditions · Information sharing · Decision making

1 Introduction

Treating and managing Discordant Chronic Comorbidities (DCCs) is a major challenge in health care [17–19]. DCCs are when two or more conditions have unrelated or even conflicting treatment plans. For example, depression, arthritis, and end-stage renal disease are discordant to type-2 diabetes [18,21]. Patients with DCCs must often coordinate between multiple providers and each provider prioritizes the specific condition they are treating. These competing priorities make it difficult for patients to know how to create a treatment plan that is best for their particular situation [18]. For example, a patient with type-2 diabetes and arthritis may work with one provider to control their diabetes symptoms while simultaneously working with another provider to control their arthritis

© ICST Institute for Computer Sciences, Social Informatics and Telecommunications Engineering 2022
Published by Springer Nature Switzerland AG 2022. All Rights Reserved
H. Lewy and R. Barkan (Eds.): PH 2021, LNICST 431, pp. 346–362, 2022.
https://doi.org/10.1007/978-3-030-99194-4_22

symptoms. As such, changes in the treatment plan for diabetes can negatively impact the maintenance of arthritis. This exposure to disease and treatment interaction requires a patient with DCCs to have a lifetime engagement with the healthcare system. There is a continuous need to change strategies as a patient goes through unstable cycles, with an attempt to find a new normal [18]. In fact, these periods of stability are often quite short for patients with DCCs, since treatment for one condition may be contraindicated by treatment for another condition.

There is a body of work in the Human-Computer Interaction (HCI) and Personal Informatics, that emphasizes the design and implementation of tools, models, and frameworks to support the management of chronic conditions. For example, i) a holistic framework describing patients' complex and diverse cancer journeys from diagnosis through survivorship [10,13], ii) a five-stage model (Stage-based Model of Personal Informatics Systems) for understanding how people use personal informatics tools and barriers people face in each stage [15], iii) a lived informatics model for personal informatics that captures the practices of self-trackers to help change behavior, encourage or maintain an activity, or motivate individuals to self-track [8], and iv) a tool, the mobile diabetes detective (MODD), designed to facilitate reflection and problem-solving in diabetes self-management [16]. However, these current approaches and tools are limited to helping patients manage a single chronic condition and do not support patients with DCCs [18,24]. Furthermore, these current technology tools and models do not consider the complex interactions and unstable disease changes experienced by patients with DCCs.

We provide three main contributions in this paper: i) we investigate the health management challenges of patients with DCCs, including the perspectives of healthcare providers, ii) we propose a conceptual model that represents a process of sense-making and decision making for treating DCCs and seeks to address the challenges of managing DCCs, and iii) we discuss design implications that address complexities of DCCs care.

2   Background

Current studies have explored and designed models that inform and support the design of tools that track, monitor individual patients' behaviors, and promote sense-making and decision-making among patients and healthcare providers. However, these models are not capturing the complexity of DCCs. Here, we discuss the examples of those models and their limitations when it gets to care of complex interacting conditions.

First we discuss Personal Health Informatics models and tools that support decision-making and adherence. A model of shared decision-making consists of four key elements: i) at least two participants (i.e., the physician or multiple clinicians, patient, and family members) are involved in the decision-making process; ii) participants engage in all steps of the treatment decision-making process; iii) information is shared prior to the shared decision-making, and iv) both participants agree to the decision. The model highlights three major constructs [4]. The first construct is information sharing between clinicians (i.e. treatment options, risks, benefits, and patients' histories). The second construct is equal participation/contribution to the treatment priorities by patients and their providers, and in some instances, family, caretakers, or other healthcare providers also contribute to this discussion process [4]. At the end of the discussion, options are presented, including those that are not being considered for a patient to pursue. Finally both patients and providers agree on the best course of action. During the setting and implementation of this course of action, goal setting and self-efficacy constructs play a major role. For example, they are being used to design tools that facilitate patient engagement. [1,2]. Patient engagement tools include self-monitoring and receiving behavioral reminders [22]. Patients can now be engaged by self-management technological tools (heart rate monitors, blood glucose monitors and medication reminders) [5,13,16].

The second consideration for models in HCI and personal health informatics is Li et al.'s five-stage model. Inspired by the TTM, Li et al. developed a model that characterizes how people transition between five stage (i.e., preparation, collection, integration, reflection, and action) of their personal informatics tracking needs and describes the iterative nature of these information tracking stages and the barriers that prevent transitions [15]. This model was later expanded to include two phases of reflection, and discovery and maintenance [15]. These new phases allowed individuals to ask different types of questions in each phase. However, the model did not adequately account for the daily activities of self trackers. To address this challenge, Epstein et al. expanded the five stage model and created "a lived informatics model of personal informatics" which adequately characterizes the integration of self-tracking into everyday life by individuals. A set of studies in diabetes care are exploring the design and implementation of social technological interventions that i) support patients in tracking and collecting relevant information [6], ii) facilitate reflection and problem-solving, and iii) help patients make healthy dietary and exercise choices [5].

Third, Mamykina et al. [16] used their self-reflection and problem-solving tool (MODD) to develop a diabetes self-management model with steps that include i) identifying problematic glycemic control patterns, ii) exploring behavioral triggers, iii) selecting alternative behaviors, and iv) implementing these behaviors while simultaneously monitoring behaviors for improvement.

Finally, in cancer management, Hayes et al. proposed four stages of caring for cancer patients [10]. These stages include: i) screening and diagnosis, ii) initial information seeking, iii) acute care and treatment, and iv) no evidence of disease or chronic disease management. This work has informed the design of interventions including the *"cancer journey framework"* and associated *"my journey campus"* intervention used to help patients with breast cancer navigate through their healthcare needs from diagnosis to survivorship [13]. My journey campus provides a list of tools that i) accompany people on their healthcare journeys, ii) accommodate shifts in patients' needs, and iii) motivate patients and increase patients' energy levels and goals in the different stages of their journey [10].

In this section, we show that there are personal health informatics models that strive to i) inform the strategies and tool designs used to empower patients in becoming active agents of their health; ii) help engage patients in activities that promote exercise, diet, socializing, medication management, and symptom reporting while also helping patients monitor their own physical and emotional status and make incremental goals; and iii) support patients with chronic diseases with setting and adjusting their treatment plans. While existing models focus on people's readiness to change and provide actionable steps for different stages, we have yet to see work that focuses on people's ability to reengage and iterate when complications occur due to complicating events that are common with DCCs, such as multiple contradicting recommendations and interactions between goals. Future work is needed to explain how people can simultaneously handle multiple decisions within and across different stages of behavioral change. Furthermore, the increase in multimorbidities, especially when the conditions are conflicting (DCCs), require healthcare and healthcare systems to shift their traditional focus from individual conditions to approaches that account for a patient's multiple health needs [14,17,23]. This paper introduces such a model.

3 Methods

3.1 Data Collection

In prior work, [18,19] we conducted two studies to understand the challenges of caring for and supporting the care of discordant chronic comorbidities. In the first study [18], we distributed questionnaires and conducted a photo-elicitation interview (PEI) with patients with DCCs. We investigated how patients with DCCs navigate the care and treatment of their complex health conditions and uncovered challenges faced by patients with type-2 diabetes. Fifteen participants completed the study (participants were recruited until we reached data saturation [9]). The participants i) were between the ages of 25–65, ii) expressed an interest in the study and were willing to take photographs and participate in interviews, and iii) self-reported as having type-2 diabetes and at least one additional chronic condition, such as arthritis or depression or both.

In the second study [19], we conducted interviews and focus groups with healthcare providers attending to patients with DCCs. In this study healthcare providers included; physicians, health coaches, nurses, psychiatrists, clinical and social workers, and pharmacists. The interview focused on gaining a deeper understanding of healthcare providers' perspectives on DCC patient care. The focus groups focused on the challenges identified during the interviews and brainstorming strategies and opportunities to effectively support the complex care of DCCs. Eight healthcare providers participated in the interview study. Seven of these providers participated in a focus group study. Only healthcare providers who self-reported treating type-2 diabetes and common DCCs associated with type-2 diabetes (e.g., depression, chronic kidney disease, or arthritis) participated in the study. Given difficulty in recruiting healthcare providers, eight (N = 8) participants is an acceptable number for these types of studies

[7,12]. The Institutional Review Board (IRB) at our university approved the both studies.

3.2 Analysis

The research team employed a variety of techniques to analyze the results from the two studies. First, to understand patients and providers perspectives about the DCCs care needs, we used a thematic analysis [3] and affinity diagramming [11] to analyze patient and provider data. We systematically segmented the data from each study and broke the audio transcripts into exemplary quotes, each of which contained a key thematic point. Our team of six (for patients study) and three (for providers study) inductively organized these quotes into new categories to identify major themes.

From the patient study, five themes emerged from our analysis of the data. The second study, highlighted five themes. Themes from the patient study and provider study were further categorized into subcategories and were used to create a codebook that generated final codes. The research team refined the codebook and conducted iterations of data analysis. In each iteration, we discussed the codes and the respective excerpts and created new ones, resulting in the following three themes: i) information gathering and comprehension, ii) decision making when determining treatment plans, and iii) implementing treatment plans. For details about the methods, participant selection, and study design, please see [18] for the patients' study and [19] for the healthcare providers' study.

4 DCC Challenges

In this section, we describe the challenges that are specific to patients with DCCs based on our work with patients with DCCs [18] and their healthcare providers [19]. We summarize these challenges in three distinct stages identified in our prior work: i) information gathering and comprehension, ii) decision making when determining treatment plans, and iii) implementing treatment plans. See (Fig. 1) Below we discuss these stages in detail, all statements come from the prior work.

4.1 Information Gathering and Comprehension

Patients must constantly take in new information and determine if it necessitates a conversation with one or more of their providers. The new information may come in the form of new symptoms or diagnoses. For example, if a patient experiences new information (a symptom), it may be severe enough to prompt a patient to report it to their provider, resulting in a treatment plan change; however, sometimes a symptom may simply be an inconvenience to the patient and the patient may determine that reporting the information to a provider would not be worth the risk of upsetting the current balance. Other reasons patients intentionally do not to share information with providers include that

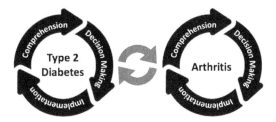

Fig. 1. Treating multiple conditions in isolation can lead to unexpected interactions. (*In the iterative analysis of the patients' and providers' data, we observed that changes in the treatment plan for one condition often negatively impact the control of the other condition. Leading three-stage management (i.e., information gathering and comprehension, decision making when determining treatment plans, and implementing treatment plans) cycle for each of their conditions.*)

the information might negatively impact their insurance coverage, or because the patient believes the provider would not be interested in knowing the information. There are also times when patients unintentionally neglect to share relevant information. This is typically because patients have difficulty with clinical terms and procedures and cannot remember all the relevant information.

Regardless of the reason why, providers view the patient altering or omitting details as frustrating the provider's ability to accurately assess the health and treatment plans of their patient. Providers also complain that information is sometimes shared in an unhelpful manner. For example, the information may be presented in the form of a large disorganized pile of paper records from past doctors' office visits. This practice also frustrates providers.

4.2 Decision Making and Setting Treatment Plans

To better manage DCCs, patients and their providers have to prioritize different conditions to set achievable goals. However, setting these priorities can be challenging. One primary challenge is that different healthcare providers have different treatment preferences. In particular, healthcare providers typically feel that the condition they are treating should be the priority. For example, a healthcare provider who treats patients for diabetes asserted that mental health issues cannot be addressed until a patient's diabetes is under control. Whereas another healthcare provider insisted that mental health issues keep patients from taking care of their physical health, so mental health should be the priority. These different views result in conflicts in the decision-making process [18,21].

Another issue is treatment plan (i.e., prescriptions such as drugs, lifestyle, assistive devices, and therapies) interactions complicate prioritization. Complex interactions cause adverse effects in patients with DCCs, such as rapid and severe changes in symptoms. Although providers recognized this complexity, they pointed to several reasons it was difficult to overcome. First, the rapid changes in symptoms and disease progression interfere with providers' abilities to observe and prioritize treatments for their patients. Second, providers are constrained for time and do not have enough time to thoroughly evaluate their patients and make informed treatment decisions. Third, patients react differently to each combination of treatment plans, so providers use trial and error with each patient. This is much harder when a patient is treating multiple conditions. Finally, providers are not able to easily consult their patients' other providers located in other healthcare systems, which inhibits providers from reconciling their patients' treatment, including therapies and prescription medicines. This is especially true for patients and providers in our studies, where mental health providers reside in different healthcare organizations than physical health providers.

Finally, even when a treatment plan is set, the cost of managing DCCs is higher and patients are not always able to afford and complete the treatment plan prescribed to them. Providers and patients agree that the cost of managing DCCs is higher [18,19]. Costs often interfered with providers' abilities to help some patient's complete treatment plans. Patients are greatly burdened by the costs of their prescribed treatment plans.

4.3   Implementing Treatment Plans

Patients with DCCs often have a complex treatment plans (i.e. medications, therapy, procedures and tests). This complexity increases patients' chances of getting overwhelmed and some patients even experience worse treatment outcomes, which in turn affect patients' abilities to implement or adhere to such prescriptions. Healthcare providers think that this non-adherence is made worse when providers prescribe treatment plans without considering the potential conflicts with prescriptions written by their other providers or the burden it imposes on patients. Even if treatment plans for different conditions did not conflict, patients are often overwhelmed with the quantity and complexity of treatment protocols.

When implementing an agreed upon treatment plan, patients are also frustrated by constant side effects. When confronting the struggle of balancing the complex and sometimes conflicting advice from multiple providers, patients also face an additional barrier such as coping with constantly changing symptoms and drug interactions imposed by another DCC. Healthcare providers also think that patients are not capable of implementing complex treatment plans. This issue arises when the patient tries implementing a treatment plan and new and often worse symptoms emerge. This issue also arises because a patient's mental capability or energy levels are too low to proceed with a complex treatment plan. Moreover, patients also sometimes experience negative side effects when implementing a new plan. Thus, a patient must be on the lookout for both positive and negative changes in their health. These changes may necessitate the patient to terminate a current treatment plan and return to the decision-making stage and alter the treatment plan.

Another challenge in treatment implementation and adherence results from patients' support networks. We noticed conflicting perception between patients and providers regarding the impact of patients' support networks. Healthcare providers claim that patients' support networks are a significant cause of patients' poor treatment decisions and lifestyle choices and often compromise patients' willingness to medicate. For example, some healthcare providers think that some patients refuse to implement a prescribed treatment plan or undergo the recommended procedure because of the miss-information patients receive from their support networks. However, patients find the informational support they get from their support network helpful. Patients learn from their peers' experiences–both what worked and what did not work for them. The healthcare providers were particularly against their patients learning from and changing their treatments based on the opinions of their peers because every patient with DCC has unique experiences. Current studies suggest that some patients can be experts about their conditions [8]. Patients (peers) can provide perspectives as experts from their unique experience and knowledge [20].

5   Discordant Chronic Condition Care (DC³) Model

In a prior section, we show how care and management of DCCs requires simultaneous coordination of multiple aspects of a patient's health in which one change in management of one disease may negatively impact another disease. This added complexity can potentially lead to shorter times of stability and longer periods of detective work and changing treatment plans. Alongside the challenge of implementing a complex treatment plan, it can be difficult for patients with DCCs to even track down the underlying source of a particular symptom, given their multiple conditions and numerous medications and management tasks. For patients with a single disease (e.g. diabetes or cancer), the diagnosis process is often simplified: it's either yes or no. While patients with DCCs always need to ask "but which one?". If a patient has DCCs, they need to deal with the confusion created by disease interactions and conflicting advice between multiple healthcare providers. In addition, providers often want the patient to prioritize the condition they are treating, and there are no mechanisms for helping the patient prioritize different aspects of their treatment across conditions or providers. Indeed, prioritization is often ad-hoc and haphazard. Further, patients are frequently used as the conduit for de-facto communication between providers, resulting in frustration on all sides. We use these observations to introduce the Discordant Chronic Condition Care (DC³) model (Fig. 1). The DC³ model recognizes DCCs complexities and incorporates key strategies for i) assessing and addressing the complexity of DCCs care, ii) adapting to an individual's varying goals and needs, and iii) working closely with healthcare providers who understand the disease and the patients who are living with DCCs.

The DC³ model identifies 3 major stages:

- Comprehension: a patient encounters a new symptom, condition, information or advice that requires an interpretation and contextualization to their

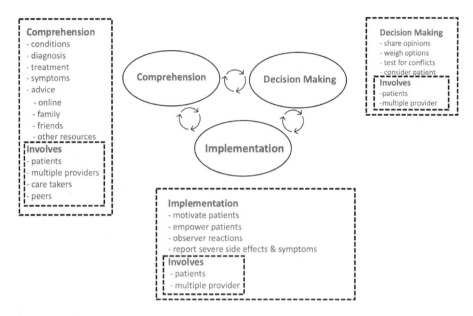

Fig. 2. DC³ model for DCCs. (*We use the information presented by patients with DCCs* [18] *and their health providers* [19] *to develop diagram that simulates three stages of management (DC³ model): i) information comprehension, ii) treatment plan decision making, and iii) treatment plan implementation. Other additions to the diagram include accounting for all stakeholders (patients, providers, and patients' support networks (friends, family, and peers)) and the iterative nature of the DCCs care process)*

current health condition. This process of interpreting the new input often requires the patient to communicate with providers to fully understand the implications and decide if a change in treatment should be considered. The comprehension stage identifies a need to support patients in recording any potentially relevant information (Takeaway #1), and support providers in filtering that information to focus on the most urgent and relevant (Takeaway #2). This will help address the challenges caused by the complex information patients collect. Further, this process of supporting patients and providers may include identifying information sources and multiple facts for all of the patient's conditions and sharing of that information with and among multiple healthcare providers.

– Decision making: based on the understanding of the new information, the patient and providers must decide if they will modify the current treatment plan. Additional information may be sought (e.g. further tests), and a cost/benefit analysis performed. Patients may decide the potential risks of changing their treatment plans are too severe, such as upsetting their other conditions and balancing the conflicting advice from multiple providers. The decision making stage suggests a need to i) help patients navigate conflicting advice and prioritize different aspects of their treatment plans (Takeaway #3) and ii) support patients and providers in recording, reviewing, and starting/stopping treatment plans including therapies and prescription medicines (Takeaway #4). This will allow patients to prioritize their daily tasks intelligently and spend time on high-value treatment plans. It should provide patients an avenue to identify what types of decisions require professional consultation and what types of decisions can be initiated and implemented by the patient themselves. Further, it allows patients and providers to keep track of treatment plans including therapies and prescription medicines that were stopped and why they were stopped.

– Implementation: after a new plan is formulated, the patient needs support in executing the plan, including monitoring the outcome of the changes and communicating that information to their multiple providers. A change in health status may move the patient to the first stage where the cycle may begin again. The implementation stage needs to: First, help patients break down larger treatment goals into smaller, achievable tasks reflecting the patient's capabilities to help patients address the difficulty of adhering to complex treatment plans (Takeaway #5). Second, consider a patient's unique cognitive capability, energy level, and external resources available to that patient to implement a plan. This will help patients who are failing to adhere to their treatment plan because of negative side effects or severe mental, physical or environmental limitations (Takeaway #6). Third, support patients to digest and process new information received from their support network and seek a second opinion from a healthcare professional. This will help reduce any negative contributions of patients' support networks in patient non adherence (Takeaway #7). Finally, costs should be brought to the forefront so that a patient and their healthcare providers can reduce the risk of a patient failing to afford an agreed upon treatment plan or procedure (Takeaway #8).

6   Discussion

Throughout this paper, we present results from two studies that led to the DC³ model. This section compares the DC³ model with some existing models and frameworks and discusses how the DC³ model might be used to influence the design of tools to support patients with DCCs.

6.1   Comparison of DC³ Model

The DC³ model suggests a lens for designers looking to support individuals with multiple complex needs and can be differentiated from others in the following ways:

First, the DC³ model focuses on the fact that two or more single diseases go in parallel and have complex interactions. The DC³ model could help designers focus on disease interactions that complicate DCCs care. This is not the case in the care and support of single chronic diseases. It is true that some single chronic diseases are extremely difficult to manage because of conflicts between symptoms. For example, with respect to epilepsy, patients are confronted with choosing between having seizures or having the ability to think fast. Likewise, patients with Parkinson's may have to choose between feeling nauseous or having better motor skills. Despite that, if a patient has a single disease, they are aware of such conflicts. However, if a patient has DCCs, they need to deal with the confusion created by disease interactions and conflicting advice between multiple healthcare providers.

Secondly, compared to other models - such as the cancer management models [10], the journey framework [13], a lived informatics model of personal informatics [8], and TTM - the DC^3 model suggests strategies necessary to generate a rich understanding of when a patient needs change. The model also suggests the input on how designers might develop solutions to match an individual's needs. The DC^3 model does not specify endpoints of diagnosis and cure, or pre-contemplation and termination of behavior, as patients with DCCs will likely live the rest of their lives with these conditions. Instead, the model contains the general cycle of information seeking, decision making, and implementation present in the diabetes model, and also recognizes that there are multiple diseases to manage. The detective work involved must balance many potentially conflicting factors. For this reason, patients may stay in one stage for an extended period of time, or even backtrack to a prior stage before being able to move on to the next stage. The DC^3 model represents the complexity and time-consuming process of continuously having to comprehend new symptoms, information, and advice. In addition, the DC^3 model also accounts for the modification of treatment plans, including how to prioritize and implement different plans that may come from different providers, while monitoring for changes in the progression and symptoms of a condition. Furthermore, The DC^3 model emphasizes the need to communicate amongst multiple providers throughout this process.

6.2   Implications for Design

DCCs care is already complex, but is further worsened by multiple actors. Doctors are zooming in on certain aspects of the disease and trying to optimize that part only. They can lose focus of how the other conditions are impacting their patients and they need support in focusing on their patients' complex needs. Take as an example, the geographic aspects of a map. Maps guide us by telling us where to go; maps orient us by pointing us in certain directions; and maps place us in context and tell us what is around us. Here we discuss how the DC^3 model could inform the design of tools to support providers and patients with DCCs in seeing beyond a singular disease. These design suggestions include creating tools: for a single stage, to transition between stages, to simplify complexities, and to coordinate the treatment plans prescribed by multiple healthcare providers.

Tools for a Single Stage
The DC^3 model could be used to design tools to support patients with multiple conditions in individual stages of the management process. In the comprehension

stage, tools could help patients organize information across multiple conditions instead of focusing on a single condition or type of data. Tools that collect symptoms, condition information and common treatments for different conditions should be created. These tools should not separate this information based on different conditions. Instead, these tools should present all of the information and symptom in a way that makes sense to a patient. In essence, we advocate for providing a view of the entire patient instead of individual conditions. Thus, when a patient reports/records a new symptom, it can be placed in the context of their other symptoms, regardless of which condition caused the symptom. Focusing on the conglomeration of symptoms and other information associated with a patient's multiple conditions reduces the probability of a patient or provider making a change for one condition without considering how that change might impact a patient's other conditions.

In the decision-making stage, tools could be created that help patients collect all of the different treatment recommendation made by their various providers and evaluate them simultaneously. While a single provider might not recommend too many adjustments to a treatment plan at once, as the combination of treatment adjustments across providers might be too much for the patient to execute. Further, by collecting all of the treatments together in one place, patients and providers can be attuned to look for possible interactions across recommendations for different conditions. Finally, in the implementation stage, tools should be created to help patients track their progress for the entire plan, and not just individual components.

Tools for Transitions Between Stages

In addition to developing tools to help with the challenges of individual stages, tools that help patients transition from one stage to the next would be extremely valuable. Patients with complex conditions can bounce back and forth between stages when trying to determine or implement an appropriate plan. For example, a patient who has noticed a new symptom and goes to a provider to adjust their treatment plan, may be asked to record other information. This information may be used to identify whether an adjustment may impact another condition. This can take the patient back to the comprehension phase. Similarly, a patient and their provider might alter the treatment plan, only to discover, after implementation of the plan, a negative impact on one of the patient's conditions. Tools are needed to help quickly communicate with all providers and adjust the plan, without a patient having to wait days or weeks to see their various providers. In the comprehension stage, the communications with and among providers is challenged when patients alter or omit details when communicating their other providers' recommendations. Providers are also frustrated and unable to accurately assess the health and treatment plans of their patient, because their patients share information in a disorganized and unhelpful manner. We recommend the design of tools to support patients in recording any potentially relevant information (Takeaway #1), and to support providers in filtering that information into the most urgent and relevant items of information (Takeaway #2).

Tools to Simplify the Complexity

Patients with DCCs are differentiated from patients with a single condition in that all of the stages and transitions are complicated by the presence of conditions which may work against each other. In the implementations stage, patients struggled with complex treatment plans, were overwhelmed and often experienced worse treatment outcomes.

We recommend the design of tools to help patients breakdown larger treatment goals into smaller, achievable tasks reflecting the patient's capabilities (Takeaway #8). These complicated interactions need to be simplified so patients can easily flag them (to discuss with providers), and better understand how a treatment for one condition may impact another. Similar to having drug interaction lists that are commonly available [26], patients should have access to treatment interaction lists tailored to their conditions. This would allow potential negative interactions to be flagged contemporaneous to the provider recommending a particular diet or lifestyle change. This would allow the provider to consider if there is another recommendation that could be made without exacerbating the other condition (e.g. swimming for exercise instead of walking when a patient has arthritis).

Furthermore, in the implementation stage, the cost of implementing multiple treatment plans brings in another complexity and consequently hinders a patient's ability to adhere to the treatment plans. The financial aspect should also be included in the tools. For example, when setting treatment plans, the tool should bring the cost to the forefront so that a patient and their healthcare providers lessen the risk of a patient failing to afford a treatment plan or procedure (Takeaway #5). The tools should include what is covered by a patient's insurance and what activities can be obtained through local community groups. The tools should also include less expensive options, such as lifestyle changes opposed to expensive medications. The benefits of alternative less expensive treatment plans, such as lifestyle changes, could result in multiple positive outcomes. In fact, for DCCs, (with type-2 diabetes) not only could lifestyle lower the costs but also reduces the risk of harmful medication side effects (i.e. hypoglycemia and weight gain).

However, for DCCs lifestyle changes may have barriers too. When a patient has arthritis, increasing physical activity may be another challenge. This is another example of how treatment interactions force patients and providers to prioritize treatment plans. This situations is worse when a treatment plan interaction causes adverse side effects, and rapid and severe changes in symptoms. Tools should help the patient and providers prioritize their treatment plans and strike a balance, since the patient may need to take multiple medications. Doing so requires careful monitoring to ensure that a patient complies with the goal set with his or her provider, so to avoid worse complications. If complications occur, tools must support patients in stopping certain plans. For example, a tool meant to support patients and providers in prioritizing treatment plans should also support patients and providers in recording, reviewing and starting/stopping treatment plans. Further, these tools should also ensure that the reason for each prescription (symptom and disease) is recorded for easier review in the future, as well as linking symptoms to potential drug side effects, especially when starting a new prescription or changing a dosage (#4).

Tools for Coordinating with Multiple Providers

The care of DCCs relies on a shared understanding of a patient's complex information. Tools that help patients coordinate communication amongst their various providers are desperately needed (as suggested in the "Transitions Between Stages" section above). While EHR can be an adequate communication tool for providers that reside in the same health system, many patients with DCCs see providers in different health systems. When this occurs, providers often rely on patients to be the conduit for communication, yet patients struggle with this role [18]. A tool that facilitates communication between providers could help prevent bad treatment choices and alleviate the frustrations experienced by both patients and providers. These tools could be similar to monitoring tools suggested in [25]. In addition, when the information is shared, these tools should have a capability to support multiple healthcare providers and patients to collaboratively digest and process new information as well as seek professional verification of the new information (Takeaway #7).

In the decision-making stage, a major concern is that different healthcare providers have different treatment preferences. Tools should be created to help patients navigate conflicting advice and prioritize different aspects of their treatment plans (Takeaway #3). We also would like to emphasize the importance of shared decision making. Tools must be created to facilitate shared decision making and allow one provider to i) gain a realistic understanding of the patient's current health status (comprehension), ii) evaluate a patient's unique cognitive capability, energy level, and external resources available to implement a plan (#6), and ii) seek the perspective of other providers attending to the same patient. For patients with DCCs, tools can also provide an overview of the patient's severe symptoms resulting from multiple interacting chronic conditions as well as progressive symptoms that may become problematic at a later time. Tools should be designed to explore each of these scenarios and best characterize patients' current situations and how their health is likely going to evolve over time before making a treatment recommendation.

We need to recognize that patients with DCCs struggle to make decisions due to conflicting treatment paradigms and conflicting professional advice. We also need to recognize that designs can help these people make better decisions despite the multiple and often conflicting recommendations they receive. How can we help these patients sort through all this information so they can formulate a plan and try that plan? Some may decide to consult their other doctors' views about a decision. Some patients may want to know the time elapse before they begin to see a change. Patients need to be aware of potential side effects and reactions, and should be informed on the recommended steps if such events occur. Most technologies used to support patients do not account for any of the above. Patients should be empowered to have these conversations and bring this knowledge to their healthcare providers.

7 Conclusion

In this paper, we present results from two studies focused on challenges that patients with DCCs and their providers face when managing multiple conditions which may have conflicting treatment plans. Challenges revolve around having multiple conditions with multiple providers, complex treatment plans in which a change in the treatment of one condition can worsen another condition, and limitations on what patients can accomplish. We use these empirical results to develop the DC^3 model intended to support the design of systems to assist in the care and treatment of DCCs. Contrary to existing chronic disease care models, DC^3 focuses on the complexity of prioritizing multiple treatment goals and explicitly acknowledges the somewhat erratic nature of DCCs in which there is not always a clear trajectory or end. DC^3 also highlights the multiple stakeholders, emphasizing the difficulties patients often have with communicating and negotiating between multiple providers who may not be sensitive to the impact their recommendations may have on other aspects of the patient's health. Finally, DC^3 recognizes that attaining a "stable state" for patients with DCCs is difficult, fraught with lengthy detective work and experimentation. This experimentation can set patients back, forcing them to revisit their plans (in consultation with multiple providers) in search of a new normal.

References

1. Bandura, A.: Self-efficacy: toward a unifying theory of behavioral change. Psychol. Rev. **84**(2), 191 (1977)
2. Bandura, A.: Social Foundations of Thought and Action, Englewood Cliffs 1986)
3. Braun, V., Clarke, V.: Using thematic analysis in psychology. Qual. Res. Psychol. **3**(2), 77–101 (2006)
4. Charles, C., Gafni, A., Whelan, T.: Decision-making in the physician-patient encounter: revisiting the shared treatment decision-making model. Soc. Sci. Med. **49**(5), 651–661 (1999)
5. Connelly, K., Siek, K.A., Chaudry, B., Jones, J., Astroth, K., Welch, J.L.: An offline mobile nutrition monitoring intervention for varying-literacy patients receiving hemodialysis: a pilot study examining usage and usability. J. Am. Med. Inform. Assoc. **19**(5), 705–712 (2012)
6. Consolvo, S., Klasnja, P., McDonald, D.W., Landay, J.A., et al.: Designing for healthy lifestyles: design considerations for mobile technologies to encourage consumer health and wellness. Found. Trends® Human-Comput. Interact. **6**(3–4), 167–315 (2014)
7. Daugherty, J., Waltzman, D., Popat, S., Groenendaal, A.H., Cherney, M., Knudson, A.: Rural primary care providers' experience and usage of clinical recommendations in the CDC pediatric mild traumatic brain injury guideline: a qualitative study. J. Rural Health **37**(3), 487–494 (2021)
8. Epstein, D.A., Ping, A., Fogarty, J., Munson, S.A.: A lived informatics model of personal informatics. In: Proceedings of the 2015 ACM International Joint Conference on Pervasive and Ubiquitous Computing, pp. 731–742 (2015)

9. Guest, G., Namey, E., Chen, M.: A simple method to assess and report thematic saturation in qualitative research. PLoS ONE **15**(5), e0232076 (2020)

10. Hayes, G.R., Abowd, G.D., Davis, J.S., Blount, M.L., Ebling, M., Mynatt, E.D.: Opportunities for pervasive computing in chronic cancer care. In: Indulska, J., Patterson, D.J., Rodden, T., Ott, M. (eds.) Pervasive 2008. LNCS, vol. 5013, pp. 262–279. Springer, Heidelberg (2008). https://doi.org/10.1007/978-3-540-79576-6_16

11. Holtzblatt, K., Beyer, H.: Contextual Design: Design for Life. Morgan Kaufmann, Burlington (2016)

12. Hopp, F.P., Hogan, M.M., Woodbridge, P.A., Lowery, J.C.: The use of telehealth for diabetes management: a qualitative study of telehealth provider perceptions. Implement. Sci. **2**(1), 1–8 (2007)

13. Jacobs, M., Clawson, J., Mynatt, E.D.: A cancer journey framework: guiding the design of holistic health technology. In: Proceedings of the 10th EAI International Conference on Pervasive Computing Technologies for Healthcare, pp. 114–121. ICST (Institute for Computer Sciences, Social-Informatics and Telecommunications Engineering) (2016)

14. Jaen, C.R., Stange, K.C., Nutting, P.A.: Competing demands of primary care: a model for the delivery of clinical preventive services. J. Fam. Pract. **38**(2), 166–174 (1994)

15. Li, I., Dey, A., Forlizzi, J.: A stage-based model of personal informatics systems. In: Proceedings of the SIGCHI Conference on Human Factors in Computing Systems, pp. 557–566 (2010)

16. Mamykina, L., et al.: Structured scaffolding for reflection and problem solving in diabetes self-management: qualitative study of mobile diabetes detective. J. Am. Med. Inform. Assoc. **23**(1), 129–136 (2016)

17. Mankoff, J., Kuksenok, K., Kiesler, S., Rode, J.A., Waldman, K.: Competing online viewpoints and models of chronic illness. In: Proceedings of the SIGCHI Conference on Human Factors in Computing Systems, pp. 589–598 (2011)

18. Ongwere, T., Cantor, G., Sergio, R., Shih, P.C., Clawson, J., Connelly, K.: Design hotspots for care of discordant chronic comorbidities: patients' perspectives. In: Proceedings of the Nordic Conference on Human-Computer Interaction. ACM (2018)

19. Ongwere, T., Cantor, G.S., Clawson, J., Shih, P.C., Connelly, K.: Design and care for discordant chronic comorbidities: a comparison of healthcare providers' perspectives

20. Pfeiffer, P.N., Heisler, M., Piette, J.D., Rogers, M.A., Valenstein, M.: Efficacy of peer support interventions for depression: a meta-analysis. Gen. Hosp. Psychiatry **33**(1), 29–36 (2011)

21. Piette, J.D., Kerr, E.A.: The impact of comorbid chronic conditions on diabetes care. Diabetes Care **29**(3), 725–731 (2006)

22. Rejeski, W.J., Fanning, J.: Models and theories of health behavior and clinical interventions in aging: a contemporary, integrative approach. Clin. Interv. Aging **14**, 1007 (2019)

23. Ritchie, C.S., Zulman, D.M.: Research priorities in geriatric palliative care: multimorbidity. J. Palliat. Med. **16**(8), 843–847 (2013)

24. Sinnott, C., Mercer, S.W., Payne, R.A., Duerden, M., Bradley, C.P., Byrne, M.: Improving medication management in multimorbidity: development of the multimorbidity collaborative medication review and decision making (my comrade) intervention using the behaviour change wheel. Implement. Sci. **10**(1), 1–11 (2015)

25. Sultan, M., Kuluski, K., McIsaac, W.J., Cafazzo, J.A., Seto, E.: Turning challenges into design principles: telemonitoring systems for patients with multiple chronic conditions. Health Inform. J. **25**(4), 1188–1200 (2019)
26. Wang, M.Y., Tsai, P., Liu, J.W.S., Zao, J.K.: Wedjat: a mobile phone based medicine in-take reminder and monitor. In: Ninth IEEE International Conference on Bioinformatics and BioEngineering, BIBE'09, pp. 423–430. IEEE (2009)

Assistive Technologies

Lessons Learned in Developing Sensorised Textiles to Capture Body Shapes

Leonardo A. García-García[1]([⊠]) [iD], George Valsamakis[1],
Niko Münzenrieder[1,2] [iD], and Daniel Roggen[1] [iD]

[1] Sensor Technology Research Centre, University of Sussex, Brighton BN1 9QT, UK
l.a.garcia-garcia@sussex.ac.uk
[2] Faculty of Science and Technology, Free University of Bozen-Bolzano,
39100 Bozen, Italy

Abstract. Motivated by the need to replace plaster casts or image acquisition approaches to capture body shapes to create orthoses, we explored the feasibility of using smart textile sleeve enhanced with arrays of stretch and bend sensors. The sensors' data is interpreted by an ad-hoc optimisation-based shape inference algorithm to come up with a digitised 3D model of the body part around which the sleeve is worn. This paper summarises the state of the art in the field, before illustrating the approach we followed and lesson's learned in developing smart textile sleeves and the associated data processing algorithms. The unique approach we followed was to realise from the ground up the sensing elements, their integration into a textile, and the associated data processing. In the process, we developed a technology to create stretch and bend sensing elements using carbon black and ecoflex, improving curvature detection; we also found ways to interconnect large arrays of such sensors, digitise their data, and developed several mathematical optimisation models for the inference of the sleeve shape from the sensor readings.

Keywords: Sensing sleeve · Smart textile · Body monitoring · Shape reconstruction · Flexible sensors

1 Introduction

New methods for the fabrication of personalised orthoses and prosthesis have been developed in recent years [7]. The increasing interest in developing personalised medical devices has prompted the application of technologies such as 3D printing or CNC machining to achieve this goal [1, 15]. However, body acquisition systems has not advanced in the same pace, being 3D scanning [5,6] or photogrametric methods [1, 7] the most used for creation of 3D models of the body. These systems can be faster, but they do not have a better accuracy or reliability than casting methods [5]. Therefore, new technologies such as smart textiles are required to obtain more accurate models of the body shape. The development of

© ICST Institute for Computer Sciences, Social Informatics and Telecommunications Engineering 2022
Published by Springer Nature Switzerland AG 2022. All Rights Reserved
H. Lewy and R. Barkan (Eds.): PH 2021, LNICST 431, pp. 365–380, 2022.
https://doi.org/10.1007/978-3-030-99194-4_23

flexible sensors has giving rise to the development of smart textiles with ubiquitous sensors for human motion monitoring [2,3,14], posture tracking [9], ECG signal analysis [16], or for shape measurement [8,12]. Despite of this, there is no register a functional textile to measure body shape.

Efforts for posture tracking includes optical fibre integrated in garments [4], inductive sensors for posture monitoring [9], stainless steel yarns [11], silicone with FBG sensors for lower back movement tracking [17]. Although the use of arrays stretchable sensors have been proposed [13,14], these have been limited to identify postures on the back.

The work here discussed is part of a project that focused on the development of a system for body shape sensing using a smart textile and a shape inference algorithm. The system aims to acquire body's shape to help in the fabrication of prostheses and orthoses. The device has been conceived as a smart textile enhanced with and array of bend/stretch sensors. The ends of each sensors is visualised as a node with coordinates in a $\mathbb{R}^3$ space. The coordinates of each node changes when the textile is worn, and this variation is proportional to the strain or bending angle of each sensor. A simulation of the sensors' array has been developed for the shape optimisation that includes a target and an inference meshes of n number of nodes that matches the number of the ends of the sensors, then gradient descent algorithm is used to optimise the inference shape to the target mesh. The system will help in the generation of accurate 3D models of the human body.

This paper presents the practical lessons learned during the ongoing work carried out to develop a smart sensing stretchable sleeve for body shape sensing. These lessons are here documented to show the progress and drawbacks made during the development with the intention to lead the way of those considering working on wearable technologies with similar characteristics. Section 2 presents a description of the system and shows the prototypes generated during the research, whil the algorithm used for the shape optimisation is presented in Sect. 3. Section 4 discusses issues presented during the development of the sleeve and the algorithm, finishing with the conclusions and future work in Sect. 6.

2   Shape Sensing Sleeve

The underlying principle of the shape reconstruction sleeve is the integration of flexible sensors in a stretchable textiles that will be able to measure localised changes in a stretchable textile as this goes from a rest state to a final stretched state. In this project this principle has been investigated with five different prototypes, each one with an array of sensors placed on a stretchable textile.

2.1   Stretchable Sleeve with Commercial Strain Sensors

The first iteration was formed by a commercial sleeve (Rymora Calf Compression Sleeves, Rymora Sports, UK) with 8 rings (Fig. 1); each ring had 8 commercial conductive rubber sensors of 20 mm length by 2 mm (Adafruit, USA). Firstly each sensor was connected to 0.19 mm enamelled copper wires on each end using conductive epoxy (CW2400, CircuitWorks, Chemtronics, Netherlands). The rings where then formed by attaching 8 sensors to an acrylic fettuccina yarn (Yeoman Yarns, Leicester, UK) with mouldable glue (Sugru, U.K.) separated 5 mm from each other. This resulted in non-stretchable sections of 16.12 ± 1.32 mm between each sensor. The rings where then placed on the sleeve 13.80 ± 1.55 mm apart from each other using adhesive and sewing the rigid areas to the sleeve. The array was connected to an interface software formed by four multi channel analogue multiplexers (CD74HC4067) plugged to an Arduino Uno board and the data was interface to the PC with MATLAB for data acquisition.

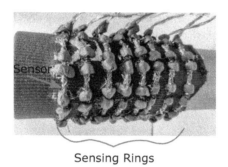

Sensing Rings

Fig. 1. Sensing sleeve with off-the-shelf sensors. The sensing sleeve is formed by 64 sensors arranged in 8 rings of 8 sensors each one.

2.2 Stretchable Sleeve with a Single Ring and Conductive Elastomer Strain and Bend Sensors

A second prototype was formed by a in house designed and fabricated stretchable sensors attached to a sleeve. This sensing device had a single ring formed with stretch and bend sensors made of Conductive Elastomer (CE). The composite material was created with silicone elastomer Ecoflex (00-30 Smooth-on, Pennsylvania, United States), Carbon Black (CB) (Vulcan P, Cabot, Boston, Massachusetts, United States), and heptane. Theses components were mixed with in the following ratios, 10 : 1.3 : 8. CB and heptane were mixed using a magnetic stirrer for 0.5 h, then Ecoflex part B was added and stirred for 5 h and Ecoflex part A was added and stirred for further 0.25 h. The solution was then degassed to remove all the air trapped during the mixing process and poured in 3D printed moulds. The 3D printed moulds were 20 mm long by 5 mm width by 2 mm thick. Each mould was prepared with fetuchina yarn to join the sensors. To prevent the material for the bend sensors from stretching, an extra piece of fetuchina yarn was added. Enamelled copper wires (0.19 mm) were placed on each end of each mould once the solution was poured to create the interfacing contacts for the sensors.

2.3   Stretchable Sleeve with a Single Ring and CE Strain and Bend Sensors Interfaced with Filament Wires

The third iteration was the same as the second prototype described in Sect. 2.2, but this time the copper wires for contacting the sensors were substituted for filament wires. The substitution was done enhance the interfacing, preventing the loosing of the contacts after stretching the sensors. Filament wires were selected after load and cyclic load test performed to CE interfaced with 5 different contacting methods [10].

2.4   Sleeve with a Long Array of CE Sensors and Filament Wires

A fourth prototype was build by designing an array of 70 CE sensors. The sensors are made of carbon black conductive nano particles embedded in a Ecoflex silicone matrix, and the fabrication process is the same as the one described in Sect. 2.2. A 3D printed mould was specially designed to generate four long stripes of sensors that will become four rings. The rings are connected to each other by a row of bend sensors. Each ring is comprised by a long stripe of five stretch alternated with five bent sensors connected in series, i.e. two sensors share a single interface. This reduced the number of interfacing wires to number of sensors $(n) + 1$. The formed rings will measure changes in the perimeter of the cross section of the shapes where the sleeve is put on. The rings were joint with 3 rows of 10 inter-rings bend sensors connected in parallel to measure changes perpendicular to the cross section; each end of these sensors was interfaced with filament wire (Fig. 2). The sensors are 1.5 mm thick and 5 mm with lengths of 16 mm for bending sensors and 13 mm for strain sensors. The sensors are formed by the same mixture, and although the stretch sensors is only the piezoresistive material, the bend sensors were formed using two pieces of jute twine string fibre with the sensors' length which are covered in ecoflex and placed at the bottom of the moulds. This resulted in a thin layer of the piezoresistive material covering the surface which will generate changes in resistance proportional only to bending and not when stretching.

2.5   Sleeve with a Long Array of CE Sensors and Conductive Thread

The last prototype was created following the same process and configuration as the fourth prototype (Sect. 2.4), but the interfacing of the sensors was done using nylon thread coated with silver. This was used as textiles had demonstrated higher adhesion force to ecoflex [10]. This method improved the interfacing, resulting in less change in resistance due to the interfacing of the contacts. A data acquisition board was specially designed to acquire the data from the fourth and fifth prototype. The sleeve was interfaced to a PCB (Fig. 3) that has 6 circuits connected to a microcontroller system (Teensy 3.2). The measurements from the rings are acquired by four circuits with two 16 channel analogue multiplexers, two Op Amp, and a digital potentiometer. The values of the bend sensors

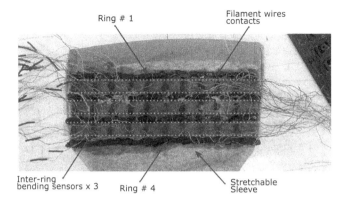

Fig. 2. Long array sleeve. The sensing sleeve is formed by 70 sensors arranged in 4 rings of 10 sensors each one and interconnected through three rows of bending sensors. The sensors in this prototype have been interfaced with filament wires.

connecting the rings are read by two circuits built with two 16 channels analogue multiplexers, one digital potentiometer, and one Op Amp. The multiplexer alternates each sensor to form a voltage divider with the digital potentiometer, which adjusts its value to the sensor resistance values for accurate results. The microcontroller is interfaced over a USB serial line. The data is acquired, stored, and processed in MATLAB.

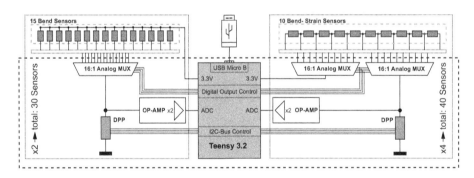

Fig. 3. Read out circuit. Made of 6 individual circuits: two 16 channels analogue multiplexers, 1 digital potentiometer, and 2 Op Amps to read the data from each ring. The other 2 circuits read data from 30 inter-ring bend sensors using a 16 channel analogue multiplexer, 1 digital potentiometer, and 2 Op Amps.

3   Shape Reconstruction

The sleeve sensor data is processed to infer the shape it is worn on (target shape) using the differences between sensors at rest and when conformed to an arbitrary shape. We used the reconstruction and simulations to explore the challenges in inferring the target shape given no prior knowledge other than the sleeve structure and sensors' readings. The number of sensors per ring, sensors reading accuracy and the errors, adds complexity to this challenge. The simulation is used to evaluate the reconstruction with higher number of sensors, different parameters and possibilities for error correction. A virtual model was developed and simulated to evaluate this process. The model is used to simulate draping over target shapes with varied morphology features and retrieve simulated sensor readings. The optimisation algorithm developed infers the target shape using only these measurements.

At first, simple target shapes were used, cylinders and cones. In the first approach using this algorithm [12], conical shapes were measured using the first iteration of the sleeve using only stretch sensors. Afterwards, we expanded the concepts further [8] to incorporate reading of bend sensor in the optimisation algorithm on shapes with arbitrary features such as curves, cross section twists, and lumps. In the latter, weighting factors for the reading of the bend sensor were incorporated and analysed, showing that certain target shapes benefited by adjusting these factors.

3.1 Reconstruction and Simulation Approach

The approach taken for the real and the simulated virtual sleeve is shown in Fig. 4. The steps for draping the virtual sleeve on STL models introduced the challenge to reproduce the way the physical sleeve is worn on a shape. This is because the level of detail in the reconstruction is limited by the number of sensors on the sleeve. This is important for the comparison of the end low-resolution result with the high-resolution STL model or real body limb.

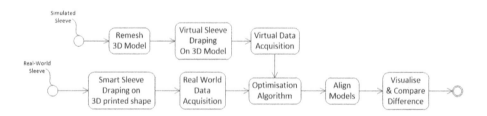

Fig. 4. Inference and simulation process.

While in the simulation the target shape is generated using a STL file, in the experimental part the sensors' data is passed to the optimisation function, producing the final set of points representing the target shape. From the optimisation stage onward, the process is common for both versions of the sleeve

3.2 Simulation Methodology

The following steps are followed to perform simulations:

1. Remesh and import target shape: The target shape is imported as a point cloud (Fig. 5).
2. Alignment and scaling: The target sleeve starts as a set of points of a cylindrical shape at a scale larger than the target shape. It is then centered to the centre of mass of the target shape and scaled.
3. Drape target sleeve over target shape: Using a number of estimation methods to adhere to the real sleeve constraints.
4. Optimise: Run minimisation algorithm to obtain an inferred sleeve that best matches the elongations and bends of the target sleeve.
5. Align and compare: Compare node Euclidean differences of the inferred sleeve vs. the target sleeve for evaluation.

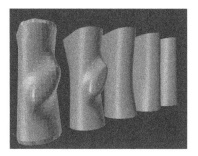

Fig. 5. Target shapes, remesh pre-processing for simulation.

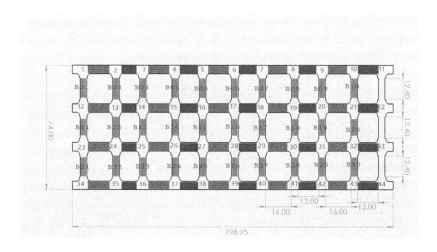

Fig. 6. Sleeve sensor structure. Bend Sensors (B and BS) in Green, Stretch sensors (SS) in yellow. (Color figure online)

The simulated model of the sleeve follows the sensor structure of the latest version of the sleeve, shown in Fig. 6. Figure 7 shows the initial, cylindrical state of the virtual sleeve, with the different edges coloured by type of sensor.

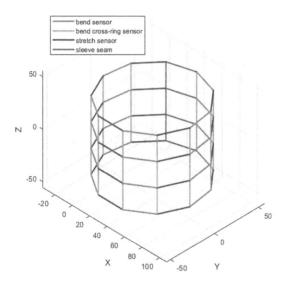

Fig. 7. Virtual sleeve in it's initial state.

3.3   Virtual Sleeve Alignment and Draping

This task moves points of the target sleeve from it's cylindrical form to points on the surface of the target shape. It is here referred to as conforming to shape or draping. The 2 geometries differ in the number of nodes that represent them so this is an $n \times m$ nodes task. The first objective is to align the 2 geometries, scale the target sleeve around the shape and translate to where required to cover the shape. Then, each node of the sleeve is moved to it's closest point of the shape. This process is filtered to conform to some of the constraints of the real sleeve. Figure 8 shows a 8 ring by 11 node sleeve draping over a bend shape. The corrections shown in red are examples of nodes that exceeded the maximum length between the rings.

Several other methods exist for performing this that can be explored: Iterative Closest Point, using geodesic distance instead of euclidean or using covariant distances. Other heuristics such as comparing surface normals for sets of points to detect curves could be used to improve results.

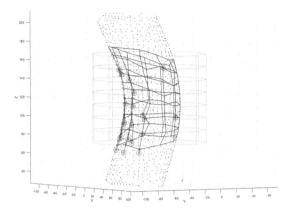

Fig. 8. An 8 by 11 sensor virtual ring (blue) draping over a bending shape (black point cloud). Outliar corrections are shown in red. (Color figure online)

3.4 Shape Inference Algorithm

This stage is oblivious to the shape and it attempts to converge a new sleeve geometry into the target sleeve by using the sensor measurements. The inference is carried out using an optimisation process based on the difference between the data obtained from the sensors when at rest and when they are in an active state (stretch or bend). The following equation that, derived in [8] is being used:

$$L = \sum_{i=1}^{E} \left(\left((e_{inf,i} - e_{tar,i})^2 \cdot \lambda_1 \right) \right.$$
$$+ (1 - \lambda_1) \cdot \left(\left((\theta_{C_{inf},i} - \theta_{C_{tar},i})^2 \cdot \lambda_2 \right) \right.$$
$$\left. + \left((\theta_{L_{tar},i} - \theta_{L_{inf},i})^2 \cdot (1 - \lambda_2) \right) \right)$$

Two weighting factors were introduced, $0 < \lambda_1 < 1$ and $0 < \lambda_2 < 1$. λ_1 assigns a higher importance to the matching lengths between the inferred shape and the sensor readings and a lower importance $(1 - \lambda_1)$ to the matching angles on the cross section; λ_2 assigns a higher importance to the angles on the cross section and the remaining value $(1 - \lambda_2)$ to the angles perpendicular to the cross section. The loss function L is minimised using a Gradient descent algorithm (BFGS Quasi-newton) to compute the partial derivative of the nodes' displacement $\left(\|x_{i_{inf}} - x_{i_{tar}}\| \right)$, with $x_i = (x_i, y_i, z_i)$; then the gradient descent adjust the coordinates to match the distances to those of the sensor readings.

Figure 9a shows the virtual sleeve at rest on a cylinder after the optimisation of the sensors' readings. Figure 9b shows the configuration of the sensors used on the sleeve, highlighting the different angles measured with the inter-ring (green) and the intra-ring (cian) bend sensors.

a)   b)

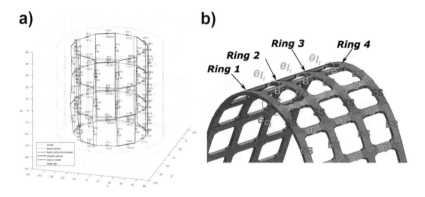

Fig. 9. a) Virtual sleeve representing the real sleeve at rest position b) Angles between sleeve edges that are being measured (Color figure online)

Noise and Error Correction. In the experiments conducted with the sleeve the data from the sensors were not always consistent and some were not producing usable results. The filtering applied to these values shifted the reconstructed shapes further than the reality. Noise and error is also produced from shape areas where interpolation or smoothing is used in between the sleeve nodes. MATLAB point cloud toolbox was used to measure this error. A combination of Iterative Closest Point and Coherent Point Drift methods were used to register the target and the optimised point clouds.

4   Results and Discussion

The developed prototypes were tested by putting them on a set of 3D printed parts with different cross sections that tests the capability of the bending and stretching of the sensors. The data obtained from these measurements was used to create the target shapes for the inference algorithm. The parts were designed in a CAD software and exported to STL to be printed. The same STL were imported into MATLAB to be used as the target shape in the inference simulation.

4.1   Textile Sleeve Evaluation

An important part of the sensors is the calibration to determine the correlation between strain/bend and change in resistance. The calibration was done with an initial state of the sleeve as a cylinder with a diameter equal to that its inner diameter without stretching the sensors. Then, the sleeves were put on cylinders with different diameters from 58 mm to 64 mm. The change in resistance $\Delta R/R_0$ was calculated for every diameter, where ΔR is the change in resistance when the sleeve is at rests (R_0) to the resistance when is on the cylinder. An initial measurement was taken at rest, then another after 10 min of being on the shapes to calculate ΔR. This procedure was performed up to 3 times for each cylinder.

Cylinders were designed in CAD and 3D printed to determine the capacity of the sleeve to measure shapes with complex round topologies on both parallel sides and cross sections. These shapes were designed in Solidworks, exported as STL for simulation and for 3D printing. Each shape have different topologies with round features that ranges from one to three different diameters in the cross sectional area, to bumps and bends on the parallel sides, as shown in Fig. 10. A cylinder with a double ellipsis was designed to test different radius on the cross section. Similarly, a cone, a double ellipsis bent cylinder, and a cone with a bump were designed to measure changes on the cross sections and on the parallel sides with different radii.

The first prototype was under constrained, limited only to detect changes in lengths. Therefore, only cylindrical and conical shapes could be measured [12]. As the sensors had a long recovery time, the sleeve was on rest and the resistance values were obtained after 10 min, then was put on the shape to calibrate/measure and another measurement was taken after 10 min, but the sensors were left to recover 24 h after put them on a greater cylinder. This is because the recovery of the sensors after stretched to 50% is $\approx$3.1 h.

Table 1. Main features of the developed prototypes.

Material	Contact method	Sensors configuration	Drawback	Failure	Accuracy
Off-the-shelf sensors	Copper wire	64 Stretch sensors	long recovery time ($\approx$3.5 h), reconstruction only of cylinders and cones	NA	0.4 mm
CBE	Copper wire	8 Stretch and bend sensors	Bend sensors affected by strain, calibration not completed	Loose contacts after 15 cycles	NA
CBE	Filament wire	8 Stretch and bend sensors	Bend sensors affected by strain, calibration not completed	Loose contacts after 40 cycles	NA
CBE	Filament wire	8 Stretch and bend sensors	Calibration not completed	Loose contacts after 300 cycles	NA
CBE	Filament wire	70 Stretch and bend sensors	Calibration not completed for inter-ring sensors	Loose contacts after 300 cycles	0.08 mm
CBE	Silver coated thread	70 Stretch and bend sensors	NA	NA	NA

CBE = Carbon Black-Ecoflex polymer. NA = No Available.

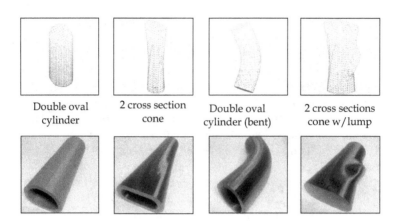

Double oval	2 cross section	Double oval	2 cross sections
cylinder	cone	cylinder (bent)	cone w/lump

Fig. 10. Geometries used for testing the capacity of the sleeve to reconstruct complex shapes.

In the case of the second prototype, the material showed a better recovery time, 15 min, with a maximum stretchability up to 700%. However, for this iteration the contacts became loose after five calibration cycles. This was the result of the difference between the stiffness of the copper wires and the stiffness of the CE, as well as the poor surface adhesion between both components [10]. This failure was observed as an increase in resistance at rest up to 10 times.

The third prototype lasted up to 40 cycles, but the sensors rendered ineffective after this. In the case of the fourth prototype, the sensors showed a better performance for strain and bend, and the sleeve managed to withstand the calibration process of the rings. However, because of the complex configuration of the sensors, the calibration of the inter-ring bend sensors was not achieved. Moreover, when taking measurements of the complex shapes, the sensors stretched substantially more in places with features like bumps or large diameters, causing the contacts to become loose. This resulted in high resistance values of the sensors when put on the shapes to be measured. The fifth prototype is ongoing with the contacts fixed using nylon thread coated with silver. Table 1 list the main features as well as the main drawbacks and failures of each prototype.

4.2 Textile Sleeve STL Results

The work performed on the textile prototypes was mainly calibration as a result of the failure of the contacts. Despite of this, the prototype one (Sect. 2.1) and prototype four (Sect. 2.4) were used to measure features on 3D printed parts described in Sect. 4.1.

The first sleeve (Sect. 2.1) was underconstrained, therefore it could be only used to with cylinders with circular cross sections. The sleeve was used to measure the diameters of two different cones with an average difference of 0.44 ± 0.22 mm. But the results shade light on how to improve the model to add more constrains to improve the shape sensing system. The prototype four (Sect. 2.4) was used to measure geometries with more complex topologies. Although the inter-ring bend sensors provided no data because of calibration issues, the data of the intra-ring bend and strain sensors was used for the reconstruction. From the topology of the sleeve sensors, the bending of the stretch sensors had to be assumed, and the principle used to assign angles was the fact that the sum of all 11 angles around each ring computes to 360°. Outlier data from the working bend sensors due to loose contacts were also filtered out, and replaced with the adjacent bend sensor of the neighbouring ring. Figure 11 depicts the selected shapes from the previous section, as reconstructed by the optimisation algorithm. The similarities with the target shape are difficult to distinguish due to lack of or interpolated angular data.

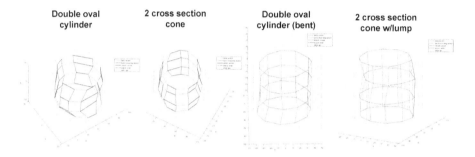

Fig. 11. Real sleeve data from prototype 4. Bend sensors are in green and red, stretch sensors in yellow or cyan, and the sleeve's seam is in grey. (Color figure online)

4.3 Virtual Sleeve on Leg Model Results

Figure 12 Shows the simulation of a leg model with a sleeve with higher number of rings and nodes. The challenge presented is draping the sleeve over the ankle and draping a 90° bend.

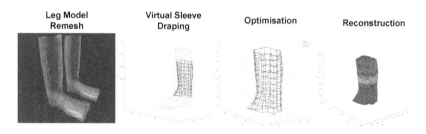

Fig. 12. Simulated reconstruction of a leg model using a 11-ring with 16 sensor nodes per ring virtual sleeve.

5   Recommendations for Smart Textiles for Body-Shape Sensing

The main limitation to address in the current research was the interfacing of the sensors, therefore a good method that prevents the sensors from becoming inoperative is needed. As it has been demonstrated, although thread has a better surface adhesion to conductive elastomer, its feasibility still to be proved. If successful, this will increase the life span of the sensors and their reliability. Similarly, the developed prototypes are structured arrays of sensors with a defined topology. In order to have better results, the arrangement of sensors has to be explored. The possibility of changing the bend/stretch sensor's order in each ring should be explored so that each intra-ring bend sensor has a stretch sensor adjacent to it on the neighbouring ring. This gives the potential to provide better results when the algorithm estimates the bending of the stretch sensors. Deploying stretch sensors in the ring cross section will also provide more data for the inference process. Similarly, an unstructured mesh of sensors to cover a higher surface area with less elements. Another possibility will be the capability of measure both strain and bend with a single structure.

6   Conclusions and Future Work

This paper has presented lessons learned fro work in progress of a shape sensing technology as means for creating a smart textile with stretchable and bendable soft sensors. Five different prototypes and the main characteristics and failures of each one were presented. Similarly, challenges in the shape inference process and algorithm for anticipating missing or erroneous data have also been presented and discussed. Future work will look for the improvement of the system by addressing the issues here presented for each prototype and to explore the feasibility of capacitive sensors.

Acknowledgement. This work was funded by EPSRC, GCRF, and NIHR. Contact number: EP/R013837/1 (SmartSensOtics).

References

1. Barrios-Muriel, J., Romero-Sánchez, F., Alonso-Sánchez, F.J., Rodríguez Salgado, D.: Advances in orthotic and prosthetic manufacturing: a technology review. Materials **13**(2) (2020). https://doi.org/10.3390/ma13020295. https://www.mdpi.com/1996-1944/13/2/295
2. Bello, H., Zhou, B., Suh, S., Lukowicz, P.: MoCapaci: posture and gesture detection in loose garments using textile cables as capacitive antennas. In: 2021 International Symposium on Wearable Computers. ACM (2021). https://doi.org/10.1145/3460421.3480418

3. Costa, J.C., Spina, F., Lugoda, P., Garcia-Garcia, L., Roggen, D., Münzenrieder, N.: Flexible sensors–from materials to applications. Technologies **7**(2), 35 (2019). https://doi.org/10.3390/technologies7020035
4. Dunne, L.E., Walsh, P., Hermann, S., Smyth, B., Caulfield, B.: Wearable monitoring of seated spinal posture. IEEE Trans. Biomed. Circuits Syst. **2**(2), 97–105 (2008). https://doi.org/10.1109/tbcas.2008.927246
5. Farhan, M., Wang, J.Z., Bray, P., Burns, J., Cheng, T.L.: Comparison of 3D scanning versus traditional methods of capturing foot and ankle morphology for the fabrication of orthoses: a systematic review. J. Foot Ankle Res. **14**(1), 1–11 (2021). https://doi.org/10.1186/s13047-020-00442-8
6. Garcia-Garcia, L.A., Rodriguez-Salvador, M.: Additive manufacturing knowledge incursion on orthopaedic device: the case of hand orthoses. In: Proceedings of the 3rd International Conference on Progress in Additive Manufacturing, (Pro-AM 2018), pp. p571–6 (2018)
7. García-García, L.A., Rodríguez-Salvador, M., Moya-Bencomo, M.D.: Development of a customized wrist orthosis for flexion and extension treatment using reverse engineering and 3D printing. In: Lhotska, L., Sukupova, L., Lacković, I., Ibbott, G.S. (eds.) World Congress on Medical Physics and Biomedical Engineering 2018. IP, vol. 68/2, pp. 609–613. Springer, Singapore (2019). https://doi.org/10.1007/978-981-10-9038-7_113
8. Garcia-Garcia, L.A., Valsamakis, G., Kreitmair, P., Munzenrieder, N., Roggen, D.: Inferring complex textile shape from an integrated carbon black-infused ecoflex-based bend and stretch sensor array. In: Adjunct Proceedings of the 2021 ACM International Joint Conference on Pervasive and Ubiquitous Computing and Proceedings of the 2021 ACM International Symposium on Wearable Computers, UbiComp '21, pp. 298–303. Association for Computing Machinery, New York (2021). https://doi.org/10.1145/3460418.3479347
9. García-Patiño, A., Khoshnam, M., Menon, C.: Wearable device to monitor back movements using an inductive textile sensor **20**(3), 905 (2020). https://doi.org/10.3390/s20030905
10. García-García, L.A., Costa, J.C., Lugoda, P., Roggen, D., Münzenrieder, N.: Copper wire based electrical contacts for direct interfacing of stretchable sensors. In: 2020 IEEE SENSORS, pp. 1–4. IEEE (2020). https://doi.org/10.1109/SENSORS47125.2020.9278749
11. Lou, M., et al.: Highly wearable, breathable, and washable sensing textile for human motion and pulse monitoring **12**(17), 19965–19973 (2020). https://doi.org/10.1021/acsami.0c03670
12. Lugoda, P., Garcia-Garcia, L.A., Richoz, S., Munzenrieder, N., Roggen, D.: ShapeSense3d. ACM (2019). https://doi.org/10.1145/3341162.3343846
13. Mattmann, C., Amft, O., Harms, H., Troster, G., Clemens, F.: Recognizing upper body postures using textile strain sensors. In: 2007 11th IEEE International Symposium on Wearable Computers, pp. 29–36 (2007). https://doi.org/10.1109/ISWC.2007.4373773
14. Tormene, P., et al.: Estimation of human trunk movements by wearable strain sensors and improvement of sensor's placement on intelligent biomedical clothes. Biomed. Eng. Online **11**(1), 1–8 (2012). https://doi.org/10.1186/1475-925x-11-95
15. Wang, Y., Tan, Q., Pu, F., Boone, D., Zhang, M.: A review of the application of additive manufacturing in prosthetic and orthotic clinics from a biomechanical perspective. Engineering **6**(11), 1258–1266 (2020). https://doi.org/10.1016/j.eng.2020.07.019. https://www.sciencedirect.com/science/article/pii/S2095809920302575

16. Yapici, M.K., Alkhidir, T., Samad, Y.A., Liao, K.: Graphene-clad textile electrodes for electrocardiogram monitoring. Sensors Actuators B: Chem. **221**, 1469–1474 (2015). https://doi.org/10.1016/j.snb.2015.07.111

17. Zaltieri, M., et al.: A wearable device based on a fiber bragg grating sensor for low back movements monitoring **20**(14), 3825 (2020). https://doi.org/10.3390/s20143825

Translating a DC³ Model into a Conceptual Tool (DCCs Ecosystem): A Case Study with a Design Team

Tom Ongwere[1]([✉]), Erik Stolterman[2], Patrick C. Shih[2], Clawson James[2], and Kay Connelly[2]

[1] University of Dayton, Dayton, USA
tongwere1@udayton.edu
[2] Indiana University Bloomington, Bloomington, USA
{estolter,patshih,clawson,connelly}@indiana.edu

Abstract. In this paper, we draw inspiration from the Discordant Chronic Comorbidity Care (DC³) model. The model recognizes the complexities of DCCs and incorporates key strategies for assessing and addressing the complexities of DCCs care. We worked with user experience design experts over several design sprints to come up with a conceptual design. It became clear early on that because of the changing DCCs care needs, there is no one-size-fits-all solution for DCCs needs. Thus, the effective care of DCCs requires a holistic approach. The holistic approach involves designers collecting multiple individual tools and mapping those tools to specific needs for DCC care and treatment, which ultimately results in the creation of an ecosystem. We discussed how this ecosystem may be optimized and personalized using machine learning to address individual DCCs needs. Furthermore, putting together these multiple sets of tools could introduce an engineering challenge. We provide strategies and recommendations for future work to address these engineering challenges and how to make a theoretical concept adaptable to technology.

Keywords: Discordant chronic comorbidities · Designing with experts · Design sprints

1   Introduction

Patients with complex needs face many challenges, such as Discordant Chronic Condition (DCCs). DCCs have unrelated or contradicting care and treatment plans, for example, depression, arthritis, or end-stage renal disease is discordant to type-2 diabetes [23]. Type-2 diabetes is often co-occurring with DCCs [22]. Thus, the effective DCCs treatment involves treating the primary condition

© ICST Institute for Computer Sciences, Social Informatics and Telecommunications Engineering 2022
Published by Springer Nature Switzerland AG 2022. All Rights Reserved
H. Lewy and R. Barkan (Eds.): PH 2021, LNICST 431, pp. 381–397, 2022.
https://doi.org/10.1007/978-3-030-99194-4_24

(Type-2 diabetes) plus varied concurrent conditions (i.e., arthritis, depression, or both) and mitigating the risks of developing additional conditions or severe symptoms [2,10,22]. In this situation, every new development in a patient's health, a new disease, treatment, or procedure often leads to new conflicts. Like single chronic diseases, effective treatment of DCCs may require prioritizing and making trade-offs. However, these treatment plans are more complex for patients with type-2 diabetes and DCCs. There may be single chronic conditions that portray characteristics similar to DCCs, (i.e., cancer or Parkinson's) by requiring individualized treatment plans, coordination of multiple providers, and consultation of multiple resources, however, these conditions often have a defined disease trajectory and may present fewer challenges than the DCCs.

Recently, a plethora of models, systems, mobile apps, and linked devices have become available to help individuals manage comorbidities [7,8,13,29]. However, these tools, theories, and models are targeted to a specific goal or disease and are therefore unable to adapt as a user's disease needs evolve over time or alter with context [20].

In this study, we worked with a design team over several design sprints (sessions) to design for complex and dynamic patient needs, especially for the patient who has DCCs. To do this, we draw inspiration from the Discordant Chronic Comorbidity Care (DC^3) model [redacted for anonymity] that recognizes the complexities of DCCs care and incorporates key strategies for i) assessing and addressing DCCs care, ii) adapting to an individual's varying goals and needs, and iii) working closely with healthcare providers who understand the disease and the patients who are living with DCCs.

We provide three main contributions in this paper: i) we show a case study of how to use design sprints in a complex design context (the case study can be a model for future studies), ii) we propose an ecosystem that seeks to address the challenges of managing DCCs, and iii) we discuss strategies to further optimize and standardize the proposed ecosystem to better address the complexities of DCCs care.

2   Background

In this section, we discuss theories and models relevant to multiple chronic conditions care. We also, present an overview of tools suggested by DC^3 model for DCCs care and support.

2.1   Theories and Models in Multiple Chronic Disease Care

In Human-Computer Interaction, Personal Informatics, and healthcare, models and theories are being used to guide people in i) deciding what information to gather, ii) deciding what tools to use, iii) discerning what needs are pertinent, and iv) participating in shared decisions. For example, Hayes et al. [5] show how cancer patients' physical and emotional needs evolve as cancer progresses over time. The journey care framework depicts the responsibilities, challenges, and personal impacts that patients face while transitioning from diagnosis through post-treatment survivorship [8]. These models have consequently informed the design of decision aids to assist patients in difficult decisions [7,8], and support clinicians in including patient preferences into illness management [7,14].

Further, theories and their applications are used in interventions targeting behavioral risk factors (e.g. smoking, [24]), encouraging health-protective behaviors (e.g., health screening, [3]), and improving adaptation to chronic and acute illness (e.g., adherence to medical advice, [17]), addressing clinical problems including depression [1], diabetes management [13], and other behaviors). These models and theories, and interventions that implement these models and theories show that specific strategies or constructs may work for one group of people while another strategy works for other populations. However, these studies do not account for patients with DCCs who have multiple and interacting experiences. These multiple and interacting experiences is the topic of this paper.

There are systems looking to address multiple needs. For instance, Health-Kits are being used to help people with multiple conditions to use different tools to navigate their situation. Health-Kits can interface with many care systems, however, they are unable to resolve conflicts that you often find in DCCs and it is usually static configuration and does not evolve over time as DCCs would require. The second consideration is a multi-component application for comorbidity support [27]. However, a multi-component system is limited to specific integrated interventions, which limits the ability of the patient with DCCs to choose tools appropriate for their care needs.

2.2 DC^3 Model and Tools

In our prior work, we explored the patients' perspectives [18,20] and providers' perspectives [19] and proposed a conceptual care model (DC^3) [21]. The DC^3 model suggested tools to support patients with DCCs in every stage of management (i.e., information comprehension, treatment plan decision making, and treatment plan implementation). They include tools: for a single-stage, to transition between care stages, to simplify complexities, and to coordinate multiple healthcare providers.

– *Tools for a single stage*
  We suggested tools to be used in a single stage to help patients organize information across multiple conditions instead of focusing on a single condition or type of data. For example, tools that help patients collect all of the different treatment recommendations made by their various providers and evaluate them simultaneously and tools to help patients track their progress for the entire plan and not just individual components.
– *Tools for transitions between stages*
  We suggested tools that help patients transition from one stage to the next, including tools that help patients quickly communicate with all providers and adjust the plan, without a patient having to wait days or weeks to see their various providers. We also included tools to support patients in recording

any potentially relevant information and to support providers in filtering that information into the most urgent and relevant items of information.

- *Tools to simplify the complexity.*
  We suggested tools to simplify complexity in care, such as, tools that help patients break down larger treatment goals into smaller, achievable tasks reflecting the patient's capabilities. We also suggested tools that support patients and providers in recording, reviewing, and starting/stopping treatment plans.
- *Tools for coordinating with multiple providers.*
  We suggested tools for supporting multiple healthcare providers and patients to collaboratively digest and process new information, as well as seek professional verification of the new information. Additionally, we suggested tools that can help patients navigate conflicting advice and prioritize different aspects of their treatment plans. Finally, we also suggested tools that provide an overview of the patient's severe symptoms resulting from multiple interacting chronic conditions as well as progressive symptoms that may become problematic at a later time.

In this paper, we take these suggestions and engage a team of professional designers/design experts through design sprints to design for the multiple and interacting experiences of DCCs.

3   Methods

This section describes three design sprints to produce ideas and a conceptual tool to support patients with DCCs in prioritizing their care and communicating with multiple providers. These design sprints were guided by the following two design questions(DQs):

- **(DQ 1)** How might a patient use this conceptual design idea to set goals and navigate their situation during the time of crisis, during times of change, and when symptoms are stable? and
- **(DQ 2)** If implemented, will this design help a patient prioritize their treatment and communicate with their multiple healthcare providers?

In our prior research [18–20], we explored the following: i) how technology might help patients with DCCs to prioritize their treatment and communicate with multiple healthcare providers, ii) how designs might help patients with DCCs set goals and navigate their situation during the time of crisis and change, and when their symptoms are stable, and iii) how we might present and foster interaction with a tool that allows patients with DCCs to do this prioritization and goal setting, and iv) what patients' experiences with a tool may be like.

We are using these findings to explore the DCCs design space and to supplement these research questions, we are introducing two specific design questions **(DQ 1 and DQ 2)**.

3.1   A Case Study

To answer our research question and design questions, we used the Design Sprint technique to engage the design experts. The idea of design sprints was first introduced by "Google Ventures" to tackle critical business problems and design viable solutions within five days [16]. A Design Sprint often consists of five stages, which include: i)understand, ii) diverge, iii) decide, iv) prototype and v) validate. [26]. Because of limited resources in this study (we did not have full time engineers to build prototypes), we set out to complete the first three stages. In the first Design Sprint (understand), we focused on introducing participants to the care needs of patients with DCCs and creating a journey map of patients' actions. A journey map is a visualization of the process that a person goes through in order to accomplish a goal [6]. In the second Design Sprint (diverge), we explored several potential design strategies and tools for DCCs care and support. We then narrowed our focus and explored a conceptual ecosystem in the third Design Sprint (decide). Each subsequent Design Sprint was dependent on the activities of the previous Design Sprint. Below we discuss these activities in further detail.

Design Sprint 1, has two parts, part A and part B. The purpose of the Design Sprint 1, part A, was to introduce the participants to the challenges of supporting and caring for patients with DCCs. The session started with an ice breaker, where participants briefly introduced themselves and talked about what their day in life is like. This was followed by the researcher giving a brief presentation about the DCCs challenges that need to be addressed through design. In the presentation, the researcher also presented the design opportunities that included tools that support patients with DCCs in every stage of their care (**see Background section for details**). After the presentation, the researcher asked the participants to read through the patient scenario that demonstrates the daily life of a patient with DCCs (**see below**).

In the Sprint 1, Part B, the researcher began the session by reviewing themes from Design Sprint 1, Part A. The researcher used the patient's scenario to reflect and solicit comments from participants. The participants then created a journey map showing how the patient and providers interacted in the study scenario. The researcher led a discussion about the features of the journey maps that stood out.

Design Sprint 2 started by the researcher reminding participants of the ideas generated in the Design Sprint 1 and ensuring everyone had a common understanding and focus of the study. The participants then brainstormed design ideas for a conceptual tool, filtered those ideas, and mapped the ideas and tools to meet the needs and pain points they identified. In Design Sprint 3, the participants combined multiple tools together to form an ecosystem and discussed how this ecosystem may work to address needs of patients with DCCs.

The first author facilitated each Design Sprint, which lasted 60–90 min. Each Design Sprint was initiated by an ice breaker, followed by a presentation (sprint 1 part A) or reflection (for sprint 1 part B, sprint 2, and sprint 3), and then the probe.

Probe: Jeff, is dealing with type-2 diabetes, arthritis, and severe depression. All of which present continuously changing disease episodes and drug interactions. Jeff needs to set and monitor his treatment goals and to learn about other activities to improve his health. Jeff also needs to monitor and communicate his current level of function. To do these activities effectively, Jeff will need to consult and coordinate his care with multiple providers.

This probe was followed by leading question:

"How might designs help Jeff set goals and navigate their situation during the time of crisis and change, and when their symptoms are stable?".

In addition, as the participants started each Design Sprint, the researcher used the suggested tools for DCCs care (which are described in Background section) to narrow the scope of the participants' ideation and design focus. The participants used the shared miro-board (an online visual collaboration platform for teamwork [11]) to record, share, brainstorm, and sketch conceptual ideas/designs with each other.

All the materials (including the zoom recordings and miro-board sketches) for each Design Sprint was collected for analysis by the researcher and for preparation for the next Design Sprint. The researcher's analysis process was guided by DQ4 and DQ5.

3.2 Scenario

Here we provide, a summary of the scenario, a full summary is one and a half pages and is available in our website (http://tongwere.com/category/project/). The scenario describes the life experience of Jeff (patient with DCCs). Jeff is restless, experiences sad moods and fatigue such that his mobility and independence are affected. When symptoms come up (or interactions), Jeff gets a recommendation from his provider (Dr. Zoo) to see a psychiatrist, Dr. Depreux. Jeff calls Dr. Depreux, who gives him some directions, but Jeff is also dealing with type-2 diabetes symptoms. And he ends seeing another provider, Dr. Beetis-his diabetes doctor who gives him another directive. Dr. Beetis didn't have a full understanding of Jeff's arthritis and refers Jeff to Dr. Arthur. So, Jeff calls Dr. Arthur and gets additional directions. And slowly, Jeff's care process becomes complicated and expensive.

3.3 Participants

We recruited a total of five (N = 5) user experience (UX) designers. Three (N = 3) work with health-related firms, one (N = 1) works with a top non-profit IT corporation, and the remaining participant is a freelance user experience designer. One of the five designers leads a large team of designers and engineers, another is a senior user experience designer, and the remaining three participants are UX designers researchers (Table 1).

This study was approved by our University's Institutional Review Board (IRB).

Table 1. Participants

Participant	Experience	Job title
P1	5+ years	UX Designer
P2	5+ years	UX Designer
P3	5+ years	UX Designer
P4	8+ years	Senior UX Designer
P5	10 + years	leads a large team of designers and engineers

3.4 Analysis

The first author did the thematic analysis after each design sprint and then met with the research team to decide what results we are going to use in the next design sprint. The analysis process began as soon as each design sprint concluded and continued up to when all design sprints were completed. The analysis and design process was iterative, the result of the one sprint informed the results of the succeeding sprint. For sprint one, parts A and B, we extracted all the answers and evaluated those answers. In part B, we started by leading experts in reflecting on items they have suggested in part A. Six(6) sub-themes emerged out of that analysis. We iterated on these themes to create two(2) major themes (problems and pain points, and interactive solutions for DCCs care and support). After Design Sprint 2, we analyzed the data collected and four major themes emerged and were further iterated. This iteration resulted in a focus on an ecosystem in Sprint 3. When the three design sprints concluded, we analyzed the data and extracted four (4) sub-themes. We further iterated on these themes and came up with two main themes: i) critical components of an ecosystem for DCCs support, and ii) considerations for an ecosystem for DCCs support.

4 Findings

In this section, we highlight the findings of the three design sprints and talk about how these findings influenced our design iterations. Because of limited space and page limits, we are not discussing them in detail. We will discuss the process of design sprints (case study) in the discussion section.

4.1 Design Sprint 1: (Understand)

In design sprint 1, part A, the researcher, and participants highlighted problems and pain points they found to be prominent and that should be addressed. In part B, we reviewed and reflected on the identified pain points, the participants then created a journey map showing how the patient and providers interacted in the study scenario. The participants used the journey map to emphasize the pain points in the patient care process and to ensure there is some continuity in their view of DCCs care needs. They also discussed technologies and other

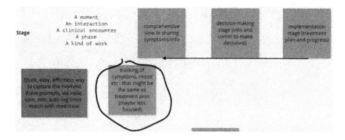

Fig. 1. Narrowing the design problems and design insights (*Figure showing the needs of the patients with DCCs that experts believe to be prevalent. These needs occur during patients' clinical encounters, data collection and sharing, treatment decision making, and implementation of those treatment plans. The figure emphasizes the moments of the patient's life and barriers they face and solutions to those barriers, for example, communication, mood swings/depression, conflicting and overwhelming treatment plans & medications.*)

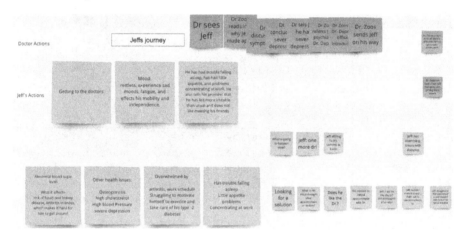

Fig. 2. DCCs Journey Map [6] (*Showing a visual presentation of the process that a patient with DCCs goes through in order to get help. This process includes i) a patient's symptoms, ii) a patient's treatment plan, iii) a patient's interactions with health care systems, iv) barriers affecting those interactions, and vi) support strategies and tools to help a patient navigate their care*)

design ideas that could support patients in navigating their care process. We show some of those pain points in (Fig. 1) and the journey map in (Fig. 2).

4.2 Design Sprint 2: (Diverge)

In Design Sprint 2, participants expanded and reflected on the problems and pain points, and interactive solutions for DCCs care and support themes they identified in Sprint 1 part A and part B. Participants discussed how addressing DCCs issues requires engaging patients in multiple different ways and patients need to be proactive for it to be effective. Some strategies may work for one patient but not work for other patients. We show in (Fig. 3) some of those DCCs support resources.

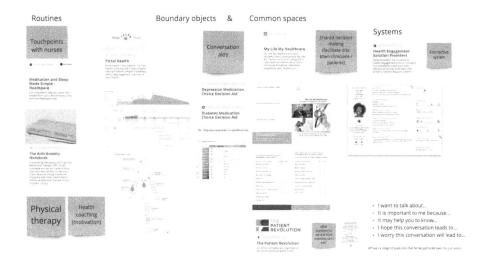

Fig. 3. DCCs Support resources, projects and tools *(A figure showing DCCs support resources and tools that the participants discussed, including i) tools to visualize and communicate patients' symptoms, ii) shared decision aids, iii) tools to flag conflicts and treatment plan interactions, and iv) models to combine and moderate the operation of the care tools)*

4.3   Design Sprint 3: (Decide)

In Design Sprint 3, the participants considered two ways to design for DCCs needs. One way was to focus on a single stage of DCCs care and build a tool for that stage. The second way consisted of mapping out an ecosystem to address the care of patients with DCCs. Because multiple things need to be considered when caring for DCCs, all participants agreed to focus on designing an ecosystem. Designing an ecosystem for DCCs involved participants taking different tools and learning how to put them together to address the individual needs of patients with DCCs. (Fig. 4) shows components that make up the DCCs ecosystem. Here we briefly present i) critical components of an ecosystem for DCCs support, and ii) considerations for an ecosystem for DCCs support.

4.4   Critical Components of an Ecosystem for DCCs Support

Participants discussed how each of these parts fit together to address the needs of patients with DCCs. For examples, P1 explains that:

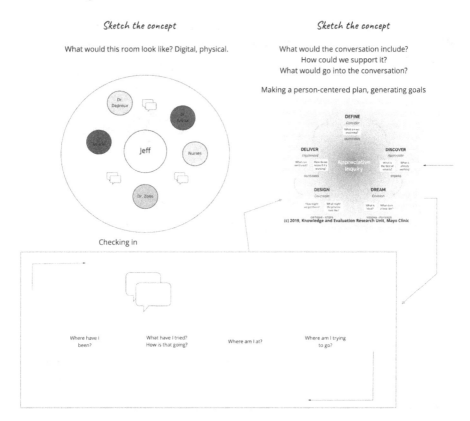

Fig. 4. Critical components of DCCs ecosystem *(A figure showing some components that make an ecosystem, including i) patients at the center of their support network, ii) a tool that helps a patient set goals and prepare for doctors office visits, iii) a model to guide doctor-patient discussion and goal-setting process, and iv) a tool to evaluate a patient's progress)*

> "In case of when [patient] had a range of questions that he has gathered over the past week . . . So that to [participant] is kind of attaches to that moment of conversation . . . a boundary object or a conversation tools can support that conversation."

Another tool that relates to similar needs is a shared decision aid, P2 explained how

> "[A doctor] can like invite a patient and think through, like what they want to talk about what's important to them what they want the clinician to know and their hopes and worries for the conversation"

4.5 Considerations for an Ecosystem for DCCs Support

Our experience engaging experts shows that the process of designing for the DCCs ecosystem is a complicated one. Here we provide a sample of the participants' concerns. For example, the participants found that there are a lot of parts to be moved around.

> *"we have to bring things all together, one part should focus on helping a patient self-reflect . . . This one part should deal with their emotions, another [part] enables patient [to] get answers from other people".-* P2

Nonetheless, the participants discussed about introducing models to tie all these items together. One of the participants suggested using the Appreciative Inquiry Model, saying

> *"And then you have to do, your conceptual kind of thing . . . and use the Appreciative Inquiry to guide that thinking"* - P5

In this situation, patients may end up using multiple tools a day. There is a need for a tool to help patients choose the tools appropriate for a given context. For example, one participant explained

> *"If you have to describe the daily life scenario of [patient], from the morning when he gets up, to the night [when] he goes to bed, interacting with this in . . . different kind of scenarios."* - P4

5 Discussion

The Design Sprint participants (n=5) generated a diverse range of ideas for supporting patients with DCCs. Here we discuss the using design sprints in research and the design space for DCCs.

5.1 A Case Study of Using Design Sprints in Research

This work was a case study on how to engage the design team in design for a complicated situation. We show how we engaged designers, who are less familiar with the DCCs population, in the design process for identifying pain points. We **provided a conceptual map on how to think about processes of designing for a complicated situation**. First, every designer must understand the problems associated with a complex situation. Secondly, in our case study, we originally wanted the experts to design tools, but then experts wanted to create an ecosystem. This changed our conceptualization of what a good solution was. Future researchers should be open to the direction of the research changing slightly because you might find something really surprising that might be beneficial. However, it is challenging to keep participants on task without suppressing their creativity. In our case study, some of discussions that went off track ended up leading to very positive, creative outcome, while other discussions did not. **Future researchers need to explore how to master the**

balance of being open to something while not allowing discussion to go too far off course. We recommend the following strategies, First, nudge the discussions within the sessions, this might be harder to manage within the session. The time between design sprints (which are normally 90 minutes), gives researchers the flexibility to reflect where discussions went off course and time to figure-out how to bring the discussion back on task. This same break also gives researchers time to reevaluate whether participants came up with something creative that should be further pursued and explored more fully. It is also good practice to ensure researchers have time to discuss the Design Sprint session with their fellow researchers before they make decisions about the next session. The second recommendation is to refer to focus group management techniques, where there are people who dominate and people are more quiet. Researchers should be careful to engage everyone and not make anyone feel left out. However, if some participants are in really productive conversation, engaging a participant who has been quiet at that moment might derail the conversation. Researchers need to allow those discussions to finish before they try to bring the quiet people into the discussion. Finally, avoid asking participants open ended questions. Instead, focus on re-engaging participants by asking more targeted questions to direct the discussion. For example, *"do you know how you might improve this solution?"*

5.2 Design Space for DCCs

Here we recommend three design directions, tools to empower patients make and implement treatment goals, tools to record and communicate the DCCs needs, and the DCC Ecosystem.

Tools to Empower Patients to Make and Implement Treatment Goals
In DCCs care, we need to understand that there is no generic, one-size-fits-all solution for DCCs patients. Machine learning algorithms can be used to observe the interaction and learn the patient's preferences. To do this, we need to first identify the baseline to i) understand what patients care about and why, ii) observe the behavior of patients and understand their needs with data, and iii) be able to prompt patients at the right time. Thus, a feedback loop between patients and the system needs to be created and this loop needs to evolve. A second consideration is the use of human input. For example, we should allow a patient to decide what information is valuable enough to record and prompt the patient to record the information at the appropriate times. We understand, there is a lot of literature justifying why some patients don't take medication when they should. With that said, reminders alone may not solve the problem and some patients will not record or take medications even when they are reminded. **We need to explore systems that address all types of patients (patients who respond to reminders and patients that do not respond reminders).**

For example, designers should focus on helping patients understand what is good for them. Such tools must; i) be empathetic, ii) provide the evidence necessary for the patient to make effective decisions or show patients what happened in the past when a similar situation occurred, iii) explain to patients why they are not feeling well and the benefits of the choices available to a patient, and iv) prepare patients to pose questions to their providers and understand interactions coming from multiple treatment plans. A patient should be placed at the center of every design and designers have to understand that every time the system generates a recommended action – a patient's needs must come first.

Tools to Record and Communicate the DCCs Needs

Patients with DCCs experience severe symptoms and multiple issues. To the best of our knowledge, there is no system robust enough for these patients to record and communicate their issues to multiple providers. The current healthcare system is relying upon the patient to personally communicate their issues, and that is not fair, efficient, or accurate. Current studies confirm this argument. For example, the Jacobs et al. [8] study on breast cancer patients showed that oncologists and surgeons were interested in understanding the emotional health of their patients, however, these patients hesitated to share this information. Ongwere et al., showed that patients did not share all of their information because they assumed that providers may not be interested in some aspects of their life, some patients were fearful of judgment and other patients forgot terms that were used by their various providers [20]. Tools are being used to help patients record and share their information. For example, online journals are used to track patients' information. However, the challenges associated with this type of tool are the challenges of recording, filtering, and communicating that information across multiple providers. There are health video blogs that allow individuals with chronic illnesses to share their stories, experiences, and knowledge with the general public [12]. There are also web-based personal health records that can be used by patients to collect and manage their health information (e.g., medical history, past surgeries, medications, and allergies), request self-referrals, and store a record of their consultations [28]. However, these systems employed data entry methods that limit the range and content of patient-entered information related to medical history, medications, laboratory tests, diagnostic studies, and immunizations [9]. The findings of this case study raise new questions about the modalities of recording and sharing DCCs information with multiple providers.

First, because of their DCCs, we must understand that not every patient is the same and may not relate similarly to the modality. Some patients with DCCs may be visual, some may prefer writing or text, and others may want a voice. Researchers should recognize that patients with DCCs are diverse and should be provided with diverse modalities to record and share their information. Further, these modalities may also be impacted by the events in a patient's life. **Future research could explore how to provide a suitable tool for a patient to record and share their information when in crisis/overwhelmed and when they are stable.** For example, i) the research could explore the design of smart systems that can switch the modality based on the situation of an individual patient with DCCs, and ii) research could also identify ways to help patients emotionally prepare for interaction when in crisis and also when stable.

The DCC Ecosystem

The effective support and care for patients with DCCs should be consistent with the patient's values, desires, and goals. The DCCs care and support should be feasible and flexible to accommodate shifts in a patients' life and must be tailored so it makes intellectual, emotional, and practical sense to a patient. Studies are looking to help patients and healthcare providers set the care goals that are tailored to each patient's needs. For example, the use of decision aids help clinicians share information about the options and their consequences during the clinical encounter [4]. The decision aids help clinicians tailor care and reduce the burden of treatment on patients with DCCs and help patients reflect on their values and goals with their healthcare providers. Some tools such as motivational interviewing help create conversations about the options and their relative merits and downsides [25].

For DCCs, any modification to a patient's treatment plan often introduces new complications to patients' care [20]. If a patient wants to make a modification to their treatment, the research could explore how to bring into the forefront the issues that may matter to a patient in making that switch. More specially, research must visualize what it would be like to stop or introduce a new treatment plan. There are apps that are designed to help visualize patients' health histories and symptom maps, with a focus on people living with complex conditions [15]. Patients may visualize and communicate their histories and symptoms maps. However, communicating with a provider alone might not necessarily lead a patient to change their behavior or solve a problem. Sometimes a patient may be struggling to get around their mood and other patients may be scared of change. If there is a need to switch a treatment plan, a tool must show how that process would look like. Further, a tool must have an interactive interface where a patient could visualize how minimizing one behavior may affect their quality of life. Thus, identifying the pain points and making all potential issues tangible to a patient can help them in a crisis. Such a tool may take a real-time log of a patient's thoughts. Such a tool may also monitor whether a patient is not going to relapse and should show a patient's current trajectory. There are systems that are already addressing such multiple needs. For example, Health-Kits and multi-components applications. However, patients need to be supported in identifying the combination of tools that work best for their involving and complex needs. **Future research should explore how DCCs can be addressed, by combining existing single condition tools and systems and how to guide patients with DCCs in identifying the combination of systems and tools that make an ecosystem that is appropriate for their situation.** Further, putting together multiple sets of tools could be a challenge. For example, some of the tools could be owned by private companies looking to make profits, others may be very difficult to integrate. **Future research could**

explore how to address this engineering challenge and how to make a theoretical concept adaptable to technology.

6   Conclusion

In this study, we show how design experts explored the DCCs problems space, and discussed and refined strategies to address the problems they identified. The design experts focused on discussing the ideas for conceptual tools that make patients the center of the design. For example, they strongly suggested the need for i) tools that frame feedback around patients' experiences rather than framing feedback around statistical risks, ii) tools to visualize a patient's progression and motivate patients using gamification, and iii) tools that are capable of providing a view of all the patient's conditions, instead of individual conditions. When a patient reports a condition, the participants suggest that it should be placed in the context of their other conditions regardless of which condition caused the symptom. Experts decided that the best way to address the DCCs was to combine tools to form an ecosystem. When conducting design sprints, the following strategies worked for us; First, introducing participants to design space in the first meeting and laying a solid foundation. The second item was analyzing and reflecting on the design trajectory after every Design Sprint session. This allowed us to answer design questions (DQ 1 and DQ 2) and formulate discussion points to be used at the next Design Sprint session. Finally, having designers keep an open mind and allowing them the flexibility to explore fresh conceptual design ideas. However, this may result in experts diverging from designing for the original problem/need. There is a need for a high level of management to keep experts focused on the original problem.

Acknowledgement. It is with true pleasure that we acknowledge the contributions of our design experts Daria Loi, Kevin Shaw, Timothy Kelly, Janette Shew, and Ginny Hong. Thank you for generously sharing your time, experience, and other resources for this project.

References

1. Ancker, J.S., Witteman, H.O., Hafeez, B., Provencher, T., Van de Graaf, M., Wei, E.: "You get reminded you're a sick person": personal data tracking and patients with multiple chronic conditions. J. Med. Internet Res. **17**(8), e4209 (2015)
2. Ballegaard, S.A., Hansen, T.R., Kyng, M.: Healthcare in everyday life: designing healthcare services for daily life. In: Proceedings of the SIGCHI Conference on Human Factors in Computing Systems, pp. 1807–1816. ACM (2008)
3. Becker, M.H.: The health belief model and sick role behavior. Health Educ. Monogr. **2**(4), 409–419 (1974)
4. Butler, M., Ratner, E., McCreedy, E., Shippee, N., Kane, R.L.: Decision aids for advance care planning: an overview of the state of the science. Ann. Intern. Med. **161**(6), 408–418 (2014)

5. Hayes, G.R., Abowd, G.D., Davis, J.S., Blount, M.L., Ebling, M., Mynatt, E.D.: Opportunities for pervasive computing in chronic cancer care. In: Indulska, J., Patterson, D.J., Rodden, T., Ott, Max (eds.) Pervasive 2008. LNCS, vol. 5013, pp. 262–279. Springer, Heidelberg (2008). https://doi.org/10.1007/978-3-540-79576-6_16

6. Howard, T.: Journey mapping: a brief overview. Commun. Design Q. Rev. 2(3), 10–13 (2014)

7. Huh, J., Ackerman, M.S.: Collaborative help in chronic disease management: supporting individualized problems. In: Proceedings of the ACM 2012 Conference on Computer Supported Cooperative Work, pp. 853–862. ACM (2012)

8. Jacobs, M., Clawson, J., Mynatt, E.D.: A cancer journey framework: guiding the design of holistic health technology. In: Proceedings of the 10th EAI International Conference on Pervasive Computing Technologies for Healthcare, pp. 114–121. ICST (Institute for Computer Sciences, Social-Informatics and Telecommunications Engineering) (2016)

9. Kim, M.I., Johnson, K.B.: Personal health records: evaluation of functionality and utility. J. Am. Med. Inform. Assoc. 9(2), 171–180 (2002)

10. Lagu, T., et al.: The impact of concordant and discordant conditions on the quality of care for hyperlipidemia. J. Gen. Intern. Med. 23(8), 1208 (2008)

11. Lee, L.J.: Tools: MIRO real-time board, visual collaborations and tools, easy screen sharing and presentation (2020)

12. Liu, L.S., Huh, J., Neogi, T., Inkpen, K., Pratt, W.: Health vlogger-viewer interaction in chronic illness management. In: Proceedings of the SIGCHI Conference on Human Factors in Computing Systems, pp. 49–58 (2013)

13. Mamykina, L., et al.: Structured scaffolding for reflection and problem solving in diabetes self-management: qualitative study of mobile diabetes detective. J. Am. Med. Inform. Assoc. 23(1), 129–136 (2016)

14. Mamykina, L., Nakikj, D., Elhadad, N.: Collective sensemaking in online health forums. In: Proceedings of the 33rd Annual ACM Conference on Human Factors in Computing Systems, pp. 3217–3226. ACM (2015)

15. McCurdy, K.: Visual storytelling in healthcare: why we should help patients visualize their health. Inf. Vis. 15(2), 173–178 (2016)

16. Nashrulloh, M., Setiawan, R., Heryanto, D., Elsen, R.: Designing software product with google ventures design sprint framework in startup. In: Journal of Physics: Conference Series, vol. 1402, p. 022084. IOP Publishing (2019)

17. Naylor, M.D., Van Cleave, J.: Transitional care model. Transitions Theory: Middle-range and Situation-specific Theories in Nursing Research and Practice, pp. 459–465. Springer, New York (2010)

18. Ongwere, T., Cantor, G., Martin, S.R., Shih, P.C., Clawson, J., Connelly, K.: Too many conditions, too little time: designing technological intervention for patients with type-2 diabetes and discordant chronic comorbidities. In: Workshop on Interactive Systems in Health Care (2017)

19. Ongwere, T., Cantor, G.S., Clawson, J., Shih, P.C., Connelly, K.: Design and care for discordant chronic comorbidities: a comparison of healthcare providers' perspectives (2020)

20. Ongwere, T., Cantor, G.S., Martin, S.R., Shih, P.C., Clawson, J., Connelly, K.: Design hotspots for care of discordant chronic comorbidities: patients' perspectives. In: NordiCHI, pp. 571–583 (2018)

21. Ongwere, T., Stolterman, E., Clawson, J., Shih, P.C., Connelly, K.: Design for discordant chronic comorbidities (DCCS): a DC^3 model (2021)

22. Pentakota, S.R., et al.: Does diabetes care differ by type of chronic comorbidity?: An evaluation of the Piette and Kerr framework. Diabetes Care **35**(6), 1285–1292 (2012)
23. Piette, J.D., Kerr, E.A.: The impact of comorbid chronic conditions on diabetes care. Diabetes Care **29**(3), 725–731 (2006)
24. Prochaska, J.O., Velicer, W.F.: The transtheoretical model of health behavior change. Am. J. Health Promot. **12**(1), 38–48 (1997)
25. Rollnick, S., Miller, W.R., Butler, C.: Motivational Interviewing in Health Care: Helping Patients Change Behavior. Guilford Press, New York (2008)
26. Sari, E., Tedjasaputra, A.: Designing valuable products with design sprint. In: Bernhaupt, R., Dalvi, G., Joshi, A., K. Balkrishan, D., O'Neill, J., Winckler, M. (eds.) INTERACT 2017. LNCS, vol. 10516, pp. 391–394. Springer, Cham (2017). https://doi.org/10.1007/978-3-319-68059-0_37
27. Setiawan, I.M.A., et al.: An adaptive mobile health system to support self-management for persons with chronic conditions and disabilities: usability and feasibility studies. JMIR Form. Res. **3**(2), e12982 (2019)
28. Wang, M., Lau, C., Matsen, F.A., Kim, Y.: Personal health information management system and its application in referral management. IEEE Trans. Inf. Technol. Biomed. **8**(3), 287–297 (2004)
29. Zulman, D.M., Kerr, E.A., Hofer, T.P., Heisler, M., Zikmund-Fisher, B.J.: Patient-provider concordance in the prioritization of health conditions among hypertensive diabetes patients. J. Gen. Intern. Med. **25**(5), 408–414 (2010). https://doi.org/10.1007/s11606-009-1232-1

Towards Enhancing the Multimodal Interaction of a Social Robot to Assist Children with Autism in Emotion Regulation

Marcelo Rocha[1]([✉]), Pedro Valentim[1], Fábio Barreto[1], Adrian Mitjans[2], Dagoberto Cruz-Sandoval[3], Jesus Favela[2], and Débora Muchaluat-Saade[1]

[1] MÍdiaCom Lab - UFF, Niterói, Brazil
`{marcelo_rocha,pedroalvesvalentim,fbarreto,debora}@midiacom.uff.br`
[2] CICESE, Ensenada, Mexico
`favela@cicese.mx`
[3] Computer Science and Engineering, UC San Diego, San Diego, USA
`dcruzsandoval@eng.ucsd.edu`

Abstract. Assistive robots are expected to become ubiquitous by transforming everyday life and are expected to be widely used in healthcare therapies. SARs (Socially Assistive Robots) are a class of robots that are at an intersection between the class of assistive robots and that of interactive social robots. SARs are being explored to assist in the diagnosis and treatment of children with ASD (Autism Spectrum Disorder). A SAR called EVA has been used to assist non-pharmacological interventions based on verbal, non-verbal communication and social interaction. The EVA robot can currently speak, listen and express emotions through looking. Towards offering immersive therapies for autistic children, this work enhances EVA's capabilities to recognize user emotions through facial expression recognition and also to create light sensory effects in order to make the therapy more attractive to users. A therapy session was developed through a serious game where the child should recognize the robot's emotions. During the game, EVA recognizes the child's facial expression to check his/her learning progress. We invited a neurotypical 6-year-old child to play the game, with the consent of her parents, and recorded videos of the game session. Those videos were evaluated by 48 expert physicians and psychologists in therapies for ASD using the Technology Acceptance Model (TAM). They considered our work useful and agreed it would help them doing their job more effectively.

Keywords: Socially Assistive Robots (SAR) · Multimodal interaction · Serious game · Emotion regulation · Autism Spectrum Disorder (ASD)

1 Introduction

Robotic technologies are no longer used only in factories and have been increasingly used to assist people perform activities of daily living. Assistive robots

H. Lewy and R. Barkan (Eds.): PH 2021, LNICST 431, pp. 398–415, 2022.
https://doi.org/10.1007/978-3-030-99194-4_25

have been used to improve the quality of life in society and are becoming more and more common [28]. Robots are used in our lives as assistive devices and robotics is a method capable of enhancing the physical and cognitive abilities of humans [7]. Robots can help with housework or assist people with some type of physical disability. However, advances have emerged in a new field of robotics where the objective is not only to provide assistance, but to provide stimuli to humans through interaction with the robot [27]. Robots are expected to become ubiquitous by transforming everyday life and are expected to be widely used in healthcare therapies. SARs (Socially Assistive Robots) [7] are a class of robots that are an intersection between the class of assistive robots (of the types that provide user assistance) and that of interactive social robots (those that communicate with the user through social and not physical interaction). SARs have been used in various types of healthcare therapies, such as non-pharmacological interventions, which can improve the quality of life for patients and those around them [18]. A Socially Assistive Robot called EVA [4,32] has been used to assist non-pharmacological interventions based on verbal, non-verbal communication and social interaction with patients with dementia and Alzheimer's disease (AD). A user study with five patients with (AD) was conducted and showed that EVA was effective in engaging therapy participants. The EVA robot can currently speak, listen and express emotions through looking.

The development and use of interactive technologies for individuals with ASD (Autism Spectrum Disorder) has also been growing rapidly. Those technologies can enrich interventions, facilitate communication, support data collection and have the potential to improve the assessment and diagnosis process of individuals with ASD [12]. In [26] there is a proposal for a robotic coaching platform for social training, motor and cognitive capabilities. The robot used in this work is the NAO robot, which has been widely used in social therapy with children with ASD. As the NAO is a humanoid robot, it looks like a human without being one, and it can provide audio and visual stimuli. All these characteristics are favorable for interaction with ASD children, who tend to prefer simplified stimuli to avoid focusing on details. The work [30] compares the results from robot-based interventions with those from human-based applied to children with ASD and intellectual disabilities. In [6], positive results of the interaction of children with ASD with a robot are presented, indicating a greater incidence of eye contact, proximity and interaction than the interactions between children and a human. There is evidence supporting the claim that autistic children prefer robots to humans [13,14,21]. The results of these studies indicate that robots can generate several positive effects in this type of therapy and that human-robot interaction can help to solve the problems that occur in human-human interaction. Deficits in social and communication skills in patients with autism encompass a number of other disabilities, such as difficulty in recognizing body language or demonstrating eye contact with whom they talk to and problems in expressing their own emotions and understanding those of others [6].

In order to enhance robot capabilities to interact with users, multimodal interaction can be very useful. Besides voice interaction, which is frequently used by SARs such as EVA, video interaction could be provided to help capture user emotion, for example. In addition, sensory effects could be used to create immersive therapies and make them more attractive to users, specially children.

Towards offering immersive therapies for autistic children, this work enhances EVA's capabilities to recognize user emotions through facial expression recognition and also to create light sensory effects in order to make the therapy more attractive to users. The idea is to use the interactive robot as the first stage of an emotion recognition therapy for children with ASD.

We developed a therapy session through a serious game where the child should recognize the robot's emotions. During the game, EVA recognizes the child's facial expression to check his/her learning progress. We invited a neurotypical 6-year-old child to play the game, with the consent of her parents, and recorded videos of the game session. Those videos were evaluated by expert physicians and psychologists in therapies for ASD using the Technology Acceptance Model (TAM). We made a statistical analysis to compare evaluation results between expert and beginner ASD therapists.

The remainder of this paper is structured as follows. Section 2 discusses related work. Section 3 presents EVA's architecture and main functionalities. Section 4 presents our extensions to EVA. Section 5 discusses the autism therapy session that we have implemented. Section 6 presents an evaluation done by ASD therapists. Section 7 concludes this paper and presents future work.

2   Related Work

SARs have become popular tools in interventions with patients with ASD. Robots have been used in special education schools and care centers for autistic people. In [11], a framework was developed to engage children with ASD in sensory interactions. They used two robots, the first called Romo and the second was a small humanoid robot. They were capable of producing visual and audio stimuli. The Romo robot could express its emotions through three components: movement, facial expressions and sound effects. The framework was used as a tool for emotion regulation therapies and worked as follows. The patient interacted with the robot through a game, which ran on a notebook. The game uses three key states, which are the user's emotion state, the penguin character's emotion state, and a fixed predetermined goal emotion state towards which the penguin steers the user. To build a relationship with the user, the penguin first dynamically allocates a temporary goal state that approximates the user's state, then it gradually moves that temporary goal state closer to the predetermined goal to facilitate emotion regulation. Thus, based on the continuous interaction with the penguin character, the algorithm tries to guide the user towards the desired target state. The participant was then guided, progressively, through the robot's social behavior (movement/facial expression/sound effects) until the final facial expression. The results of a user study confirmed the viability of the framework as a tool for regulating emotion.

In [25], a mobile robot was developed and used to investigate its potential in stimulating social interactions in children with autism. Those stimuli were provided through games or therapeutic activities. During sessions with the robot, specialists in autism observed some capabilities in patients who had never been seen in other therapies, indicating that the robot could assist those specialists in finding new capacities in children with autism, creating more effective therapies, adapted to each patient.

A proposal to use a robot, which is capable of measuring the social behavior of a child with ASD during an interaction, was made in [9]. That proposal uses a wearable device to detect the child's smile. Although the device allows a smile to be detected even without the child facing the robot, the use of a wearable device can be uncomfortable, especially for children with ASD who tend to have tactile hypersensitivity.

The authors in [2] present an interactive robotic system that provides emotional and social behaviors for multisensory therapy for children with ASD. The system uses two robots, one of which is capable of expressing emotions through facial expressions and the other demonstrates its emotions using body language and gestures. The authors' proposal is that the robots go through a maze-like scenario and during the circuit find objects that stimulate the five senses, i.e. sight, hearing, smell, taste and touch. The idea is that children can learn from robots to deal with sensory overload.

A study using two robots was conducted in [8]. The aim was to examine the robot's behavior and whether or not it affected the behavior of children with ASD. Evidence was found that the robot's behavior does affect the child's social behavior, both in human-human interaction and in human-robot interaction.

The use of sensory effects has also been applied for autism therapies. In [19] there is a proposal for an adaptive physical environment that allows children with severe autism to successfully interact with multimodal stimuli. This environment generates stimuli of various types (visual, aural, and vibrotactile) in real-time. In [34] a system of sensory devices is presented to support therapists of children with ASD. The Sensor Box could be handled by children and was capable of generating a series of sensory stimuli, such as sounds and light effects.

A large-scale elastic multisensory surface that allows users to make music when tapping and touching on top of the canvas was developed in [3]. On this surface, users could play sounds of different musical instruments. BendableSound is a system using a Kinect sensor, speakers, and an ultra-short throw projector placed behind a spandex fabric.

Previous studies [17] point to a link between playing action games and cognitive and perceptual improvement. However, that improvement is not only associated with playing action games. Different types of games can improve different cognitive aspects. In [20] an implementation of the Stroop game with light sensory effects was made for the Brazilian digital TV system. A serious game (SG) was developed to train the selective attention of the elderly through the Stroop effect. The game displays on the screen the name of a color written with another color, then, the user through the TV remote control buttons, selects the correct color to answer. The light sensory effect is used for helping the elderly user with the correct answer.

Through the use of games it is possible to provide interactivity, increase mental activity and promote social interaction between various users. The work in [24] describes the development of an SG that can be used by children with ASD in order to improve communication and social interaction. In [1] an SG for children with ASD was proposed with the aim of investigating the effects of a game as a play therapy. Through an empirical study, conventional games (non-computer block-games) were compared with the proposed SG. Evidence showed an improvement in the social interaction of children, in the process of collaboration between them and a decrease in solitary games.

The emotional development of a child involves the ability to understand his/her own feelings as well as those around him/her. For a child with ASD, the process of understanding and expressing feelings is very difficult. An SG was designed in [31] with the aim of helping children with ASD, through an imitation process, to recognize different facial expressions.

Unlike the previously mentioned studies, our work extends the multimodal interaction capabilities of a SAR, integrating sensory effects and facial expression recognition in a single robot-based platform. The authors of [2,8,9,11,25] propose the use of robots for therapies with children with ASD, without offering the possibility of capturing the child's facial expression through video. In [3,19,34] sensory effects are used for ASD therapies, including light effects, but they do not use a robot-based platform. The studies [1,17,20,24,31] deal with SG, however, this work proposes an SG offered by the robot. These points are summarized in Table 1.

Table 1. Related work comparison

Related work	Use a robot	Light sensory effects	Voice recognition	Use facial expression	Serious game	Facial expression recognition
[2]	✓	–	–	✓	–	–
[8,11]	✓	–	–	✓	✓	–
[9]	✓	–	–	–	–	✓
[25]	✓	✓	–	✓	✓	–
[19]	–	✓	✓	–	–	–
[3]	–	✓	–	–	–	–
[34]	–	✓	✓	✓	–	–
[1,17,24]	–	–	–	–	✓	–
[20]	–	✓	–	–	✓	–
[31]	–	–	–	–	✓	✓
Our Work	✓	✓	✓	✓	✓	✓

3   EVA: An Open-Source Social Robotics Platform

EVA (Embodied Voice Assistant) is an open-source robotics platform. EVA provides most of the resources to build a fully functional social robot at an affordable cost, and design and create interactions for specific contexts and populations. EVA's repository provides all the elements to make your own social robot, such as 3D models, software, and guidelines to assemble it using open-hardware solutions such as the Raspberry Pi and Arduino-based card-boards. The basic version of the EVA robot includes a voice interface (microphone array and speaker) and a 5-inch touchscreen to display a set of basic facial expressions and manage the robot's basic features. Furthermore, EVA integrates a ring of LEDs in its chest to display light animations. In addition to the above elements, the intermediate version (see Fig. 1) includes two servo-motors to provide 2 degrees of freedom (DOF) to the robot's head and a depth camera (Intel RealSense) for tasks involving computer vision. The complete (mobile) version includes a mobile platform based on TurtleBot to explore more complex body gestures and mobility features. Although these three versions have been proposed by the creative and development team, makers and research teams can create, combine, or add new elements to create their new EVA-based solutions.

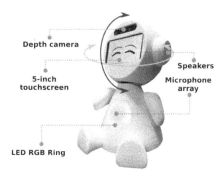

Fig. 1. Intermediate version of EVA

3.1   Software Architecture

The software architecture of EVA includes two main modules. The first one is a graphical interface accessible using the touchscreen directly. The operator uses it to configure and manage the basic features, such as Wi-Fi connection, deploy pre-programmed interaction, network information, restart, and shutdown. The second one, called Core Module, has all the logic and core features of EVA, including back-end components: server, behavioral controller; and front-end components: operator console, WoZ design, programming, and configuration. Figure 2 illustrates EVA's main software components, which are detailed as follows.

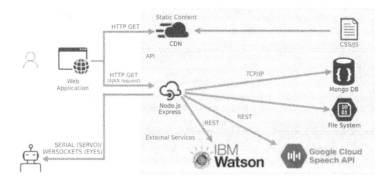

Fig. 2. EVA's main software components [16]

Core Module. The back-end components of the Core Module are responsible for the logic and operation of EVA. These components are the core of the EVA and implement tasks such as: running a server to establish communication between the operator and robot; controllers to interact with the sensors and actuators; and directly managing the database. The back-end components have been developed with NodeJS, Python, and C++.

Server Controller. This component enables a web server that deploys a REST API used by the front-end components to manage and configure EVA's features and behavior. The server controller manages the request and handles those which are related to configuration and storage. Those requests related to EVA's features, operation, and behavior are sent to the behavioral controller.

Behavioral Controller. This is the main component of EVA. It enacts the behavior (utterances, gestures, movements, facial expressions, light animations) of the robot controlling the actuators (speaker, display, servo-motors, and ring of LEDs). Furthermore, it manages and processes the inputs of the sensors (microphone, camera) in order to enact the specific response or behavior of the robot. The component uses third-party cognitive services from Watson (Text-to-Speech, Vision) and Google (Speech, Dialogflow) to process inputs from sensors and outputs to actuators. Moreover, open-source solutions can be integrated, such as Vosk (speech recognition), Mimic (Text-to-Speech), and Padatious (Natural Language Understanding).

The front-end components of the Core module deploy user interfaces to configure and manage the behavior and features of the social robot. The frond-end has been developed using the framework AngularJS. The description of each front-end component is provided as follows.

Operator Console. The operator can manage the behavior of the robot directly using this component. The operator console includes modules to send personalized utterances, enact facial expressions, make personalized and pre-programmed movements, and deploy light animations. Using this module, a user can operate the robot in real-time.

WoZ Design. Wizard of Oz (WoZ) is one of the most popular techniques to conduct early interactions to design and define future autonomous interactions. The EVA platform considers the importance of this approach and provides a component to design and deploy this kind of interaction. The component allows creating WoZ interactions using (pre)defined utterances, sounds, music tracks, pre-programmed facial expressions, and gestures (movements). These interactions are stored in the database for future uses.

Visual Programming. In addition to the WoZ module, the platform EVA includes this component to design and deploy autonomous interactions. The user can design the interaction scripts defining the flow (sequence, conditions, loops) using a visual programming language (VPL). This includes the definition of actions such as utterances, voice recognition, time to response, atom responses (utterances, sounds, facial expressions, gestures, light animations), or composed responses - a combination of atom responses. These autonomous interactions are stored in the database for future applications.

Configuration. The configuration module is used to define the robot's name (wake-word), voice (language, gender), and voice recognition (language). Supported languages are based on Watson (TTS, STT) and Google Cloud Speech. Moreover, we can include credentials to use third-party cognitive services.

4   Extending EVA's Multimodal Interaction

As we mentioned previously, the EVA robot is able to conduct a personalized session through interaction scripts. These scripts can be easily created using a VPL designed exclusively for EVA [16]. VPL is not concerned with the syntactic details of a conventional programming language, it was created to facilitate the construction of interaction scripts allowing people who are not specialized in programming to create their own scripts.

With the use of a graphical tool, building a script is done in a simple way, simply dragging and dropping the control components into the application window. The language has several components, including those that control the flow of script execution, counters, timers, conditional controls and the robot's speech and listening controls. Executing the interaction script, the robot can interact with the user, obtaining information through listening and expressing itself through speech, facial expressions, body gestures and light animations.

This work uses the EVA platform and extends its core and front-end capabilities for user interaction with video capture and sensory effects. Particularly, we used the basic version of EVA in our work. We extended VPL to include light sensory effects into therapy scripts, so that EVA can communicate with a smart bulb using a Wi-Fi interface to turn it on or off. We also extended VPL to capture the user emotion through facial expression recognition, therefore, an integrated camera is used to take the user's picture and analyze his/her facial expression to identify if he/she is happy, sad, angry or neutral. Section 4.1 presents our proposal for including light sensory effects and Sect. 4.2 discusses our proposal for facial expression recognition.

4.1   Light Sensory Effects

The first component added to the language was *Light*, which gives the robot the ability to control lighting. With the addition of this component, EVA can turn on the light, turn it off and select the desired color. The color selection can be done with the help of an RGB color palette. At the moment a *Light* component is inserted into a script, a configuration window appears and the script developer can select the light color and bulb status, which can be turned on or off.

All lighting control is done through a TCP connection between the robot and the smart bulb. A Xiaomi Yeelight smart bulb was used for our implementation. The control commands use a JSON string that must contain the lamp identifier, the type of command and its parameters. All command strings must end with "\r\n". These parameters are defined when the *Light* component is inserted into the script. Figure 3 shows the connection scheme between EVA and a smart bulb with identifier equal to 1 and IP address 192.168.1.105.

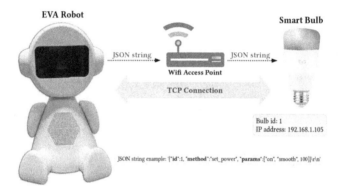

Fig. 3. EVA controlling a smart bulb

4.2   Facial Expression Recognition

Being able to identify the user's emotion through the recognition of facial expressions and using this information within the application is an important facility, which expands the power of the robot's interaction with the user [33]. For this purpose, a second extension was added to VPL giving the robot the ability to recognize facial expressions. A new component was created and added to the visual programming language, named *User Emotion*. It uses the services of an external module developed in Python. Both the Python module and the EVA software run on the same device, a Raspberry PI 4.

Communication between the module and the robot takes over a TCP connection. When started, the face recognition module creates a TCP server that keeps waiting for the connection with the robot. After establishing the connection, the facial recognition module activates the webcam, thus initiating the image capture and facial expression inference processes. At the end of the procedure, the module returns to the TCP client (EVA), a string containing the identified expression. The facial recognition module can return the following expressions: "NEUTRAL", "ANGRY", "DISGUST", "FEAR", "SURPRISE", "HAPPY" and "SAD". In order to obtain the user's facial expression, the robot, through the *User Emotion* component, sends a request to the Python facial recognition module. The process works as illustrated in Figure 4.

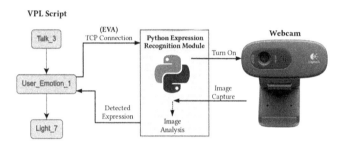

Fig. 4. Communication between EVA and the Facial Expression Recognition module

We have done tests to evaluate the accuracy of the facial expression module to recognize user's emotion when "HAPPY", "ANGRY" and "SAD". We chose those three facial expression types, because they are the ones that can currently be expressed by EVA and will be used in the therapy session we implemented as going to be discussed in the following section. We implemented a program with EVA to recognize 30 facial expressions and two users have tested this program with 5 expressions of each type "HAPPY", "ANGRY" and "SAD". Therefore, considering 30 facial expression recognition events, EVA correctly recognized 24, obtaining an accuracy of 80%. Considering only the "HAPPY" expression, EVA's accuracy was 100%. The tests were performed by two adults. Thus, we considered it as a satisfactory result that can be used in practice.

5   Serious Game for Autism Therapy

In order to serve as the object of evaluation of our proposal, we developed a serious game [1] using the robot's programming language. This game is aimed at assisting in emotion regulation therapies for children with ASD.

During the game design phase, we talked to an ASD expert therapist to discuss our ideas. The therapist recommended us to only emphasize correct answers given by a child. EVA should not say, for example, "your answer is wrong" to the child. On the other hand, EVA should compliment the child when the given answer is fine. This procedure is used in interventions in Applied Behavior Analysis called Discrete Trial Training (DTT) [29]. DTT is a practice that uses instructions with repeated teaching attempts, where each shot presents an answer and a reinforcement to that answer, if appropriate. It is a fully structured training, with a clearly defined beginning and end. This type of discrete experimental intervention increases the likelihood of correct patient responses based on error-free learning. The interaction between therapist and child must be carried out in an environment without distractions, with clear, concise and objective instructions and immediate reinforcement for each correct answer.

We designed a game with three stages. The first stage is called *game of colors*, in which the child is asked to match the colors that are presented by the robot using light sensory effects. In the second stage, called *game of emotions*, the robot presents several facial expressions, while the child tries to identify them. In the third stage, called *imitation game*, the child needs to imitate the robot's emotions with his/her own facial expressions.

Each stage includes three questions. If the child gives an incorrect response, he/she is provided with a new chance to try the correct answer. Stage 1 follows the flowchart shown in Fig. 5.

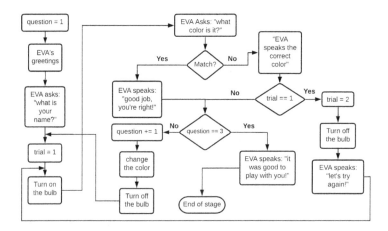

Fig. 5. Flowchart of stage 1 of the game

Using the robot's TTS (Text-to-Speech) feature, a greeting text is transformed into speech and the game starts with the robot greeting the child. Then, the robot listens, waiting for the child's response and through the STT resource (Speech-to-Text) the participant's name is captured, transformed into a string and stored in a variable. Then, the robot, using the *Light* component proposed in this work, presents the first color, lighting the bulb and asking the child to name its color. At this point, using the VPL's conditional testing feature, the child's response, already transformed into a string, is compared with the string that represents the correct answer. If the child gets it right, the robot congratulates him/her and checks if it has reached the maximum number of questions, if not, a new color is selected and the process of presenting is repeated by presenting

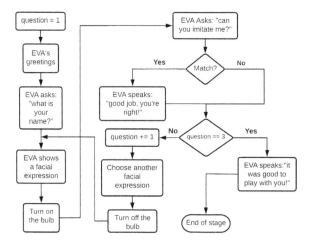

Fig. 6. Flowchart of stage 3 of the game

a new color. If the child makes a mistake, the robot speaks the correct name of the color and gives another opportunity for the child to try again. After three questions, the robot gives a final greeting and the game ends.

Stage 2 follows the same logic as stage 1, but now the child has to recognize the robot's emotions. Therefore, instead of presenting the colors and turning on the bulb, the robot presents emotions through its own gaze expressions. Three emotions are represented: *happy, anger and sadness.*

In stage 3, the logic of the game changes as shown in Fig. 6 . The robot shows a facial expression and asks the child to imitate it. Unlike the previous stages where the robot takes the child's voice as input, in this stage, the robot obtains the child's response by recognizing his/her facial expression using the *User Emotion* component proposed in this work. The robot captures the child's expression and checks if he/she provided the correct response. EVA congratulates the child when his/her imitation is recognized correctly. Three facial expressions are presented in a match.

6   Proposal Evaluation

In order to evaluate our proposal, we used the Technology Acceptance Model (TAM) [15]. This instrument is widely used for evaluating technology applied to healthcare [10]. TAM is based on a questionnaire that assesses Intention to Use the technology by evaluating Perceived Usefulness (PU), "the degree to which a person believes that using a particular system would enhance his or her job performance"; and Perceived Ease-Of-Use (PEOU), "the degree to which a person believes that using a particular system would be free from effort" [5].

As suggested by [22], the game was tested by a Brazilian neurotypical 6-year-old child with the consent of her parents for participating in the experiment. The robot spoke Portuguese in the therapy session. As not all physical parts of the robot were already available, we connected a TV to the Raspberry Pi to show the robot's eyes to the child. However, at the moment, we already have the robot fully built with all the parts that make it up[1]. We recorded videos of the child playing each game stage with EVA[2,3,4], with the consent of her parents. Figure 7 shows the child playing game stage 3.

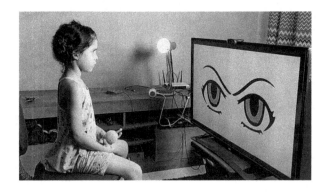

Fig. 7. Child playing the imitation game

We have adapted a TAM questionnaire for our evaluation and asked healthcare professionals and students to watch those videos and complete the questionnaire. The results are shown in Table 2. Questions for evaluating perceived usefulness (PU) and easy-of-use (PEOU) used a likert scale varying from (1) completely disagree to (5) completely agree.

A group of 48 adult users, aging from 19 to 61 years old, including healthcare professionals and students, such as physicians, psychiatrists, psychologists, nurses, psychopedagogues, educators, speech therapists, and occupational therapists, have evaluated our proposal. All of them have given their consent to participate in the experiment, otherwise they would not be able to watch the videos and answer the questionnaire. We considered professionals with two or more years of experience in taking care of children with ASD as experts and the ones with less than two years of experience, including students, as beginners [23]. Four participants were excluded from the experiment because they had not specified their graduation course. Therefore, our final group was divided into 24 experts in ASD and 20 beginners in ASD. Table 2 shows the average (AVG) and standard deviation (SD) results for PU and PEOU questions, considering the whole group of 44 participants (All) and also specific subgroup results (experts and beginners). Average results greater than or equal to 4,0 indicate participants

---

[1] https://bit.ly/3kNt4u3.
[2] https://bityli.com/0ceIRU.
[3] https://bityli.com/IhTkIc.
[4] https://youtu.be/PU8BLwTkGaw.

Table 2. TAM questionnaire and results

Technology Acceptance Model - TAM		All		24 Experts		20 Beginners		Mann-Whitney	
Perceived Usefulness (PU)		AVG	SD	AVG	SD	AVG	SD	U	p-exactly
PU1	The use of technology helps me to do my job	4,39	0,72	**4,46**	0,72	4,30	0,73	206,5	0,217
PU2	The EVA interactive robot would be useful to assist me in therapies for autism spectrum disorder (ASD)	4,23	1,16	**4,25**	1,11	4,20	1,24	238,5	0,486
PU3	The EVA interactive robot would hinder my therapy sessions for autism spectrum disorder (ASD)	2,32	1,39	**2,08**	1,18	2,60	1,60	196	0,154
PU4	The color recognition game would be useful to assist me in therapies for autism spectrum disorder (ASD)	4,25	1,06	**4,29**	1,08	4,20	1,06	218	0,308
PU5	The game to recognize emotions would be useful to assist me in therapies for autism spectrum disorder (ASD)	4,39	0,97	**4,54**	0,88	4,20	1,06	186	0,105
PU6	The game to mimic the emotions of the robot would be useful to assist me in therapies for autism spectrum disorder (ASD)	4,39	0,97	**4,46**	0,88	4,30	1,08	227	0,385
PU7	The EVA interactive robot could help me increase the effectiveness of therapies for autism spectrum disorder (ASD) in recognizing emotions	4,25	1,10	**4,33**	1,13	4,15	1,09	202	0,190
PU8	The EVA interactive robot could be useful in other types of therapies	4,59	0,90	**4,58**	1,02	4,60	0,75	222	0,341
Perceived Ease-Of-Use (PEOU)									
PEOU1	A child with ASD would easily interact with the robot through voice	3,82	1,04	**3,75**	1,11	3,90	0,97	223	0,350
PEOU2	The light effect makes the therapy session with children with ASD LESS attractive	2,57	1,35	**2,71**	1,46	2,40	1,23	207	0,224
PEOU3	**Sound effects make the therapy session with children with ASD MORE attractive**	**4,05**	**1,14**	3,79	1,18	**4,35**	**1,04**	**169,5**	**0,048**
PEOU4	I think it would be easy to use the robot in my therapy sessions with children with ASD	4,14	1,00	**4,00**	1,10	4,30	0,86	205	0,210
PEOU5	I would need a lot of effort to use the robot in my therapy sessions with children with ASD	2,30	1,32	**2,17**	1,24	2,45	1,43	213,5	0,268

completely/partially agree with the question, and results less than or equal to 3,0 indicate they completely/partially disagree with it.

Analyzing the obtained PU results, we can conclude that most experts agree that Eva would be useful to help them during therapy sessions (PU1, PU2, PU3 and PU8). Notice that PU3 is a negative question where the opposite answer (disagree) is desired and obtained. Experts also agree that the extensions proposed in our work are useful and would help them doing their job more effectively (PU4, PU5, PU6 and PU7).

Considering PEOU results, most experts agree it would be easy to use EVA in their ASD therapy sessions (PEOU4) without much effort (PEOU5). On the other hand, some experts indicated that patients may have difficulty to interact with EVA using voice (PEOU1), depending on the level of social communication compromising they have. Most experts disagree that light effects makes the therapy less attractive (PEOU2), which is a promising result. On the other hand, considering sound effects, experts also have few concerns about it (PEOU3).

We did a statistical analysis using the Mann-Whitney nonparametric test to compare TAM responses between the groups of experts and beginners for each question. Table 2 shows U and p-exactly one tail results in the last column. A one-tailed test is appropriate if we want to determine if there is a difference between groups. We only found a statistical difference in PEOU3 (U = 169,5; $p < 0,05$), where beginners found sound effects make the therapy session more attractive than experts. In all other questions beginners and experts agree on their answers. Analyzing TAM results, we conclude that EVA is useful and easy to use according to healthcare professionals.

Participants have also given suggestions to improve our work, such as: asking the child's age before starting the therapy, including a test phase before the game starts, increasing the time the smart bulb stays turned on, implementing a tablet or smartphone version for EVA, implementing EVA as an avatar, including activities with music, improving the robot's expressions including its mouth besides its eyes, providing games to recognize vowels, consonants and numbers, providing simple math and Portuguese questions, and personalizing the therapy session according to the child. Those suggestions are considered future work.

6.1   Limitations

The accuracy of the robot's facial recognition module depends mainly on two factors: the correct positioning of the child in front of the camera and the lighting conditions in the room. It is necessary for the child to be positioned properly so that his/her face can be captured from the front. It is also very important that the room is well lit.

Another limitation that we noticed, when using the EVA platform, is that there is a delay in the audio capture process in the step that precedes the STT (Speech-to-Text) step. The robot system cannot capture the child's speech instantly after executing the Listen component. Thus, it is necessary to wait, up to two seconds, for the system to be ready to capture the child's voice.

A limitation of our study is that we have used a TV set and not the robot itself to interact with the child in the experiment. We are currently requesting the Ethics Research Committee Approval to conduct future tests with children with ASD. We hope to run those tests in a near future.

7   Conclusion

This work presented an extension of the EVA robot designed for Autism Spectrum Disorder (ASD) therapies. Our proposal enhanced EVA's capabilities for multimodal interaction using light sensory effects with a smart bulb and facial expression recognition with a webcam to recognize children's emotions.

We developed a serious game with three stages that can help emotion regulation therapies for children with ASD. The first stage is a game where the child has to match light colors. The second stage is a game where the child has to match the robot's emotions. And the third stage asks the child to imitate the robot's emotions with his/her own facial expressions. The game was evaluated by 44 healthcare professionals using the TAM model. Results were very promising indicating that they considered our proposal useful and easy to use in therapy sessions for ASD children.

As future work, we intend to show video or images on the screen of the robot. It could be useful for showing people's emotions as part of the game. We are also going to extend EVA's script language to include our extensions for light effects and user emotion recognition to facilitate creating and editing therapy sessions. During the game scripting process, we missed a component in the VPL that could generate random numbers. It is our goal to extend the language by adding this type of component. For some types of scripts, the use of a graphical programming interface does not seem to be the best option. It would be interesting if therapy session scripts could also be written in pseudocode or in XML and could be imported into the robot system. Another idea is to integrate the robot into other mulsemedia applications. In this case, the robot would work as an avatar and could interact with the player using voice, giving tips and motivating the participant, promoting more engagement.

Acknowledgment. This work was partially supported by CNPq, FAPERJ, CAPES, CAPES Print and INCT-MACC.

References

1. Barajas, A.O., Al Osman, H., Shirmohammadi, S.: A serious game for children with autism spectrum disorder as a tool for play therapy. In: 2017 IEEE 5th International Conference on Serious Games and Applications for Health (SeGAH), pp. 1–7. IEEE (2017)
2. Bevill, R., et al.: Multisensory robotic therapy to promote natural emotional interaction for children with ASD. In: 2016 11th ACM/IEEE International Conference on Human-Robot Interaction (HRI), p. 571 (2016). https://doi.org/10.1109/HRI.2016.7451861
3. Cibrian, F.L., Peña, O., Ortega, D., Tentori, M.: BendableSound: an elastic multisensory surface using touch-based interactions to assist children with severe autism during music therapy. Int. J. Hum. Comput. Stud. **107**, 22–37 (2017)
4. Cruz-Sandoval, D., Favela, J.: A conversational robot to conduct therapeutic interventions for dementia. IEEE Pervasive Comput. **18**(2), 10–19 (2019). https://doi.org/10.1109/MPRV.2019.2907020
5. Davis, F.D.: Perceived usefulness, perceived ease of use, and user acceptance of information technology. MIS Q. 319–340 (1989)
6. Fachantidis, N., Syriopoulou-Delli, C.K., Zygopoulou, M.: The effectiveness of socially assistive robotics in children with autism spectrum disorder. Int. J. Dev. Disabil. **66**(2), 113–121 (2020)
7. Feil-Seifer, D., Mataric, M.: Defining socially assistive robotics. In: 9th International Conference on Rehabilitation Robotics, ICORR 2005, pp. 465–468 (2005). https://doi.org/10.1109/ICORR.2005.1501143
8. Feil-Seifer, D., Mataric, M.: Robot-assisted therapy for children with autism spectrum disorders. In: Proceedings of the 7th International Conference on Interaction Design and Children, pp. 49–52 (2008)
9. Hirokawa, M., Funahashi, A., Pan, Y., Itoh, Y., Suzuki, K.: Design of a robotic agent that measures smile and facing behavior of children with autism spectrum disorder. In: 2016 25th IEEE International Symposium on Robot and Human Interactive Communication (RO-MAN), pp. 843–848 (2016). https://doi.org/10.1109/ROMAN.2016.7745217
10. Hu, P.J., Chau, P.Y., Sheng, O.R.L., Tam, K.Y.: Examining the technology acceptance model using physician acceptance of telemedicine technology. J. Manag. Inf. Syst. **16**(2), 91–112 (1999)

11. Javed, H., Park, C.H.: Interactions with an empathetic agent: regulating emotions and improving engagement in autism. IEEE Robot. Autom. Mag. **26**(2), 40–48 (2019). https://doi.org/10.1109/MRA.2019.2904638
12. Kientz, J.A., Goodwin, M.S., Hayes, G.R., Abowd, G.D.: Interactive technologies for autism. Syn. Lect. Assistive Rehabil. Health-Preserving Technol. **2**(2), 1–177 (2013)
13. Lee, J., Takehashi, H., Nagai, C., Obinata, G.: Design of a therapeutic robot for interacting with autistic children through interpersonal touch. In: 2012 IEEE RO-MAN: The 21st IEEE International Symposium on Robot and Human Interactive Communication, pp. 712–717 (2012). https://doi.org/10.1109/ROMAN.2012.6343835
14. Lee, J., Takehashi, H., Nagai, C., Obinata, G., Stefanov, D.: Which robot features can stimulate better responses from children with autism in robot-assisted therapy? Int. J. Adv. Robot. Syst. **9** (2012). https://doi.org/10.5772/51128
15. Marangunić, N., Granić, A.: Technology acceptance model: a literature review from 1986 to 2013. Univ. Access Inf. Soc. **14**(1), 81–95 (2014). https://doi.org/10.1007/s10209-014-0348-1
16. Mitjans, A.A.: Affective computation in human-robot interaction. Master thesis, Centro de Investigación CientÍfica y de Educación Superior de Ensenada, Baja California (2020). http://cicese.repositorioinstitucional.mx/jspui/handle/1007/3283
17. Oei, A.C., Patterson, M.D.: Enhancing cognition with video games: a multiple game training study. PLoS ONE **8**(3) (2013). https://doi.org/10.1371/journal.pone.0058546
18. Olazarán, J., et al.: Nonpharmacological therapies in Alzheimer's disease: a systematic review of efficacy. Dement. Geriatr. Cogn. Disord. **30**(2), 161–178 (2010). https://doi.org/10.1159/000316119
19. Pares, N., Masri, P., Van Wolferen, G., Creed, C.: Achieving dialogue with children with severe autism in an adaptive multisensory interaction: the "mediate" project. IEEE Trans. Visual Comput. Graph. **11**(6), 734–743 (2005)
20. de Paula, G., Valentim, P., Seixas, F., Santana, R., Muchaluat-Saade, D.: Sensory effects in cognitive exercises for elderly users: stroop game. In: 2020 IEEE 33rd International Symposium on Computer-Based Medical Systems (CBMS), pp. 132–137 (2020). https://doi.org/10.1109/CBMS49503.2020.00032
21. Robins, B., et al.: Human-centred design methods: developing scenarios for robot assisted play informed by user panels and field trials. Int. J. Human Comput. Stud. **68**(12), 873–898 (2010)
22. Salleh, M.H.K., Miskam, M.A., Yussof, H., Omar, A.R.: HRI assessment of ASKNAO intervention framework via typically developed child. Procedia Comput. Sci. **105**, 333–339 (2017)
23. Samonte, M.J.C., Guelos, C.M.C., Madarang, D.K.L., Mercado, M.A.P.: Tap-to-talk: Filipino mobile based learning augmentative and alternative through picture exchange communication intervention for children with autism. In: Proceedings of the 2020 The 6th International Conference on Frontiers of Educational Technologies, pp. 25–29 (2020)
24. Sandoval Bringas, J.A., Carreño León, M.A., Cota, I.E., Carrillo, A.L.: Development of a videogame to improve communication in children with autism. In: 2016 XI Latin American Conference on Learning Objects and Technology (LACLO), pp. 1–6 (2016). https://doi.org/10.1109/LACLO.2016.7751751
25. Santatiwongchai, S., Kaewkamnerdpong, B., Jutharee, W., Ounjai, K.: Bliss: using robot in learning intervention to promote social skills for autism therapy. In: Proceedings of the International Convention on Rehabilitation Engineering & Assistive

Technology. i-CREATe 2016, Singapore Therapeutic, Assistive & Rehabilitative Technologies (START) Centre, Midview City, SGP (2016)

26. Santos, L., Geminiani, A., Schydlo, P., Olivieri, I., Santos-Victor, J., Pedrocchi, A.: Design of a robotic coach for motor, social and cognitive skills training toward applications with ASD children. IEEE Trans. Neural Syst. Rehabil. Eng. **29**, 1223–1232 (2021)

27. Shibata, T.: An overview of human interactive robots for psychological enrichment. Proc. IEEE **92**(11), 1749–1758 (2004). https://doi.org/10.1109/JPROC.2004.835383

28. Shibata, T.: Therapeutic seal robot as biofeedback medical device: qualitative and quantitative evaluations of robot therapy in dementia care. Proc. IEEE **100**(8), 2527–2538 (2012). https://doi.org/10.1109/JPROC.2012.2200559

29. Smith, T.: Discrete trial training in the treatment of autism. Focus Autism Other Dev. Disabil. **16**(2), 86–92 (2001)

30. So, W.C., et al.: Who is a better teacher for children with autism? Comparison of learning outcomes between robot-based and human-based interventions in gestural production and recognition. Res. Dev. Disabil. **86**, 62–75 (2019)

31. Tan, C.T., Harrold, N., Rosser, D.: Can you copyme? An expression mimicking serious game. In: SIGGRAPH Asia 2013 Symposium on Mobile Graphics and Interactive Applications, SA '13. Association for Computing Machinery, New York (2013). https://doi.org/10.1145/2543651.2543657

32. Tentori, M., Ziviani, A., Muchaluat-Saade, D.C., Favela, J.: Digital healthcare in Latin America: the case of Brazil and Mexico. Commun. ACM **63**(11), 72–77 (2020)

33. Valentim, P.A., Barreto, F., Muchaluat-Saade, D.C.: Possibilitando o reconhecimento de expressões faciais em aplicações Ginga-NCL. In: Anais Estendidos do XXVI Simpósio Brasileiro de Sistemas Multimídia e Web, pp. 53–56. SBC (2020)

34. Zubrycki, I., Granosik, G.: Designing an interactive device for sensory therapy. In: 2016 11th ACM/IEEE International Conference on Human-Robot Interaction (HRI), pp. 545–546. IEEE (2016)

MPredA: A Machine Learning Based Prediction System to Evaluate the Autism Level Improvement

Masud Rabbani[1]([✉]), Munirul M. Haque[2], Dipranjan Das Dipal[1],
Md Ishrak Islam Zarif[1], Anik Iqbal[1], Amy Schwichtenberg[3], Naveen Bansal[4],
Tanjir Rashid Soron[5], Syed Ishtiaque Ahmed[6], and Sheikh Iqbal Ahamed[1]

[1] Ubicomp Lab, Department of Computer Science, Marquette University, Milwaukee, WI, USA
masud.rabbani@marquette.edu
[2] R.B. Annis School of Engineering, University of Indianapolis, Indianapolis, IN, USA
[3] College of Health and Human Sciences, Purdue University, West Lafayette, IN, USA
[4] Department of Mathematical and Statistical Sciences, Marquette University, Milwaukee, WI, USA
[5] Telepsychiatry Research and Innovation Network Ltd, Dhaka, Bangladesh
[6] Department of Computer Science, University of Toronto, Toronto, ON, Canada

Abstract. This paper describes the developmental process of a machine learning-based prediction system to evaluate autism Improvement level (MPredA), where the concerned user (parents or clinical professionals) can evaluate their children's development through the web application. We have deployed our previous work (mCARE) data from Bangladesh for prediction models. This system can predict four major milestone parameter improvement levels of children with ASD. In this four-broad category, we have classified into four sub-milestones parameters for each of them to predict the detailed improvement level for each child with ASD. This MPredA can predict 16 milestone parameters for every child with ASD. We deployed four machine learning algorithms (Decision Tree, Logistic Regression, K-Nearest Neighbor, and Artificial Neural Network) for each parameter with 1876 data of the children with ASD to develop 64 prediction models. Among the 64 models, we selected the most accurate 16 models (based on the model's accuracy and evaluation scores) to convert pickles file for the MPredA web-based application. For the prediction system, we have determined the most ten important demographic information of the children with ASD. Among the four-machine learning algorithms, the decision tree showed the most significant result to build the MPredA web-based application. We also test our MPredA -web application by white box testing and get 97.5% of accuracy with real data.

Keywords: Autism Spectrum Disorder (ASD) · Milestone Parameter (MP) · Prediction of MP Improvement · Demography of children with ASD · Importance of demography

© ICST Institute for Computer Sciences, Social Informatics and Telecommunications Engineering 2022
Published by Springer Nature Switzerland AG 2022. All Rights Reserved
H. Lewy and R. Barkan (Eds.): PH 2021, LNICST 431, pp. 416–432, 2022.
https://doi.org/10.1007/978-3-030-99194-4_26

Aberration

Autism Spectrum Disorder (ASD): Behavioral development disability among the children at an early age
Milestone Parameter (MP): The list of early age children's behavioral achievement

1 Introduction

In 1943, Kanner first identified the disorder in the children's behavior [1], and later this neurodevelopmental disorder [2] is known as Autism Spectrum Disorder (ASD). Now, this ASD is a global problem [3], and people of all societal levels suffer from ASD [4]. About 1%–1.5% of children have been suffering from ASD in developed countries [5]; for example, in the United States, 1 out of 54 children have ASD symptoms [6, 7]. Though in developed countries, we have a statistic of the ASD number, in developing countries, especially in low-and-middle-income countries, this scenario is not as good as than developed countries. In developing countries, sometimes they do not properly understand the ASD, and there ASD number is largely unknown. [8] So, children with ASD do not get the proper and early treatment in those countries. In the globe, about 46% of children with ASD do not get the proper diagnosis after identifying the ASD symptoms. [8] Sometimes, parents think this is their curse from GOD. [9, 10] They blame themselves for their previous sin and having a child with ASD. This superstitious belief of the people makes this disorder more complex for children with ASD. [11] But proper ASD knowledge of parents, early identification of ASD [12], and starting of the treatment process, [13] developing attitude towards the children [14] help to develop the children with ASD. And it is scientifically proved that the society's positive point of view towards the family with ASD children and demography of the children with ASD have a significant impact on the children's (with ASD) development.[15, 16] In this study, based on this concept (demography's impaction on children with ASD development), we have developed a machine-learning-based web application that can predict the milestone parameter (four major types) depending on children's demography (ten demographical data).

Currently, most of the innovative work (by deploying technology) and tools are for early identification, recognition of ASD [12, 17, 18], or diagnosis in different phases of the treatment process [2]. There is no such tool that can predict the improvement level (milestone parameter) based on the children's demography. This tool will be helpful for both the clinical professional and the parents or primary caregiver to know earlier the children's developmental or improvement level based on their demography. However, there has a little research-based work on proving the demographical importance on the children (with ASD) [2]. This will be the first research-based (by machine learning models with real data set) web tool, where both caregiver or care-practitioner can give their children's baseline data and the demographic information to get the real-time predicted improvement level of their children based on their provided data.

The main novelty of this work is that parents can update or develop their demography if they learn earlier the improvement level of their children (with ASD) based on their current demography or which demography is the most important for their children's (with ASD) development. In this study, we broadly classify and predict the 16 different milestones parameters level into four major categories of (i) daily living skills, (ii) communication, (iii) motor skills, and (iv) socialization. Based on our previous work (mCARE) [19] data, we have selected the most ten important demographical data types to build robust machine learning models. Then we used these models to develop the web-based MPredA. Therefore, MPredA can predict the milestone parameter improvement level of children with ASD with minimal error. Since currently, we rarely have an accurate system or state-of-the-art system that can predict this improvement level; for this reason, we have a plan to deploy this system in our future project to observe the MPredA's scientific contribution.

The rest of the paper is organized as follows. Section 2 summarizes some related works. Section 3 describes the methodology of MPredA for predicting the milestone parameters. Section 4 illustrates the experimental studies. Finally, Sect. 5 concludes the paper.

2   Related Works

Recently some research-based work has been developed to inform the demographical importance of developing children with ASD. The approach proposed in [20] is machine learning-based research work, where a set of demographical-based machine learning models developed to predict the children's (with ASD) development. In this work, four machine learning algorithms have been deployed to build the models to predict the children's (with ASD) "Daily Living Skills" improvement level. They recommend ten important demographical data, which are very significant to the children's development. Based on the findings in this study, we have extended the data set for four major milestone parameters with 1876 data and built 64 machine learning models. Among these models, we selected the best 16 models to develop our web-based MPredA system.

Another machine learning-basedwork has been developed by Tarik et al.[2] to measure the developmental delays of children with ASD by deploying the home videos in Bangladesh. They used a 2-classification layer of Neural Network with 85% of accuracy to predict the "risk scores" for the children with ASD. This prediction-based work is also helpful for the early detection of autism remotely. Though this work used the Bangladeshi data, the authors' used the US data to train the model. This makes the model culturally divergent. Maenner et al. [21] evaluated the ADDM status of children with ASD based on the machine learning model by deploying the word and phrases during the children's developmental evaluation period.

3   Machine Learning Based Prediction System for Autism Level Improvement (MPredA)

MPredA has been proposed and developed a web-based application [22] that can easily predict the developmental level based on the children's demographic information. It consists of several steps, which are described as follows. Figure 1 is the flow chart of the steps of MPredA.

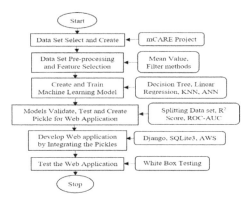

Fig. 1. Outline of research design.

3.1 Select and Create Data Set

This study has deployed the mCARE (Mobile-based Care for children with Autism Spectrum Disorder using Remote Experience Sampling Method) project [19] data. We had approval from the Marquette University Institutional Review Broader (Protocol number HR-1803022959) for deploying the data which had been collected from four centers in Bangladesh. In this study, we have used the "test group" patients' data, who had been monitored and intervened by the clinical coordinators for one year. These data had been collected by the mCARE system [23], and the patient distribution among the four centers for the test group has been shown in Table 1.

Table 1. Test group patient distribution among the four centers.

Serial	Center name	Patient distribution
		Test group (n = 150)
1	The National Institute of Mental Health (NIMH) [24]	50
2	The Institute of Pediatric Neuro-disorder & Autism (IPNA) [25]	50
3	Autism Welfare Foundation (AWF) [26]	25
4	Nishpap autism foundation [27]	25

Since MPredA's machine learning models have been developed based on the children's demography, Table 2 shows the participants' demography in the mCARE project.

From Table 2, we can observe that in mCARE, there had a total of 45 demographic information in 10 broader categories. From this 45 demography, in this study, we have selected ten important demography (details selection process in step 2) for building the machine learning-based training models. Besides the demographic information, we need the specific milestone parameters' baseline level (at the study's starting point) and improvement level (at the ending point) by the corresponding demographic information.

Table 2. Test group participants (n = 150) demographic information.

Serial	Demographics	Participant, n (%)	Serial	Demographics	Participant, n (%)
1	Patients' age: 2–6 6–9	37 (24.7%) 113 (75%)	6	Father's occupation: Service Business Cultivation Other Unemployed	70 (46.7%) 45 (30.0%) 1 (0.7%) 7 (4.7%) 23 (15.3%)
2	Gender: Male Female	124 (82.7%) 26 (17.3%)	7	Mother's occupation: Student Unemployed Housewife Service Business Cultivation Maid Other Not applied	0.0 (0.0%) 0.0 (0.0%) 124 (82.7%) 17 (11.3%) 4 (2.7%) 0 (0.0%) 1 (0.7%) 1 (0.7%) 3 (2.0%)
3	Educational opportunity for the patients: Never went to school Went to usual academic school but failed to continue study Went to specialized school but failed to continue study Currently he/she is going to usual academic school Currently he/she is going to specialized academic school	34 (22.7%) 22 (14.7%) 4 (2.7%) 12 (8.0%) 78 (52.0%)	8	Family expenditure per month (in thousand taka)[a]: <15 K 15–30 K 30–50 K >50 K	19 (12.7%) 44 (29.3%) 31 (20.7%) 56 (37.3%)
4	Father's educational Level: Primary Secondary Undergraduate Graduate Postgraduate	29 (19.3%) 23 (15.3%) 23 (15.3%) 29 (19.3%) 46 (30.7%)	9	Family size: Nuclear Extended	113 (75.3%) 37 (24.7%)

(continued)

Table 2. (*continued*)

Serial	Demographics	Participant, n (%)	Serial	Demographics	Participant, n (%)
5	Mother's educational Level: Primary Secondary Undergraduate Graduate Postgraduate Student	19 (12.7%) 37 (24.7%) 25 (16.7%) 32 (21.3%) 37 (24.7%) 0.0 (0.0%)	10	Living area: Urban Semiurban Rural Slum	120 (80.0%) 15 (10.0%) 15 (10.0%) 0.0 (0.0%)

a. US $1 = 84.70 Taka (as of June 22, 2021).

For that reason, we have developed a total of 16 data sets (based on the milestone parameters) in four main categories of (i) Daily Living Skill, (ii) Communications, (iii) Motor Skills, and (iv) Socialization. For these 16 data sets, in MPredA, we have built 64 machine learning training models (four machine learning models for each data set). We have deployed our 150 test group participants to build these data set, and in total, we got in total 1875 instances (data) for the 16 data set. Table 3 shows the 16 data sets (Four types of Milestone Parameters) with the data set size, n (participants number for building each data set).

3.2 Data Set Preprocessing and Feature Selection

After creating the 16 data sets, in this step, we preprocessed the data set by the following steps:

Data Cleaning: We have observed some noisy data (filled by negative value) in our dataset, which had no impact on the machine learning models. We removed these noisy data. After that, we found some missing, especially the age and family expenditure columns. We deployed the most popular method, "the attribute mean value" [28, 29], to handle these missing values.

Feature Extraction and Binarization: This is a very critical step in building our data sets to deploy in machine learning algorithms. Initially, our data set had some non-numeric columns (13 out of 19 columns) with more than one feature in one column (for example, in father education, there had all educational level's information of the mothers in one column). In this step, we did the feature extraction and binarization process simultaneously and covert data set on 45 (according to the Table 2 demographic information) columns with an only numerical value ('0' for negative and '1' for positive value). Besides these, we also applied the MinMaxScaler [30] to convert all the features in the range of 0 to 1; this conversion is very important to increase the machine learning algorithms' performance [31, 32].

Feature Selection: After getting the extraction features (total 45) from the previous step, we deployed the "Filter Method" [33, 34] to select the most important features

Table 3. MPredA data sets with participants number for building the predictive training models.

Serial	Milestone type and parameter	Number of patient (n)	Serial	Milestone type and parameter	Number of patient (n)
Daily living skills			Motor skills		
1	Asks to use toilet	105	9	Draws circle freehand while looking at example	136
2	Brushes teeth	140	10	Glues or pastes 2 or more pieces together	130
3	Buttons large buttons in front, in correct buttonholes	109	11	Jumps with both feet off floor	104
4	Urinates in toilet or potty	112	12	Runs smoothly without falling	119
Communication			Socialization		
5	Listens to a story for at least 15 min	100	13	Answers when familiar adults make small talk (eg. If asked 'how are you_' says 'fine')	120
6	Modulates tone of voice, volume, and rhythm appropriately (eg. Does not consistently speak too loudly, too softly or in a monotone)	100	14	Keeps comfortable distance between self and others in social situations	134
7	Points to at least 5 body parts when asked	116	15	Talks with others about shared interests (eg. Sports, tv shows, cartoons)	126
8	Says month and day of birthday when asked	116	16	Use words to express emotions (eg. 'I am happy', 'I am scared')	109

(continued)

Table 3. (*continued*)

Serial	Milestone type and parameter	Number of patient (n)	Serial	Milestone type and parameter	Number of patient (n)
Total		1876			

from our extracted data sets. We have deployed four popular feature selection approaches (univariate selection [35], feature important [35], correlation matrix with heatmap [36], and information gain [37]) under the filter method. We selected the most ten important features from the 45 features of our data sets based on the results of these four feature selection approaches. Figure 2 shows the results of the most important features from univariate selection [35], feature important [35] approaches.

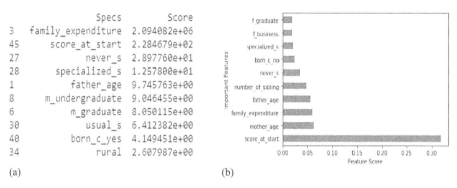

	Specs	Score
3	family_expenditure	2.094082e+06
45	score_at_start	2.284679e+02
27	never_s	2.897760e+01
28	specialized_s	1.257800e+01
1	father_age	9.745763e+00
8	m_undergraduate	9.046455e+00
6	m_graduate	8.050115e+00
30	usual_s	6.412382e+00
40	born_c_yes	4.149451e+00
34	rural	2.607987e+00

(a)   (b)

Fig. 2. Most ten important features of the data set are based on (a) Univariate selection and (b) Feature important approaches.

We combine the result from the four feature selection methods and select the following features: (i) baseline data, (ii) family expenditure, (iii) father age, (iv) mother age, (v) father occupation as a businessman, (vi) mother as a housewife, (vii) children's education in a specialized school, (viii) mother's education level (undergraduate), (ix) living in urban, and (x) number of siblings. We also have valid these selected features by analyzing our data.

Data Set Quality Assurance: According to [38], the lower R-value (co-officiant value between two columns) indicates the higher classification accuracy. We randomly selected two columns from our data set (whole data set with 1876 instants) and got R = 0.01 which very much lower value (close to zero) that indicates an excellent data set quality according to the categorical overlap evaluation method [38].

3.3   Build Machine Learning Models

For developing the web-based prediction application for predicting the milestone parameter of the children with ASD, we have deployed four supervised classification algorithms

(Decision Tree (DT) [39], Logistic Regression (LR) [40], K-Nearest Neighbor (KNN) [41], and Artificial Neural Network (ANN) [42]) to build the machine learning-based prediction models. In this step, we developed 64 machine learning models for a total of 16 milestone parameters. We validated the models by determining the models' accuracy with the train-test split method [43], where we have used 80% data for the training data set and 20% for the testing data set. Then we evaluated the models by two methods: (i) R^2 value [44] and (ii) ROC-AUC value [45]. The summary of all models' accuracy with evaluation score has been shown in Table 4.

Table 4 shows all models' accuracy with the evaluation scores. Here every row represents every milestone parameter, and we show the four separate machine learning models' results in the same row. The accuracy of each model has been shown by percentage, and the evaluation scores (by r2 scores and ROC-AUC value) are also mentioned with the accuracy.

3.4   Analyze the Models and Create Pickles

From the 64 prediction models, we have selected the best 16 models for 16 milestone parameters based on the models' accuracy and evaluation scores (Bold in Table 4). Based on the accuracy and performance of the models, we have selected the best models for each milestone parameter and created 16 pickles file [46]. These pickle files have been deployed to build the web-based Prediction System to Evaluate the Autism Level Improvement (MPredA).

3.5   Create and Test the Web Application

We have used the best 16 pickle files for developing the web application to predict the milestone parameter improvement level based on the children's (with Autism) demography. These pickles have been run on the Amazon web Service (AWS) [47] server to predict the 16 milestones parameters. The website front-end was designed and implemented by Django [48]. We have used the SQLite3 database [49] to store the data in this web application. The web application of MPredA is available on the web named as "MPredA" [22]. After developing the web application, we have tested the web application by "White Box" [50] testing. Our expert user and phycologist test the web application in this testing phase. For the 16-milestone parameters, initially, we randomly selected 80 input sets (5 for each parameter) and separated them for testing purposes. We observed our web application has 78 correct results from 80 sets of inputs in the testing phase, which is 97.5% accuracy.

4   Experimental Analysis

4.1   Experimental Setup

MPredA has been developed under the environment on Apple M1 chip with 8-core CPU, 8-core GPU, and 16-core Neural Engine with 8.0 GBytes of RAM running on Big Sur operating system. For developing the machine learning models, we have deployed four

Table 4. Summary of the accuracy with evaluation scores of all prediction models based on the demography for four milestone parameters.

	Parameter types	DT	LR	KNN	ANN
Daily living Skills Daily living Skills aily Living Skill	Asks to use toilet	86% $R^2 = 0.21$ roc_auc = 0.77	90% $R^2 = -.11$ roc_auc = 0.68	**90% $R^2 = 0.53$ roc_auc = 0.84**	84% $R^2 = -.09$ roc_auc = 0.622
	Brushes teeth	**96% $R^2 = 0.46$ roc_auc = 0.75**	96% $R^2 = -.04$ roc_auc = 0.51	96% $R^2 = -.04$ roc_auc = 0.91	93% $R^2 = 0.09$ roc_auc = 0.81
	Buttons large buttons in front, in correct buttonholes	**91% $R^2 = 0.54$ roc_auc = 0.83**	91% $R^2 = -.10$ roc_auc = 0.77	82% $R^2 = 0.27$ roc_auc = 0.83	82% $R^2 = -.53$ roc_auc = 0.9
	Urinates in toilet or potty	96% $R^2 = 0.62$ roc_auc = 0.98	**1.0% $R^2 = 1.0$ roc_auc = 1.0**	91% $R^2 = -.10$ roc_auc = 0.51	86% $R^2 = 0.03$ roc_auc = 0.60
Communication	Listens to a story for at least 15 min	**85% $R^2 = 0.39$ roc_auc = 0.86**	80% $R^2 = 0.19$ roc_auc = 0.35	76% $R^2 = 0.03$ roc_auc = 0.77	80% $R^2 = 0.13$ roc_auc = 0.74
	Modulates tone of voice, volume, and rhythm appropriately (eg. Does not consistently speak too loudly, too softly or in a monotone)	**95% $R^2 = 0.78$ roc_auc = 0.93**	80% $R^2 = 0.17$ roc_auc = 0.88	90% $R^2 = 0.58$ roc_auc = 0.90	55% $R^2 = 0.11$ roc_auc = 0.67
	Points to at least 5 body parts when asked	83% $R^2 = 0.33$ roc_auc = 0.83	79% $R^2 = 0.06$ roc_auc = 0.78	**92% $R^2 = 0.67$ roc_auc = 0.94**	63% $R^2 = 0.05$ roc_auc = 0.66
	Says month and day of birthday when asked	**92% $R^2 = 0.66$ roc_auc = 0.91**	92% $R^2 = -.09$ roc_auc = 0.73	92% $R^2 = 0.40$ roc_auc = 1.0	71% $R^2 = 0.13$ roc_auc = 0.68

(*continued*)

Table 4. (*continued*)

	Parameter types	DT	LR	KNN	ANN
Motor Skills	Draws circle freehand while looking at example	85% $R^2 = 0.38$ roc_auc = 0.8	**93% $R^2 = 0.58$ roc_auc = 0.91**	71% $R^2 = -.52$ roc_auc = 0.70	93% $R^2 = -.25$ roc_auc = 0.87
	Glues or pastes 2 or more pieces together	92% $R^2 = 0.57$ roc_auc = 0.95	**96% $R^2 = 0.46$ roc_auc = 0.98**	85% $R^2 = 0.38$ roc_auc = 0.83	81% $R^2 = 0.21$ roc_auc = 0.78
	Jumps with both feet off floor	**1.0% $R^2 = 1.0$ roc_auc = 1.0**	90% $R^2 = 0.22$ roc_auc = 0.65	91% $R^2 = 0.39$ roc_auc = 0.67	81% $R^2 = 0.10$ roc_auc = 0.81
	Runs smoothly without falling	**98% $R^2 = 0.48$ roc_auc = 0.75**	96% $R^2 = -.04$ roc_auc = 0.26	95% $R^2 = -.04$ roc_auc = 0.41	92% $R^2 = -.11$ roc_auc = 0.32
Socialization	Answers when familiar adults make small talk (eg. If asked 'how are you_' says 'fine')	**92% $R^2 = 0.62$ roc_auc = 0.94**	79% $R^2 = 0.06$ roc_auc = 0.72	75% $R^2 = -.03$ roc_auc = 0.70	67% $R^2 = 0.10$ roc_auc = 0.57
	Keeps comfortable distance between self and others in social situations	**93% $R^2 = 0.71$ roc_auc = 0.92**	81% $R^2 = -.23$ roc_auc = 0.65	81% $R^2 = 0.04$ roc_auc = 0.78	81% $R^2 = 0.04$ roc_auc = 0.63
	Talks with others about shared interests (eg. Sports, tv shows, cartoons)	88% $R^2 = 0.51$ roc_auc = 0.89	92% $R^2 = 0.64$ roc_auc = 0.86	**1.0% $R^2 = 1.0$ roc_auc = 1.0**	73% $R^2 = 0.20$ roc_auc = 0.79
	Use words to express emotions (eg. 'I am happy', 'I am scared')	91% $R^2 = 0.54$ roc_auc = 0.83	**1.0% $R^2 = 1.0$ roc_auc = 1.0**	68% $R^2 = -0.32$ roc_auc = 0.61	86% $R^2 = 0.34$ roc_auc = 0.76

supervised classifiers ((i) tree.DecisionTreeClassifier [51], (ii) LogisticRegression class [52], (iii) KneighborsClassifier [53], and (iv) keras.Sequential [54]) from the sklearn library [55] of Python [56]. We have used the 6.2.0 Jupyter Notebook [57] in 4.10.1 Anaconda Navigator [58]. For developing the web application, we have deployed Django 3.2.4 [48] framework with Amazon Web Service (AWS) [47]. The web application of MPredA is available on the web named as "MPredA" [22].

4.2 Experimental Result

For predicting the milestone parameters, the caregiver or care-practitioner has to give two types of information the MPredA web application [22]. The first type of input is the baseline data of the children (with ASD) in 16 milestone parameter fields (in four major categories). Figure 3 shows the screenshot of an anonymous children's (with ASD from mCARE dataset) baseline data for four major milestone parameter categories.

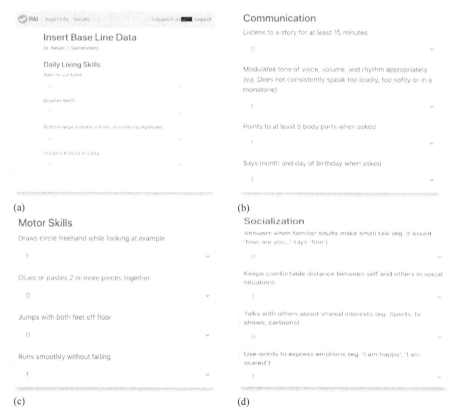

Fig. 3. A screenshot from MPredA web application to input the children's baseline data: (a) Daily living skills, (b) Communication, (c) Motor skills, and (d) Socialization.

After proving the baseline data, the caregiver or care-practitioners must input the selected (ten) demographical information into the system. Figure 4(a) shows the demographical input form of the MPredA web application. Then MPredA web application parses these data to the pickles at the AWS server and shows the children's predicted milestone improvement level data by the result page. Figure 4(b) shows the result page of MPredA web application based on the data provided by Fig. 3 and Fig. 4(a) children's data.

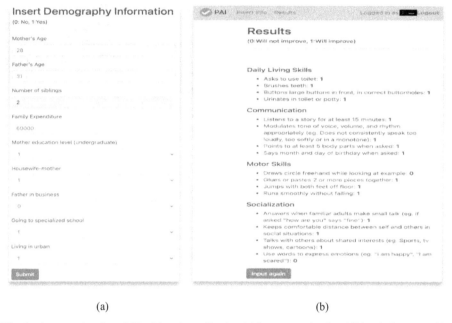

(a)   (b)

Fig. 4. A screenshot from MPredA web application (a) input page for the children's demographic information, (b) result page from MPredA web application.

4.3 Discussions

The experiment result presented in the above section shows how MPredA can predict the improvement level of milestone parameters of children with ASD. This mHealth research-based web application can be used by both the primary caregiver and also the care practitioner. They can use this application at the starting of the treatment process to know the development level (milestone parameter) based on the children's demography. And this web application can be used both in the home and in the clinical setting to determine the children's milestone parameter improvement level. However, the user of this application can determine all 16 milestone parameters' improvement level at a time by giving all baseline data (showed as previous experience result), or they can determine only one milestone parameter in one run by giving only the baseline data that they want to determine the improvement level and leaving the other baseline data blank. Since we determine the improvement level of the milestone parameters by running separate pickle files with a separate machine learning model, it will not have any impact if any user leaves blank on the baseline data or wants to determine only one milestone improvement level in one run of the application. The main advantage of this application is determining the improvement level of a children's (with ASD) milestone parameter without any clinical intervention. It can be done at the starting point of the treatment process. And parents can know their children's improvement level based on their demography as early; they can update or change their demography to develop their children's milestone parameters. In this study, we have worked on 16 milestone parameters in four major categories, which are very common in children with ASD. This data set size is another challenging issue in our work, as the real data in this area is very rare to collect. But in this study, we have tried to give more focus on the data integrity and quality to get the more accurate result to determine the milestone parameter improvement level.

5 Conclusion

In case to predict the milestone parameter improvement level, MPredA will be the first web application based on the children's (with ASD) demography. We have used four robust machine learning algorithms with real patient data to build the prediction models in this system. The model used for developing MPredA-web applications is the most accurate and competitive (selected 16 models among the 64 models). Among the four machine learning classifiers, we have observed a decision tree as an effective and accurate classifier for this kind of data. As we have an excellent accuracy of all models and the web application (97.5% accuracy with white box testing), this machine learning-based application will be a mental health development tool for children with ASD. For the web application, the caregiver can learn the importance of their demography for their children's development, and they can update or develop their demography based on their children's development; whereas the care-practitioners can know the improvement level of children before starting the treatment process and they can take the proper treatment or therapy based on the prediction result. Though this type of real data set is very rare, we have the challenge of building the machine learning models with this limited data set. It is expected that we will deploy this system with the same data set to build a recommendation system for the development of children with ASD.

Acknowledgement. This study has been partially supported by an NIH grant (1R21MH116726–01). The authors are thankful to 4 specialist autism health care centers and institutions in Bangladesh: The Institute of Pediatric Neuro-disorder & Autism (IPNA) Bangladesh, The National Institute of Mental Health (NIMH), Autism Welfare Foundation (AWF), and Nishpap Autism Foundation and their respective departments for their continuous support throughout this study.

Conflicts of Interest. None declared.

References

1. Kanner, L.: Autistic disturbances of affective contact. Acta Paedopsychiatr. **35**(4), 100–136 (1968)

2. Tariq, Q., et al.: Detecting developmental delay and autism through machine learning models using home videos of Bangladeshi children: development and validation study. J. Med. Internet Res. **21**(4), e13822 (2019)

3. Wallace, G.L., et al.: Real-world executive functions in adults with autism spectrum disorder: profiles of impairment and associations with adaptive functioning and co-morbid anxiety and depression. J. Autism Dev. Disord. **46**(3), 1071–1083 (2016)

4. W. H. Organization. Autism spectrum disorders. https://www.who.int/news-room/fact-sheets/detail/autism-spectrum-disorders. Accessed 30 June 2021

5. Sealey, L., et al.: Environmental factors in the development of autism spectrum disorders. Environ. Int. **88**, 288–298 (2016)

6. DiGuiseppi, C.G., et al.: Demographic profile of families and children in the Study to Explore Early Development (SEED): case-control study of autism spectrum disorder. Disabil. Health J. **9**(3), 544–551 (2016)

7. S. A. Autism Statistics and Facts. autism speaks. https://www.autismspeaks.org/autism-statistics-asd. Accessed 9 June 2021

8. Happé, F.G., Mansour, H., Barrett, P., Brown, T., Abbott, P., Charlton, R.A.: Demographic and cognitive profile of individuals seeking a diagnosis of autism spectrum disorder in adulthood. J. Autism Dev. Disord. **46**(11), 3469–3480 (2016)

9. Gona, J.K., et al.: Parents' and professionals' perceptions on causes and treatment options for autism spectrum disorders (ASD) in a multicultural context on the Kenyan coast. PLoS ONE **10**(8), e0132729 (2015)

10. N. A. A. MOM. "Is Autism a Gift or a Curse?. https://notanautismmom.com/2018/12/20/perspective/. Accessed 30 June 2021

11. Sommer, M., et al.: False belief reasoning in adults with and without autistic spectrum disorder: Similarities and differences. Front. Psychol. **9**, 183 (2018)

12. Zwaigenbaum, L., et al.: Early identification of autism spectrum disorder: recommendations for practice and research. Pediatrics **136**(Supplement 1), S10–S40 (2015)

13. C. f. D. Control and Prevention.Treatment and intervention services for autism spectrum disorder (2019)

14. Liu, Y., et al.: Knowledge, attitudes, and perceptions of autism spectrum disorder in a stratified sampling of preschool teachers in China. BMC Psychiatry **16**(1), 1–12 (2016)

15. Liu, K., Zerubavel, N., Bearman, P.: Social demographic change and autism. Demography **47**(2), 327–343 (2010)

16. King, M.D., Fountain, C., Dakhlallah, D., Bearman, P.S.: Estimated autism risk and older reproductive age. Am. J. Public Health **99**(9), 1673–1679 (2009)

17. Zwaigenbaum, L., Bryson, S., Garon, N.: Early identification of autism spectrum disorders. Behav. Brain Res. **251**, 133–146 (2013)

18. Barbaro, J., Halder, S.: Early identification of autism spectrum disorder: current challenges and future global directions. Curr. Dev. Disord. Rep. **3**(1), 67–74 (2016)

19. Haque, M.M., et al.: Grant report on mCARE: mobile-based care for children with Autism Spectrum Disorder (ASD) for Low-and Middle-Income Countries (LMICs). J. Psychiatry Brain Sci. **6** (2021)

20. Haque, M.M., et al.: Informing developmental milestone achievement for children with autism: machine learning approach. JMIR Med. Inf. **9**(6), e29242 (2021)

21. Maenner, M.J., Yeargin-Allsopp, M., Van Naarden Braun, K., Christensen, D.L., Schieve, L.A.: Development of a machine learning algorithm for the surveillance of autism spectrum disorder. PLoS ONE **11**(12), e0168224 (2016)

22. U. Lab. MPredA: A machine learning based prediction system to evaluate the autism level improvement. http://mpreda.ubicomp.us/. Accessed 4 July 2021

23. Haque, M.M., et al.: Towards developing a mobile-based care for children with autism spectrum disorder (mCARE) in low and middle-income countries (LMICs) like Bangladesh. In: 2020 IEEE 44th Annual Computers, Software, and Applications Conference (COMPSAC), pp. 746–753. IEEE (2020)

24. O Solution. National Institute of Mental Health (NIMH). The National Institute of Mental Health. Accessed 29 June 2021

25. IPNA: The Institute of Pediatric Neuro-disorder and Autism. http://ipnabsmmu.edu.bd/. Accessed 29 June 2021

26. Awfbd. Autism Welfare Foundation. https://awfbd.org/. Accessed 29 June 2021

27. Nishpap. Nishpap Autism Foundation. https://nishpap.org/. Accessed 29 June 2021

28. Acuña, E., Rodriguez, C.: The treatment of missing values and its effect on classifier accuracy. In: Banks, D., McMorris, F.R., Arabie, P., Gaul, W. (eds.) Classification, clustering, and data mining applications, pp. 639–647. Springer, Berlin, Heidelberg (2004). https://doi.org/10. 1007/978-3-642-17103-1_60

29. Zhu, X., Zhang, S., Jin, Z., Zhang, Z., Xu, Z.: Missing value estimation for mixed-attribute data sets. IEEE Trans. Knowl. Data Eng. 23(1), 110–121 (2010)

30. s.-l. developers. MinMaxScaler. https://scikit-learn.org/stable/modules/generated/sklearn.pre processing.MinMaxScaler.html. Accessed 29 June 2021

31. Singh, D., Singh, B.: Investigating the impact of data normalization on classification performance. Appl. Soft Comput. 97, 105524 (2020)

32. Jo, J.-M.: Effectiveness of normalization pre-processing of big data to the machine learning performance. J. Korea Inst. Electron. Commun. Sci. 14(3), 547–552 (2019)

33. Sánchez-Maroño, N., Alonso-Betanzos, A., Tombilla-Sanromán, M.: Filter methods for feature selection – a comparative study. In: Yin, H., Tino, P., Corchado, E., Byrne, W., Yao, X. (eds.) IDEAL 2007. LNCS, vol. 4881, pp. 178–187. Springer, Heidelberg (2007). https://doi. org/10.1007/978-3-540-77226-2_19

34. Shaikh, R.: Feature selection techniques in machine learning with Python. https://toward sdatascience.com/feature-selection-techniques-in-machine-learning-with-python-f24e7d a3f36e. Accessed 29 June 2021

35. Liang, R.: Feature selection using Python for classification problems. https://towardsda tascience.com/feature-selection-using-python-for-classification-problem-b5f00a1c7028. Accessed 29 June 2021

36. Gu, Z., Eils, R., Schlesner, M.: Complex heatmaps reveal patterns and correlations in multidimensional genomic data. Bioinformatics 32(18), 2847–2849 (2016)

37. Azhagusundari, B., Thanamani, A.S.: Feature selection based on information gain. Int. J. Innovative Technol. Exploring Eng. (IJITEE) 2(2), 18–21 (2013)

38. Oh, S.: A new dataset evaluation method based on category overlap. Comput. Biol. Med. 41(2), 115–122 (2011)

39. Safavian, S.R., Landgrebe, D.: A survey of decision tree classifier methodology. IEEE Trans. Syst. Man Cybern. 21(3), 660–674 (1991)

40. R.E. Wright: Logistic regression (1995)

41. Peterson, L.E.: K-nearest neighbor. Scholarpedia 4(2), 1883 (2009)

42. Wang, S.-C.: Artificial neural network. In: Interdisciplinary computing in java programming, pp. 81–100. Springer, Boston (2003). https://doi.org/10.1007/978-3-662-44725-3_5

43. Vabalas, A., Gowen, E., Poliakoff, E., Casson, A.J.: Machine learning algorithm validation with a limited sample size. PLoS ONE 14(11), e0224365 (2019)

44. Moriasi, D.N., Arnold, J.G., Van Liew, M.W., Bingner, R.L., Harmel, R.D., Veith, T.L.: Model evaluation guidelines for systematic quantification of accuracy in watershed simulations. Trans. ASABE 50(3), 885–900 (2007)

45. Peterson, A.T., Papeş, M., Eaton, M.: Transferability and model evaluation in ecological niche modeling: a comparison of GARP and Maxent. Ecography 30(4), 550–560 (2007)

46. Brownlee, J.: Save and load machine learning models in Python with scikit-learn. https://machinelearningmastery.com/save-load-machine-learning-models-python-sci kit-learn/. Accessed 29 June 2021

47. AWS. Amazon web Service. https://aws.amazon.com/. Accessed 29 June 2021

48. Django. Django makes it easier to build better web apps more quickly and with less code. https://www.djangoproject.com/. Accessed 29 June 2021

49. SQLite. What Is SQLite?. https://www.sqlite.org/index.html. Accessed 29 June 2021

50. Ostrand, T.: White-Box testing. Encycl. Softw. Eng. (2002)

51. s.-l. developers. A decision tree classifier. https://scikit-learn.org/stable/modules/generated/sklearn.tree.DecisionTreeClassifier.html. Accessed 29 June 2021

52. s.-l. developers. Logistic Regression (aka logit, MaxEnt) classifier. https://scikit-learn.org/stable/modules/generated/sklearn.linear_model.LogisticRegression.html. Accessed 29 June 2021

53. s.-l. developers. Classifier implementing the k-nearest neighbors vote. https://scikit-learn.org/stable/modules/generated/sklearn.neighbors.KNeighborsClassifier.html. Accessed 29 June 2021

54. fchollet. The Sequential model. https://keras.io/guides/sequential_model/. Accessed 29 June 2021

55. Varoquaux, G., Buitinck, L., Louppe, G., Grisel, O., Pedregosa, F., Mueller, A.: Scikit-learn: Machine learning without learning the machinery. GetMobile: Mob. Comput. Commun. **19**(1), 29–33 (2015)

56. P.S. Foundation. python. https://www.python.org/. Accessed June 2021

57. P. Jupyter, Jupyter. https://jupyter.org/. Accessed 29 June 2021

58. Anaconda, I.: Anaconda Navigator. https://docs.anaconda.com/anaconda/navigator/. Accessed 29 June 2021

Technologies and Health Behavior

Gamifyhealth: A Generic Software Framework for Health Behavioral Change

Grace Lee$^{(\boxtimes)}$ and Christine Julien

Department of Electrical and Computer Engineering, University of Texas at Austin, Austin, USA
{gracewlee,c.julien}@utexas.edu

Abstract. Many serious games integrate sensed health data to drive behavior change. However, game developers create each game individually, leading to fragmentation, where a new game is created for each new combination of health data and game story. We present GamifyHealth, a generic software framework that integrates sensors for measuring health data with games that encourage health behavior change. We start by identifying elements common to apps that gamify health across three categories: (1) the sensors that provide data; (2) gamification elements; and (3) the mapping of health data to gameplay. Based on a characterization of existing games, we create the GamifyHealth framework that supports generic and flexible development of games for health behavior change. A game can access available health data through a series of observer interfaces provided by the framework. This allows separation of code that interacts with specific sensors and code that presents the game story so that sensor developers and game developers can work independently. Because GamifyHealth provides a clear abstraction of connections from health data to gameplay, a health domain expert can focus attention on connections between sensor data and the game elements that effect behavior change. We have implemented the framework as an Android library and demonstrate its usefulness by re-implementing two existing sensor controlled digital games using GamifyHealth. Gamify-Health simplifies the code of these games and separates the logic for the game developer, the health domain expert, and the sensing integrator, making the resulting implementations more flexible and maintainable.

Keywords: Software framework · Serious games · Sensing

1 Introduction

In recent years, gamification in healthcare has been gaining momentum [19], and previous research has shown that serious games have positive effects in promoting healthy lifestyles [11]. Gamification is defined as the use of concepts that are typical of gameplay in situations that are not strictly games [4]. According to a report from IQVIA Institute for Human Data Sciences, there were over 300,000

© ICST Institute for Computer Sciences, Social Informatics and Telecommunications Engineering 2022
Published by Springer Nature Switzerland AG 2022. All Rights Reserved
H. Lewy and R. Barkan (Eds.): PH 2021, LNICST 431, pp. 435–451, 2022.
https://doi.org/10.1007/978-3-030-99194-4_27

mHealth applications available in app stores as of 2017 [1], many of which have some aspect of gamification. These gamified health apps are in almost every field of health care, ranging from apps that promote physical fitness [15], to those for medication adherence, chronic disease care, or mental health management. These apps have audiences that include people of all ages. Generically, these apps use real-time health data to influence game play. By connecting progress or points in a game to positive health behaviors as indicated by the health data, the apps aim to motivate positive health behavior change. The key components of any such app are therefore the health data sources (which are commonly sensors or self-reports from an individual), the game story and elements of game play, and the health domain knowledge that connects the data to the game.

Unfortunately, the gamified health app space is very *fragmented*, a term we use to refer to the fact that games are developed independently, and thus it is difficult to reuse code, despite the fact that apps share similar components. When the gamified app designs are completely independent, each designer determines (1) which health sensors are used to collect data; (2) which game elements and what game story are used to motivate behavior; and (3) how health data is connected to game elements. If an individual uses more than one gamified health app, the apps operate independently, from collecting data from independent sensor streams to employing motivational tools that are specific to the game design but not specific to the individual. To the best of our knowledge, there is no software framework that supports generic gamification of apps for health behavior change in a way that (1) allows sensor streams to be connected to multiple games and (2) allows different users to have entirely different game stories or game play elements for the same health behavior change purpose.

We have developed GamifyHealth, a generic software framework that enables the development of health behavior change games based on real-time sensor data at higher levels of abstractions. When using GamifyHealth, game developers and health domain experts do not have to deal with the user's health data streams directly. Health sensing experts can focus on the best ways to get real-time sensor information into a consumable format, game development experts can focus on essential aspects of game play, and health domain experts can focus on how health behavior changes can result from connecting sensor data to game elements. If multiple apps rely on the same sensed data, the same data streams can be reused. If a set of game elements that make up a game can be driven by different health data, they can be repurposed.

To enable this flexibility, Gamifyhealth provides abstractions of the common elements found in these three principle components of gamified health behavior change apps: acquiring health data from sensors, game elements that underlie serious games, and the connection between sensor data and game elements that realizes health behavior change. Our key contributions are as follows:

- To create a generic framework, we first identified common components in serious games, health data that is related to these games, and goals that the patient should achieve in order to promote health behavior change.

- We implemented the GamifyHealth framework as an Android library, which enables generic connections from real-life sensors to arbitrary game elements.
- We used the Android library implementation of the GamifyHealth framework to mock the reimplemenation of two existing sensor controlled health games.

2 Related Work

Recently, the healthcare domain has been using serious games to motivate and promote healthy behavior [23] in various domains, including heart failure [20], diabetes [14], and treatment adherence [17]. It has been shown that gamification has positive impact on self-managing health behavior [3,11].

For instance, Acticore [24] helps users learn about and train their pelvic floor muscles. A user sits on a sensor seat that connects to the app via Bluetooth. With the health data provided from the seat, Acticore displays an avatar and engages the user in games that train different aspects of the pelvic floor muscles.

FunSpeech [5] motivates children who were born deaf to practice their speech. The app takes audio as input and provides immediate feedback through mini-games that address different aspects of speech, such as pitch, intensity, and phoneme construction. In one mini-game, the user controls a helicopter with the pitch of their voice. In another, the player makes monkeys disappear by producing sounds at a specific volume for a specific duration of time.

Richard et al. [22] developed an underwater exploration game that motivates people affected by cystic fibrosis to perform airway clearance exercises. An incremental pressure sensor is attached to a Positive Expiratory Pressure device to detect the user's breathing. When the user employs correct breathing patterns as instructed, they can "swim" forward in the game, and they are also rewarded with treasures upon reaching a target "diving distance".

Heart Mountain [20] targets older patients with chronic heart diseases. Each user has an activity sensor and a smart scale to track step count and whether they weighed themselves on a daily basis. By achieving a daily step count goal and weighing in every day, the user earns coins and makes progress in the game.

Without a generic framework, each of these serious games is developed independently. This makes it difficult to personalize games to fit each user's preferences. For example, if a person with cystic fibrosis would rather control helicopters than explore underwater, a different app would have to be developed, although the code for the helicopter game and breathing sensors have already been developed by existing teams. With a generic framework, the sensor portion of the app and the game elements would be decoupled, allowing gamified health apps to be tailored towards each user without increasing workload of developers.

Multiple prior efforts have provided different lists of what are considered common elements in gamification. Garett and Young [7] provided a list of some common gamification elements in health care, such as points, leaderboards, progress status, and badges/medals. In this paper, we took the common gamification elements and grouped them based on the similarities of their structure and purpose. In other words, we abstract the commonality of the different but similar elements into components of the software framework.

There have been a few other software frameworks or middlewares aimed at supporting digital interventions using sensor data or gamification. For instance, Koutsouris et al. developed a platform that merges the user's activity in real life with a real game that they play in [16]. UNITY-Things [25] is a software framework specifically designed to link Arduino-enabled devices with the UNITY game engine, instead of supporting connections between generic devices and games.

Göbel et al. [8] designed a technical framework for exergames that also allows the integration of sensors into the game. They also provide a user interface that allows health domain experts to configure the game to fit the user's health needs. In contrast, our work focuses on a different problem; GamifyHealth is a software framework that provides generic functionalities, as well as abstract components for developers to plug in their code to create any sensor-connected game they envision.

The Ayogo Model [13] explicitly incorporates health domain experts into the game design process; similar to our software framework, in the Ayogo Model, health domain experts identify health behavior goals that are tailored towards a chronic illness. However, our contributions are focused on how to simplify the process of developing a full stack game, whereas the Ayogo Model focused on how to design and develop a game that taps into a user's ability to self manage.

3 The GamifyHealth Framework

We next describe our contributions via the GamifyHealth framework in two stages. First, we explore existing serious games for health behavior change to identify common components connecting real-time sensing, game elements, and health behavior change. Using these constructs, we then present the design of the GamifyHealth framework and its application programming interfaces (APIs).

3.1 Common Components in Games for Health Behavior Change

To identify generic components across games for health behavior change, we studied several games, including (1) health behavior change related games from the six editions of the Gamification & Serious Game Symposiums that include mobile games and sensors[1]; (2) games published in other conferences or journals; and (3) some popular games available in app stores. We first provide an overview of the 13 games we reviewed, then look at them across our three dimensions.

- Ludicross [2]: the player's forced exhalations, measured by a spirometer, drive a virtual car around a race track.
- FunSpeech [5]: the app's collection of mini-games all take sound as input; the player is asked to make or sustain sounds to achieve game goals.

---

[1] https://gsgs.ch/.

- Mission:Schweinehund [10]: in this gardening-themed game, upon achieving daily step count goal or completing in-game physical activities, the user gets materials to help tend and grow a virtual garden.
- Project SMART [12]: elementary school students move along a virtual journey by being physically active as measured by accelerometers or self-reports.
- Monster Manor [13]: children log their blood glucose to earn virtual currency that they use to purchase virtual items needed to progress through the game.
- Type 2 Travelers [13]: players log medication and glucose monitoring activities to earn virtual currency to personalize an avatar and unlock new game levels; the game also includes social interaction with other patients.
- Picture It [13]: this game integrates an activity monitor and helps promote weight loss and healthy habits in patients preparing for bariatric surgery.
- Hand washing game for nurses [18]: sensors on a sink or alcohol dispenser measure time spent near these areas to determine if users complied to hand hygiene standards. Each user's compliance is shown in a leaderboard.
- Heart Mountain [20]: users climb a virtual mountain and earn coins and awards by achieving a daily step count and weigh in; the player's avatar dynamically reflects the player's success in the game's healthy habits.
- Underwater exploration [22]: users can swim forward to explore underwater in the game and earn treasures by doing airways clearance exercises.
- Acticore [24]: an avatar cheers the user on and provides feedback for doing pelvic floor muscle exercises on a "Sensor Seat".
- Stay Fit Longer [26]: by completing a set of daily quests involving physical and cognitive activities, users can earn daily rewards.
- Stellar Spine: scoliosis braces for children are outfitted with a Bluetooth-enabled sensor; achieving a prescribed number of hours of wear time daily allows the child to collect stars and eventually construct constellations.

We organized the common components into three categories: components for sensing health data, game elements, and components that bridge the two.

Integrating Sensing of Health Data in Serious Games. A wide variety of sensors are integrated into games in order to encourage health behavior change. Depending on the purpose of a game, the health data may be collected in a variety of ways: data may be pulled directly from wearable devices or sensors in a user's home; it may be retrieved from a cloud server that belongs to another service, or the data may be input manually by the user. Table 1 lists the 13 games we reviewed and indicates their mechanism for integrating sensor information.

Identifying Game Elements for Health Behavior Change. In our review of existing games, we identified several key constructs that are commonly connected to sensed health data in games. These include some mechanism for assigning "points" in the game, displaying leaderboards that engender healthy competition, mechanisms for indicating progress towards some goal, and badges or other collectibles that indicate achievement [7]. In addition, games commonly involve some story line and potentially random challenges [9].

Table 1. Sensing integration and gamification elements in studied games

Game	Direct Sensor	Cloud Service	User Input	Goals	Progress	Points	Leaderboard	Avatar
Ludicross [2]	✔			✔				
FunSpeech [5]	✔			✔	✔			
Mission:Schweinehund [10]	✔			✔	✔	✔		
Project SMART [12]	✔	✔	✔	✔		✔		
Monster Manor [13]		✔	✔	✔	✔			
Type 2 Travelers [13]		✔	✔	✔	✔			✔
Picture It [13]		✔	✔	✔		✔		✔
Hand washing game for nurses [18]	✔					✔		
Heart Health Mountain [20]		✔		✔	✔	✔	✔	✔
Underwater exploration game [22]	✔	✔				✔		
Acticore [24]	✔			✔	✔			
Stay Fit Longer [26]		✔	✔		✔	✔		
Stellar Spine	✔			✔		✔		

Connecting Health Data to Game Elements. Serious games for health behavior change also have health goals that guide users to achieve an objective identified by a healthcare professional. For the games in our review, users commonly have to complete goals in real life in order to push the game forward, or receive awards. In other words, goals integrate live health data to game elements. Table 2 shows the goal mapping for each of the games in our review.

Many goals also have a time aspect. For instance, one FunSpeech's minigames asks the user to produce specific sounds for a given length of time [5]. The underwater exploration game instructs users to exhale continuously for a specific duration [22]. Users earn rewards by doing daily tasks in Heart Mountain [21].

3.2   The Design of the GamifyHealth Framework

A software framework provides generic functionalities that allow developers to plug in their code to create personalized programs. As such, a framework implements some concrete components but leaves others as abstract, to be reified by developers who use the framework. In GamifyHealth, we envision three categories of developers as shown in Fig. 1: (1) sensing integrators; (2) game developers; and (3) health domain experts. These three types of developers have decidedly different areas of expertise and different interests in the resulting game.

Integrating Sensing of Health Data in Serious Games. Building on the mechanisms identified above, GamifyHealth supports three modes of data inte-

Table 2. Connecting health data to game goals

Game	Example Data → Goal
Ludicross [2]	perform measured forced exhalation → make car progress around a race track
FunSpeech [5]	emit a sound at the specified time → earn fish in game
Mission:Schweinehund [10]	complete in-game workouts → earn materials in game storyline
Project SMART [12]	physical activity → progress on virtual journey
Monster Manor [13]	input blood glucose → earn coins
Type 2 travelers [13]	log medication and glucose monitoring → earn coins, unlock levels, interact with others
Picture it [13]	achieve activity and adhere to healthy goals → update avatar and earn currency
Hand washing game for nurses [18]	achieve hand hygiene compliance → move up leaderboard
Heart mountain [20]	achieve step goal and weigh in → advance game levels and earn coins
Underwater exploration game [22]	correctly complete breathing exercise → advance in game progress
Acticore [24]	complete training schedule → avatar comments on the performance
Stay fit longer [26]	complete daily quests → earn coins
Stellar spine	achieve daily brace wear-time goal → earn stars and learn about constellations

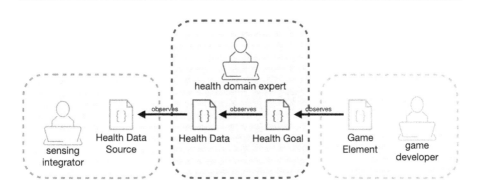

Fig. 1. Separation of concerns in GamifyHealth by developer expertise

gration: direct sensing, data collection from a server, and manual user input. All three of these mechanisms are unified under a single abstract `HealthDataSource` component in the framework, shown in Listing 1 (lines 2–12).

Listing 1. Sensing Integration Interfaces

```
1   package com.example.healthgamifylib
2   abstract class HealthDataSource(val name: String) : Subject() {
3     var value: Any = -1
4     override fun notifyObservers() { for (o in observers) { o(value) } }
5     // template method implements 2 step algorithm: update the value and notify observers
6     fun updateValue(): Unit {
7       updateHealthDataFromSource()
8       notifyObservers()
9     }
10    // this method is overridden by sensor integrator
11    abstract fun updateHealthDataFromSource() : Unit
12  }
13  abstract class Subject {
14    var observers: MutableList<(Any?) -> Unit> = mutableListOf()
15    fun registerObserver(whatToCall: (Any?) -> Unit) : Unit {
16      observers.add(whatToCall)
17    }
18    fun removeObserver(whatNotToCall: (Any?) -> Unit) : Unit {
19      observers.remove(whatNotToCall)
20    }
21    abstract fun notifyObservers() : Unit
22  }

24  import com.example.healthgamifylib.HealthDataSource
25  class MyDataSource(name: String) : HealthDataSource(name){
26    override fun updateHealthDataFromSource(){
27      // sensor-specific implementation written by sensor integrator
28    }
29  }
```

Each `HealthDataSource` exposes a `value` that stores the value of the collected data. The `HealthDataSource` component relies on the *Observer* pattern [6], where the health data source itself is an observable component, and other components in the game (the observers) can observe changes to the data value stored in the data source. To realize this in the GamifyHealth framework, the `HealthDataSource` extends the `Subject` abstract class (shown in Listing 1 in lines 13–22), which manages the registered observers. The `HealthDataSource` implements a *template method* called `updateValue` (lines 6–9 in Listing 1) which retrieves the updated health data from the data source and then notifies any registered observers. The `updateValue` method is final so that derived classes cannot override it and change the template.

The developer integrating health sensing into a game constructed with the GamifyHealth framework does not need to concern themselves at all with the observation of the value. Instead, the sensor integrator simply does the following:

- create a class derived from `HealthDataSource` for the specific sensor
- as part of fulfilling the contract of the extension, write the implementation for `updateHealthDataFromSource` (for example, as lines 24–29 in Listing 1)
- define how `updateValue` in the new `HealthDataSource` is called, whether periodically on a timer or triggered by new data available from a sensor, etc.

Game Elements for Health Behavior Change. The second type of developer is the game developer, responsible for the user's perception of the game

Listing 2. Game Developer Interfaces

```
package com.example.healthgamifylib
abstract class Points (var maxValue: Int) : Observer {
  var value: Int = 0
}
interface Observer {
    fun update(value: Any?) : Unit
}

import com.example.healthgamifylib.Points
class MyPoints(maxValue: Int) : Points(maxValue) {
  override fun update(value: Any?) {
    // game-specific implementations of what happens when points change
    // written by the game developer
  }
}
```

Listing 3. Health Domain Expert Interfaces: The Health Data Class

```
package com.example.healthgamifylib
open class HealthData(val healthDataSource: HealthDataSource) : Subject(), Observer {
  var value: Any = -1
  var timestamp: Date? = null
  open override fun update(value: Any?) {
    this.value = value as Int
    this.timestamp = LocalDateTime.now()
  }
  override fun notifyObservers() { for (o in observers) { o(value) } }
}
```

play. A significant portion of this person's effort is focused on the visual and story elements of the game; the GamifyHealth framework allows this person to not have to consider health sensing details. GamifyHealth supports a variety of game elements that can observe the health goals defined by the health domain expert in Fig. 1 (e.g., a daily step goal or a wear-time goal or a forced exhalation target). We describe the implementation of these goals in the next subsection. However, as one example of such a game element, consider the concept of **Points**. Listing 2 shows the abstract **Points** class, which is an observer of some other component (i.e., a goal). The game developer simply provides a definition of the **Observer**'s **update** method; every time the observed goal's value changes, the **update** method is called, and the associated element in the game also changes, based on the developer's definition of the method. Ultimately, this **update** method (e.g., line 11 in Listing 2) is passed as the observer to the observed goal's **registerObserver** method. This connection is made by the health domain expert, who connects health data sources to game elements. These processes are described next. In addition to these **Points**, game developers will implement progress measures, leaderboards, and the other game elements we identified previously. Their implementations mirror that of **Points**.

Connecting Health Data to Game Elements. The health domain expert is responsible for: (1) health data, which abstracts away from the specific sensors that collect data and (2) health goals, which expose hooks for gamification. A **StepCount** class might be an instance of **HealthData**, while a **FitBit**

or a `WithingsTracker` may be a `HealthDataSource` that can be observed by `StepCount`. The `HealthData` component (Listing 3) is a simple observer of a `HealthDataSource`. `HealthData` provides a simple implementation of the `update` method in the `Observer` contract. However, this class is also open for extension if a derived `HealthData` needs to convert from a lower level sensed data type into a higher level one. For instance, in Stellar Spine, the sensor captures body temperature, which is converted into a boolean indicating whether the brace is being worn or not, depending on a comparison to expected body temperature.

The `HealthData` component is also observable; in particular, it is observed by goals. To show how GamifyHealth supports defining goals, we provide examples of the `WindowGoal` and `RepeatingWindowGoal` in Listing 4. These directly respond to the fact that many goals in the games we reviewed are associated with completing a task for a duration (e.g., a sustained forced exhalations) or within a duration (e.g., achieving a daily step count).

Each `WindowGoal` (lines 2–35 in Listing 4) has a `window` to store the length of the duration and a `goalAchieved` to store whether the goal has been achieved within the window. For example, line 10 of Listing 4 checks whether the `value` of the embedded `HealthData` object has reached or exceeded the `targetValue`. This is a common pattern seen in existing games, but a health domain expert can also extend `WindowGoal` and override the `update` method to provide a different logic for evaluating reaching the goal.

Upon creation, a `WindowGoal` schedules a `StartWindow` task and an `EndWindow` task. `StartWindow` sets `goalAchieved` to `false` and registers as an observer of the `HealthData`. `EndWindow` unsubscribes from the `HealthData` and calls `finalizeGoal` (line 16), whose main purpose is to notify the `WindowGoal`'s observers when the player fails to achieve the goal (when the player achieves the goal, any registered observers are notified immediately). The developer can also optionally override the `finalizeGoal` method.

To support goals that repeat, GamifyHealth uses `RepeatingWindowGoal`. Its `repetitions` variable stores the number of `WindowGoals` to create, `streak` stores the target streak the player is aiming to achieve, and `currentStreak` stores the number of consecutive achieved goals, as calculated upon the end of each `WindowGoal` (lines 49–53). For example, if the player needs to complete a daily goal for a week, but misses the goal on the 5th day, then `repetitions` would have a value of 7, and after the 7th day ends, the `currentStreak` is 2 (days 6 and 7). To make sure that the previous `WindowGoal` closes before a new `WindowGoal` is created, `RepeatingWindowGoal` passes a `ReentrantLock` to each `WindowGoal` (lines 65 and 59). The `WindowGoal` locks the `ReentrantLock` at the beginning of `StartWindow` and unlocks at the end of `EndWindow`.

For a `Points` classes to observe a `RepeatingWindowGoal`, the game developer registers `Points`'s `update` method as an observer of `RepeatingWindowGoal`. The `RepeatingWindowGoal` registers the observers to each of the `WindowGoals` it creates (Listing 4, lines 60 and 66). The `notifyObserver` method updates its observers of the `currentStreak` when `streak` is achieved (Listing 4, line 51).

Listing 4. Health Domain Expert Interfaces: The Health Goal Classes

```
package com.example.healthgamifylib
open class WindowGoal(var targetValue: Int, var observedData: HealthData,
                      var start: Date, var window: Duration, val lock: ReentrantLock) :
                          Subject(), Observer {
  private val timer = Timer()
  var goalAchieved: Boolean = false
  // satisfying the Subject contract
  override fun notifyObservers() { for (o in observers) { o(goalAchieved) } }
  // satisfying the Observer contract; can be overridden for more tailored behavior
  open override fun update(value: Any?){
    if(!goalAchieved && value >= targetValue) {
      goalAchieved = true
      notifyObservers()
    }
  }
  // finalizeGoal can be overridden if player is not penalized for not achieving the goal
  open fun finalizeGoal() { if(!goalAchieved) { notifyObservers() } }
  private inner class StartWindow() : TimerTask() {
    override fun run() {
      lock.lock()
      goalAchieved = false
      observedData.registerObserver(this@WindowGoal::update)
    }
  }
  private inner class EndWindow() : TimerTask() {
    override fun run() {
      observedData.removeObserver(this@WindowGoal::update)
      finalizeGoal()
      lock.unlock()
    }
  }
  init {
    timer.schedule(StartWindow(), start)
    timer.schedule(EndWindow(), start + window)
  }
}
open class RepeatingWindowGoal(targetValue: Int, observedData: HealthData,
                               start: Date, window: Duration,
                               var repetitions: Int, var streak: Int = 0) : Subject() {
  var embeddedWindowGoal : WindowGoal
  val timer: Timer = Timer()
  val goalArray = mutableListOf<Boolean>()
  var repetitionsCompleted = 0
  val lock = ReentrantLock()
  var currentStreak = 0
  override fun notifyObservers() { for (o in observers) { o(streak) } }
  private inner class UpdateWindowGoal() : TimerTask() {
    override fun run() {
      goalArray.add(embeddedWindowGoal.goalAchieved)
      if(emeddedWindowGoal.goalAchieved) {
        currentStreak++
        if (currentStreak >= streak){ notifyObservers() }
      }
      else { currentStreak = 0 }
      notifyObservers()
      repetitionsCompleted++
      if(goalArray.size < repetitions) {
        newStart = start + goalArray.size * window
        embeddedWindowGoal = WindowGoal(targetValue, observedData, newStart, window, lock)
        for (o in observers) { embeddedWindowGoal.registerObserver(o) }
      }
    }
  }
  init { // this creates and starts the first repetition of the window goal
    embeddedWindowGoal = WindowGoal(targetValue, observedData, start, window, lock)
    for (o in observers) { embeddedWindowGoal.registerObserver(o) }
    timer.schedule(UpdateWindowGoal(), start + window, window)
  }
}
```

4   Case Study on the Framework

We have implemented a prototype of our framework design as an Android library[2]. We re-implemented two of the games from our review to use this framework. In these mock implementations, we do not focus on the graphical interfaces associated with game play and instead focused on implementing the pipeline shown in Fig. 1. We seek to answer the following research questions:

- How do the GamifyHealth generic constructs manifest themselves in real games for health behavior change?
- Can the GamifyHealth framework be used to integrate real-world sensing into games for health behavior change?
- Do the GamifyHealth framework representations of health goals support the needs of real games?

4.1   Case Study Game 1: Heart Mountain

Heart Mountain [21] is a sensor controlled digital game for patients with heart failure. Players are challenged to complete a daily step goal, capture their weight with a digital scale, and progress by answering quizzes about heart failure.

Integrating Sensing of Health Data in Heart Mountain. Each player has two physical sensors: an activity tracker and a smart scale, both of which are connected to the Withings server. The game downloads each player's data from the Withings server. Listing 5 shows the `WTActivityTracker` class that the Heart Mountain sensor integrator would write. Upon initialization, the sensor integrator is responsible for authenticating the user with their Withings account (e.g., by showing a login modal). Then the sensor integrator defines an update period for the data; when the timer fires, the task calls the base class's `updateValue` method, which in turn calls `updateHealthDataFromSource` to retrieve the data from the Withings API, followed by a call to notify any observers.

Game Elements for Health Behavior Change in Heart Mountain. For the game developer, the most important elements are (1) the user's points, in terms of both hearts and coins; (2) the user's avatar, whose appearance changes based on the player's collection of hearts; and (3) the player's progress up the heart mountain. Hearts and coins are straightforward extensions of the `Points` class, with simple implementations of the `update` method. The avatar is squarely in the game developer's expertise and can be updated based on updates to the hearts value. Finally, progress in the game can be inferred from an array of accomplished goals that the game developer can easily create and store. The majority of the work of the game developer for the Heart Mountain game would be focused on the user interface and graphics associated with the user experience.

---

[2] https://github.com/UT-MPC/HeartHealthMountain-Kotlin/tree/pervasiveHealth.

Listing 5. Heart Mountain: Sensing Integration

```
package com.example.heartmountain
class WTActivityTracker(name: String, val updateInterval: Int) : HealthDataSource(name) {
  inner class NewValue(): TimerTask(){
    override fun run() {
      updateValue()
    }
  }
  override updateHealthDataFromSource(){
    /** make API call to Withings server to retrive step data **/
    value = /** retrieved step data **/
    timer.schedule(NewValue(), LocalDateTime.now() + updateInterval)
  }
  init {
    /** authenticate user to Withings backend **/
    val timer = Timer()
    timer.schedule(NewValue(), LocalDateTime.now() + updateInterval)
  }
}
```

Listing 6. Heart Mountain: Connecting Sensing to the Game

```
package com.example.heartmountain
class MainApplication() : Application() {
  override fun onCreate() {
    // update interval of one day
    val updateInterval = 86400
    // create a type of Points, called Heart, with maxValue 1000
    val heart = Heart(1000);
    // create the withings scale data source
    val withingsScale = WTScale(name = "Withings Scale", updateInterval = updateInterval)
    // create a HealthData around the Withings scale data source
    val weighed = HealthData(healthDataSource = withingsScale)
    // create a repeating window goal for the daily weigh in
    val dailyWeighIn = RepeatingWindowGoal(targetValue = 1, observedData = weighed,
                                           start = startDate, window = updateInterval,
                                           repetitions = 30, streak = 25)
    // register the game construct heart as an observer of the goal
    dailyWeighIn.registerObserver(heart::update)
    /** something similar for the step goal **/
  }
}
```

Connecting Health Data to Game Elements in Heart Mountain. The health domain expert plays a pivotal role in connecting health behaviors as measured by data sources to game elements that motivate health behavior change. In Health Mountain, in particular, the health domain expert needs to define two types of HealthData: (1) daily steps and (2) daily weigh-in. They would then also define the RepeatingWindowGoals the player is expected to achieve, i.e., hitting a target number of steps and simply stepping on the scale each day.

However, the health domain expert is not expected to be an expert programmer, and the GamifyHealth framework seeks to ease their programming burden as much as possible. In many cases the health domain expert does not need to extend the framework but rather only need instantiate instances of existing HealthData and WindowGoal classes. Listing 6 shows an example of creating these connections in the Heart Mountain game.

Listing 7. Stellar Spine: Game Developer Interfaces

```
1  package com.example.stellarspine
2  import com.example.healthgamifylib.Points
3  class Stars(maxValue: Int) : Points(maxValue) {
4    // each constellation is a variable number of stars
5    val constellations = /** collection of constellations **/
6    var constellationsCollected: Int = 0
7    var stars: Int = 0
8    var starsUsed: Int = 0
9    override fun update(value: Any?) {
10     val braceWorn = value as Boolean
11     if(braceWorn) {
12       stars++
13       val starsAvailable = stars - starsUsed
14       if(starsAvailable >= constellations[constellationsCollected].stars) {
15         starsUsed += constellations[constellationsCollected].stars
16         constellationsCollected++
17       }
18     }
19   }
20 }
```

4.2 Case Study Game 2: Stellar Spine

Stellar Spine is designed to encourage children with scoliosis to wear a brace for a certain amount of time per day. Stellar Spine uses Bluetooth to read data from a temperature sensor embedded in a brace that the child wears around their chest. The temperature sensed is used to determine if the brace is worn or not, based on the value's similarity to expected body temperature. In Stellar Spine, players earn stars for every day they reach their target wear time. These stars construct constellations, and players learn facts about the stars and constellations.

Integrating Sensing of Health Data in Stellar Spine. The sensor integrator for Stellar Spine needs to create a HealthDataSource class that sets up Bluetooth bonding with the device embedded in the brace. The design of the Bluetooth connection for Stellar Spine was intentional with respect to ensuring battery longevity for the sensor in the brace; therefore the update method is triggered manually via a button on the brace combined with a simultaneously performed explicit refresh in the app. As a result, instead of updating the HealthDataSource periodically, the updateValue method needs to be triggered explicitly from the game's API. Once triggered, the base class's updateValue method can call the derived class's updateHealthDataFromSource, which can then retrieve the data from Bluetooth and format it into an array of temperature values. These correspond to the average temperature sensed in 15 min intervals since the last retrieved update. This array is stored in the HealthDataSource's value.

Game Elements for Health Behavior Change in Stellar Spine. The primary game elements for Stellar Spine are the stars, for which we created a class Stars that derives from Points. It stores the number of stars the user has earned, as well as the constellations that the stars form. Listing 7 shows

Listing 8. Stellar Spine: Health Domain Expert Interfaces

```
package com.example.stellarspine
import com.example.healthgamifylib.HealthData
class WearTime(source: HealthDataSource) : HealthData(source) {
  val bodyTemp = 37
  override fun update(value: Any?){
    // value from source is array of temperature values
    val valueAsArray = (value as? Array<*>)?.filterIsInstance<Int>()
    var sum: Int = 0
    for(i in valueAsArray) {
      if (bodyTemp - 1 < i < bodyTemp + 1) { sum = sum + 1 }
    }
    // each temperature represents a 15 minute window
    value = sum * 15
  }
}
```

the mock implementation for this class. When **update** is called, if the value propagated from the daily wear goal is **true**, the player collects a new star. Subsequently, if this new star means the player has collected enough stars for the next constellation, the data structures are updated. The game developer can use this information to update the game interface, e.g., displaying the new constellation.

Connecting Health Data to Game Elements in Stellar Spine. The Stellar Spine mock game has two details that fall in the purview of the health domain expert: (1) converting temperature values to wear time values in a **HealthData** class and (2) defining the repeating wear time goal. To solve the first, the health domain expert creates a class derived from **HealthData** called **WearTime** that observes the brace sensor's **HealthDataSource**. If the temperature sensed is close to body temperature, **WearTime**'s value is incremented. Because the brace sensor's **HealthDataSource** contains an array of temperature values, this converts to an array of times, measured in 15 min intervals. This is shown in Listing 8.

The health domain expert must also create a repeating window goal that has a target wear time equivalent to the "prescription" given to the player. If the player achieves that amount of wear time in a day, then the player achieves the goal and is awarded the daily star (as shown in Listing 7).

5   Conclusions and Future Work

We presented GamifyHealth, a generic software framework that supports flexible development of serious games for health behavior change by providing abstractions in three categories: (1) sensors that provide data that drives the game (e.g., health data); (2) elements of gameplay (e.g., points); and (3) the mapping of health data to gameplay. The separation of these three categories allows sensing integrators, game developers, and health domain experts to work independently, which also allows sensor streams to be connected to multiple games.

We implemented the framework as an Android library. To support other operating systems, a future implementation of the framework could be a multiplatform Kotlin implementation, which would allow GamifyHealth to work on all platforms that Kotlin supports, which includes iOS. We demonstrated the usability of GamifyHealth by creating mock implementations of two existing games, Heart Mountain and Stellar Spine. We are currently extending the mock implementations to develop full implementations of the two games, so that the original code and the code implementing GamifyHealth can be further compared. We are also implementing a hybrid of the two games, i.e., health data used in Heart Mountain connected to the game elements of Stellar Spine, to further explore the potential of GamifyHealth.

References

1. Aitken, M., Clancy, B., Nass, D.: The growing value of digital health: evidence and impact on human health and the healthcare system (2017)
2. Bingham, P.M., Lahiri, T., Ashikaga, T.: Pilot trial of spirometer games for airway clearance practice in cystic fibrosis. Respir. Care **57**(8), 1278–1284 (2012)
3. Charlier, N., Zupancic, N., Fieuws, S., Denhaerynck, K., Zaman, B., Moons, P.: Serious games for improving knowledge and self-management in young people with chronic conditions: a systematic review and meta-analysis. J. Am. Med. Inf. Assoc. **23**(1), 230–239 (2015). https://doi.org/10.1093/jamia/ocv100
4. Deterding, S., Dixon, D., Khaled, R., Nacke, L.: From game design elements to gamefulness: defining "gamification". In: Proceedings of the 15th International Academic MindTrek Conference: Envisioning Future Media Environments, MindTrek 2011, p. 9–15. Association for Computing Machinery, New York, NY, USA (2011). https://doi.org/10.1145/2181037.2181040
5. Florent, G., et al.: Funspeech: Promoting speech production in young children with hearing disabilities. In: International Conference on Gamification and Serious Game (2019)
6. Gamma, E., Helm, R., Johnson, R., Vlissides, J.M.: Design Patterns: Elements of Reusable Object-Oriented Software, 1st edn. Addison-Wesley Professional, Boston (1994)
7. Garett, R., Young, S.D.: Health care gamification: a study of game mechanics and elements. Technol. Knowl. Learn. **24**, 341–353 (2018)
8. Göbel, S., Hardy, S., Wendel, V., Mehm, F., Steinmetz, R.: Serious games for health: Personalized exergames. In: Proceedings of the 18th ACM International Conference on Multimedia, MM 2010, pp. 1663–1666. Association for Computing Machinery, New York, NY, USA (2010). https://doi.org/10.1145/1873951.1874316
9. Hamari, J., Koivisto, J., Sarsa, H.: Does gamification work? - a literature review of empirical studies on gamification. In: 2014 47th Hawaii International Conference on System Sciences, pp. 3025–3034 (2014). https://doi.org/10.1109/HICSS.2014.377
10. Höchsmann, C., Infanger, D., Klenk, C., Königstein, K., Walz, S.P., Schmidt-Trucksäss, A.: Effectiveness of a behavior change technique-based smartphone game to improve intrinsic motivation and physical activity adherence in patients with type 2 diabetes: Randomized controlled trial. JMIR Ser. Games **7**(1), e11444 (2019)

11. Johnson, D., Deterding, S., Kuhn, K.A., Staneva, A., Stoyanov, S., Hides, L.: Gamification for health and wellbeing: a systematic review of the literature. Internet Interv. **6**, 89–106 (2016)
12. Julien, C., Castelli, D., Bray, D., Lee, S., Burson, S., Jung, Y.: Project smart: a cooperative educational game to increase physical activity in elementary schools. Smart Health **19**, 100163 (2021)
13. Kamel Boulos, M.N., et al.: Digital games for type 1 and type 2 diabetes: underpinning theory with three illustrative examples. JMIR Ser. Games **3**(1), e3390 (2015)
14. Klingensmith, G.J., et al.: Evaluation of a combined blood glucose monitoring and gaming system (Didget®) for motivation in children, adolescents, and young adults with type 1 diabetes. Pediatr. Diabetes **14**(5), 350–357 (2013)
15. Knight, E., Stuckey, M.I., Prapavessis, H., Petrella, R.J.: Public health guidelines for physical activity: is there an app for that? A review of android and apple app stores. JMIR mHealth uHealth **3**(2), e4003 (2015)
16. Koutsouris, N., Kosmides, P., Demestichas, K., Adamopoulou, E., Giannakopoulou, K., De Luca, V.: Inlife: a platform enabling the exploitation of IoT and gamification in healthcare. In: 2018 14th International Conference on Wireless and Mobile Computing, Networking and Communications (WiMob), pp. 224–230 (2018). https://doi.org/10.1109/WiMOB.2018.8589153
17. Whiteley, L., Brown, L., Lally, M., Heck, N., van den Berg J: A mobile gaming intervention to increase adherence to antiretroviral treatment for youth living with HIV: development guided by the information, motivation, and behavioral skills model. JMIR Mhealth Uhealth. **6**, e8155 (2018). https://doi.org/10.2196/mhealth. 8155,https://mhealth.jmir.org/2018/4/e96
18. Lapão, L., Marques, R., Gregorio, J., Pinheiro, F., Povoa, P., Mira da Silva, M.: Using gamification combined with indoor location to improve nurses' hand hygiene compliance in an ICU ward. Stud. Halth Technol. Inform. **221**, 3–7 (2016). https://doi.org/10.3233/978-1-61499-633-0-3
19. Lister, C., West, J.H., Cannon, B., Sax, T., Brodegard, D.: Just a fad? Gamification in health and fitness apps. JMIR Ser. Games **2**(2), e3413 (2014)
20. Radhakrishnan, K., et al.: Abstract 13122: sensor-controlled digital game may improve weight monitoring among older adults with heart failure. circulation **142**(Suppl.3), A13122–A13122 (2020). https://doi.org/10.1161/circ.142.suppl.3. 13122
21. Radhakrishnan, K., et al.: Usability assessment of a sensor-controlled digital game for older adults with heart failure. Innov. Aging. **3**, S8192 (2019)
22. Richard, W., Tobias, K.: Prototyping a virtual reality diving game to support breathing exercises to treat cystic fibrosis. In: International Conference on Gamification and Serious Game (2019)
23. Sardi, L., Idri, A., Fernández-Alemán, J.L.: A systematic review of gamification in e-health. J. Biomed. Inform. **71**, 31–48 (2017)
24. Sebastian, I.: Ani: how to turn a muscle into a motivating character. In: International Conference on Gamification and Serious Game (2019)
25. Svanæs, D., Scharvet Lyngby, A., Bärnhold, M., Røsand, T., Subramanian, S.: Unity-things: an internet-of-things software framework integrating Arduino-enabled remote devices with the unity game engine. In: Fang, X. (ed.) HCI in Games: Experience Design and Game Mechanics, pp. 378–388. Springer International Publishing, Cham (2021)
26. Sylvain, C., et al.: Gamification to improve adherence in home-based activities for seniors. In: International Conference on Gamification and Serious Game (2019)

The Design of an Ontology-Driven mHealth Behaviour Change Ecosystem to Increase Physical Activity in Adults

Stéphanie Carlier[1]([✉]) [iD], Maya Braun[2] [iD], Annick De Paepe[2] [iD],
Geert Crombez[2] [iD], Femke De Backere[1] [iD], and Filip De Turck[1] [iD]

[1] IDLab, Department of Information Technology, Ghent University - imec,
Technologiepark Zwijnaarde 126, 9052 Ghent, Belgium
stephanie.carlier@ugent.be
[2] Department of Experimental Clinical and Health Psychology,
Faculty of Psychology and Educational Sciences,
Henri Dunantlaan 2, 9000 Ghent, Belgium

Abstract. The global pandemic and the resulting lock-downs have indicated the importance of regular physical activity for both mental and physical wellness. Many mHealth applications to increase physical activity exist, they however continue to fail to achieve their objective. The need arises for a more theoretically-grounded approach that considers the dynamic nature of the individual. To create a system that is context-aware and personalised, an interdisciplinary approach is needed and regular input of stakeholders and end-users is of the essence. This expert knowledge is captured into an ontology, centred on the Health Action Process (HAPA) model for behaviour change. This paper describes the requirements for the design of such a mobile health Behaviour Change System for increased physical activity in adults and emphasises the need for personalisation on the level of the user, action and coping planning and motivational level.

Keywords: Knowledge representation · Ontology · Health care · User-centric · Personalisation · Decision support system · Human-computer interaction · Health behaviour change

1 Introduction

The past two years, as we stayed more at home than ever, habits and hobbies had to be replaced and reinvented. Due to the global pandemic and lock-downs, physical activity was reduced to a minimum, as shops and sport centres were closed and working from home became the norm. Nonetheless, physical activity remained important for both mental and physical health [5,8,10]. Non-communicable diseases (NCDs) such as cardiovascular diseases, cancer, chronic respiratory disease, and type-2 diabetes, are worldwide responsible for 41 million

H. Lewy and R. Barkan (Eds.): PH 2021, LNICST 431, pp. 452–468, 2022.
https://doi.org/10.1007/978-3-030-99194-4_28

deaths each year, equivalent to 71% of total deaths [32]. Harmful habits such as physical inactivity, alcohol abuse, and unhealthy diets all increase the risk of dying from a NCD. Now more than ever it is important to form healthy active habits to reduce the risk factors of unhealthy habits. Interventions that aim to reduce these risks can decrease premature deaths by one-half to two-thirds [33].

Mobile health Behavioural Change (hBC) interventions, e.g., to quit smoking or to increase physical activity, have the potential to modify these risks as they have the potential for high reach [33]. As the number of available mHealth applications keeps rising, these applications have yet to reach their full potential to become essential tools for change in the healthcare sector [23]. Mobile health Behaviour Change Support Systems (hBCSS), which have hBC as their objective, often show to be effective, however, comprehensive evaluation of their long-term effectiveness is often lacking and sustained engagement levels outside studies are low [33]. hBCSSs have been successful for e.g., stress, anxiety and promotion of healthier lifestyles [1], but the evidence base for mHealth apps is still in its infancy [23]. Even though these apps can spark interest at first, few manage to retain the attention and are often abandoned after a few uses [27]. Most downloaded mHealth apps are often not even opened, with around 26% that are never used a second time and continued use remains extremely rare [19,23]. Additionally, recent studies show that wearables, e.g., pedometers, are only worn for a limited amount of time: around 32% stop wearing them after 6 months, while 50% stops after 1 year [24]. Another obstacle is that most health apps are disease specific and do not take the needs of diverse stakeholders into account, which could lead to early abandonment if this diversity is not properly addressed [23].

To create an effective mobile hBCSS, it is necessary to go beyond researching the average person in the average context and to take into account some of the basic tenets of human behaviour: individuals are dynamic beings who attune their behaviour as a function of varying contexts. Moreover, because theory-based interventions are more effective than others, it is also recommended to model the knowledge that resides in the theoretical frameworks to drive behaviour change.

This paper presents the requirements for the design of an ontology-driven intelligent Decision Support System for the personalised and context-aware promotion of physical activity in adults. The remainder of this paper will first discuss relevant background information in Sect. 2. Next, in Sect. 3, the interdisciplinary approach to build the ontology and designing the Decision Support System is explained, while underlining the importance of different sources of expert knowledge. Section 4 lists the findings that followed from the several workshops with stakeholders that were organised to date. Following from these findings, requirements for the system and interaction with the end-users were defined, which are detailed in Sect. 4.

2   Background

In order to create an Intelligent Decision Support System to increase physical activity, insight is needed into what theoretical frameworks can be used as the

backbone of the system. The following subsections will first elaborate on the
added value of ontologies, followed by the chosen model for behaviour change
and indication of the significance of previous research.

2.1   Ontologies

Knowledge can be modelled in various ways [2]. In recent years, behavioural
scientist have began to use computerized knowledge-based systems to represent
domain-knowledge more formally and to use this knowledge to solve complex
problems [15]. A key component in a knowledge-based system is an ontology,
which describes concepts in a certain domain, together with their relationships
and attributes. This structuring of knowledge facilitates the communication,
collaboration and integration of complex problems in a multidisciplinary manner.
Furthermore, by combining an ontology with intelligent algorithms, it is possible
to reason over the information available in that knowledge domain to gain new
knowledge and insights.

2.2   The HAPA Model

Increasing levels of physical activity (PA) is much harder than initially
expected [11]. As many mHealth applications remain unsuccessful in creating
sustainable behaviour change [14,18], the need arises for more theory-based interventions, both to better understand the processes of behaviour change and to
improve the efficacy of the interventions [3,17].

   One of the most comprehensive models for behaviour change is the "Health
Action Process Approach" (HAPA) model, shown in Fig. 1 [28]. The model
describes behaviour change in two layers. On a first stage layer, it distinguishes
people based on their intentions and behaviour concerning a specific health
behaviour goal: (1) pre-intenders have not yet formed an intention, (2) intenders
have formed an intention without acting on it, and (3) actors have formed an
intention and translated that intention into action.

   The processes that are relevant for each stage and particularly for stage
transitions are described in the continuum layer of the model. The HAPA model
describes (1) motivational, e.g. risk perception, outcome expectancies, and (2)
self-regulatory factors, e.g. action planning, and their role in the process of
behaviour change. The two layers of the HAPA make it suitable for both basic
research and intervention development [28]. It is also well-grounded in fundamental and experimental research and meets criteria that have been identified
as relevant for good theory [6], and a theory diagram has been created for it [12].

   Perhaps most importantly, HAPA encompasses the entire cycle of goal-
directed action. It includes motivational processes, leading to a behavioural
intention, and volitional, self-regulation processes, which bridge the gap between
intention and actual behaviour. Research showed that self-regulation strategies,
in which participants select their own goals and how to reach them, i.e. action
planning, explore solutions for possible obstacles, i.e. coping planning, and keep

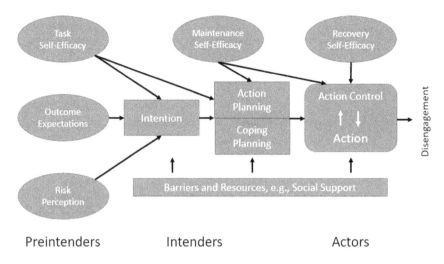

Fig. 1. The Health Action Process Approach (HAPA) model.

track of their change, i.e. action control or self-monitoring, are effective in bridging the intention-behaviour gap [29].

2.3 MyPlan: Action and Coping Planning

As part of previous research, the eHealth interventions, 'MyPlan 2.0' [9] and 'MyDayPlan' [7] support individuals in setting goals and developing and implementing plans for healthy lifestyles. MyPlan 2.0 [9] focuses on creating weekly action plans, while participants using MyDayPlan [7] were asked to create daily action plans. These interventions are based on the HAPA model and investigated the efficacy and processes underlying the promotion of PA in various settings [9,25,31] and various populations [9,16,26,31]. In these interventions, individuals are their own expert: free to set their own goals and formulate their own action and coping plans while being guided by a series of questions and clarifying examples. This approach has proven to be effective but has several disadvantages [7]. The use and quality of the defined plans vary, as users are free to formulate them as they see fit. A plan is considered to be of high quality when it is instrumental to the formulated goal and highly specific [21]. Lower quality of action or coping plans is predictive of less goal attainment [25]. Related, some participants report experiencing difficulties in formulating plans [7]. This indicates the need for more contextualised and personalised support in this planning process.

3 Methodology: An Interdisciplinary Approach

This research is part of an interdisciplinary project at Ghent University, Belgium, involving researchers from the field of Computer Science, Health and Behavioural

Sciences and Movement and Sport Sciences. To capture the knowledge in the ontology that drives the context-aware and personalised decision support system, knowledge from these different domains needs to be combined and modelled. Intelligent self-learning algorithms from the field of Computer Science need to be fed expert knowledge from the Health and Behavioural Sciences field.

Figure 2 gives an overview of the process to design the Health Behaviour Change System for increasing physical activity. The ontology and the Decision Support System are designed using an iterative approach. The system will be periodically validated by stakeholders to solve potential gaps and make sure the system is tailored to the needs of the end-users.

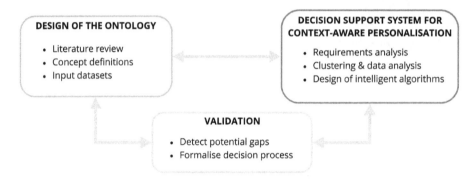

Fig. 2. The Health Behaviour Change Support System is designed using an iterative interdisciplinary approach, exploiting regular validation possibilities to fix potential gaps in the system. Different sources of expert knowledge are consulted during the design of the ontology and the Decision Support System.

The following paragraphs elaborate on the interdisciplinary approach by discussing the different sources of expert knowledge that are consulted during the project.

3.1   Data Analysis

This research aims to use an iterative approach, where close interaction with domain experts and end-users is essential. Information and data collected from previous studies, end-users and stakeholders form a valuable source of information to learn what needs improvement, but also to identify already existing habits or patterns. These existing data sets are thus used for data analysis for both the ontology and the Decision Support System. Moreover, new data collection and data analysis will continue to take place as needed throughout the project.

First, for the design of the ontology, information extracted from the data sets collected from previous studies, such as MyPlan [9] and MyDayPlan [7], has been used to gain insight into action and coping planning. The drafted plans illustrate the types of physical activity people often choose to do, the goals they set, the obstacles they face, and their respective solutions. The data from these studies was used to create a list of necessary concepts and information that needs to be captured in the ontology. Second, a literature review will be conducted to identify and analyse relevant existing ontologies and how they can be integrated in our ontology.

Third, for the design of the Decision Support System, more studies using the questionnaires from MyDayPlan and MyPlan will be conducted. This data contains extensive information of the user, such as a demographic questionnaire and the International Physical Activity Questionnaire- Long Form (IPAQ-LF), which has shown to be a reliable measurement tool for measuring habitual physical activity [4,7,9,13]. New data, together with previously collected data can be fed to clustering algorithms to identify hidden relationships between concepts or profiles of users. This allows users to receive personalised support from the start.

3.2   Panel of Experts

To capture the necessary knowledge from all the involved research domains, a panel of experts from these domains has been composed. The role of the panel of experts has been to help shape the vision of this system from concept to actual requirements, which are translated into an architecture for the system and form the foundation of the ontology.

First, for the design of the ontology, assignments and workshops have been held to help identify the necessary concepts and topics that need to be captured in the ontology. These topics range from general concepts, such as time, to domain-specific information, such as the medical background of the user. For example, if you want to provide personalised suggestion for an individual with chronic back pain, information regarding physical activity for patients with low back pain needs to be captured within the ontology. To create the ontology, the co-design method by F.Ongenae et al. [20] is applied. Via role-playing and decision-tree workshops ontology concepts and rules or axioms are defined.

Second, for the Decision Support System, intelligent algorithms that are able to make personalised suggestions to the user are embedded into the system. But before these can be created, the requirements of the system need to be defined. To do so, the required functionality of the system was defined during multiple Requirement Analysis workshops with the panel of experts. During these workshops the experts were asked to define how the user can interact with the application and why. This was done by defining user stories in the form of *As a user I want to be able to ... as to ...* These workshops resulted into use cases that define the interaction of the user with the system. A concrete example of some of these use cases was illustrated in the scenario in Sect. 5.1.

3.3   Focus Groups

Finally, for the validation of both the ontology and the Decision Support System, different focus groups, consisting of end-users and other stakeholders, will be composed. Workshops and interviews with the focus groups are essential to evaluate the completeness of the ontology or system. Moreover, as the ontology takes shape and the functional requirements are defined, workshops with focus groups are held to formalise the decision processes that drive the personalised and context-aware Decision Support System.

4   Findings

This section gives an overview of our findings to date. These findings are the result from (1) the data analysis that has been conducted on the collected data sets from the MyPlan [9] and MyDayPlan [7] studies and (2) the workshops that were held so far with the panel of experts on the concepts of the ontology and the requirements analysis of the Decision Support System. First, the conclusions that can be made regarding the ontology are presented. Next, an overview of important decisions made during the requirement analysis is given. Finally, several opportunities for personalisation are discussed.

4.1   Building the Ontology

The studies regarding MyPlan [9] and MyDayPlan [7] have shown that to form action or coping plans with enough instrumentality and specificity, more support is needed in the form of personalised suggestions regarding the user's current context. Daily, users were prompted to fill in a questionnaire, which guided them through the process of creating action and coping plans. However, they did not receive any guidance or support as to what the content of those plans could or should be. No suggestions were made and all questions were free-text format, which often resulted in action and coping plans that remained too vague or were irrelevant. The objective of the system is to counteract this by making suggestions for their plans that make sense for that specific user on that specific moment. However, providing these personalised suggestions is not an easy feat, as the meaningfulness can change in function of time, context or person.

Formalisation of the HAPA model as a generic model exists and an ontology has been built, which is used as the starting point for the ontology [12]. As the concepts defined in the HAPA model, such as action and coping planning, remain vague and limited, the ontology will need to be extended to take into account the profile and context of the user to make meaningful suggestions. For example, Fig. 3 shows a part of the HAPA ontology extended with an example of some domain-specific concepts and concrete instances on the lowest level of the ontology. These HAPA concepts, such as *action* and *coping planning* remain vague and need to be defined further to be used for personalised support. The example shows a possible action plan of a person, Ada, to go biking and indicates possible barriers for this plan could be rain or fatigue. To define these domian-specific concepts and instances, existing ontologies such as ACCIO [20], modelling basic to psychological, sociological to biological profile information

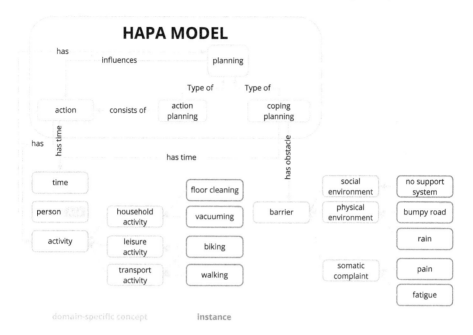

Fig. 3. An example of the HAPA model ontology (partial) extended with domain-specific concepts and instances necessary to formulate a possible action plan for the specific person, Ada. A relevant action plan to suggest to Ada is a leisurely bike ride. Possible barriers for her not to go on a bike ride, are fatigue and rain. The yellow arrows indicate the concepts and relationships necessary to suggest this plan.

or the PACO ontology [22], modelling physical activity are researched to be integrated into our ontology.

Furthermore, the panel of experts was responsible to identify these topics that needs to be modelled in the ontology. Together with the results of the data analysis, this information is used to extend the ontology to create an ontology that can provide this level of personalised support, is future-proof, and in the long run, can support all types of end-users.

4.2 Requirements Analysis

During the Requirement Analysis workshops, the panel of experts defined how the user can interact with the system by defining user stories. These workshops uncovered several important design decisions that impact the ontology and Decision Support System.

First, not all physical activities are deemed equal when it comes to planning. Certain activities require to be planned more in advance than others, based on the necessary preparation time, transport, duration or other factors. For example, an activity such as swimming requires that you have your swimming gear on you and it takes time to get to the pool. Moreover, people might prefer to plan activities in advance if they take a significant amount of time out of your schedule. For example, a mother of two young children might need to schedule time to exercise in advance, so other tasks can be planned around it. Therefore the need arises for a distinction between a weekly plan and daily plans. At the start of each week, the user is prompted to create their action plans for the week and each morning, the user is reminded of what they planned for the day and receive the suggestion to make additional action plans for that day. The weekly plan forms the backbone of the system, whereas the usage of daily action plans keeps the user "on track" to reach their weekly goal.

Second, although the aim is to create a personalised and context-aware system, the user still makes the final decision. Multiple suggestions for action and coping plans are offered to the user based on their current context and history, but in the end the user decides which of the suggestions they want to focus on. Similarly, for the weekly plan, suggestions are made regarding timing and types of action plans, but the user has the autonomy to decide when and what activities to add to their schedule.

Finally, people are unique and context changes over time. Whereas the action and coping planning can support the user as they start the process of behaviour change as an intender, this might not be the case when a habit starts to form. Therefore, there is a need to include other techniques to motivate the user throughout the entire process, such as gamification. As people are unique, multiple opportunities arise to extend the personalisation to different levels of the system, which will be explained in the next subsection.

4.3   Levels of Personalisation

Multiple levels of personalisation are needed: First, the system needs to keep track of the progress or regress of behaviour change within the entire cycle of goal-directed action. Any techniques or support delivered to the user should be tailored to the phase to which the individual belongs, i.e., pre-intender, intender, or actor. Often, this type of personalisation occurs only once, namely at the beginning of the intervention, i.e. static tailoring. As the individual will change their behaviour during the intervention, i.e. increase or decrease their physical activity, the system should be able to dynamically adapt to the shifting phases of the individual.

In such a complex intelligent Decision Support System, many opportunities for personalisation arise. To exploit these opportunities, several levels of personalisation are provided, as shown in Fig. 4. To validate their impact on the system and the user's behaviour change process, multiple user studies will be conducted, to incrementally test the influence of a more personalised support system.

First, on the level of the user, the distinction is made between person-similar and person-specific personalisation. For the former, users receive personalised support based on information extracted from users with a similar profile. The latter is implemented on the level of the individual by using reinforcement learning which is capable of making suggestions based on the individual's previous

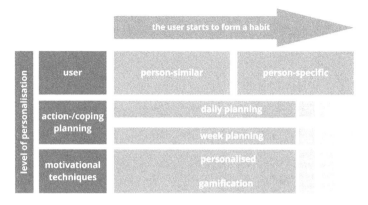

Fig. 4. The system should adapt to the user as they evolve or relapse throughout the process. To do so, personalisation is offered on (1) the level of the user, offering person-similar and person-specific personalisation, (2) the level of the action and coping planning by introducing a fade-out of support and (3) the level of motivational techniques in the form of personalised gamification.

actions. At the start of the process, when the user starts using the system, person-similar personalisation allows the user to receive personalised support from the start. As they progress and the system learns who the user is, more person-specific personalisation will be applied.

Next, personalisation is provided on the level of action and coping planning. Users will be supported during the drafting of these plans providing personalised suggestions for these plans based on their current context. An example is explained in Sect. 5.1 Scenario. Moreover, the use of action and coping plans should fade out as the user progresses or be reinstated if the user relapses.

Finally, applied motivational techniques, such as gamification should be personalised as the system detects if the user is in a slump and requires extra motivational support. The Hexad Player Type [30] model defines the player type of the user and what gamification elements they might respond to. Nevertheless, the used gamification should be dynamic and allow the user to change player types throughout the process and therefore offer different game elements or fade-out when support becomes less essential.

5   System Design

Based on the findings from the workshops with the panel of experts and the data analysis of previously collected data sets, requirements of the system were defined. First, the ontology that will be build needs to contain enough detail to provide meaningful suggestions to specific users. Next, the distinction between weekly and daily plans is made, giving the user autonomy over the final decision to include specific action or coping plans. Finally, multiple levels of personalisation will be realised to offer continued support to the user throughout the entire behaviour change cycle.

The following paragraphs will first discuss an example scenario that shows how this support will be offered. To conclude, a high level overview of the system's most important building blocks will be given.

5.1   Example Scenario

The following paragraphs describe a scenario to illustrate how the future system can support the user by providing personalised suggestions for action and coping plans. The scenario indicates how personalised support is provided weekly as well as daily, based on the user's current context information, such as calendar or weather and many more.

Profile. Margaux is a 28-year-old female living in the centre of Ghent with her boyfriend. She has a sedentary office job, which requires her to unexpectedly work late on some days. During the weekends she likes to visit museums or exhibitions but has otherwise mostly sedentary hobbies, such as reading and board games. She is generally in good health. To stay active, she cycles to work, but as this is only a short trip, she likes to increase her daily physical activity.

She has been using the Intelligent Decision Support System for a few weeks to help her formulate action and coping plans to increase her physical activity. Her current goal is to achieve around 60 min of physical activity a day.

Scenario. On Sundays, she uses the system to help her make a plan for the coming week, using that week's agenda as a starting point. The system learned from her behaviour during the previous weeks that Tuesday afternoons, Saturday, and Sunday mornings are moments she often succeeds in pursuing her plans. Based on this knowledge and her preferences, the system suggests to go swimming twice this week and to take a few walks. Margaux agrees with this suggestion, as shown in Fig. 5, without adding extra activities.

On Monday morning, Margaux receives a notification with her scheduled activities for the day, as shown in Fig. 6. Planned for today is a short lunch walk. The system asks her if there are possible obstacles that might stop her from going on a walk. As the weather forecast said to expect rain and Margaux has been indicating that she failed to exercise due to too little time, the system suggests these as possible hindrances. Margaux thinks the rain might be her biggest obstacle today, to which the system suggests to take an umbrella with her to work or to schedule another indoor activity for today. Margaux feels brave today, so she takes an umbrella to work. Luckily, the brisk walk in the rain under her umbrella cleared her head during an otherwise stressful day at work.

By Thursday, her week has been so hectic she had to cancel swimming and failed to do any exercise apart from her short lunch walk on Monday. As usual, in the morning, she receives a notification with her plans for the day, as shown in Fig. 7. The system knows she has not been reaching her set goals and apart from the already planned lunch walk, suggests some more action plans for that day. Margaux decides to try and be more active throughout the day by taking

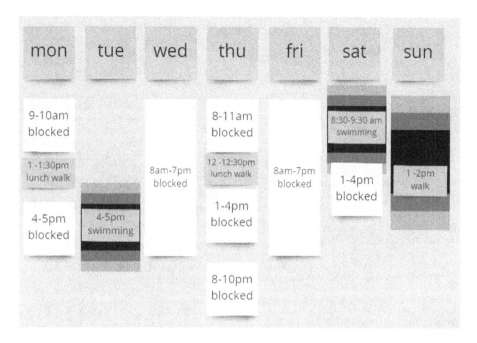

Fig. 5. Based on Margaux's calendar of the coming week (white) and information on her behaviour previous weeks, the system knows what moments are ideal for exercising (green). The system uses this information to make several suggestions for physical activities in this week (pink). (Color figure online)

the stairs when possible. To shake off the stressful week, she decides to do yoga in the evening. She adds coping plans for the selected action plans and starts her day.

5.2 Overview

The effectiveness or relevance of different instantiations of action or coping plans may vary widely as a function of the person, context and time. In other words: what works for one person might not work for another. The constructs in theoretical models, such as the HAPA model remain generic and abstract and thus require specific operationalisation or instances that work for the individual. For example, the instance of an action plan "During lunch, I will take a walk outside" should be accompanied by an instantiation of a coping plan that makes sense for this specific action plan, such as "if it rains, I will use an umbrella". The intelligent decision support system will support the user in this process by providing personalised suggestions based on the individual's current context and history.

The system shall consist of 3 major components, as shown on Fig. 8: a mobile application that supports the user in formulating their own action and coping plans. Next, an ontology that captures relevant concepts and their relationships.

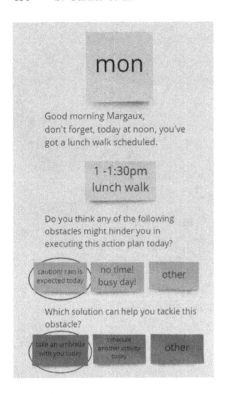

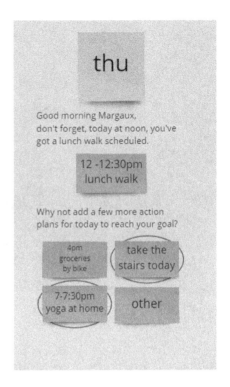

Fig. 6. Margaux receives a notification with today's plans (pink). The system suggests possible obstacles that could hinder her in completing those plans (green) based on her current context. Next, the system suggests possible solutions for the chosen obstacle (orange). (Color figure online)

Fig. 7. By Thursday, Margaux has failed to keep up with the activity goal, so the system suggests some more action plans (pink) that can help her be more active throughout the day. (Color figure online)

The ontology, centred on the HAPA model, forms the backbone of the system, supporting the user in formulating personalised and context-aware action and coping plans. The final component, the Decision Support System, forms the connection between the ontology and the application. It has the responsibility, based on the user's profile information and current context information, to decide which information, extracted from the ontology, is best used at that moment to provide personalised suggestion to the user for finalising their action or coping plan.

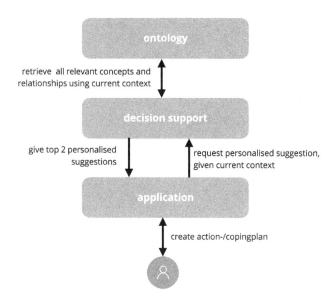

Fig. 8. The system consists of 3 major components: an ontology, modelling the expert knowledge, the decision support module that decides which information from the ontology is currently relevant and finally, an application that interacts with the end user by gathering context data and offering personalised suggestions to the user while making action or coping plans.

6 Conclusions

Mobile health Behaviour Change Support Systems show the potential to alter unhealthy habits that increase the risk of non-communicable diseases. However, they lack long-term effectiveness and sustained user engagement as these intervention fail to consider the dynamic nature of their target audience.

We propose an ontology-driven Intelligent Decision Support system, that uses the theoretical HAPA framework as backbone to increase physical activity and form a healthy sustainable habit. To design the system, an interdisciplinary approach is taken, combining knowledge from the field of Computer Science and Health and Behavioural Sciences.

From the workshops and data analysis of previously collected data sets, several requirements for such a system were defined. For the ontology, we learned that there is a need to model information on the level of the individual, i.e. the instances, to be able to formulate action and coping plans tailored to specific individuals. These plans should be offered to the user as suggestions, giving the user freedom in the final decision. To create sustainable behaviour change, the distinction is made between a weekly plan, to encourage the user to be physically active regularly and a daily plan, to keep the user on schedule to reach their weekly goal. Finally, to sustain the motivation of the user, there is a need for personalisation on multiple levels of the system. On the level of the user, person-similar personalisation is supported by person-specific personalisation as the user progresses, taking into account groups of similar users as well as the personal growth of the individual. Throughout this progress, action and coping planning should be tailored to the user's current context, fading out support as the user starts to form a healthy habit. Finally, motivational techniques such as gamification should be personalised to the user to detect possible slumps or should fade when support is not needed.

Acknowledgements. This research is funded by an interdisciplinary research grand of the Special Research Fund of Ghent University, Belgium (BOF-IOP, BOF.24Y.2020.0012.02).

References

1. Alahäivälä, T., Oinas-Kukkonen, H.: Understanding persuasion contexts in health gamification: a systematic analysis of gamified health behavior change support systems literature. Int. J. Med. Inform. **96**, 62–70 (2016). https://doi.org/10.1016/j.ijmedinf.2016.02.006
2. Bimba, A.T., et al.: Towards knowledge modeling and manipulation technologies: a survey. Int. J. Inf. Manag. **36**(6), 857–871 (2016). https://doi.org/10.1016/j.ijinfomgt.2016.05.022
3. Brosschot, J.F., Van Dijk, E., Thayer, J.F.: Daily episodes of worrying and stressors increase daytime- and nighttime cardiac activity. Psychol. Health **19**(SUPPL. 1), 29 (2004). https://doi.org/10.1080/0887044031000141199, https://www.tandfonline.com/doi/abs/10.1080/0887044031000141199
4. Craig, C.L., et al.: International physical activity questionnaire: 12-country reliability and validity. Med. Sci. Sports Exerc. **35**(8), 1381–1395 (2003). https://doi.org/10.1249/01.MSS.0000078924.61453.FB, https://pubmed.ncbi.nlm.nih.gov/12900694/
5. Creese, B., et al.: Loneliness, physical activity, and mental health during COVID-19: a longitudinal analysis of depression and anxiety in adults over the age of 50 between 2015 and 2020. Int. Psychogeriatr. **33**(5), 505–514 (2021). https://doi.org/10.1017/S1041610220004135, https://pubmed.ncbi.nlm.nih.gov/33327988/
6. Davis, R., Campbell, R., Hildon, Z., Hobbs, L., Michie, S.: Theories of behaviour and behaviour change across the social and behavioural sciences: a scoping review. Health Psychol. Rev. **9**(3), 323–344 (2015). https://doi.org/10.1080/17437199.2014.941722, https://pubmed.ncbi.nlm.nih.gov/25104107/
7. Degroote, L., Van Dyck, D., De Bourdeaudhuij, I., De Paepe, A., Crombez, G.: Acceptability and feasibility of the mHealth intervention 'MyDayPlan' to increase physical activity in a general adult population. BMC Public Health **20**(1) (2020). https://doi.org/10.1186/s12889-020-09148-9
8. Dwyer, M.J., Pasini, M., De Dominicis, S., Righi, E.: Physical activity: benefits and challenges during the COVID-19 pandemic (2020). https://doi.org/10.1111/sms.13710, https://www.ncbi.nlm.nih.gov/pmc/articles/PMC7323175/
9. van Dyck, D., Herman, K., Poppe, L., Crombez, G., de Bourdeaudhuij, I., Gheysen, F.: Results of MYPLAN 2.0 on physical activity in older Belgian adults: randomized controlled trial. J. Med. Internet Res. **21**(10) (2019). https://doi.org/10.2196/13219, https://pubmed.ncbi.nlm.nih.gov/31593541/

10. Goethals, L., Barth, N., Guyot, J., Hupin, D., Celarier, T., Bongue, B.: Impact of home quarantine on physical activity among older adults living at home during the COVID-19 pandemic: qualitative interview study. JMIR Aging **3**(1), e19007 (2020). https://doi.org/10.2196/19007, https://aging.jmir.org/2020/1/e19007

11. Hallal, P.C., et al.: Global physical activity levels: surveillance progress, pitfalls, and prospects (2012). https://doi.org/10.1016/S0140-6736(12)60646-1, https://pubmed.ncbi.nlm.nih.gov/22818937/

12. HAPA: OSF | 24. Health Action Process Approach - FINAL.pdf. https://osf.io/znmvc/

13. Kim, Y., Park, I., Kang, M.: Convergent validity of the international physical activity questionnaire (IPAQ): meta-analysis, March 2013. https://doi.org/10.1017/S1368980012002996, https://pubmed.ncbi.nlm.nih.gov/22874087/

14. Kohl, L.F., Crutzen, R., De Vries, N.K.: Online prevention aimed at lifestyle behaviors: a systematic review of reviews. J. Med. Internet Res. **15**(7) (2013). https://doi.org/10.2196/jmir.2665, https://pubmed.ncbi.nlm.nih.gov/23859884/

15. Larsen, K.R., et al.: Behavior change interventions: the potential of ontologies for advancing science and practice. J. Behav. Med. **40**(1), 6–22 (2016). https://doi.org/10.1007/s10865-016-9768-0

16. Loh, W.W., Moerkerke, B., Loeys, T., Poppe, L., Crombez, G., Vansteelandt, S.: Estimation of controlled direct effects in longitudinal mediation analyses with latent variables in randomized studies. Multivariate Behav. Res. **55**(5), 763–785 (2020). https://doi.org/10.1080/00273171.2019.1681251, https://www.tandfonline.com/doi/abs/10.1080/00273171.2019.1681251

17. Michie, S., et al.: From theory-inspired to theory-based interventions: a protocol for developing and testing a methodology for linking behaviour change techniques to theoretical mechanisms of action. Ann. Behav. Med. **52**(6), 501–512 (2018). https://doi.org/10.1007/s12160-016-9816-6, https://pubmed.ncbi.nlm.nih.gov/27401001/

18. Milne-Ives, M., LamMEng, C., de Cock, C., van Velthoven, M.H., Ma, E.M.: Mobile apps for health behavior change in physical activity, diet, drug and alcohol use, and mental health: systematic review. JMIR mHealth uHealth **8**(3) (2020). https://doi.org/10.2196/17046, https://pubmed.ncbi.nlm.nih.gov/32186518/

19. Miyamoto, S.W., Henderson, S., Young, H.M., Pande, A., Han, J.J.: Tracking health data is not enough: a qualitative exploration of the role of healthcare partnerships and mhealth technology to promote physical activity and to sustain behavior change. JMIR mHealth uHealth **4**(1) (2016). https://doi.org/10.2196/mhealth.4814, https://pubmed.ncbi.nlm.nih.gov/26792225/

20. Ongenae, F., et al.: An ontology co-design method for the co-creation of a continuous care ontology. Appl. Ontol. **9**(1), 27–64 (2014). https://doi.org/10.3233/AO-140131

21. van Osch, L., Lechner, L., Reubsaet, A., de Vries, H.: From theory to practice: an explorative study into the instrumentality and specificity of implementation intentions. Psychol. Health **25**(3), 351–364 (2010). https://doi.org/10.1080/08870440802642155, https://pubmed.ncbi.nlm.nih.gov/20204939/

22. PACO: Physical Activity Ontology - PACO - Classes | NCBO BioPortal. https://bioportal.bioontology.org/ontologies/PACO/?p=classes&conceptid=root

23. Peiris, D., Jaime Miranda, J., Mohr, D.C.: Going beyond killer apps: building a better mHealth evidence base. BMJ Glob. Health **3**(1), e000676 (2018). https://doi.org/10.1136/bmjgh-2017-000676, http://gh.bmj.com/, http://gh.bmj.com/lookup/doi/10.1136/bmjgh-2017-000676

24. Piwek, L., Ellis, D.A., Andrews, S., Joinson, A.: The rise of consumer health wearables: promises and barriers. PLoS Med. **13**(2), e1001953 (2016). https://doi.org/10.1371/journal.pmed.1001953, https://journals.plos.org/plosmedicine/article?id=10.1371/journal.pmed.1001953

25. Plaete, J., Crombez, G., Van Der Mispel, C., Verloigne, M., Van Stappen, V., De Bourdeaudhuij, I.: Effect of the Web-based intervention MyPlan 1.0 on self-reported fruit and vegetable intake in adults who visit general practice: a quasi-experimental trial. J. Med. Internet Res. **18**(2) (2016). https://doi.org/10.2196/jmir.5252

26. Poppe, L., et al.: Efficacy of a self-regulation-based electronic and mobile health intervention targeting an active lifestyle in adults having type 2 diabetes and in adults aged 50 years or older: two randomized controlled trials. J. Med. Internet Res. **21**(8) (2019). https://doi.org/10.2196/13363, https://pubmed.ncbi.nlm.nih.gov/31376274/

27. Sardi, L., Idri, A., Fernández-Alemán, J.L.: A systematic review of gamification in e-Health (2017). https://doi.org/10.1016/j.jbi.2017.05.011, https://pubmed.ncbi.nlm.nih.gov/28536062/

28. Schwarzer, R., Lippke, S., Luszczynska, A.: Mechanisms of health behavior change in persons with chronic illness or disability: the health action process approach (HAPA). Rehabil. Psychol. **56**(3), 161–170 (2011). https://doi.org/10.1037/a0024509, https://pubmed.ncbi.nlm.nih.gov/21767036/

29. Sniehotta, F.F.: Towards a theory of intentional behaviour change: plans, planning, and self-regulation (2009). https://doi.org/10.1348/135910708X389042, https://pubmed.ncbi.nlm.nih.gov/19102817/

30. Tondello, G.F., Wehbe, R.R., Diamond, L., Busch, M., Marczewski, A., Nacke, L.E.: The gamification user types Hexad scale. In: CHI PLAY 2016 - Proceedings of the 2016 Annual Symposium on Computer-Human Interaction in Play, pp. 229–243. Association for Computing Machinery Inc, New York, October 2016. https://doi.org/10.1145/2967934.2968082, http://dl.acm.org/citation.cfm?doid=2967934.2968082

31. Van Dyck, D., Plaete, J., Cardon, G., Crombez, G., De Bourdeaudhuij, I.: Effectiveness of the self-regulation eHealth intervention 'MyPlan1.0'. on physical activity levels of recently retired Belgian adults: a randomized controlled trial. Health Educ. Res. **31**(5), 653–664 (2016). https://doi.org/10.1093/her/cyw036, https://pubmed.ncbi.nlm.nih.gov/27422898/

32. WHO: World Health Statistics Monitoring Health for SDGs. Technical report (2018). World Health Organization, Geneva (2018). Licence: CC BY-NC-SA 3.0 IGO

33. Zhao, J., Freeman, B., Li, M.: Can mobile phone apps influence people's health behavior change? An evidence review. J. Med. Internet Res. **18**(11), e287 (2016). https://doi.org/10.2196/jmir.5692

The SharedHeart Approach: Technology-Supported Shared Decision Making to Increase Physical Activity in Cardiac Patients

Cindel Bonneux[1]([✉]), Dominique Hansen[2], Paul Dendale[3], and Karin Coninx[1]

[1] Faculty of Sciences, HCI and eHealth, UHasselt-tUL, Agoralaan,
3590 Diepenbeek, Belgium
{cindel.bonneux,karin.coninx}@uhasselt.be
[2] Faculty of Rehabilitation Sciences, UHasselt, Agoralaan, 3590 Diepenbeek, Belgium
dominique.hansen@uhasselt.be
[3] Faculty of Medicine and Life Sciences, UHasselt, Agoralaan,
3590 Diepenbeek, Belgium
paul.dendale@uhasselt.be

Abstract. After a cardiac event, patients typically enroll in a cardiac rehabilitation program in a rehabilitation center, where physiotherapists guide them in overcoming their fear to move and increasing physical activity. Effectively changing patients' health behaviour and bringing the newly formed habits to their home environment remains challenging. At home, patients experience difficulties interpreting exercise targets and monitoring physical activity. To bridge the gap between supervised rehab in the center and regular exercise in daily life, we propose a shared decision making (SDM) approach SharedHeart that supports patients in changing their health behaviour and transferring the knowledge and healthy habits to their homes. We developed 3 applications that support patients and physiotherapists in following a SDM approach: (1) a tablet app to record the patient's sports preferences, (2) a caregiver dashboard to create and follow up on a patient-tailored exercise plan during and in between SDM encounters, and (3) a mobile app to report and follow up on physical activity at home. In this paper, we present the results of our survey investigating physiotherapists' application of SDM in their current practice and perceived usefulness of SDM and supporting tools. Next, we discuss our proposed SDM approach on the conceptual level and the guideline-based design of the supporting IT applications. We conclude by highlighting how our approach and tools align with physiotherapists' needs.

Keywords: Shared decision making · Physical activity · Cardiac rehabilitation · Patient empowerment · eHealth

Published by Springer Nature Switzerland AG 2022. All Rights Reserved
H. Lewy and R. Barkan (Eds.): PH 2021, LNICST 431, pp. 469–488, 2022.
https://doi.org/10.1007/978-3-030-99194-4_29

1   Introduction

After an acute ischemic heart disease event, secondary prevention (including cardiac rehabilitation) is recommended by evidence-based guidelines to improve functional capacity, prognosis, and quality of life [2,23,25,28]. Cardiac rehabilitation (CR) is a comprehensive, multidisciplinary program composed of several key components, such as medication, healthy nutrition, smoking cessation, stress management, education, and physical activity. It has been proven that CR is effective in improving quality of life, and reducing both morbidity and mortality. Despite these demonstrated benefits, CR remains underused in current practice [19,22]. The EUROASPIRE surveys [8] concluded that only 40% of cardiac patients reached the physical activity target at 6 months after hospital discharge. In our current research, we focus on improving cardiac patients' adherence to physical activity with support of IT tools, while still being embedded in a multidisciplinary CR program. The research findings on the use of the digital SDM tools in this context are likely to be generalizable to a broader rehabilitation context.

1.1   Current Practice

In Europe, the cardiac rehabilitation program is typically divided in three subsequent phases. *Phase I* starts when the patient is hospitalized after an acute cardiac event, and focuses on early mobilization and brief introductory counseling. At hospital discharge, patients proceed to *Phase II*, which is usually a supervised ambulatory outpatient CR program in a hospital or rehabilitation center. Here, patients are supported by a multidisciplinary team in managing and reducing their risk factors for about three months. During the rehabilitation sessions, they focus on increasing the patient's physical activity. Patients are guided by physiotherapists while performing exercises on for example stationary bikes, treadmills, and arm bikes [19,22]. Unfortunately patients regularly skip rehabilitation sessions due to varying reasons, such as personal feelings and beliefs (e.g. embarrassment about exercising in group), system and service barriers (e.g. contradictory advice from the healthcare team), and logistic limitations (e.g. lack of transport and parking) [21]. Moreover, patients are instructed to exercise at home on days that they do not go to the rehabilitation center. Given their age and often sedentary lifestyle, most cardiac patients are not accustomed to performing non-supervised exercise training at home [24] and have fear to exercise. Behaviour change is a complex process, requiring people to restructure their priorities, and daily and social routines [17]. However, patients lack guidance on how to integrate exercise into their daily life and how to exercise independently at home [24]. When patients finish the outpatient CR program, they advance to *Phase III*, the lifetime maintenance or long-term outpatient CR phase, where the support of the multidisciplinary team is reduced. Patients have to maintain their physical fitness and perform additional risk factor reduction more independently [19,22]. Patients often experience difficulties in transferring the knowledge and habits formed during supervised rehabilitation in the center to the unsupervised rehabilitation at home. It is a challenge for them to interpret their overall rehabilitation targets, identify the physical activities they should do, and monitor their progress over time [24].

1.2 Telerehabilitation

Telerehabilitation can provide a possible solution to cope with the low attendance rates at rehabilitation sessions and the low long-term adherence to recommendations. In telerehabilitation, patients are not restricted to the hospital or rehabilitation center, but rehabilitate remotely at home supported by interactive applications and technology. Reviews [4,11] concluded that telerehabilitation can be a feasible and effective add-on or alternative compared to conventional in-hospital cardiac rehabilitation, and has the potential to support patients in adhering to the recommended level of physical activity. However, telerehabilitation solutions need to be personalized and tailored to the patient's individual condition and needs [10]. Patient involvement is a prerequisite for good clinical practice. In this regard, research has shown that shared decision making has the potential to improve patient satisfaction, adherence, and psychological and physical well-being (e.g. quality of life, anxiety, and depression) [15]. Patients prefer to share decisions or at least give their opinion about treatment before the physiotherapist makes a decision [9]. However, the rather paternalistic model where caregivers decide for their patients is still dominating in practice [7,9]. Accordingly, in most telerehabilitation systems targeting physical activity, patients have only limited input in their exercise prescription and plan.

1.3 Shared Decision Making

Shared decision making is an approach that combines the patient's personal preferences, goals, values, and context with the clinical evidence and expert opinions to make an informed decision [18,27]. To design and develop a personalized telerehabilitation solution targeting physical activity, we propose to incorporate shared decision making (SDM) as a means to involve and empower cardiac patients in the process of constructing an exercise plan. In this context, from the patient's perspective, their current habits, sport preferences, and physical disabilities or limitations should be considered. For example, a dog lover will prefer going for a walk with his/her dog over cycling. On the other hand, the evidence-based guidelines for physical activity and the expertise of the caregivers guiding the patient in the rehabilitation center should be taken into account when making decisions about the patient's physical activity.

1.4 Our Proposed SharedHeart Approach

In this paper, we propose SharedHeart, a technology-supported shared decision making approach for physical activity. Given the fact that currently most healthcare decisions are made by caregivers [7,9], we investigated physiotherapists' current practices of SDM and perceived usefulness of SDM and using SDM tools in a survey. Using our SharedHeart platform, patients and their physiotherapists set up goals together to construct a tailor-made exercise plan in order to get patients involved to make their own decisions. As such, we want to bridge the gap between supervised and unsupervised rehabilitation and improve long-term adherence to physical activity recommendations. The SharedHeart platform is composed of three applications: (1) a tablet application to record the patient's preferences for physical activity, (2) a caregiver dashboard to create and follow up on a patient-tailored exercise plan during and in between SDM encounters, and (3) a mobile application for the patient to report and follow up on physical activity at home. The caregiver dashboard was designed by applying the guidelines of Bonneux et al. [6] for the design of SDM tools targeting health behaviour change. We conclude by highlighting some directions for future research.

2 Physiotherapists' Opinion About Shared Decision Making

In general, shared decision making is not yet applied extensively in clinical practice [7,9]. When designing tools to support caregivers in SDM, important factors influencing uptake of these tools are caregivers' willingness to do it and their acceptance of SDM tools. Given the focus of this paper on physical activity in phase II cardiac rehabilitation (CR), we assessed physiotherapists' current practice of SDM and their perceived usefulness of shared decision making and SDM tools for physical activity in the context of phase II CR. We conducted a custom-made survey with ten physiotherapists working in the rehabilitation center (i.e. ReGo) of Jessa Hospital (Hasselt, Belgium). In the rehabilitation center, cardiac patients are supported by a multidisciplinary team, consisting of cardiologists, physiotherapists, dietitians, psychologists and social nurses in recovering from a cardiac incident. The rehabilitation program for a patient lasts three months and consists of 45 multidisciplinary sessions (individual and in group). The physiotherapists that participated in the survey had varying experience in CR, ranging from physiotherapists guiding cardiac patients during their exercise training half a day per week to daily, to a trainee and the head of the rehabilitation center.

Given the target audience of the survey, we only included questions in relation to SDM for physical activity and exercise training as part of phase II rehabilitation in the rehabilitation center. The survey consisted of four parts assessing physiotherapists' current practice of SDM, usefulness of topics for discussing with patients, usefulness of a tool during discussions with patients and preferences for conversations about physical activity. Questions about usefulness were 5-point Likert scale questions, ranging from not useful at all to very useful. Questions about frequencies and timing for SDM were multiple-choice questions, but also some open questions were included to gain deeper insights into physiotherapists' preferences.

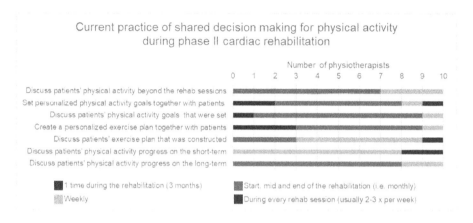

Fig. 1. Physiotherapists' current practice of shared decision making for physical activity during phase II cardiac rehabilitation.

We assessed physiotherapists' current application of SDM in their daily practice by asking them about their interaction with patients. For a selection of physical activity related topics, we collected information on how frequently they discuss these topics with their patients (i.e. perform shared decision making). The results are depicted in Fig. 1. The most frequently discussed topic is patients' short-term progress for physical activity, which is discussed by all physiotherapists at least on a weekly basis. For all other topics, several physiotherapists indicated a lower frequency of SDM (e.g. monthly or only once during the rehabilitation program). Creating a personalized exercise plan together with the patients is done the least frequently, with only one physiotherapist discussing it on a weekly basis, six physiotherapists discussing it monthly, and the remaining three physiotherapists only discussing it once during the rehabilitation.

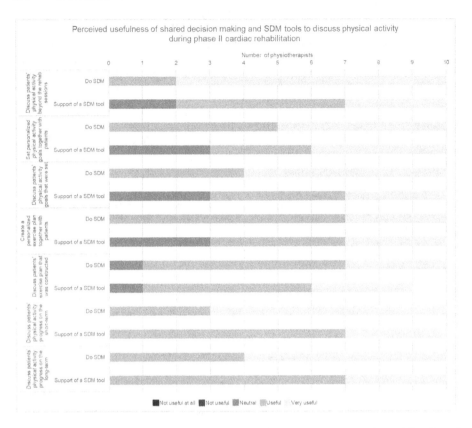

Fig. 2. Physiotherapists' perceived usefulness of shared decision making (SDM) and using a SDM tool to discuss physical activity during phase II cardiac rehabilitation.

Secondly, for the same set of physical activity related topics, we assessed physiotherapists' perceived usefulness of 1) shared decision making (i.e. discussing these topics with their patients) and 2) receiving support of a SDM tool during these discussions. The results are depicted in Fig. 2. In general, physiotherapists perceived for all topics shared decision making as valuable. Only for one topic (i.e. discussing patients' exercise plans) one physiotherapist indicated neutral, but for all other topics all physiotherapists indicated that it is (very) useful to discuss them with their patients. Discussing physical activity that patients do next to their rehabilitation sessions in the center was identified as the most useful discussion topic, followed by discussing patients' short- and long-term progress and physical activity goals.

Physiotherapists' perceived usefulness of a SDM tool to support the discussion of physical activity related topics was slightly more neutral, indicated by a higher number of neutral responses. Nevertheless, no physiotherapist indicated that he/she would not find it useful to use a SDM tool. There were no topics that clearly stood out as the most or least useful to discuss with the aid of a

SDM tool. The slightly lower perceived usefulness of a SDM tool compared to doing SDM could be due to physiotherapists' current way of working and the fact that they did not have any experience with a SDM tool and we did not give them a detailed explanation of the possible features of such a tool.

Lastly, we asked physiotherapists about their preferences for timing of conversations about physical activity with their patients, i.e. when would they find it useful to have these conversations and what is the preferred frequency. Most physiotherapists (8/10) indicated that they would find it useful to discuss their patients' physical activity every week during the rehabilitation program in the rehabilitation center (i.e. the entire phase II cardiac rehabilitation). Varying reasons were indicated for this, including the importance of physical activity in the rehabilitation process, patients' need for evaluation and confirmation, easy integration into training sessions, influence on motivation and involvement, working efficiently, adapting timely and detecting problems. Some physiotherapists also noted that it is especially important to discuss the physical activity that patients do next to their rehabilitation in the center. The two other physiotherapists indicated varying moments for conversations about physical activity. One physiotherapist would prefer the combination of the first and last 6 weeks of the rehabilitation program and at the long-term follow-up. As such, the buildup and progress at home and during the rehabilitation goes in parallel with the cardiopulmonary exercise test that was done in the rehabilitation center. Another physiotherapist would prefer the combination of biweekly discussions during the rehabilitation program, with closer follow-up in the first and last 2 weeks, plus at the long-term follow-up. The physiotherapist noted that it should not be too frequent, because it should be organizationally feasible and it should be possible to detect progression or stagnation. On the other hand, it should be discussed frequently enough to increase or sustain motivation and to provide a broader reference frame for the physiotherapist.

We also assessed physiotherapists' preferences for the frequency of conversations with patients about physical activity. The frequency varied: 4 physiotherapists preferred weekly, 4 physiotherapists preferred biweekly, 1 physiotherapist preferred both weekly and biweekly and 1 physiotherapist preferred monthly. One physiotherapist noted that it could be frequent in the beginning but with a degrading frequency, ranging from every session to once a month. Reasons for these frequencies included allowing for checking up on and guiding the patient, providing patients a clear goal to train and make progression, updating the training parameters more adequately (e.g. number of repetitions and sets), stimulating patients frequently to continue exercising at home, following up patients and adjusting the training when needed, detecting problems and possible pitfalls, adapting short- and long-term goals, and keeping the overview of the patients' physical activity. Some physiotherapists noted the importance of having enough time to do the rehabilitation exercises. Furthermore, adapting exercise habits requires time. On the other side, there should be enough time for a decent discussion. For both the current and preferred frequency of SDM, the diversity in answers may be due to a physiotherapist's interpretation of a SDM moment, varying from briefly asking how the patient is doing to having a decent conversation about the patient's activity.

We want to conclude the presentation of the results of our survey by mentioning that we did not investigate explicitly how physiotherapists perceive the time they spend discussing with their patients. However, this could have an influence on their perceived usefulness of shared decision making and SDM tools.

3   Decision-Making in the SharedHeart Approach

Shared decision making (SDM) for physical activity during the supervised ambulatory outpatient cardiac rehabilitation program (phase II) is one of the key topics in our current research. To support patients in exercising at home during phase II and bridge the gap between supervised and unsupervised rehabilitation, we propose a SDM approach supported by a digital platform, SharedHeart.

3.1   Approach for the Rehabilitation Program

During phase II cardiac rehabilitation, patients come two to three times a week to the rehabilitation center to train under the supervision of physiotherapists. In the SharedHeart approach, we combine these training sessions with SDM encounters supported by digital tools. Ideally, from the first week of the supervised rehabilitation onwards, the patient has once a week a SDM consultation with a physiotherapist to discuss his/her physical activity.

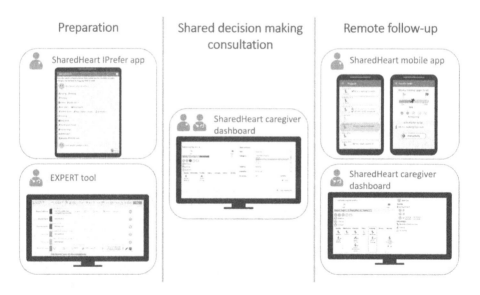

Fig. 3. An overview of the different tools that support the SharedHeart approach.

Typically the supervised rehabilitation program takes about three months. Joint goal setting with patients, discussing progress and frequent encouragement from caregivers are important factors facilitating continuation in CR programs [20]. However, physiotherapists have many patients to supervise. Both the patients and the physiotherapists would benefit from SDM tools that retain efficiency, while increasing the quality and depth of their interaction during the encounters. Therefore, in line with the survey results, we propose to have one SDM encounter every week for the first half of the supervised rehabilitation and then decrease this to one SDM encounter every two weeks. The gradual decrease in control by the physiotherapists shifts the responsibility gradually to the patient. In this way, when the patient finishes rehabilitation in the center, the currently best fitted exercise plan for the patient has been found and the patient is ready to take the full responsibility to maintain physical fitness. By following this SDM approach, our aim is to teach patients the skills for planning their physical activity, and to build strong habits during phase II of rehabilitation, that they will continue in phase III to foster long-term adherence.

In the SharedHeart approach, we integrated digital tools of the different *categories* proposed by Bonneux et al. [5]. Before the first SDM encounter, patients use *a preference elicitation application* to indicate their preferences and physiotherapists use *a clinical decision support system* to prepare for the encounter. In the encounters, patients and their physiotherapists create a personalized exercise plan for the patient with the aid of *a SDM tool that provides data and recommendations to foster communication and deliberation and guides the stakeholders through the SDM process.* Between encounters, patients use *a mobile tool providing decision support at home* and the physiotherapists use *a tool for remote follow-up.* Figure 3 gives an overview of the proposed SharedHeart approach and supporting digital applications.

3.2   Approach During a Single Encounter

At the start of the supervised rehabilitation, all information needed for shared decision making needs to be collected. From the patient's side, we need to assess his/her sports preferences, current situation (e.g. home and work situation), and physical limitations (e.g. pain or balance problems). To relieve the burden for physiotherapists, patients can indicate their preferences in the IPrefer tablet application in the waiting room. From a clinical point of view, we need the patient's latest clinical data (e.g. physiological parameters and results of cardiopulmonary exercise testing) and a tailored exercise prescription conforming to the evidence-based guidelines for physical activity. To support physiotherapists in making a guideline-based exercise prescription for the patient, we integrated the EXPERT tool [12,13], i.e. a clinical decision support system that suggests a personalized, guideline-based exercise prescription for a patient, into the SharedHeart caregiver dashboard.

In the encounters, patients and their guiding physiotherapists discuss the patient's preferences for physical activity and collaboratively construct an exercise plan for the upcoming week in the SharedHeart caregiver dashboard. To stimulate discussion and encourage exploration of new physical activities, the SDM tool provides guidance in creating the exercise plan by suggesting activities that comply with the clinical evidence on exercise effectiveness and the patient's sports preferences. At the end of each encounter, the patient goes home with a tailor-made, achievable exercise plan for next week.

Between encounters, the patient tries to adhere to the exercise plan. Encouraging health-promoting lifestyle change requires interventions that are integrated into daily life and provide support when and where people make decisions [17]. Therefore, we developed a mobile, persuasive telerehabilitation application that motivates patients to exercise and enables them to follow up on their exercise plan that was prepared in the SDM setting. Physiotherapists can also remotely follow up on the data that their patients collect in the SharedHeart caregiver dashboard.

One or two weeks after the previous SDM encounter, the patient has a new SDM encounter with the physiotherapist in which they discuss how the patient experienced the past days (e.g. How active was the patient? Did the patient adhere to the program?). This discussion is supported by the SharedHeart caregiver dashboard that visualizes the data collected in the patient mobile application. Based on the patient's recent performance and updated preferences and constraints, the exercise prescription is adapted and the plan for next week is constructed. This process repeats until the currently best fitting exercise prescription and exercise plan for the patient have been found.

4   The Design of the SharedHeart Platform

The SharedHeart digital platform augments the proposed SDM approach. In this section, we discuss the design of these applications and we highlight their contribution to shared decision making. The SharedHeart caregiver dashboard is the main application (as depicted in Fig. 3), supporting SDM during the encounters between the physiotherapist and the patient. The caregiver dashboard offers support in collaboratively setting exercise targets, creating an exercise plan and discussing progress. In the application, we applied the seven *principles* of Bonneux et al. [6] for the design of SDM tools for health behaviour change. In the context of our application, the behaviour change goal is being more physically active. The design principles of Bonneux et al. are depicted in *italics*. Next to using the caregiver dashboard during the SDM encounter, physiotherapists can also use it to prepare for their next encounter with the patient and to follow up on the patient's progress between visits. The IPrefer tablet application supports the preference elicitation before the first consultation, whereas the SharedHeart mobile application supports the patient in following up on the decisions that were made during the encounter.

4.1   Goal-Setting for Physical Activity

A key aspect in shared decision making for health behaviour change is *encouraging collaborative goal-setting*. In the context of physical activity for cardiac rehabilitation, the goal can be expressed as an exercise prescription. Physiotherapists can use the EXPERT tool [12,13] to generate a personalized exercise prescription for their patients. An example of a typical exercise prescription for a patient is as follows: "exercise at moderate intensity 3 to 5 times a week for 20 to 60 min per session and for at least 24 weeks". Prior to the first SDM encounter, the physiotherapist prepares the initial exercise prescription for the patient using the EXPERT tool. This exercise prescription is discussed with the patient during the encounter. The EXPERT tool often defines ranges in the exercise prescription (e.g. 20–60 min of physical activity for 3–5 times per week). These can be discussed with the patient to come to a feasible exercise prescription for the patient. Furthermore, it is possible that the exercise prescription is too hard and thus not feasible for the patient at a certain point in the rehabilitation program. In this case, the physiotherapist can update the exercise prescription during the SDM encounter. In the follow-up encounters, the exercise prescription can be updated based on the patient's progress and changes in risk profile, to make it more challenging for the patient.

The patient's current status (e.g. most recent parameter values and physical fitness) is shown in the risk profile bar in the SharedHeart caregiver dashboard and the target situation is represented by the patient's exercise prescription. As such, the design principle of Bonneux et al. [6] *give an overview of the current status, the target situation, and the available options* is met, but not combined into a comprehensive overview. As the available options, we can consider the ranges of the exercise prescription but also the ways to achieve the exercise prescription (as discussed in Sect. 4.2).

4.2   Creating an Exercise Plan

Patients experience difficulties in translating a generic exercise prescription to a concrete exercise plan fitting their needs. Also, interpreting exercise targets is a challenge for a number of patients. Patients need support when making decisions in their daily life related to their health condition, but physiotherapists are often not able to perform this demanding task. Moreover, patients should be encouraged to do lifestyle physical activity (e.g. taking the stairs, gardening and cleaning), additional exercise or both on days that they do not attend cardiac rehabilitation sessions [3]. Supporting patients in performing physical activity on these days is essential [26]. It is not a trivial task for physiotherapists to include all these aspects in their daily practice. Therefore, we provide patients and physiotherapists *support in making an action plan*, by constructing and following up on a patient-tailored exercise plan that includes both the training sessions in the rehabilitation center and the physical activities that the patient performs at home, as depicted in the exercise plan (i.e. nr 3 in Fig. 4). The information that is difficult for patients to understand (e.g. the exercise prescription) and the preference-sensitive decisions that should be made (e.g. the exercise plan) are the central components of this SDM screen.

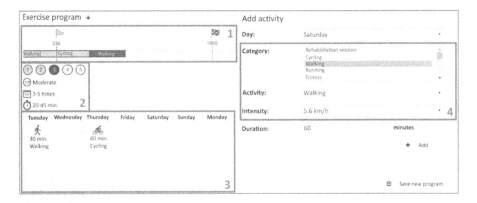

Fig. 4. During the SDM encounters, the patient and physiotherapist collaboratively construct an exercise plan by choosing activities (nr 4). The calendar view (nr 3) and patient-tailored progress bar (nr 1) provide an overview of respectively the plan and the associated progress towards the exercise targets. Also, the patient's exercise prescription is shown (nr 2).

To foster discussion of the exercise plan and improve patient understanding of the exercise prescription and associated targets, we offer multiple complementary visualizations when constructing the exercise plan (Fig. 4). These visualizations were designed to encourage physiotherapists to collaboratively decide upon the patient's physical activity. The exercise plan for the upcoming week is displayed in a weekly calendar (nr 3), which is a well-known representation format that can be easily understood by patients. In addition, the progress that will be made by the activities of the composed plan is visualized in a tailor-made progress bar (nr 1). The flags in the progress bar denote the personalized weekly exercise targets calculated based on the patient's parameters and exercise prescription. To support patient understanding and encourage exploration of different activities, there is an indication of how much each activity contributes to achieving the targets, allowing the physiotherapist to *demonstrate the effects of behaviour change*. The overview of the patient's prescription with an indication of how many training sessions will be completed by the composed plan (nr 2) links the exercise prescription to the exercise plan.

Research has demonstrated that patients prefer to choose their exercises from a range of exercise options [20]. Accordingly, the SharedHeart caregiver dashboard offers a patient-tailored list of recommended activity categories (nr 4) based on the patient's ranking of sports activities as compiled in the IPrefer tablet application. For each activity category, multiple activities and variations are available (e.g. different speeds or intensities). For example, the category walking entails two specific activities: walking and Nordic walking. For each of these, there are different variations, including different walking speeds and conditions (e.g. with a dog). The list of available categories, activities, and variations was constructed by selecting relevant activities from the Compendium of Physical Activities [1]. Since the focus of SharedHeart is on exercise training, no general lifestyle activities, such as cleaning and gardening, were included. To help physiotherapists and patients in choosing the appropriate variation (e.g. walking speed) for the patient, there is an indication of how well the specific activity variation matches with the patient's profile based on the patient's exercise prescription and the table of Vanhees et al. [29]. The recommendations for sports activities and intensities support the physiotherapist in *providing suggestions or tips* to the patient.

Next to the exercise prescription, the EXPERT tool offers patient-tailored safety advice to optimise medical safety of exercise training [12,13]. The physiotherapists can use this advice to *provide suggestions or tips* on how to perform physical activity. In collaboration with an expert in exercise training for cardiac patients, we expanded these safety precautions with activity specific safety precautions and supplementary safety advice that can be provided based on the patient's physical limitations (pain and balance problems) that were collected in the IPrefer tablet application. During the SDM encounters, the physiotherapists can discuss the patient-tailored list of safety precautions with the patients to reduce their fear to exercise and improve their self-efficacy to perform exercise independently at home.

4.3   Reporting and Following Up on Physical Activity

The patient leaves the SDM encounter with a tailored exercise plan for the upcoming week. At home, patients use the SharedHeart mobile application to report and follow up on their physical activity (Fig. 5). The mobile application intends to keep the shared decision making process ongoing by giving cues of what was decided during the SDM encounter and offering supporting features to achieve the mutually agreed goals.

First of all, the application gives an overview of the patient's pre-constructed exercise plan that was made in the SDM setting and how well the patient adheres to it (Fig. 5A). Between encounters, patients can report which activities from the pre-constructed plan they perform and can follow up on their progress towards the weekly exercise targets in the progress visualization (Fig. 5B). Sometimes it is not possible to perform the planned activity, e.g. it is raining and the patient planned to go walking outside. When patients want to deviate from the exercise plan, they can add a new activity by selecting it from the list of recommended activities in the app, similarly as during the SDM encounter.

Cardiac patients should perform both exercise training and unstructured, lifestyle physical activity. The goal should be to carry out at least moderate intensity activities during the day (e.g. gardening, cleaning or vacuuming). At the end of the day, patients can report on their lifestyle physical activity (Fig. 5C). If the patient did not achieve the goal of at least moderate intensity activities, a tip to increase lifestyle physical activity is given. These tips are tailored to the patient's work and home situation (that was collected with the IPrefer application). Furthermore, patients can view the entire history of their self-reported physical activity in the mobile app.

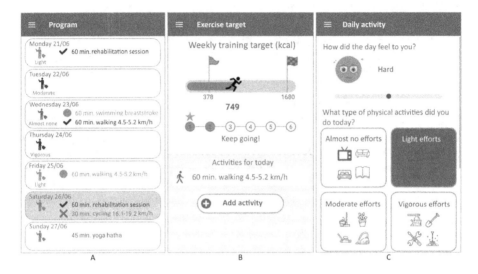

Fig. 5. During the week, patients can use the mobile application to A) follow up on their exercise plan, B) monitor their physical activity and C) report their daily activity.

Patients need knowledge to be able to take part in shared decision making [16]. To improve patients' knowledge and understanding of their condition, we offer short educational videos about cardiac rehabilitation in general and physical activity in particular. Moreover, we provide some videos tailored to the patient's exercise plan. These videos provide tips and tricks for the specific activity categories incorporated in the exercise plan. We collaborated with an experienced physiotherapist to record videos for the most prevalent activity categories (i.e. walking, biking, fitness and racket sports). Watching an educational video can raise some questions. Patients can record these questions or other concerns in the notes, so they can discuss these issues in an upcoming appointment with their physiotherapist.

4.4   Discussing Performance of Physical Activity and Progress

All information that patients enter in the SharedHeart mobile application can be consulted by the physiotherapists in the caregiver dashboard (Fig. 6A). During the SDM encounter, the physiotherapist can use the caregiver dashboard to discuss how the patient performed last week. Optionally the physiotherapist can also follow up on the patient's activity between encounters, but given the busy schedules of physiotherapists this is not mandatory for our proposed approach.

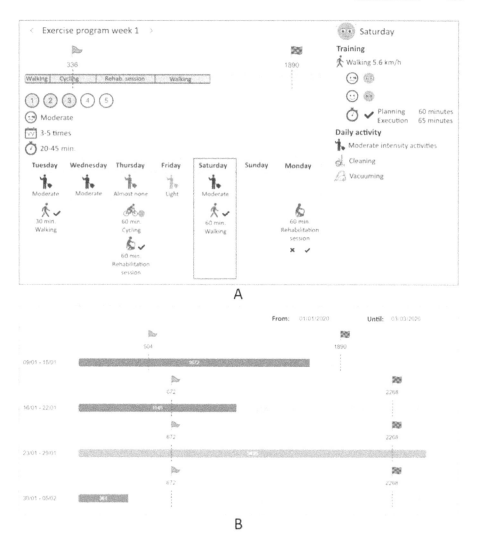

Fig. 6. During the SDM encounter, the patient's exercise of the past week is discussed. A) The calendar overview indicates how the patient adhered to the constructed exercise plan. B) The progress bars show the patient's long-term progress for physical activity.

In the discussion screen (Fig. 6A), we applied similar visualization techniques as in the construction screen (Fig. 4): a weekly calendar view and a tailor-made progress bar with exercise prescription and training sessions, both *enabling progress follow-up with visual elements* and supporting to *give feedback on performance*. The calendar view depicts the exercise plan that was constructed during the previous SDM encounter and how the patient adhered to it. The detailed information of an activity (e.g. time, tiredness, enjoyment) can be consulted as well. The progress bar shows how the activities that the patient performed contributed to achieving the exercise targets. Whereas the activities' contribution to the targets was predicted when constructing the exercise plan (Fig. 4), the exact contribution of each performed activity is appraised during the SDM discussion (Fig. 6A). By demonstrating how the different activities contributed to achieving the exercise targets, the design principle *demonstrating the effects of behaviour change* is met. Feedback is provided by means of icons (e.g. reported activities), colors (e.g. adherence to the exercise plan) and visual indications (e.g. progress towards the exercise flags).

A more fine-grained application of the principle *overview of the patient's current status, the target situation and the available options* can be found in the weekly calendar overview with an indication of the patient's adherence to the exercise plan and the accompanying progress visualization. The current situation is the amount of physical activity that the patient already did in that week. The target situation is reaching the exercise targets (i.e. depicted by the flags). The available options are the different sports activities that the patient can perform to progress towards the exercise targets.

For patients, it is not always easy to understand how their health condition progresses over time. Therefore, it is very important to *enable progress follow-up with visual elements* and *give feedback on performance*. The evolution of the weekly exercise targets and the patient's achievement of these targets is depicted in Fig. 6B. Patients can see how their exercise targets (i.e. visualized by the flags) changed over time depending on their exercise capacity; a better exercise capacity results in adaptations to the exercise prescription and increases the associated exercise targets. Moreover, the long-term follow-up supports physiotherapists in making these adaptations to the exercise prescription and associated exercise targets.

Patients often think of topics they wanted to discuss right after an encounter [14]. We offer patients the possibility to take notes in the mobile app, so they can remember more easily what they want to discuss with their caregivers. The notes can be consulted in the SharedHeart caregiver dashboard. During the SDM encounter, the notes can be used to discuss the patient's concerns, and the physiotherapist can also consult the notes when preparing for the encounter.

5   Discussion

In phase II cardiac rehabilitation, the multiple-consultation model that is needed for shared decision making is in place [16]. Patients come several times a week to the rehabilitation center for their training sessions. In the SharedHeart approach, we combine these training sessions with SDM consultations to discuss the patient's physical activity. Given the busy schedules of physiotherapists and the number of patients that they have to supervise simultaneously, a balance should be made when deciding how often physiotherapists have SDM encounters with their patients. In our survey, most physiotherapists indicated that they preferred to have weekly or biweekly conversations with their patients about physical activity during the rehabilitation program. The proposed frequency of the SharedHeart approach is in line with the physiotherapists' suggestion, i.e. weekly during the first 6 weeks and biweekly during the last 6 weeks of the rehabilitation program.

Our survey indicated that currently physiotherapists do shared decision making with patients for several topics, but the frequency is highly variant and there is still quite some room for improvement. This can be noticed by the discrepancies between physiotherapists' perceived usefulness of SDM (in Fig. 2) and the frequency that they currently perform it in their daily practice (in Fig. 1). Especially for the creation of a personalized exercise plan, there is still quite some room for improvement. The design of the SharedHeart platform revolves in particular around the follow-up of physical activity, with the personalized exercise plan as a key component. Furthermore, short- and long-term progress and goal-setting, which were considered as very useful for discussion, are the core components of the SharedHeart platform.

Based on physiotherapists' willingness to use a SDM tool to discuss physical activity with their patients, we expect that physiotherapists are willing to use the SharedHeart platform. However, when conducting the survey, we only involved physiotherapists of one rehabilitation center. Also, we did not explain the intended SharedHeart approach nor showed a similar platform supporting SDM to the physiotherapists, to prevent that they have a specific system in mind when filling in the survey. To bridge this gap, we plan to perform usability tests with patients and physiotherapists to explore the usability of the Shared-Heart platform, and their opinion about the tools. As a next step, it should be investigated what are the effects of the SharedHeart approach. We submitted a protocol (NCT05026957) and received ethical approval from the medical ethical committees of Hasselt University and Jessa Hospital to perform a randomized, controlled clinical trial (RCT) preceded by a usability study. In the RCT, 80 coronary artery disease patients will be recruited to evaluate the impact of our proposed SharedHeart approach on patients' quality of life, exercise capacity, motivation to exercise, perception of rehabilitation, and engagement in the decision making process.

6   Conclusion

In this paper, we presented SharedHeart, a technology-supported shared decision making approach for physical activity in cardiac rehabilitation. In a survey, we investigated physiotherapists' current practice of SDM and their perceived usefulness of SDM and using SDM tools to discuss physical activity during phase II CR. Next, we described the SharedHeart approach and illustrated the design of the SharedHeart platform by demonstrating how the seven guidelines for SDM tools for behaviour change of Bonneux et al. [6] were applied in the SharedHeart caregiver dashboard.

Our proposed SharedHeart approach and accompanying applications focus only on SDM for physical activity. However, cardiac rehabilitation is a comprehensive program composed of several key components, including education, nutrition counseling, physical activity, smoking cessation, stress management and medication intake [22]. For all components of the CR program that include a behaviour change, shared decision making can be a good way to increase patient motivation and involvement. With our work, we hope to provide other researchers an example of what a technology-supported SDM approach can look like and how an accompanying SDM tool can be designed. We hope that our current research provides a starting point for investigating SDM in telerehabilitation solutions to cope with the current challenges faced in cardiac rehabilitation and inspires other researchers in investigating technology-supported shared decision making for preference-sensitive decisions in diverse patient populations.

Acknowledgements. This research was funded by the Special Research Fund (BOF) of Hasselt University (BOF18DOC26), FWO-ICA project EXPERT network (G0F4220N) and the EU funded project H2020 IA CoroPrevention (848056).

References

1. Ainsworth, B.E., et al.: 2011 compendium of physical activities: a second update of codes and met values. Med. Sci. Sports Exerc. **43**(8), 1575–1581 (2011)
2. Authors/Task Force Members, Steg, P.G., James, S.K., Atar, D., Badano, L.P., et al.: ESC Guidelines for the management of acute myocardial infarction in patients presenting with ST-segment elevation: the task force on the management of ST-segment elevation acute myocardial infarction of the European Society of Cardiology (ESC). Eur. Heart J. **33**(20), 2569–2619 (2012). https://doi.org/10.1093/eurheartj/ehs215
3. Ayabe, M., et al.: The physical activity patterns of cardiac rehabilitation program participants. J. Cardiopulm. Rehabil. Prev. **24**(2), 80–86 (2004)
4. Batalik, L., Filakova, K., Batalikova, K., Dosbaba, F.: Remotely monitored telerehabilitation for cardiac patients: a review of the current situation. World J. Clin. Cases **8**(10), 1818 (2020)
5. Bonneux, C., Rovelo, G., Dendale, P., Coninx, K.: A comprehensive approach to decision aids supporting shared decision making in cardiac rehabilitation. In: Proceedings of the 13th EAI International Conference on Pervasive Computing Technologies for Healthcare, pp. 389–398. ACM (2019)
6. Bonneux, C., Ruiz, G.R., Dendale, P., Coninx, K.: Theory-informed design guidelines for shared decision making tools for health behaviour change. In: Ali, R., Lugrin, B., Charles, F. (eds.) PERSUASIVE 2021. LNCS, vol. 12684, pp. 259–274. Springer, Cham (2021). https://doi.org/10.1007/978-3-030-79460-6_21
7. Couët, N., et al.: Assessments of the extent to which health-care providers involve patients in decision making: a systematic review of studies using the option instrument. Health Expect. **18**(4), 542–561 (2015)
8. De Bacquer, D., et al.: EUROASPIRE IV and V surveys of the European observational research programme of the European society of cardiology: poor adherence to lifestyle recommendations in patients with coronary heart disease: results from the EUROASPIRE surveys. Eur. J. Prev. Cardiol. (2021). https://doi.org/10.1093/eurjpc/zwab115
9. Dierckx, K., Deveugele, M., Roosen, P., Devisch, I.: Implementation of shared decision making in physical therapy: observed level of involvement and patient preference. Phys. Ther. **93**(10), 1321–1330 (2013). https://doi.org/10.2522/ptj.20120286

10. Dinesen, B., et al.: Personalized telehealth in the future: a global research agenda. J. Med. Internet Res. **18**(3), e53 (2016). https://doi.org/10.2196/jmir.5257

11. Frederix, I., Vanhees, L., Dendale, P., Goetschalckx, K.: A review of telerehabilitation for cardiac patients. J. Telemed. Telecare **21**(1), 45–53 (2015). https://doi.org/10.1177/1357633X14562732

12. Hansen, D., Coninx, K., Dendale, P.: The eapc expert tool. Eur. Heart J. **38**(30), 2318–2320 (2017). https://doi.org/10.1093/eurheartj/ehx396

13. Hansen, D., et al.: The European association of preventive cardiology exercise prescription in everyday practice and rehabilitative training (EXPERT) tool: a digital training and decision support system for optimized exercise prescription in cardiovascular disease. Eur. J. Prevent. Cardiol. **24**(10), 1017–1031 (2017). https://doi.org/10.1177/2047487317702042

14. Henselmans, I., Heijmans, M., Rademakers, J., van Dulmen, S.: Participation of chronic patients in medical consultations: patients' perceived efficacy, barriers and interest in support. Health Expect. **18**(6), 2375–2388 (2015)

15. Joosten, E.A.G., Defuentes-merillas, L., De Weert, G., Sensky, T., Van Der Staak, C., De Jong, C.: Systematic review of the effects of shared decision-making on patient satisfaction, treatment adherence and health status. Psychother. Psychosomat. **77**(4), 219–26 (2008)

16. Joseph-Williams, N., Elwyn, G., Edwards, A.: Knowledge is not power for patients: a systematic review and thematic synthesis of patient-reported barriers and facilitators to shared decision making. Patient Educ. Couns. **94**(3), 291–309 (2014). https://doi.org/10.1016/j.pec.2013.10.031

17. Klasnja, P., Consolvo, S., McDonald, D.W., Landay, J.A., Pratt, W.: Using mobile & personal sensing technologies to support health behavior change in everyday life: lessons learned. In: AMIA Annual Symposium Proceedings, vol. 2009, p. 338. American Medical Informatics Association (2009)

18. Kon, A.A.: The shared decision-making continuum. Jama **304**(8), 903–904 (2010). https://doi.org/10.1001/jama.2010.1208

19. Mampuya, W.M.: Cardiac rehabilitation past, present and future: an overview. Cardiovasc. Diagn. Ther. **2**(1), 38–49 (2012). https://doi.org/10.3978/j.issn.2223-3652.2012.01.02

20. Moore, S.M., Kramer, F.M.: Women's and men's preferences for cardiac rehabilitation program features. J. Cardiopulm. Rehabil. Prev. **16**(3), 163–168 (1996)

21. Neubeck, L., Freedman, S.B., Clark, A.M., Briffa, T., Bauman, A., Redfern, J.: Participating in cardiac rehabilitation: a systematic review and meta-synthesis of qualitative data. Eur. J. Prev. Cardiol. **19**(3), 494–503 (2012). https://doi.org/10.1177/1741826711409326

22. Piepoli, M.F., et al.: Secondary prevention in the clinical management of patients with cardiovascular diseases. Core components, standards and outcome measures for referral and delivery: a policy statement from the cardiac rehabilitation section of the European association for cardiovascular prevention & rehabilitation. Endorsed by the committee for practice guidelines of the European society of cardiology. Eur. J. Prev. Cardiol. **21**(6), 664–681 (2014). https://doi.org/10.1177/2047487312449597

23. Roffi, M., et al.: 2015 ESC Guidelines for the management of acute coronary syndromes in patients presenting without persistent ST-segment elevation: task Force for the management of acute coronary syndromes in patients presenting without persistent ST-segment elevation of the European society of cardiology (ESC). Eur. Heart J. **37**(3), 267–315 (2016). https://doi.org/10.1093/eurheartj/ehv320

24. Sankaran, S., Luyten, K., Hansen, D., Dendale, P., Coninx, K.: Have you met your mets?: enhancing patient motivation to achieve physical activity targets in cardiac tele-rehabilitation. In: Proceedings of the 32Nd International BCS Human Computer Interaction Conference, HCI 2018, pp. 48:1–48:12. BCS Learning & Development Ltd., Swindon (2018). https://doi.org/10.14236/ewic/HCI2018.48

25. Smith, S.C., et al.: AHA/ACCF secondary prevention and risk reduction therapy for patients with coronary and other atherosclerotic vascular disease: 2011 update. Circulation **124**(22), 2458–2473 (2011). https://doi.org/10.1161/CIR.0b013e318235eb4d

26. Stevenson, T.G., Riggin, K., Nagelkirk, P.R., Hargens, T.A., Strath, S.J., Kaminsky, L.A.: Physical activity habits of cardiac patients participating in an early outpatient rehabilitation program. J. Cardiopulm. Rehabil. Prev. **29**(5), 299–303 (2009)

27. Stiggelbout, A.M., et al.: Shared decision making: really putting patients at the centre of healthcare. BMJ **344**, 28–31 (2012). https://doi.org/10.1136/bmj.e256

28. Task Force Members, Montalescot, G., Sechtem, U., Achenbach, S., Andreotti, F., et al.: 2013 ESC guidelines on the management of stable coronary artery disease: the task force on the management of stable coronary artery disease of the European Society of Cardiology. Eur. Heart J. **34**(38), 2949–3003 (2013). https://doi.org/10.1093/eurheartj/eht296

29. Vanhees, L., et al.: Importance of characteristics and modalities of physical activity and exercise in the management of cardiovascular health in individuals with cardiovascular risk factors: recommendations from the EACPR (part II). Eur. J. Prev. Cardiol. **19**(5), 1005–1033 (2012)

CovidAlert - A Wristwatch-Based System to Alert Users from Face Touching

Mrinmoy Roy, Venkata Devesh Reddy Seethi, and Pratool Bharti[✉]

Northern Illinois University, Dekalb, IL 60115, USA
{mroy,devesh,pbharti}@niu.edu

Abstract. Worldwide 219 million people have been infected and 4.5 million have lost their lives in ongoing Covid-19 pandemic. Until vaccines became widely available, precautions and safety measures like wearing masks, physical distancing, avoiding face touching were some of the primary means to curb the spread of virus. Face touching is a compulsive human behavior that can not be prevented without constantly making a conscious effort, even then it is inevitable. To address this problem, we have designed a smartwatch-based solution, CovidAlert, that leverages Random Forest algorithm trained on accelerometer and gyroscope data from the smartwatch to detect hand transition to face and sends a quick haptic alert to the users. CovidAlert is highly energy efficient as it employs STA/LTA algorithm as a gatekeeper to curtail the usage of Random Forest model on the watch when user is inactive. The overall accuracy of system is 88.4% with low false negatives and false positives. We also demonstrated the system viability by implementing it on a commercial Fossil Gen 5 smartwatch.

Keywords: Covid-19 · CovidAlert model · Sensors · Machine learning · STA/LTA algorithm · Hand to face transition dataset · Smartwatch

1 Introduction

Compulsive human behaviors and habits such as face touching cause self inoculation of germs/viruses that may lead to the contraction of influenza or a viral disease [1]. Needless to say, they have the potential to cause severe harm to individual and public health. As witnessed in the ongoing Coronavirus disease 2019 (Covid-19) pandemic, so far 219 million people have got infected while 4.5 million people have lost their lives globally [2]. Up until vaccines were widely available, safety precautions such as wearing masks, maintaining physical distance, and avoiding face touching were the primary means to reduce the spread of virus in the ongoing pandemic [3]. Although a person could make a conscious effort to wear the mask regularly, it is not comfortable to use them continuously for longer periods of time [4]. Face touching is a repetitive habit often done unconsciously

© ICST Institute for Computer Sciences, Social Informatics and Telecommunications Engineering 2022
Published by Springer Nature Switzerland AG 2022. All Rights Reserved
H. Lewy and R. Barkan (Eds.): PH 2021, LNICST 431, pp. 489–504, 2022.
https://doi.org/10.1007/978-3-030-99194-4_30

that makes it difficult to overcome such habit [5]. Therefore, correction of such behavior requires an intervention tool that is readily accessible, accurate, fast enough to detect face touching in real time, and provides convenience of use.

It is important to remember that face touching is often unanticipated that emphasizes the solution to be pervasive and convenient to use for a longer period [6]. With the recent technological advancements and ever increasing popularity across all age groups, smartwatches are a right fit to base the desired solution. Modern smartwatches are equipped with larger memory, storage, and sensors such as accelerometer and gyroscope, that has made them increasingly capable of handling machine learning applications onboard without requiring the need to interface between a smartphone or a cloud computing system to offload computation-intensive tasks. This opens an avenue to integrate and deploy human activity recognition (HAR)-based algorithms on the wrist that can track the user's hand movement in near real time and raise an alarm. A smartwatch can raise an alarm in various forms such as with a visual notification, audio cue, or through the sense of touch. Out of the three possible ways, haptic feedback (through sense of touch) such as vibration can immediately draw the attention of user right before their attempt to touch the face [7]. A gentle and short vibration is also immune to external noise and lighting conditions [8], and less distracting to other people around. In this work, we explore the challenges and their solutions in designing a smartwatch-based alarm system that can alert the user right before face touching.

2   Challenges and Contributions

Although the current work appears like a classic application of human activity recognition (HAR) system, it has its own unique challenges. First and foremost, generally a HAR system requires the activity to be detected once it is performed, but in the current work, touching the face must be detected right before its completion as it may be too late by then. Hence, the system must be designed to detect the activities while in transition. Second, collecting and tagging the sensory data when the activity is in transition requires considerably more complex manual work than completed activities. Third, error in activity detection must be low especially the false negatives (predicting not touching the face when it actually happens) as it can be catastrophic. Even though false positive error is undesirable, it has lesser consequences than false negatives. Fourth, to make this system practical it ought to be very efficient to execute on a resource scarce device without depleting much of their energy.

To overcome these challenges, we have used a pervasive wrist-worn device that beeps and vibrates when the transition of hand to face activity is detected. We used a medical-grade pervasive device, Shimmer [9], to collect the sensory data to train and test our proposed system. Additionally, we exhibited a working demo of our system on a consumer-grade Fossil smartwatch. The major contributions of our work are as follows.

- Designed a wristwatch-based alarming system that alerts the user from touching their face. The overall accuracy of our system is 88.4% for train-test-split and 70.3% for leave-one-out approach.
- Employed a highly efficient STA/LTA algorithm to reduce the system energy consumption significantly by only activating the Random Forest model when the user's hand is in active state.
- Prepared a transitional dataset [10] manually tagged with the ground truth activities. We believe our sensory dataset is first of its kind and will be very useful for the HAR research community.
- Explored polynomial interaction of statistical features and reported the most important ones.
- Implemented the system on off-the-shelf commercial Fossils smartwatch to validate the practicality.

3 Related Works

Human activity recognition (HAR) applications are exceedingly popular in tracking personal health with the evolution of modern commercial smartwatches. Currently, Apple and Android watch users can precisely track various activities, including stand, walk, run and other physical exercises throughout the day. In research, smartwatch-based HAR system have been explored for elderly assistance [11], detection of self-harming activities in psychiatric facilities [12], distracted driving [13], smoking activities [14], speed detection [15] and more. In this section, we have discussed only recent works related to face touching activities in the context of Covid-19 pandemic.

In response to the global health emergency of Covid-19 outbreak, several researchers have designed wearable devices based on HAR solutions to reduce the spreading of harmful viruses by preventing face touching activities. Among several recent works, D'Aurizio et al. [16] is able to estimate hand proximity to face and notify the user whenever a face touch movement is detected. They have discussed two different approaches - using only accelerometer and the combination of accelerometer and magnetometer. The study showed that using accelerometer and magnetometer together decreases the false positive rate from 38.1% to 3.2% in face touch detection. Although their solution improves the false positive rate to an impressive 3.2%, it requires the user to constantly wear a magnetic necklace that might not be readily accessible/acceptable to the users limiting its practical usage. Additionally, this work doesn't discuss false negative rates which are much more crucial than false positive rates. While high false positive rate might annoy users by raising false alarms, high false negative rates can be catastrophic as system will not raise alert even in case of face touching event.

Another work in this context was published by Kakaraparthi et al. [17] where they have designed an ear-worn system to detect facial touches. The system uses signals from thermal image and electromyography (EMG) sensors to train a deep learning model and achieved 83.4% accuracy in detecting face touching and 90.1% accuracy in face zone detection. Physiological signal from EMG sensor and thermal features are merged to train a Convolutional Neural Network (CNN) for the classification. While their system has achieved high accuracy, it requires the user to wear it on ear constantly which is not very pervasive or comfortable. Also, the system is reliant on another device for hosting the deep learning models that might introduce communication latency.

Authors of Sudharsan et al. [18] leveraged the combination of four sensors: accelerometer, gyroscope, pressure, and rotation vector for continuous monitoring of arm to detect face touching activity. One class classification models of this study, achieves the highest 0.93 F1 score using only accelerometer data, and Convolutional Neural Network models achieves 0.89 F1 score using accelerometer and gyroscope data. Since, their system is trained and tested on only four persons data, it requires performance analysis on larger dataset. Additionally, power consumption is not discussed which is very crucial for the viability of the application.

In [7], Michelin et al. proposed a wearable system that alerts user when they attempt to touch their face. Their system streams data from inertial sensors on a wristband and employs a 1D-Convolutional Neural Network (CNN) that achieved 92% accuracy to detect face touching activities. Additionally, the authors compared user response times from three sensory feedback modalities: visual, auditory, and vibrotactile and observed that vibrotactile feedback had shortest response time of 427.3 ms. However, the study did not discuss the challenges of real-life implementation and feasibility of implementing computationally intensive CNN algorithms on resource-constrained wrist-worn devices.

Overall, we observed in recent works that they are short in at least one of the following categories - pervasiveness of device, discussion over false negative rates, energy-efficient algorithms, real-life implementation, and size of dataset. In this work, we have attempted to fill these gaps by leveraging an efficient STA/LTA [19] and Random Forest [20] algorithms on smartwatch to design a system that can accurately detect the face touching activities while managing energy efficiency.

3.1   Dataset Preparation

In this section, we describe different parts of data collection procedure including wearable sensors, sensing modalities, sampling rate, data annotation and recorded relevant activities. Our dataset is publicly made available on GitHub [10].

Wearable Device. We used Shimmer wearable sensing device [9] for collecting sensory data while tied on the subject's wrist. It has ample processing power along with several multi-modal sensing units. Shimmer is integrated with TI MSP430 microcontroller with 24 MHz CPU and 16 KB RAM. It contains 11 channels of 12 bit A/D with 32 GB memory resources and 3.7 V, 450 mAh re-chargeable lithium polymer battery. It uses class 2 Bluetooth 2.1 for live streaming sensory data to a smartphone. The device and the Android application used to capture sensory data is shown in Fig. 1.

Participant Recruitment. We obtained permission from the Institutional Review Board at Northern Illinois University (NIU) to facilitate the experiment.

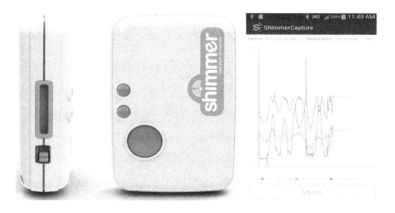

Fig. 1. Shimmer device (on left), screenshot of Shimmer Capture Android application (on right).

We recruited 10 participants (2 female and 8 male) from NIU. All participants were healthy individuals and gave their written consent before data collection. On average, our participants belonged to an age group of $(34 \pm 11$ years) and had an average height of $(170 \pm 12$ cm). Since we conducted the experiment during the ongoing pandemic, we strictly followed the Covid-19 protocols such as wearing masks, sanitizing frequently touched spaces, and maintaining social distancing. However, these protocols did not affect the procedures of our study. At the beginning of each data collection session, we secured the Shimmer device on the participant's preferred wrist. Shimmer device has been used extensively in healthcare-related research studies [21,22]. We leveraged the tri-axial accelerometer (captures acceleration in x-, y-, and z-direction) and tri-axial gyroscope (captures angular velocities in yaw, roll, and pitch directions) from the Shimmer device. The accelerometer sensor in Shimmer cancels the gravitational effects and captures low noise acceleration for the accelerometer. We sampled both sensors with a sampling rate of 102.4 Hz to obtain high-resolution data.

To estimate if we have collected enough data from participants, we conducted a study based on principal component analysis (PCA) [23] on the 340 statistical polynomial features generated from accelerometer and gyroscope data (please refer to Sect. 4.3 for details on feature generation). Briefly, PCA takes features as input and builds a covariance matrix where the eigenvalues represent principal components (PCs). Usually, the higher the variance in dataset, the more the variance is distributed among PCs and the lower the variance percentage captured by the first principal components. We can generate n upto number of PCs that are mutually orthogonal from a dataset with n features. We plotted the Fig. 2 by taking data from 1 to 10 participants (on x-axis) and the variance percentage of the first principal component (on y-axis). It was observed that variance percentage decreased from 1 participant data to 2 participants data and remained constant up to 8 participants data. It shows that adding more participants doesn't increase the variance in the dataset significantly. Therefore, we used 10 participants to capture higher variance as seen in real-life data.

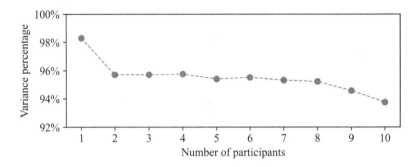

Fig. 2. Maximum percentage of variance captured by the first principal component when combining data from different number of participants.

Sensory Data Collection and Annotation. We collected data from 10 participants in two categories: face touching and no-face touching. Activities under these two categories are delineated in Table 1. While face touching activities consist of touching different parts of the face such as nose, mouth, left eye, and right eye; the no-face touching category comprised of scratching head, picking up an item on the floor, reaching for a shelf, and maintaining a stance (sitting, standing, and walking). Participants repeated each activity in three stances: sitting on chair, standing, and walking. Hence, each participant participated in 24 sessions to capture data from 8 activities across all 3 stances. In each session, participants repetitively engaged in an activity for at least 30 s or until they repeated same activity 18 times. Participants were allowed to choose their sequence of activities to complete the 24 sessions. On average, they took 15–20 min to complete 24 sessions. We encouraged the participants to take breaks during or at the end of each session, and in break time, data collection was paused and resumed soon after. We also asked them to engage in natural activities in any way they wished, such as listening to music, watching a video, or conversing with someone. We ensured that participants acted naturally, resulting in a dataset as close to the real world as possible. Annotating the sensory data with their ground truth activity was challenging since the main goal is to detect the face touching activity before it gets completed, i.e., in the transition. To do so, we streamed the sensory data from the Shimmer device to an Android smartphone using the Shimmer Capture application [9] on the phone using shimmer capture application (as shown in Fig. 1). We adopted a semi-supervised annotation technique to capture the ground truths. Hence, we developed a Python application to annotate each session on the fly whether the participant was in transition or engaged in the activity. The application takes our annotations and aligns them with the raw data files by matching their timestamps. We present an example for "touching left eye while standing" activity in Fig. 3. The figure

Table 1. Face touching and no-face touching activities in our data collection protocol.

No-face touching	Face touching
Scratch head	Touching left eye
Pick item from an overhead shelf	Touching right eye
Pick item from the ground	Touching nose
Stance (sitting, standing, walking)	Touching mouth

highlights the regions of interest with gray and pink hues, which denote that the participant's hand is transitioning to touch the left eye and the hand is in contact with the left eye. It is crucial to detect a face touching activity before it happens. Therefore our novel annotation approach makes our dataset superior to the datasets in previous studies that don't have annotations for transition to face. Since our dataset captures the transition to touch and contact phases, researchers can choose to train their models only on transition data. We made our dataset publicly available in GitHub [10].

Post data collection, we cleansed the data by discarding 2.5 s of raw data from the start and end of each session. As a next step, we visually inspected all samples by plotting the raw data from the accelerometer and the gyroscope overlayed with transition and contact phases (as shown in Fig. 3). We promptly deleted samples detected with inconsistencies in annotations. Finally, we extracted only transitional data to train and evaluate our system.

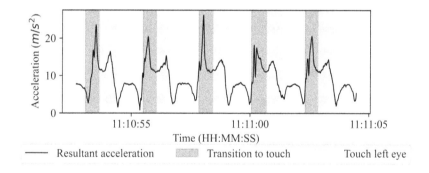

Fig. 3. Resultant acceleration plotted for touching left eye while standing. The gray and pink hues indicate transition to touch and contact phases, respectively. (Color figure online)

4   Our Proposed Method

In this section, we introduce the system workflow for CovidAlert and explain the functions of each module in detail. As shown in Fig. 4, our system streams raw accelerometer and gyroscope data from the Shimmer device and passes it to the STA/LTA triggering algorithm, which acts as a gatekeeper and is in continuous reception mode. The rationale behind STA/LTA algorithm is that when the arm is not moving, it can not touch the face. The triggering algorithm measures the energy of signals using resultant acceleration to determine if the participant's arm is in active or dormant state. If the dormant state is detected, signals are blocked and do not pass forward. However, when an active state is detected, STA/LTA allows the data to pass to Random Forest (RF) module for final classification. If and when the trained RF algorithm anticipates that the user's hand is transitioning to face touch, system alerts the user with the haptic feedback. STA/LTA algorithm is much less computationally extensive than the RF, and effectively it saves significant energy by minimizing the usage of RF algorithm.

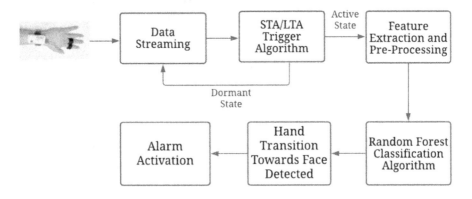

Fig. 4. System workflow of CovidAlert.

4.1   Data Streaming

The role of data streaming module is straight forward. It continuously captures the tri-axial accelerometer and gyroscope sensory data from Shimmer device and passes it to the STA/LTA triggering algorithm. The sampling frequency of both sensors are fixed at 102.4 Hz.

4.2   STA/LTA Triggering Algorithm

One of the biggest challenges in implementing any sophisticated ML solutions on smartwatch is its excessive energy consumption [24]. If we simply implement our ML-based solution on the smartwatch, it will most likely deplete the battery in 3–4 h, making the solution impractical for real-life usage. To make the solution viable, we employed Short-Time-Average/Long-Time-Average (STA/LTA) algorithm as a gatekeeper in our system which selectively decides when to use the ML algorithm instead of always utilizing it. The motive behind STA/LTA is to save the smartwatch energy by not using ML models when the person's arm is in dormant state. It determines the active/dormant state by using short time and long time windows. STA/LTA algorithm is used in seismology to detect the intensity of earthquakes [19]. In healthcare application, Bharti et al. [12] have leveraged the algorithm to detect self-harm activity in psychiatric facilities.

Taking a real-life scenario where a student attends a lecture, as long as the student is seated with no hand movements, the STA/LTA does not trigger. But, as soon as the student moves their hand to touch the face, the STA/LTA triggers an active state and opens the gate for the ML algorithm for activity recognition. In this manner, STA/LTA module regulates the usage of computationally intensive activity recognition modules and optimizes our CovidAlert to be highly energy-efficient for resource-scarce smartwatches.

The algorithm takes resultant acceleration (A_{xyz}) as input and calculates the mean (μ) of acceleration, over the Long Term Window (T_{lta}) as $L_a = \mu(A_{res}[T_{lta}])$. Similarly, the mean of acceleration, for the Short Term Window, (T_{sta}) as $S_a = \mu(A_{res}[T_{sta}])$. When a person's arm remains dormant, both long and short term window has similar energy, hence the ratio typically ranges close to 1. On the other hand, if the person's arm move suddenly, energy of short term window increases compared to long term window. This means $S_a >> L_a$ or $S_a/L_a >> 1$. When the ratio becomes greater than 1, the triggering algorithm identifies that person is in active state and allows the signals to pass on ML algorithms for final classification. While, length of long term window ranges around 30–60 s, typically short term window length is 0.5–1 s.

4.3   Preprocessing and Feature Extraction

In this module, we process the raw data to adapt it for machine learning classifier in three stages: 1) segmenting the raw data in sliding windows 2) computing relevant statistical features on segmented windows that have enough discriminative information to classify face/no-face touching activities 3) generating additional polynomial features from the interaction of features computed in stage 2.

In the first stage, we experimented with different window sizes in the range of 0.2–0.8 s. The correct window size is critical in this work because a longer window may fail as users can comfortably touch their faces within one window. Again, if the window is too small, it may not capture the relevant patterns and cause larger false positive errors that may annoy the user. To find the optimal window size, we trained an RF algorithm for different window sizes and reported their accuracies in Fig. 5. We observed the accuracy of RF increased from 82.1% for 0.2 s window upto 86.5% for 0.4 s window. The highest accuracy was achieved, 88%, for 0.7 s. However, we still opted for 0.4 s window as it was large enough to capture slow transitions and small enough to capture swift movements without overlapping with other activities. We then segmented transition parts from each activity in 0.4 length segments. Simply processing raw data from each window requires a large and complex machine learning/neural network algorithms to uncover the hidden patterns that demands higher computing resources. Smartwatches, however, cannot handle such complex models due to their limited processing and battery resources. Therefore, we chose 9 simple but relevant statistical features

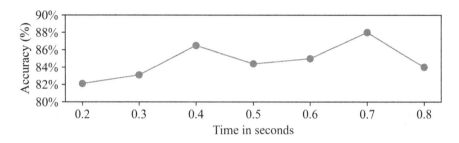

Fig. 5. Performance of RF algorithm for window sizes in the range of 0.2–0.8 s.

(listed in Table 2) that are emblematic to the raw data. Out of the 9 core features, the first 6 features are generic for HAR applications features such as minimum, maximum, mean, 25th percentile, 75th percentile, and standard deviation [25]. These 6 features together can effectively communicate the range of values in each axis of the signal. Next, we wanted to use features that represented the qualities of distribution. For this reason, we used skewness and kurtosis that measure the deviation of the data from normal distribution and the tailedness of the data. These two features together give us information about outliers in the given sample and the presence of sudden movements. Finally, we incorporated auto correlation sequence as a feature which finds the correlation with a given vector itself. The correlation score can be used to identify static activities such as standing and sitting and periodic activities such as walking. These statistical features were computed for the three axes of two sensors i.e., accelerometer and gyroscope that generated $9 \times 2 \times 3 = 54$ features.

We also generated polynomial features that project the feature space into higher dimensions by learning a polynomial function of degree 2. This generates interactive features by taking pairs of features at a time that helps discover any non-linear interactions occurring in different features. As a result, we obtained 1540 polynomial features from the 54 statistical features. Finally, we ranked the features according to random forest feature importance and selected a smaller subset of features with comparable accuracy.

4.4   Random Forest (RF) Classifier

We first experimented with different machine learning algorithms with all 1540 polynomial features. We evaluated each algorithm using 80:20 train-test-split and leave-one-out strategies. In train-test-split, 80% data is used in training the model and 20% for evaluation. On the other hand, leave-one-out selects one participant at a time for testing and remaining nine participants data for training and repeats this process for all ten participants in our dataset. The final accuracy score for leave-one-out is the mean of accuracies for all ten participants. We present the accuracies for logistic regression, gaussian support vector machine, decision tree, random forest (RF), and extreme gradient boosting (XGBoost) in Fig. 6. Train-test-split and leave-one-out metrics are shown in Fig. 6. While

Table 2. Nine statistical features and their descriptions.

Feature	Description
Minimum value, maximum value, mean	$\min(x)$, $\max(x)$, $\mu = \text{mean}(x)$
25th percentile	$Q1 =$ Feature value dividing first and second quartiles
75th percentile	$Q3 =$ Feature value dividing third and fourth quartiles
Standard deviation	$\sqrt{\sum (x_i - \mu)^2 / N}$
Skewness	$\sum (x_i - \mu)^3 / N \times \sigma^3$
Kurtosis	$\sum (x_i - \mu)^4 / N \times \sigma^4$
Auto correlation sequence	Correlation of x with delayed sample of x

both RF and XGBoost exhibit superior performance than other classifiers, RF is easier to train and faster compare to XGBoost, hence we picked RF for this study.

RF is one of the simplest but powerful machine learning algorithm. It is an efficient ensemble learning algorithm widely used in numerous recent research studies and real-life applications [26]. RF is an extension of the bagging method that combines several randomized decision trees to create a forest of trees. Each tree in the forest completes the prediction task individually and the predicted class with the most votes are selected as the model prediction. The algorithm is versatile enough to deal with both classification and regression tasks. Since, RF is combination of decision trees, it has a set of hyperparameters to tune for optimizing the performance such as number of trees, maximum number of features used for single tree, minimum number of samples required for a leaf, depth of tree and more. The most important part of training a RF algorithm is to find the optimal hyperparameters which can be done quickly and effectively by using randomized grid search technique [27].

In this work, we trained an RF algorithm to classify between face/no-face touching activities. First we divided our dataset into training and testing where 80% data is used in training the model and 20% for evaluation purpose. Then, 5 fold cross validation with randomized grid search is applied for finding the best set of parameters having the best performance score. The optimal parameters were found as bootstrap random sampling = False, maximum depth of tree = 10, minimum samples required for a leaf = 5, minimum samples required to split a node = 20 and number of trees in a forest = 150. We also extracted feature importance learned by RF to measure the contribution of each feature while making the final decision.

Table 3. Selected hyperparameters for RF using randomized grid search.

Hyperparameter	Value
Maximum depth of tree	10
Minimum samples per leaf	5
Minimum samples to split a node	20
Number of trees in forest	150
Bootstrap random sampling	False

5   Results

We trained our RF classifier using the optimal hyperparameters selected from randomized grid search. These hyperparameters are listed in Table 3. We employed two evaluation strategies: train-test-split with 80%–20% train to test split ratio and leave-one-out where repeatedly one participant data is left for the test. In train-test-split, our dataset of 4271 records (2080 no-face touch, 2191 face touch) is split into 3416 training records (1675 no-face touching, 1741 face touching) and 855 testing records (405 no-face touching, 450 face touching). The RF accuracy on the testing dataset using all 1540 features is 88.7%.

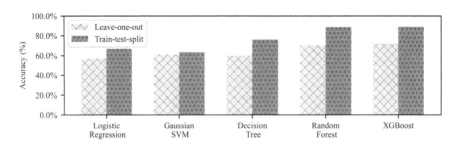

Fig. 6. Accuracy for different algorithms using leave-one-out and train-test-split evaluation strategies.

Although we achieved an impressive result, the model used a large number of features which could be energy intensive to compute especially when deployed on smartwatch. Therefore, to pick minimal number of features that are highly discriminative between the face touch and no-face touch activities, we first ranked all features using RF feature importance [20] and sorted them based on their importance scores. Then, starting from the top 10 features upto 1540 features, we iterated in the steps of 10 features, retrained RF algorithm at each step and cataloged the accuracy score as shown in Fig. 7. We found that the RF algorithm by just using the top 340 achieved 88.4% which was comparable to performance for RF when trained with all 1540 features. In case of leave-one-out approach, though overall mean accuracy is 70.3%, the highest accuracy for a single participant is reported at 87.7%. Although accuracy helps us to gauge the algorithm's efficiency, it does not show us the number of false negatives and false positives. As low false negatives are very critical to the application, to measure it, we plotted the confusion matrices in Fig. 8 for RF trained on 340 features for train-test-split and leave-one-out strategies.

The count of false negatives and false positives were higher in case of leave-one-out than in train-test-split evaluation. However, the number of test samples in leave-one-out evaluation were higher therefore we compare the false positive rate (FPR) and false negative rates (FNR) in both cases. FPR is the ratio of false positives and total negative samples. Similarly, FNR is the ratio of false negatives to total positive samples. In train-test-split, we achieved FPR and FNR of 15.5% and 10% respectively. On the other hand, leave-one-out strategy had FPR and FNR of 27% and 31.7%, respectively. As we observe that FPR is higher than FNR for leave-one-out evaluation, this is primarily due to the variance in data from different users.

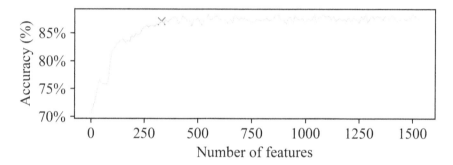

Fig. 7. Accuracy of RF taking the features sorted based on their importance scores in the increments of 10. The red cross was picked using elbow method which indicates that the top 340 features are sufficient to give good results. (Color figure online)

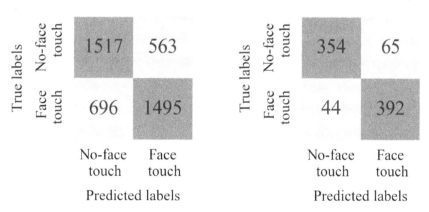

Fig. 8. Confusion matrices for RF trained on 340 important features using leave-one-out (on left) and train-test-split (on right) strategies.

6   CovidAlert Demo on Commercial Fossils Watch

We implemented CovidAlert on a commercial Fossil Gen 5 smartwatch to validate the practicality of the solution (as shown in Fig. 9). To do so, we evaluated
the duration of time taken to deplete the battery completely in three different
scenarios. In all 3 scenarios, the RF model was working without any STA/LTA
gatekeeping. The first scenario was a control test where the watch was kept on
a plain surface without any movement for the complete duration. It took 6 h
before the battery depleted. In second test, the watch was worn on wrist while
doing regular activity that took 4 h before battery was depleted. In third test, we
disabled the connection to the phone paired to the watch, and enabled airplane
mode restricting the watches Wi-Fi, and Bluetooth abilities. These restrictions
allowed the application to run for 5 h. Simply running STA/LTA algorithm on
accelerometer data allows the watch to run for 12 h before depleting the battery.
Higher usage of STA/LTA will save greater amount of energy by keeping the RF
model idle for longer period.

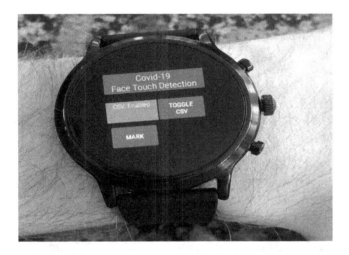

Fig. 9. CovidAlert application on Fossil Gen 5 smartwatch.

7   Conclusion and Future Works

In this paper, we described a smartwatch-based solution to classify transition of
hand to face/no-face touching activities. We employed STA/LTA algorithm to
act as a gatekeeper to significantly reduce the usage of computational extensive
RF models on the watch by keeping it idle when the user is inactive. Our system
is fast in detecting the activity in transition as it requires only 0.4 s of data
to provide its prediction. The overall system accuracy for train-test-split and
leave-one-out evaluation strategy is 88.4% and 70.3%, respectively, with low
false negatives rates. We believe our system is practical and can be used in real

life as a safety measure to protect ourselves from self-inoculation of infectious disease like Covid-19. We also implemented CovidAlert on a commercial Fossil Gen 5 smartwatch and discussed its viability.

In future, we would like to collect feedback from a larger population to improve its practicality. We also want to include more similar kinds of activities to further reduce the false negative and false positive rates. Additionally, we want our system to become smarter by prompting users to wash their hands by automatically detecting activities like a handshake or returning home from outdoors.

References

1. Macias, A.E., De la Torre, A., Moreno-Espinosa, S., Leal, P.E., Bourlon, M.T., Ruiz-Palacios, G.M.: Controlling the novel A (H1N1) influenza virus: don't touch your face! J. Hosp. Infect. **73**(3), 280–281 (2009)
2. WHO COVID-19 Dashboard, September 2021. https://covid19.who.int/
3. Gudi, S.K., Tiwari, K.K.: Preparedness and lessons learned from the novel coronavirus disease. Int. J. Occup. Environ. Med. **11**(2), 108 (2020)
4. Does wearing a mask for long periods of time affect the brain causing lethargy, headache, and dizziness because of lack of oxygen?, July 2020. https://health-desk.org/articles/does-wearing-a-mask-for-long-periods-of-time-affect-the-brain-causing-lethargy-headache-and-dizziness-because-of-lack-of-oxygen/
5. Duarte, F.: How to avoid touching your face so much, March 2020. https://www.bbc.com/future/article/20200317-how-to-stop-touching-your-face/
6. Didehbani, N.: Why we touch our faces so much – and how to break the habit, March 2020. https://utswmed.org/medblog/why-we-touch-our-faces-so-much-and-how-break-habit/
7. Michelin, A.M., et al.: FaceGuard: a wearable system to avoid face touching. Front. Robot. AI **8**, 47 (2021)
8. Exler, A., Dinse, C., Günes, Z., Hammoud, N., Mattes, S., Beigl, M.: Investigating the perceptibility different notification types on smartphones depending on the smartphone position. In: Proceedings of the 2017 ACM International Joint Conference on Pervasive and Ubiquitous Computing and Proceedings of the 2017 ACM International Symposium on Wearable Computers, pp. 970–976 (2017)
9. Burns, A., et al.: Shimmer^{TM}-a wireless sensor platform for noninvasive biomedical research. IEEE Sens. J. **10**(9), 1527–1534 (2010)
10. CovidAlert dataset (2021). https://github.com/rdverse/CovidAlert
11. Lutze, R., Waldhör, K.: Personal health assistance for elderly people via smartwatch based motion analysis. In: 2017 IEEE International Conference on Healthcare Informatics (ICHI), pp. 124–133 (2017)
12. Bharti, P., Panwar, A., Gopalakrishna, G., Chellappan, S.: Watch-dog: detecting self-harming activities from wrist worn accelerometers. IEEE J. Biomed. Health Inform. **22**(3), 686–696 (2018)
13. Goel, B., Dey, A.K., Bharti, P., Ahmed, K.B., Chellappan, S.: Detecting distracted driving using a wrist-worn wearable. In: IEEE International Conference on Pervasive Computing and Communications Workshops, pp. 233–238 (2018)
14. Shoaib, M., Bosch, S., Scholten, H., Havinga, P.J.M., Incel, O.D.: Towards detection of bad habits by fusing smartphone and smartwatch sensors. In: 2015 IEEE International Conference on Pervasive Computing and Communication Workshops, pp. 591–596 (2015)

15. Seethi, V.D.R., Bharti, P.: CNN-based speed detection algorithm for walking and running using wrist-worn wearable sensors. In: 2020 IEEE International Conference on Smart Computing, pp. 278–283. IEEE (2020)
16. D'Aurizio, N., Baldi, T.L., Paolocci, G., Prattichizzo, D.: Preventing undesired face-touches with wearable devices and haptic feedback. IEEE Access **8**, 139033–139043 (2020)
17. Kakaraparthi, V., et al.: FaceSense: sensing face touch with an ear-worn system. Proc. ACM Interact. Mob. Wearable Ubiquit. Technol. **5**(3), 1–27 (2021)
18. Sudharsan, B., Sundaram, D., Breslin, J.G., Ali, M.I.: Avoid touching your face: a hand-to-face 3D motion dataset (COVID-away) and trained models for smart-watches. In: 10th International Conference on the Internet of Things Companion, IoT 2020 Companion. Association for Computing Machinery, New York (2020)
19. Trnkoczy, A.: Understanding and parameter setting of STA/LTA trigger algorithm. In: New Manual of Seismological Observatory Practice (NMSOP), pp. 1–20. Deutsches GeoForschungsZentrum GFZ (2009)
20. Breiman, L.: Random forests. Mach. Learn. **45**(1), 5–32 (2001)
21. Greene, B.R., O'Donovan, A., Romero-Ortuno, R., Cogan, L., Scanaill, C.N., Kenny, R.A.: Quantitative falls risk assessment using the timed up and go test. IEEE Trans. Biomed. Eng. **57**(12), 2918–2926 (2010)
22. Greene, B.R., McGrath, D., O'Neill, R., O'Donovan, K.J., Burns, A., Caulfield, B.: An adaptive gyroscope-based algorithm for temporal gait analysis. Med. Biol. Eng. Comput. **48**(12), 1251–1260 (2010)
23. Wold, S., Esbensen, K., Geladi, P.: Principal component analysis. Chemom. Intell. Lab. Syst. **2**(1–3), 37–52 (1987)
24. Weiss, G.M., Timko, J.L., Gallagher, C.M., Yoneda, K., Schreiber, A.J.: Smartwatch-based activity recognition: a machine learning approach. In: 2016 IEEE-EMBS International Conference on Biomedical and Health Informatics, pp. 426–429. IEEE (2016)
25. Casale, P., Pujol, O., Radeva, P.: Human activity recognition from accelerometer data using a wearable device. In: Vitrià, J., Sanches, J.M., Hernández, M. (eds.) IbPRIA 2011. LNCS, vol. 6669, pp. 289–296. Springer, Heidelberg (2011). https://doi.org/10.1007/978-3-642-21257-4_36
26. Oshiro, T.M., Perez, P.S., Baranauskas, J.A.: How many trees in a random forest? In: Perner, P. (ed.) MLDM 2012. LNCS (LNAI), vol. 7376, pp. 154–168. Springer, Heidelberg (2012). https://doi.org/10.1007/978-3-642-31537-4_13
27. Probst, P., Wright, M.N., Boulesteix, A.-L.: Hyperparameters and tuning strategies for random forest. Wiley Interdisc. Rev. Data Min. Knowl. Discov. **9**(3), e1301 (2019)

Towards Diagnostic Support of Hyperactivity in Adults with ADHD Using a Virtual Reality Based Continuous Performance Test and Motion Sensor Data

Tobias Delcour Jensen, Weronika Katarzyna Korbutt, Georgi Petrov Nedelev, and Brian Bemman(✉)

Department of Architecture, Design and Media Technology, Aalborg University, Rendsburggade 14, 9000 Aalborg, Denmark
bb@create.aau.dk

Abstract. Attention Deficit Hyperactivity Disorder (ADHD) is a neurodevelopmental condition that affects up to 5% of adults worldwide. Recent research has suggested that diagnostic support technologies for ADHD may be less effective for adults while many focus on identifying attention deficits, leaving assessments of hyperactivity largely to subjective criteria and observations by clinicians. In this paper, we present a virtual reality (VR) based continuous performance test (CPT) intended to provide users with an attention task, during which their physical movements are measured by the system's sensors, within an environment designed to resemble a real-world situation in which symptoms of ADHD would typically manifest. The design of this virtual environment was informed through a series of interviews and collaborative design sessions with clinicians. The VR-CPT system was tested using 20 adult participants with and without ADHD in order to determine which of any single or combined measures of motion by sensor (head-mounted display, arm controller, leg controller) and inertial variable (acceleration, velocity, angular acceleration, angular velocity) can be used to distinguish the two groups. Our results indicate that of our single measures, angular velocity across all sensors, angular acceleration of the leg controller, and velocity of the arm controller proved significant. Additionally, isolating high levels of mean motion activity, as measured by our combined inertial variables measure for a single sensor, proved insufficient at distinguishing between motion activity events corresponding to observations of physical movements considered indicative of hyperactivity and events considered non-indicative by a clinician.

Keywords: ADHD · Hyperactivity · Diagnostic support · Virtual reality · Continuous performance test · Motion sensor data

© ICST Institute for Computer Sciences, Social Informatics and Telecommunications Engineering 2022
Published by Springer Nature Switzerland AG 2022. All Rights Reserved
H. Lewy and R. Barkan (Eds.): PH 2021, LNICST 431, pp. 505–521, 2022.
https://doi.org/10.1007/978-3-030-99194-4_31

1   Introduction

Attention Deficit Hyperactivity Disorder (ADHD) is an often debilitating chronic neurodevelopmental and behavioral disorder often identified in childhood and which frequently persists into adulthood [5]. The world-wide prevalence of ADHD is estimated to be approximately 5.3% in children and adolescents and anywhere between 3–5% in adults depending on reported demographics [8]. The primary clinical signs of ADHD, namely, impulsivity, inattention, and hyperactivity, manifest differently for adults and change with time. In the case of hyperactivity, while children may engage in, for example, uncontrolled running or climbing, adults may experience restlessness [8], excessive talking, an unorganized lifestyle, or the need to be constantly busy [22]. Due to the varied nature of how adult hyperactivity may manifest, doctors risk misdiagnosis [5].

Diagnosing ADHD typically involves lengthy assessments by psychologists and doctors through various clinical assessments (e.g., observations), self-reported rating scales, interviews, and computerized assessment tools, such as continuous performance tests [14]), with recommended diagnoses frequently supported by criteria specified in e.g., the Diagnostic and Statistical Manual of Mental Disorders (DSM-5) or the International Statistical Classification of Diseases and Related Health Problems (ICD-10) for ADHD [5]. Unfortunately, many of these assessments remain subjective in nature and their use differs from clinic to clinic, making rigorous and consistent diagnosis challenging. Moreover, many of the existing assessment tools based on computerized CPTs used in practice assess attention deficits and not hyperactivity while further having varying success with adults [3,14]. In recent years, however, widely available virtual reality (VR) and motion sensing technologies have shown promising results for use in diagnosis support for ADHD due, in particular, to their ability to provide more immersive experiences [1,9] and collect more sensitive measurements of bodily movement [12,18,19], respectively. A systematic integration of both a VR-based CPT and analysis of relevant bodily movements captured by various sensor measurements of a VR system for distinguishing adult ADHD hyperactivity, however, remains a problem worth continued exploration.

In this paper, we present a VR-based continuous performance test (VR-CPT) intended to provide users with an attention task, through which their physical arm, leg, and head movements are measured by the system's sensors, within an immersive environment designed to resemble a real-world situation in which symptoms of ADHD would typically manifest. Importantly, the design of this virtual environment was informed by consultations with expert clinicians having experience in the diagnosis of ADHD in adults. In our evaluation with the VR-CPT system, we carried out two tests in order to determine: (1) which of any single or combined measures of motion by sensor (head-mounted display (HMD), arm controller, leg controller) and inertial variable (acceleration, velocity, angular acceleration, angular velocity) can be used to distinguish between participants with and without ADHD, and (2) the extent to which significant motion activity events, as measured by our combined inertial variables measure for a single sensor, align with observations of physical movements indicative of hyperactivity by clinicians. In Sect. 2, we describe the current process of clinically diagnosing ADHD and provide an overview of different technological approaches that have previously been employed in the screening and diagnosis of ADHD. Section 3 details the findings from our semi-structured interviews with expert clinicians that informed the design of our VR-CPT system environment and evaluation criteria. Section 4 explains the design of the virtual environment of our VR-CPT system based on these interviews and a series of collaborative design sessions with the same clinicians. In Sect. 5, we present the two aforementioned experiments carried out with participants with and without ADHD, and discuss our results. Section 6 concludes our findings and provides a brief discussion of possible future work.

2   Related Work

In this section, we provide an overview of ADHD clinical diagnosis and how various technologies, such as CPTs, sensors, and VR, have been used in the screening and diagnosis of ADHD.

2.1   ADHD and Clinical Diagnosis

Diagnoses of ADHD can be made along three dimensions – predominantly inattentive, predominantly hyperactive-impulsive, or combined – each of which characterizing a distinct set of symptoms [5]. Predominantly inattentive individuals have difficulty in maintaining focus, planning, and executing tasks while predominantly hyperactive-impulsive individuals are impulsive and exhibit excessive motor activity. Children diagnosed with the latter tend to run, jump, and climb constantly while adults exhibit restlessness, fidget with their hands and legs, or speak at inappropriate times in conversation. Other individuals who may not be one or the other, regularly exhibit symptoms of both inattentive and hyperactive-impulsive types. The process of diagnosing ADHD is often lengthy, subjective in nature, and varies from clinic to clinic [2,5]. Recommended diagnoses are made by clinicians following a variety of methods, including observations, self-reported rating scales (e.g., D.I.V.A. [15]), interviews, and various digital assessment technologies—the most common of these latter methods perhaps are computerized continuous performance tests (CPTs) [14]. In Europe, eventual diagnoses are supported by assessment criteria specified in the International Statistical Classification of Diseases and Related Health Problems (ICD-10) for ADHD [5] which identifies, among others, criteria such as an individual fidgeting with their hands or feet and persistent and excessive motor activity not consistent with the demands or context of society.

2.2   Relevant Diagnostic Support Technologies for ADHD

Digital technologies are increasingly being used as measures for assessment of ADHD and its symptoms [1], particularly those that relate to the motor system

[7]. Some technologies, such as computerized CPTs [14], are routinely used in practice by clinicians while others, such as various sensors and VR, have been proposed for diagnostic support for ADHD [6,11,13,16,18–21].

Computerized Continuous Performance Tests. Continuous performance tests (CPTs) are neuropsychological assessments for measuring sustained and selective attention typically by presenting an individual with a repetitive and lengthy task [14]. CPTs are commonly employed by clinicians for providing supplemental and quantifiable measurements of ADHD attention deficits, however, they are generally not applicable for diagnostic support of hyperactivity and have been shown to not be particularly effective with adults [3]. One popular commercialized example is the Conners' CPT3^{TM} [14] which uses various neuropsychological measures (e.g., omission/co-mission errors and reaction time) to aid in the identification of certain attention deficits and impulsivities. During the test, letters from A–Z are presented on a computer to users for a fixed duration of 250 ms each in six blocks each consisting of a distinct ordering of three sets of 20 letters which appear at varying inter-stimuli intervals of time (i.e., 1, 2, and 4 s) and where 'X' has a 10% probability of appearing and the remaining alphabet has a combined probability of 90%. The user is tasked with pushing the space-key on the keyboard whenever any letter except 'X' appears [1,10,14].

Sensors and Virtual Reality. Various basic sensing technologies for tracking motion (i.e., inertial sensors), such as accelerometers and gyroscopes, have shown promising potential for diagnostic support for ADHD [6,13,16,18,20]. In [18], for example, general motion sensor data collected from the dominant legs and waists of children during various physical activities was shown to be capable of distinguishing between those with and without ADHD with an accuracy of approx. 95%. Moreover, of these activities, motion data collected while completing a traditional CPT proved most significant. With respect to VR, various systems and their integrated sensors have been employed in research for diagnostic support for ADHD due primarily to their (1) recent widespread availability and low cost, (2) ability to provide immersive experiences that allow for symptoms of ADHD to arise more naturally when compared to clinical settings [1], and (3) ability to measure multiple sensory systems [11,19,21]. In early work by [21], a VR-based CPT placed in a virtual classroom was developed while systematic manipulations to visual and auditory distractions in this environment were evaluated, as these have been shown to be important factors in practice when diagnosing adolescent ADHD through a CPT [4]. In [19], researchers suggested that children with ADHD would show higher levels of hyperactivity while performing cognitive tasks within the virtual classroom [21]. Using data collected from the HMD, the children's physical body displacement in space proved significant in differentiating those with and without ADHD. In more recent work [12], researchers developed the Nesplora Aula, a VR-based CPT similarly set in a classroom environment with several distractions, and evaluated its ability to detect various attention deficits in children between 6 and 16 years old.

In follow-up work [11], the Nesplora Aquarium, based on the virtual environment in [12], was developed with assessments of adult attention and working memory in mind. In [2], the AULA Nesplora was used to discriminate between the sub-types of ADHD in children, showing promising results in discriminating between hyperactivity and impulsivity using the HMD to capture general motion activity. Despite these efforts, the actual physical movements captured by the motion activity of adults measured by such VR systems which prove significant in differentiating those with and without ADHD and whether these align or not with movements that would be indicative of hyperactivity by a clinician, have not been as well studied.

3   Clinical Interviews

In this section, we detail our interviews carried out with clinicians having expertise in the diagnosis of adults with ADHD and provide a brief discussion of our findings. We conclude with a list of subjective assessments and observations used in practice by these clinicians when diagnosing adults with ADHD hyperactivity which we have used to inform the design requirements of our VR-CPT system environment (discussed in Sect. 4) and the criteria for evaluating use of our system with respect to diagnostic support for symptoms of hyperactivity (discussed in Sect. 5).

3.1   Clinicians and Procedure

We carried out five, remote semi-structured interviews across various stages of our design process with two clinicians (Interviewee A: one 1-h long interview; Interviewee B: four 1-h long interviews) where one facilitator and two note-takers participated in each. The facilitator led the conversation using a set of pre-defined questions concerning, for example, how diagnoses of ADHD are made in the clinician's respective practice, what tools and methods are used to aid in this diagnosis, and what observations of an individual's behavior are most indicative of hyperactivity, among others. Additional interview questions and consultations were made in an attempt to increase the clinical validity of the design of our VR-CPT system and environment. Interviewee A has worked in Denmark as a neuropsychology clinician for over five years diagnosing ADHD in both adults and children, while Interviewee B is employed in the same country as a psychologist in a facility focused on diagnosing attention disorders in adults.

3.2   Clinician Criteria For Assessing Hyperactivity in Practice

Responses from both interviewees were analyzed by the two note-takers using qualitative coding and indicated that a variety of approaches to the diagnosis of ADHD in adults, in terms of both methodology and tools, are employed in practice. Both clinicians noted the importance of digital CPTs to their diagnosis process with Interviewee B noting that in their facility, adults with ADHD are

Table 1. Seven subjective assessments and observations of ADHD hyperactivity used in practice by two interviewed clinicians.

Category	Assess./Obs.	Explanation	Source	Code
Motion activity	1. Restless hands or feet	Often fidgets with hands or feet or squirms on seat	ICD-10	I1
	2. General motor activity	Persistent and excessive motor activity not modified by social context or demands	ICD-10	I2
	3. Movement & ticks	How many times they move, have ticks, etc.	Clinical	C3
	4. Excessive energy	So much energy that you always need to do something	Clinical	C4
Verbal patterns	5. Talking loudly	How loud they speak	Clinical	C5
Eye activity	6. Eye activity	How many times they look other places	Clinical	C6
	7. Head movement	How many times they look other places and move their head	Clinical	C7

observed while conducting a Conners' CPT. However, they clarified that such tools are unable to adequately assess hyperactivity and therefore diagnoses must rely on observations and subjective assessments, such as those suggested in the ICD-10 and other criteria the clinician feels are important based on their experience and expertise. Additionally, it was clear that the tools used in diagnostic support differ from clinic to clinic and often times those developed for children are used with adults. With respect to making these assessments, the interviewees reaffirmed that adults with hyperactivity may learn to control their symptoms in test environments, often making it difficult to assess. Interviewee B suggested, in particular, that such controlled behavior in test environments could potentially be addressed by testing people in situations that better approximate the real-world and everyday scenarios. The importance of employing a CPT centered on an attention-based task when assessing hyperactivity was clarified by both interviewees through the suggestion that those individuals whose impulsivity was triggered by a certain task or a situation were also more prone to exhibit hyperactive behaviours.

The findings from these interviews suggest the need for improved and reliable digital tools for measuring hyperactivity in particular as well as better clarity regarding the observations that prove useful in practice when assessing such symptoms in individuals when completing CPTs and attention-based tasks. For these reasons, we have compiled a list of the subjective assessments and observations used by the interviewees when diagnosing adults with a hyperactive-impulsivity dominant sub-type of ADHD. Some of these assessments and observations are found in the ICD-10 while others were developed by the clinicians themselves based on their own experiences in practice. Table 1 shows the seven subjective assessments and observations of ADHD hyperactivity used in practice by our two interviewed clinicians – grouped into three categories of motion activity, verbal patterns, and eye activity as well as whether each is found in the ICD-10 or comes from the clinicians themselves. Note in Table 1 that two of the assessments and observations (i.e., I1 and I2) are found in the ICD-10 questionnaire and the remaining four (i.e., C1, C2, C3, C4) were devised by the clinicians. Collectively, these assessments and observations, combined with our interview findings, are used to inform the design requirements of our VR-CPT system and its environment as well as the criteria used to evaluate use of our system with respect to diagnostic support for symptoms of hyperactivity.

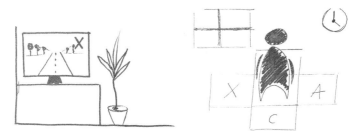

(a) CPT letters appear on the TV in a living room with the user pressing a button.   (b) CPT letters appear on the floor with the user stepping on the tile.

Fig. 1. Initial conceptual designs of the virtual CPT and environment of our VR-CPT system illustrating two different virtual environments, types of CPT, and modes of user interaction.

4   Design of the VR-CPT System and Environment

This section provides an overview of how the virtual CPT and environment of our VR-CPT system was designed in consultation with expert clinicians who provided essential feedback on initial design concepts concerning the requirements of the virtual environment, type of CPT, and mode of user interaction with the CPT.

4.1   Virtual CPT and Environment

The design process for our VR-CPT virtual environment consisted of a design sprint in which a number of basic sketches were generated and narrowed down according to the following four design requirements: (1) a CPT must be integrated tightly into the virtual environment, (2) the virtual environment must be familiar to the user, (3) the CPT and virtual environment must allow for the collection of motion data, such as head, hand, and leg movements, and (4) the type of interaction e.g., stepping, pointing, or pressing a button, must be both explicit to the user and appropriate for the CPT. Figure 1 shows two of the four narrowed down initial design concepts for the virtual CPT and environment of the VR-CPT system. Note in Fig. 1 that each initial design concept illustrates a different virtual environment, type of CPT, and mode of user interaction, with a living room and the CPT visible on a TV requiring a button press in (a) and an empty room with the CPT visible on the floor requiring stepping in (b). The other two initial design concepts featured an abstract space in which CPT letters float in the immediate field of view and require a pointing motion as well as an outdoor space in which CPT letters appear in the distant night sky as star constellations.

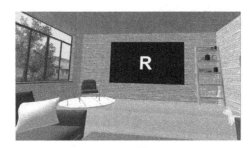

Fig. 2. Final design of the VR-CPT system environment from the point-of-view of the user showing a familiar virtual living room and the letter, 'R', from the virtual Connors' CPT displayed on the black screen visible in the mid-ground.

Collectively, these four initial design concepts were presented to the expert clinicians from Sect. 3 and through a series of consultations and collaborative design sessions, one concept, one type of CPT, and one mode of interaction i.e., the living room with letters appearing at a fixed position in the mid-ground of the user's point-of-view and a button press (shown in Fig. 1(a)), were chosen. The additional following design requirements were devised as a result: (1) the user should be in a seated position, (2) environmental distractions should be present, both in auditory and visual form, and (3) the CPT should be based on a Conners' CPT since this is the test currently employed by the clinicians. With respect to requirement (1), the clinicians noted that such a system would be better aligned with current clinical practice in which CPTs are carried out while sitting and it would be easier to see movement patterns in a position where the user is somewhat restricted in their overall body movement. Regarding requirement (2), visual and auditory distractions for the user can enhance the presence of hyperactivity symptoms during a CPT as distractions are often present in real-life situations where symptoms are more likely to manifest.

Figure 2 shows the final design and implementation of the VR-CPT system environment based on the chosen initial design concept, type of CPT, mode of interaction (i.e., Fig. 1(a)), and additional design requirements expressed by the clinicians.[1] Note in the final design that the user is seated on a sofa in a familiar living room virtual environment while letters of a virtual Connors'

---

[1] The complete code for the VR-CPT system can be found in the following repository: https://github.com/GeorgiNedelev/Hyperactivity-screening-tool-for-adults-with-ADHD.

CPT are displayed on the black screen in the mid-ground. While the CPT is being completed, there are two auditory and visual distractions (suggested by Interviewee B) which appear in the virtual environment: a cat and a bus. The cat meows and moves back and forth in the foreground from the right hand side wall to the window every 50 s while the bus drives up and down a street in the background visible from the window every two minutes with a corresponding sound of an engine.

5   Evaluation

In this section, we discuss the two experiments involving participants with and without ADHD when tasked with completing the virtual CPT using our VR-CPT system. Recall that the first experiment was carried out in order to determine which of any single or combined measures of motion by sensor (HMD, arm controller, leg controller) and inertial variable (acceleration, velocity, angular acceleration, angular velocity) can be used to distinguish between these two groups of participants. The second experiment was carried out in order to determine the extent to which significant motion activity events, as measured by our combined inertial variables measure for a single sensor, align with observations of physical movements indicative of hyperactivity by clinicians.

5.1   Sensor Data Collection

The data collected by our VR-CPT system in the two experiments include min-max normalized x, y, z vector value (excluding direction) sums for the inertial variables of acceleration (m/s), velocity (m/s), angular acceleration (deg./s), angular velocity (deg./s)[2] as measured by an Oculus Quest [17] HMD and its two handheld controllers for each of the four subjective assessments and observations of motion activity from Table 1 (i.e., restless hands or feet, general motion activity, movement and ticks, and excessive energy), leaving out the two categories of verbal patterns and eye activity. The data for each of these measurements was recorded at a maximum variable sample rate of approximately 30 samples per second, fluctuating slightly due to various hardware latencies. This means, however, that for two testing sessions with users lasting for equal durations of time, the number of data points collected may be different.

5.2   Experiment 1

Our first experiment was a two sample independent measures design where participants with and without ADHD were asked to complete the virtual CPT using

---

[2] A given three-dimensional sensor data point, p, is represented as $\langle |x|, |y|, |z| \rangle$ where $|.|$ denotes the absolute value and x, y, z are the coordinate values of the vector along their respective dimension. These non-negative coordinate values for p are summed to provide a single, instantaneous data point for each sensor which forms the basis of the data we use in the sets of combined sensor and variable measurements reported in our evaluation.

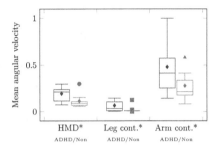

Fig. 3. Motion sensor measurements of mean angular velocity ('single sensor – single variable') from participants with and without ADHD collected by our VR-CPT system for each sensor (HMD, leg controller, and arm controller) during a virtual CPT. Asterisks (i.e., '*') denote statistically significant differences.

our VR-CPT system (discussed in Sect. 4). The purpose of this experiment was to determine whether there was any statistically significant difference between the two participant groups along the collections of data present in the following three combinations: (1) the mean values of a single measurement variable (acceleration, velocity, angular acceleration, or angular velocity) by a single sensor (HMD, arm controller, or leg controller) i.e., $4 \times 3 = 12$ 'single sensor – single variable' measurements, (2) the mean values of the sum of all measurement variables by a single sensor (i.e., three 'single sensor – all variables' measurements), and (3) the mean values of the sums of all mean measurements by all sensors (i.e., one 'all sensors – all variables' measurement). In all, we have tested 16 different measurements.

Participants and Procedure. We collected data from 20 adult volunteer participants split equally into two groups consisting of those either having a diagnosis of ADHD or not having a diagnosis of ADHD. All participants in the first group confirmed verbally that they had received a diagnosis of ADHD from a doctor or psychiatrist and all participants in the second group confirmed verbally that they had not received a diagnosis of ADHD nor had any underlying mental disorder. Eight participants with ADHD were recruited on social media groups recommended by clinicians experienced in diagnosing adult ADHD while the remaining two were recruited with the help of our interviewed clinicians (discussed in Sect. 3). The ten participants without ADHD were recruited similarly using general social media platforms. The data collected from all participants was anonymous motion sensor data concerning the movements of their head, one arm, and one leg as well as an indication of their dominant hand and diagnosis status. There was one left handed participant and the remaining 19 were right handed. An additional set of data in the form of anonymous audio-video recordings was collected from some participants who provided consent. No other personal data about the participants (e.g., age, gender, or occupation) was recorded. All data was collected in compliance with both EU GDP regulations and the participating university's protocol for carrying out non-clinical user testing with human participants.

Table 2. Independent two samples t-test results for all 16 motion sensor measurements of participants with and without ADHD collected by our VR-CPT system following the completion of a virtual CPT. Statistically significant results are indicated in boldface and with an asterisk (i.e., '*').

Measurements	t-value	p-value
Single sensor – single variable		
Acceleration HMD	1.399	0.179
Velocity HMD	1.941	0.068
Angular acceleration HMD	1.860	0.079
Angular velocity HMD	2.537	**0.021***
Acceleration leg controller	1.994	0.061
Velocity leg controller	1.555	0.137
Angular acceleration leg controller	2.263	**0.036***
Angular velocity leg controller	2.172	**0.043***
Acceleration arm controller	1.959	0.066
Velocity arm controller	2.595	**0.018***
Angular acceleration arm controller	1.737	0.099
Angular velocity arm controller	2.465	**0.024***

Measurements	t-value	p-value
Single sensor – all variables		
HMD motion activity	2.028	0.058
Leg controller motion activity	1.980	0.063
Arm controller motion activity	2.231	**0.039***
All sensors – all variables		
Overall motion activity	2.326	**0.032***

The experiment was carried out in a controlled and isolated environment over the course of seven days under the same conditions for each participant. Participants took part in the experiment individually and were asked to sign a consent form before they were permitted to begin. There were two types of consent forms allowing for either collection of anonymous audio-video recording and sensor data or only collection of anonymous motion sensor data. The participant was seated in the center of the room facing the direction of the virtual CPT, while a facilitator was located to the left of the participant and was responsible for introducing the participants to the test. Prior to the start of the test, the right controller button of the system was shown to the participants by the facilitator to ensure that they knew how to interact with the CPT, and then this controller was placed in their dominant hand. The facilitator ensured a proper fit of the HMD on the participant and the left controller was attached firmly to the leg opposite of their dominant hand. The placement of the controller positioned on the leg was due to limitations of the devices, as in some cases, if one controller hovers above the other the tracking of the controllers is lost. No irregular tracking behaviors (e.g., dropped controller or lost connection) were observed. Before each test, the point of view of the participant was reset to make sure all of the participants began with the same view. Participants were given one minute to look around in order to get familiar with their virtual surroundings and then informed of the environment by the facilitator and instructed on how to carry out the CPT. When participants felt ready, they were told to start the test by pressing the right controller button and afterwards whenever they see a letter other than 'X' on the screen. The number of stimuli presented in the CPT was reduced by half when compared to the number found in the original Connors' CPT (i.e., three blocks of 60 stimuli each) in order to minimize risk of VR sickness. Thus, the duration of each test was seven minutes, covering the time beginning from the first button press and ending with the moment the participant pressed the button on the controller for the final stimulus of the test.

Results and Discussion. All 16 mean participant motion sensor measurements were approximately normally distributed and met the additional underlying assumptions of an independent samples Student's t-test. Table 2 shows the t-test results from Experiment 1 for all 16 motion sensor measurements divided into the three measurement types (i.e., 'single sensor – single variable', 'single sensor – all variables', and 'all sensors – all variables'). Note in Table 2 that in the 'single sensor – single variable' collections of data, the mean motion sensor measurements of angular velocity for all sensors, velocity of the arm controller, and angular acceleration of the leg controller proved to be significantly different between the groups (i.e., $p < 0.05$). Moreover, the difference in mean motion activity measurements for the arm controller under the 'single sensor – all variables' collections of data also proved significant (i.e., $p < 0.04$). In contrast to previous work [19], the differences in the mean overall motion activity measurement proved to be statistically significant ($p < 0.04$). Figure 3 shows boxplots illustrating the statistically significant motion sensor measurements of mean angular velocity ('single sensor – single variable') from participants with and without ADHD collected by our VR-CPT system for each sensor (HMD, leg controller, and arm controller). For all sensors, we can see that the mean and median of mean angular velocities of participants with ADHD were higher and the spread of values was greater when compared to participants without ADHD – indicating that the participants with ADHD exhibited more varied physical movements that were generally either more active or 'sharper' in their rotations in space. What exactly these physical movements may have been will be looked at in greater detail in the following experiment.

5.3   Experiment 2

In our second exploratory experiment, we established a threshold in the motion activity ('single sensor – all variables') of participants with ADHD in order to isolate significant events and used precision and recall as measures to assess the extent to which these significant motion activity events align with observations of physical movements indicative of hyperactivity by clinicians. In our analysis, significant events are those which have motion activity above this threshold – an assumption that movements indicative of hyperactivity in individuals with ADHD have generally higher mean levels of motion activity than both movements which are not indicative of hyperactivity in these same individuals and movements that are made by individuals without ADHD.

Participants and Procedure. We collected anonymous audio-video recordings from eight of the participants with ADHD who participated in Experiment 1 and who provided consent for both the collection of anonymous motion sensor data and anonymous audio-video recording. Each recording was 7 min long, corresponding to the duration of the virtual CPT, and contained the seated profile view of the entire participant's body with the face obscured by the HMD. Recordings were provided to one of the interviewed clinicians (from Sect. 3) who agreed to participate and was asked to identify any moments in the recordings when participants exhibited signs which would indicate potential symptoms of hyperactivity, just as they would normally do in their daily practice when making a diagnosis in person. Both the types of observations (e.g., 'restless arm', 'scratches neck', or 'speaking aloud') and times at which they occurred in the recording were noted by the clinician and provided to the experimenters.

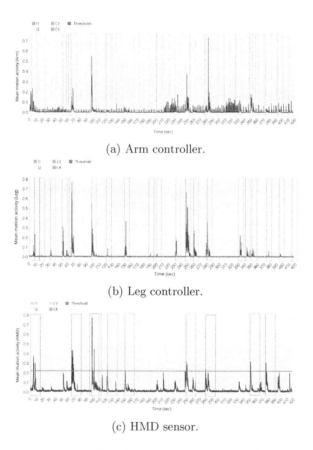

(a) Arm controller.

(b) Leg controller.

(c) HMD sensor.

Fig. 4. Mean motion activity ('single sensor – all variables') of a participant with ADHD as measured by all sensors (HMD, arm controller, leg controller) of our VR-CPT system while completing a virtual CPT. Clinician annotations of four motion activity subjective assessments and observations of ADHD hyperactivity (i.e., I1, I2, C3, and C4) are indicated with vertical colored lines and the vertical threshold is indicated with the horizontal red line. (Color figure online)

Results and Discussion. Of the eight participant recordings, our single participating clinician provided complete annotations for one participant with ADHD (due simply to time and resource constraints), so we will provide an analysis consisting of only the motion activity for this single participant. Figure 4 shows the mean motion activity of this participant as measured by the combined inertial variables measure for each of the sensors ('single sensor – all variables') from our VR-CPT system while completing the virtual CPT. In Fig. 4, we have established a vertical threshold (shown by the horizontal red line) above which indicates significant events of high mean motion activity. The vertical threshold was defined by the lowest occurring peak in the mean motion activity for each sensor that corresponds to a movement which the clinician annotated as being indicative of hyperactivity and differs from sensor to sensor. Additional horizontal thresholds were set to four second windows within which only a single motion event would be considered to occur and was defined according to the longest duration movement indicative of hyperactivity according to the clinician. Ideally, only mean motion activity events that appear both above the vertical threshold and within the horizontal thresholds would be movements identified by the clinician, however, this turns out not to be the case. Colored boxes (excluding grey) indicate significant motion activity events that align with annotations made by the clinician while grey boxes indicate significant motion activity events that do not. Some significant motion activity events which do not have any boxes (e.g., at 40 and 150 s in Fig. 4(a)) are due to sympathetic movements from other parts of the body and not due to the part of the body in which the given sensor was attached. For assessing the extent to which these movements align with significant events in motion activity, we consider the clinicians' time-stamped annotations (i.e., I1, I2, C3, and C4) as a ground truth and all events in mean motion activity above the vertical threshold and within the horizontal thresholds (i.e., the colored and grey boxes) as examples which require classification as either being 'indicative' or 'not indicative'.

Of all 35 significant arm motion activity events identified according to our thresholds, there were 12 annotated instances of indicative arm movements, resulting in a precision of $pr = 0.3428$ and recall of $r = 1$. There were 21 significant leg motion activity events and 8 annotated instances of indicative leg movements, resulting in a precision of $pr = 0.3809$ and recall of $r = 1$. There were only 10 significant HMD motion activity events and 6 annotated instances of indicative head movements, resulting in a precision of $pr = 0.6$ and recall of $r = 1$. Our relatively low levels of precision indicate that there are relatively many significant motion activity events (i.e., those having high levels of mean motion activity) but only a rather small number of these are actually physical movements indicative of hyperactivity according to our method for setting thresholds. This indicates that there are nuances to indicative physical movements that are not necessarily captured by considering only high levels of mean motion activity (as measured by our 'single sensor – all variables' measure) or motion activity within four second windows. One will further note that we have achieved perfect recall for the significant motion activity events in each sensor due to the way in which we have chosen our vertical threshold based on the clinician's annotations such that no false negatives are present. While this threshold served well in our analysis for a single participant, such thresholds would likely vary from participant to participant and need to be learned from the data in order to remain reliable. Regardless, the overall low precision indicates that hard thresholds will be unlikely to capture the nuances, either in time or level of motion activity, of indicative physical movements. Some other method, perhaps, relying on machine learning, may be better able to differentiate those significant motion activity events that are indicative from those that are not.

6   Conclusion and Future Work

This paper presented the VR-CPT system—a virtual continuous performance test and environment—designed in consultation with expert clinicians that uses motion sensor data to aid in diagnosis support for adult ADHD. In our evaluation with this system, angular velocity of all single sensor measurements (HMD, arm controller, and leg controller), velocity of the arm controller, and angular acceleration of the leg controller proved most promising in distinguishing between participants with and without ADHD. Moreover, the mean motion activity ('single sensor – all variables') of the arm controller and the overall mean motion activity ('all sensors – all variables') from participants proved significant. In our exploratory follow-up experiment, relatively low precision and perfect recall in classification indicated that setting vertical thresholds based on high levels of mean motion activity ('single sensor – all variables') may be an effective method for helping to isolate events indicative of hyperactivity from non-indicative events having low levels of mean motion activity but that such thresholds alone are insufficient in distinguishing between indicative events and non-indicative events all having high levels of mean motion activity. Collectively, these results provide further promising potential for the use of motion sensor data to support clinical diagnoses of ADHD but that distinguishing relevant physical movements from non-relevant ones remains challenging. In future work, it would be worthwhile to experiment with different virtual environments and existing distractions that might better arouse symptoms of hyperactivity. It would also be interesting to explore eye-tracking technologies and various audio analysis methods as means for investigating the non-motion activity categories of subjective clinician assessments and observations not studied here. Finally, given the amount of data collected by the VR-CPT system, it would be useful to explore different machine learning methods for providing possibly better diagnostic support of individuals with ADHD based on their physical movements, possibly through further consultation with multiple experts to provide inter-coder agreed annotations necessary for training such algorithms and making more reliable conclusions.

References

1. Areces, D., García, T., Cueli, M., Rodríguez, C.: Is a virtual reality test able to predict current and retrospective ADHD symptoms in adulthood and adolescence? Brain Sci. **9**(10) (2019). https://doi.org/10.3390/brainsci9100274
2. Areces, D., Rodríguez, C., García, T., Cueli, M., González-Castro, P.: Efficacy of a continuous performance test based on virtual reality in the diagnosis of ADHD and its clinical presentations. J. Atten. Disord. **22**(11), 1081–1091 (2018). https://doi.org/10.1177/1087054716629711
3. Baggio, S., et al.: Does the continuous performance test predict ADHD symptoms severity and ADHD presentation in adults? J. Atten. Disord. **24**(6), 840–848 (2020). https://doi.org/10.1177/1087054718822060
4. Berger, I., Cassuto, H.: The effect of environmental distractors incorporation into a CPT on sustained attention and ADHD diagnosis among adolescents. J. Neurosci. Methods **222**, 62–68 (2013). https://doi.org/10.1016/j.jneumeth.2013.10.012
5. Centers for Disease control and prevention: What is ADHD? https://www.cdc.gov/ncbddd/adhd/facts.html
6. Chen, Y., Zhang, Y., Jiang, X., Zeng, X., Sun, R., Yu, H.: COSA: contextualized and objective system to support ADHD diagnosis. In: 2018 IEEE International Conference on Bioinformatics and Biomedicine (BIBM), pp. 1195–1202 (2018). https://doi.org/10.1109/BIBM.2018.8621308
7. Cibrian, F., Hayes, G., Lakes, K.: Research advances in ADHD and technology. Synthesis Lect. Assist. Rehabil. Health-Preserv. Technol. **9**, i-156 (2020). https://doi.org/10.2200/S01061ED1V01Y202011ARH015
8. Dopheide, J.A., Pliszka, S.R.: Attention-deficit-hyperactivity disorder: an update. Pharmacother. J. Hum. Pharmacol. Drug Ther. **29**(6), 656–679 (2009)
9. Fang, Y., Han, D., Luo, H.: A virtual reality application for assessment for attention deficit hyperactivity disorder in school-aged children. Neuropsychiatr. Dis. Treat. **15**, 1517–1523 (2019). https://doi.org/10.2147/NDT.S206742
10. Folsom, R., Levin, P.: Conners' continuous performance test. In: Encyclopedia of Autism Spectrum Disorders, pp. 1179–1182 (2021). https://doi.org/10.1007/978-3-319-91280-6_216
11. Climent, G., et al.: New virtual reality tool (Nesplora Aquarium) for assessing attention and working memory in adults: a normative study. Appl. Neuropsychol. Adult 1–13 (2019).https://doi.org/10.1080/23279095.2019.1646745
12. Iriarte, Y., Diaz-Orueta, U., Cueto, E., Irazustabarrena, P., Banterla, F., Climent, G.: AULA-advanced virtual reality tool for the assessment of attention: normative study in Spain. J. Atten. Disord. **20**(6), 542–568 (2016)
13. Kam, H.J., Shin, Y.M., Cho, S.M., Kim, S.Y., Kim, K.W., Park, R.W.: Development of a decision support model for screening attention-deficit hyperactivity disorder with actigraph-based measurements of classroom activity. Appl. Clin. Inform. **1**(4), 377–393 (2010). https://doi.org/10.4338/ACI-2010-05-RA-0033
14. Keith Conners, C., Sitarenios, G., Ayearst, L.E.: Conners' continuous performance test third edition. In: Kreutzer, J.S., DeLuca, J., Caplan, B. (eds.) Encyclopedia of Clinical Neuropsychology, pp. 929–933. Springer, Cham (2018). https://doi.org/10.1007/978-3-319-57111-9_1535
15. Kooij, J.J.S., Francken, M.H.: Diagnostic interview for ADHD in adults (DIVA) diagnostisch interview Voor ADHD bij volwassenen (2010)

16. Muñoz-Organero, M., Powell, L., Heller, B., Harpin, V., Parker, J.: Automatic extraction and detection of characteristic movement patterns in children with ADHD based on a convolutional neural network (CNN) and acceleration images. Sensors **18**(11) (2018). https://doi.org/10.3390/s18113924
17. Oculus: Oculus quest (2019). https://www.oculus.com. Accessed 18 May 2020
18. O'Mahony, N., Florentino-Liano, B., Carballo, J.J., Baca-García, E., Rodríguez, A.A.: Objective diagnosis of ADHD using IMUs. Med. Eng. Phys. **36**(7), 922–926 (2014). https://doi.org/10.1016/j.medengphy.2014.02.023
19. Parsons, T.D., Bowerly, T., Buckwalter, J.G., Rizzo, A.A.: A controlled clinical comparison of attention performance in children with ADHD in a virtual reality classroom compared to standard neuropsychological methods. Child Neuropsychol. **13**(4), 363–381 (2007)
20. Ricci, M., et al.: Wearable-based electronics to objectively support diagnosis of motor impairments in school-aged children. J. Biomech. **83**, 243–252 (2019). https://doi.org/10.1016/j.jbiomech.2018.12.005
21. Rizzo, A.A., et al.: The virtual classroom: a virtual reality environment for the assessment and rehabilitation of attention deficits. CyberPsychol. Behav. **3**(3), 483–499 (2000)
22. Weiss, G., Hechtman, L., Milroy, T., Perlman, T.: Psychiatric status of hyperactives as adults: a controlled prospective 15-year follow-up of 63 hyperactive children. J. Am. Acad. Child Psychiatry **24**(2), 211–220 (1985). https://doi.org/10.1016/S0002-7138(09)60450-7

Using Topic Modelling to Personalise a Digital Self-compassion Training

Laura M. van der Lubbe[(✉)], Nina Groot, and Charlotte Gerritsen

Computer Science, Vrije Universiteit Amsterdam, De Boelelaan 1111,
1081 HV Amsterdam, The Netherlands
l.m.vander.lubbe@vu.nl

Abstract. Young adults that struggle with mental health issues experience barriers to seek help. With our online self-compassion training we try to overcome some of these barriers. To improve our training, we can personalise exercises based on topic modelling. Data from a pilot study is used to analyse and evaluate the algorithm. Overall, the algorithm has an accuracy of 54.1% for predicting the right topic. This accuracy increases to 80.4% when considering an empty prediction to be correct as well. Although this research also shows that our data makes the task of topic modelling difficult, it does prove to be a possibility to personalise the designed training.

Keywords: Self-compassion · Mental health · Personalization · Topic modelling

1 Introduction

Young adults can struggle with mental health issues due to various reasons. Mental health disorders lead to a poor quality of life and have a high contribution to the global burden of disease [11]. Although young adults are struggling with their mental health, they perceive several barriers to seek help [5]. Among these barriers are the lack of accessibility, preference for self-help instead of external help, and a lack of knowledge of what services exist.

To overcome the barriers around accessibility and self-help, an online intervention is a promising tool. It has the convenience that it is a private and flexible way of training yourself. We designed an online self-compassion training with gamification elements for young adults [7]. Self-compassion means that you are kind to yourself in difficult times, you perceive your experiences as part of the larger human experience, and that you have a mindful attitude towards difficult emotions. It has been associated with positive outcomes, such as an association with greater happiness, optimism, and positive affect [9]. Often, training courses for self-compassion are in person, in which the trainer can have interaction with the participants [3]. However, online alternatives also exist [4,10].

H. Lewy and R. Barkan (Eds.): PH 2021, LNICST 431, pp. 522–532, 2022.
https://doi.org/10.1007/978-3-030-99194-4_32

The online self-compassion training we designed is self-guided, meaning there is no professional supervision or guidance during the training. While in in-person self-compassion training such personal guidance plays an important role, we have to create an automated alternative that still provides some personalization e.g. within one of the exercises [7]. During the pilot study, that we performed to assess the user-experience of the website, we discussed the option of personalising the training content with the participants [8]. By adapting the exercises of the training to topics that participants discuss in different components of the training, it becomes possible to better suit the exercises to the needs of individual users. Therefore we have developed an algorithm for topic modelling that can be used in the improved version of our online self-compassion training.

This paper first discusses background literature on topic modelling. Next, the existing online self-compassion training is introduced and the method of the data analysis and algorithm implementation are described. Followed by the results of this analysis and the evaluation of the algorithm. Finally, we will draw conclusions on how this algorithm can be used to personalise the content of our training website, and what lessons can be learned from a technical perspective.

2   Topic Modelling

Topic modelling means finding themes in unstructured documents [2]. Different approaches and algorithms for this task exist. In [6], different ways of classifying these algorithms are described. First, the classification based on used strategy: probabilistic or non-probabilistic (or algebraic models). Non-probabilistic models use a Bag-of-Words (BoW) approach. In this approach the corpus gets converted into a term document matrix and the order of terms is neglected. The probabilistic model improves such non-probabilistic models by adding the probability sense using generative model approaches. The next classification that can be made is that of supervised and unsupervised approaches. The main difference between these two approaches is the existence of labels in the training data set [1]. Supervised modelling works with predetermined output attributes (labels). The models attempt to predict and classify the predetermined attribute, and their accuracies (alongside other performance measures) is dependent on the number of correctly classified attributes. Unsupervised modelling, on the other hand, focuses on clustering without the use of target attributes. Lastly, one can distinct whether algorithms use the sequence of words during topic modelling or use the BoW approach that does not consider this [6].

3   Method

Currently, the online self-compassion training consists of three exercises, a journal consisting of three components, and a profile page [7]. Gamification is added in the form of a story that the user progresses through. This story is about a journey that you are making: a metaphor for your self-development through learning about self-compassion. The story is a way to deliver theory to the user in a recognisable context. Moreover, to progress on your journey you have to earn kilometres, which you earn by engaging in exercises and the different journals. For each finished component you progress a certain number of kilometres, and when completing all components on a day you earn a bonus. There is a maximum progression per day, as more interaction is not considered beneficial anymore.

Initially, the story and exercises use situations written around the topics of social media, body image issues, social anxiety and troubles with friends, with as main goal reducing body image related issues of young adults. With assigning topics to previous text written by users, the choice for those situations can be personalised to the individual user. During the pilot study we discussed this possibility with users [8]. They said that they are interested in such a feature. While some users would like to practise with situations that are close to them, others noted that they would like it the other way around as that would be less personal. Moreover, users also noted that it could be beneficial to learn how to generalise the application of self-compassion, and thus it would be good to also practise with more unfamiliar situations.

Thus, the goal is to create a topic modelling algorithm that can be used to determine which topics are discussed in freely written, user created, content, which can then be used to personalise the exercises of the training. As we use predetermined topics, we cannot use existing algorithms such as those mentioned in Sect. 2. With data from the pilot study we can analyse and evaluate how the algorithm performs and how it can be embedded in the training website.

3.1 Data

In the previously mentioned pilot study, 24 users worked with the website for a limited period of time [8]. All participants were female, with a mean age of 22.5 (SD = 2.04). From these 24 users, 18 users actually entered data in the website. Of these 18 users, the data entered in the exercises and journals is saved. For this study we use the data from the gratitude and self-compassion journal, and one of the exercises called 'Practise self-compassion'. These contain texts about situations from the users' daily lives. All data is in Dutch.

In the gratitude journal users are asked to fill in something they are grateful for on that day, and characterise their answer with a short tag (max. 50 characters). Both this description as well as the tag can be used to determine the topic of the text. For the self-compassion journal users describe a situation, characterise this with a similar short tag and explain how self-compassion is used or could be used in that situation. From this journal we use the situation description and the tag. Finally, in the exercise users are asked if there is something they are struggling with and to describe this situation. Even if they are not struggling at the moment, they are asked to use a situation from their (recent) past. This description is used for the topic modelling. For the exercise no tag is available. In total, the available data contains 181 unique notes: 61 gratitude journal notes, 54 self-compassion journal notes, and 66 exercises. Not all participants contributed the same number of notes. Figure 1 shows how many notes each participant contributed.

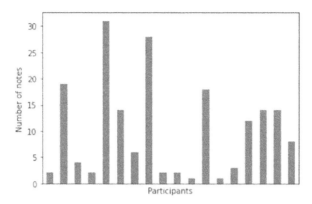

Fig. 1. Number of notes per participant

3.2 Topics and Data Labelling

In the exercises, situations around the topics of *friendship, body insecurity, social anxiety,* and *social media* are used. The choice for these topics was related to the aim of the training. However, based on the pilot study it became clear that other topics were missing [8]. The data from the interviews of the pilot study can be used to find more suitable topics.

In addition, we analysed the data to see which topics are actually discussed by the users. To do so, the data was first labelled using the four predefined labels. If none of the labels suited the text, 'no topic' was noted. When the tag matched a label, this label was noted even though the text might be less clear. When multiple topics could apply, the label that the majority of the text applied to was noted. If the text was divided equally, 'no topic' was noted. The three researchers checked the labelling and discussed any discrepancies. The labels given by the researchers are called the gold labels. After this, we studied the notes that had no label, and decided on a new set of labels based on both the data findings as well as the results from the interviews. We changed *friendship* into *relationships*, as family or romantic relationships were also discussed. We changed *body insecurity* to *body image* as this suits better with positive message about your body. The new set of labels is: *social anxiety, social media, relationships, body image, school, job,* and *emotions.* Where emotions is a topic that covers all texts where emotions, moods or feelings have an important role. Although *social media* was not used by any of the participants, we do keep it as a topic as there is already content on the website with that topic.

3.3 Algorithm

For all predefined topics, related words were gathered using the Related Words website[1] that gives a list of words that are related to a given search term. We

---

[1] https://relatedwords.org/.

created our related word lists based on the terms: 'social media', 'social anxiety', 'job', and 'emotions' for the eponymous topics, and 'body' for the *body image* topic, 'relationship' and 'friend' for the *relationship* topic, and 'school' and 'test' for the *school* topic.

For the related word lists we first included the topic name itself. Next, we excluded words from the related word list that are clearly unrelated to our topic, such as names of people or events, drugs and disorders. For most topics we looked only at the first 50 terms. For the term 'friend', we only looked at words for friends or family members. For the term 'test', we only looked at terms related to grading in the school context. For the term 'social media' we included some currently popular social media platforms that are not included yet on the Related Words website. The related word lists contain 51 words for *social media*, 62 words for *body image*, 32 words for *social anxiety*, 116 words for *relationships*, 52 words for *job*, 88 words for *school*, and 51 words for *emotions*.

Data Preprocessing. Before analysing the data, we remove any names mentioned in the data to ensure anonimity. In most cases, the names are replaced by an X to make the text still readable for the labelling process. The texts and tags are translated to English with the Google Translate API[2]. These English texts and tags are used for the further preprocessing.

The texts are preprocessed with the help of the Natural Language Toolkit (NLTK) for Python[3]. To do this, the text is first tokenized. With this tokenization, the text is separated into words (tokens). All remaining tokens with more then two characters are saved, other tokens are removed as they are not valuable. Using the NLTK stopwords list we remove stopwords from the remaining tokens. Stopwords are words that are frequently used in human language. They are removed because they often do not add much value to a sentence. The final step is lemmatizing the words and verbs. This means that verbs are turned into their present tense and plural words are put in their singular form.

The tags in the data and the related word lists are preprocessed the same way. Due to this preprocessing, some tags might be deleted. In the preprocessing of the related words we also remove words that appear multiple times for the same topic. This can happen when multiple words included the same term, and after splitting the terms in single words these duplicate words are removed.

Topic Modelling. The algorithm that is developed looks at the overlap between the prepared text and tag and the prepared related words of each topic. First, it counts the number of related words that are present in the prepared text. Each overlap adds one point to the similarity score of the topic. When a word is used multiple times, each occurance is counted. Next, it is checked whether the related words overlap with the tag (if present). If this is the case, 3 points are added to the similarity score. Finally, the topic label itself is tokenized and

---

[2] https://pypi.org/project/google-trans-new/.
[3] https://www.nltk.org/.

it is checked whether the words from that tokenized label overlap with the tag. If this is the case, the similarity score is increased with 6 points.

The higher increments for an overlap with the tag are based on the fact that the tag is the shortest description of the note, so in general it has a higher likelihood of being a description of the topic of the text. When the tag overlaps with the name of the topic, this likelihood is even higher.

Once the similarity score is determined for each topic, the predicted topic is chosen. For this, we first check if the highest similarity score is higher than a threshold value. During the evaluation we will choose the right threshold value. If the highest score is above the threshold value, and this similarity score is only calculated for one topic, this topic is predicted. In other cases, the algorithm cannot be sure about the topic and thus predicts multiple topics. When evaluating the algorithm we look at the combinations of topics that are predicted and their gold labels. If we can find patterns in this, these patterns can be used to make rules about the final prediction of the algorithm. If not, the algorithm will predict 'no topic' when multiple topics score equally.

The algorithm needs to predict at most one topic for every text written by users for one of the data sources mentioned in Sect. 3.1. This topic will be saved for that text, but can later be manually changed by the user (choosing from the predefined set of topics).

3.4 Algorithm Evaluation

To analyse the algorithm, we look at the accuracy with which it predicts the labels. To calculate this, the number of correctly predicted labels is divided by the total number of predictions. The higher the accuracy, the better. However, this accuracy is not everything. We also need to look at what goes wrong. In our application we consider it less problematic if the algorithm predicts 'no topic' instead of a wrong topic. Users will be able to manually add or edit a topic labelling if they want. However, if they do not correct mistakes, it is better if mistakes are avoided to prevent wrong displays of frequently used topics. Thus, we also calculate the accuracy of correct predictions and 'no topic' predictions compared to the total number of predictions. However, this accuracy cannot be used to improve the model, as that would mean that a 100% accuracy could be achieved by simply always predicting 'no topic'. Therefore we use the first accuracy to determine the best threshold for the points to be considered a labelling and to study the multiple label predictions to determine the final predictions.

4   Results

4.1   Data Analysis

As shown in Table 1, most of the entries have no label. Furthermore, it can be seen that *social media* has not been used as a topic in any of the data. In the gratitude journal only *friendship* is discussed, which is the topic with the most

Table 1. Numbers of notes labelled with initial labels

	Social anxiety	Social media	Friendship	Body insecurity	No topic
Gratitude	0	0	16	0	45
Journal	3	0	2	4	45
Exercise	4	0	5	5	52
Total	*7*	*0*	*23*	*9*	*142*

Table 2. Numbers of notes labelled with extended labels

	Social anxiety	Social media	Relationships	Body image	Job	School	Emotions	No topic
Gratitude	0	0	24	2	3	4	1	27
Journal	3	0	6	5	8	11	13	8
Exercise	4	0	6	5	5	10	26	10
Total	*7*	*0*	*36*	*12*	*16*	*25*	*40*	*45*

positive wording. Table 2 shows the number of counted labels when the extended set of labels is used. Still, a quarter of the texts is not labelled.

Most of the notes without a label are small notes. Figure 2 shows that the number of texts without a tag reduces if you use a threshold for the minimum number of words in a text (without preprocessing). When using a threshold of 10 the number of unlabeled texts halves, when using a threshold of 20 it reduces to 29% of the original number of unlabeld texts and with a threshold of 30 this is only 18%. However, the other line shows that the total number of texts also reduces, at a higher rate than the unlabeled data. To include as much data as possible, we will use all notes. However, we will compare it with different thresholds to see if this effects the accuracies.

We counted the words appearing in the prepared texts of the different topics, and looked at the words that were used most frequently and more than five times. As there are no texts classified for *social media*, also no words could be found. Table 3 shows that most words are clearly unrelated to the topic, such as 'n't' or 'good'. However, the word 'colleague' makes sense for *job* as well as the word 'felt' for *emotions*. 'Felt' should have been changed to 'feel' in the lemmatization. However, as 'felt' is also a noun, it was not recognized as a verb. Both 'felt' and 'colleague' are added to the related word list.

4.2   Results on Topic Modelling

First, we predict topics for each note with a points threshold of 1. If multiple topics have the highest score, we predict them all. Now we can see if there can be a pattern found in the predictions of multiple topics and their gold label. When looking at the combinations, such a pattern cannot be found. Thus, we choose that if multiple labels are predicted, the predicted label is 'no topic'.

Table 3. Gold labels and words that appear >5 times, * included in related word list

Gold label	Words
Body image	good (n = 6)
Social Anxiety	n't (n = 6)
Relationships	grateful (n = 14), good (n = 8), girlfriend* (n = 8), nice (n = 7), n't (n = 8), feel (n = 8)
Job	today (n = 7), colleague (n = 7), work* (n = 12), feel (n = 10), job* (n = 6), would (n = 7), make (n = 6), mistake (n = 6), n't (n = 7), say (n = 6), message (n = 6)
School	today (n = 8), school* (n = 7), lot (n = 6), exam* (n = 7), n't (n = 6)
Emotions	could (n = 7), feel* (n = 17), felt (n = 7), good (n = 8), get (n = 7), n't (n = 6)

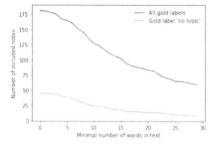

Fig. 2. Number of notes when using a minimum number of words

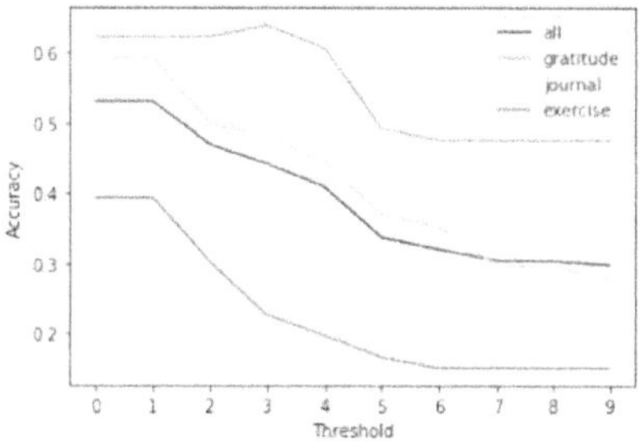

Fig. 3. Accuracies for predicted labels using threshold 1–10

Next, we test thresholds 1-10 to see which threshold has the best accuracy when using the determined prediction rule for multiple labels. From Fig. 3 it is clear that a threshold of 1 provides the best overall accuracy. Table 4 shows the accuracies that are predicted with this 1-point threshold. Both for the gratitude and journal notes the accuracy is higher than the average accuracy, but for the exercises this is lower. A difference between the gratitude/journal notes and the exercises is that the exercises do not have a tag. The accuracy of the 106 notes with a tag is 62.3%, the accuracy of the 75 notes without a tag[4] is 42.7%. Based on a Student's t-test we can conclude that this difference is significant (p-value = 0.0090).

We also analysed if using a minimum of words in the original text has an effect on the accuracy, which can be found in Table 4 as well. Overall, this does not seem to have an effect as most of the accuracies are similar. Only for gratitude there is a big difference when using only notes that have >20 words. This category also loses 65.6% of its notes when using only >20 words.

---

[4] 66 exercises notes + 9 gratitude/journal notes where the tag is removed in the preparation process

Table 4. Accuracies of different components with different word thresholds. Accuracy in brackets is accuracy including 'no topic'-predictions as correct predictions

Accuracy	All (n = 181)	>10 words (n = 127)	>20 words (n = 83)	>30 words (n = 55)
All	54.1% (80.4%)	54.3% (79.5%)	59.0% (77.1%)	58.2% (74.5%)
Gratitude	62.3% (77.0%)	69.4% (77.8%)	80.9% (85.7%)	63.5% (72.7%)
Journal	61.1% (85.2%)	62.5% (85.0%)	58.6% (82.8%)	54.5% (81.8%)
Exercises	40.9% (78.8%)	37.2% (76.5%)	45.4% (66.7%)	59.1% (68.2%)

Table 5 shows the number of notes for each topic that did not get the right prediction. The highest number of incorrect predictions are made for notes with the gold label *emotions*. However, this is also the biggest category. Relatively, the most incorrect predictions are made for gold label *social anxiety*.

Table 5. Incorrect predictions for each gold label

Gold label	Including 'no topic'	Excluding 'no topic'
Emotions	27 (67.5%)	10 (25.0%)
Relationships	20 (55.5%)	5 (13.9%)
No topic	9 (20.0%)	9 (20.0%)
Body image	8 (66.7%)	3 (25%)
School	8 (32.0%)	4 (16.0%)
Social anxiety	6 (85.7%)	3 (42.9%)
Job	5 (31.2%)	2 (12.5%)

As explained in Sect. 3.4, in our application it is better when the algorithm predicts 'no topic' instead of a wrong topic. Therefore we also calculated the accuracy when including the 'no topic'-predictions as correct predictions, again using point threshold 1. The accuracies are shown in brackets in Table 4. In Table 5 it can be seen that still the most incorrect predictions are made for gold label *emotions*, but also for *no topic*. Relatively, *social anxiety* has the most incorrect predictions.

5   Conclusion and Discussion

The goal of this paper is to explore the possibility of using topic modelling to personalise the experience of users of our self-compassion training website. Based on the accuracy of the model it seems that to some extent it is possible to predict the topic for different texts from users. Especially when you consider a 'no topic'-prediction as a correct prediction as well. This makes sense in our application as users would be able to change or add the label manually afterwards.

For our topic modelling algorithm we choose to work with a similarity score for words and related words. Other approaches would be to use machine learning. The analysis of the data showed that on word level there are hardly any words that are characteristic for specific topics. It is thus unclear if using such approaches would make sense.

We observe that the preprocessed data loses meaning. Often the topic of a text is found by the human reader in the combination of sentences and wordings. For example a sentence like 'I have a bad headache and my shoulders are stiff due to my stress about my upcoming exam.' will be preprocessed into the words: 'bad', 'headache', 'shoulder', 'stiff', 'due', 'stress', 'upcoming', and 'exam'. Based on only this text, the algorithm will predict both the topics *school* and *body image*, as it includes the word 'shoulder' and 'exam'. However, when only looking at the prepared text it is also harder for the human reader to decide what topic this text is about. It is thus interesting to explore whether a different preprocessing could help the algorithm to perform better. However, as the data is divided over many different topics, the remaining data is limited in its size and thus it is hard to draw conclusions on this. Another note that needs to be made, is that little changes in the preprocessing could have an effect on the accuracy of the algorithm. For translating, we use an API. If something in this API changes, the texts and thus the outcomes could be different. Also, spelling errors or ambiguous words effect the outcomes of the algorithm.

Participants of the pilot were not aware of any of the topics, they were completely free when writing their notes. The data therefore is very comparable to how it will be in the actual evaluation study of our training website. This holds for the content of the data, but also for the form (length of texts, writing errors etcetera). The only difference might be that in the new version of the training the minimum length of texts will be increased based on the average lengths found in the pilot data. We could have used more data, for example from our database of situation texts, but as this data is written with the topics in mind this would not be representable for the texts of the users.

With this simple form of topic modelling we can make sure that to some degree there can be personalization in the training. We plan to include a word cloud with the topics that have been predicted by the algorithm. Moreover, we will use it to ask users if they want to practise with a situation close to them (from one of their frequently discussed topics) or something less personal (from one of the topics they do not discuss (often)). In conclusion, with the topic modelling algorithms described in this paper, it becomes possible to personalise parts of the self-compassion training that the algorithm is developed for. With the proposed uses of this, the user-experience of the training will be increased.

References

1. Berry, M.W., Mohamed, A., Yap, B.W.: Supervised and Unsupervised Learning for Data Science. Springer, Heidelberg (2019). https://doi.org/10.1007/978-3-030-22475-2
2. Blei, D.M.: Probabilistic topic models. Commun. ACM **55**(4), 77–84 (2012)

3. Ferrari, M., Hunt, C., Harrysunker, A., Abbott, M.J., Beath, A.P., Einstein, D.A.: Self-compassion interventions and psychosocial outcomes: a meta-analysis of RCTs. Mindfulness **10**(8), 1455–1473 (2019)
4. Finlay-Jones, A., Kane, R., Rees, C.: Self-compassion online: a pilot study of an internet-based self-compassion cultivation program for psychology trainees. J. Clin. Psychol. **73**(7), 797–816 (2017)
5. Gulliver, A., Griffiths, K.M., Christensen, H.: Perceived barriers and facilitators to mental health help-seeking in young people: a systematic review. BMC Psychiatry **10**(1), 1–9 (2010)
6. Kherwa, P., Bansal, P.: Topic modeling: a comprehensive review. EAI Endors. Trans. Scalable Inf. Syst. **7**(24) (2020)
7. van der Lubbe, L.M., Gerritsen, C., Klein, M.C., Hindriks, K.V., Rodgers, R.F.: Designing a gamified self-compassion training. In: 22st Annual European GAMEON® Conference: Simulation and AI in Computer Games (2021)
8. van der Lubbe, L.M., Gerritsen, C., Klein, M.C., Hindriks, K.V., Rodgers, R.F.: A pilot study of a gamified self-compassion training. In: 22st Annual European GAMEON® Conference: Simulation and AI in Computer Games (2021)
9. Neff, K.D., Rude, S.S., Kirkpatrick, K.L.: An examination of self-compassion in relation to positive psychological functioning and personality traits. J. Res. Pers. **41**(4), 908–916 (2007)
10. Talbot, F., Thériault, J., French, D.J.: Self-compassion: evaluation of a psychoeducational website. Behav. Cogn. Psychother. **45**(2), 198 (2017)
11. Ustün, T.: The global burden of mental disorders. Am. J. Public Health **89**(9), 1315–1318 (1999)

EAT@WORK: Designing an mHealth App for Promoting Healthy Eating Routines Among Dutch Office Workers

Sibo Pan[1], Xipei Ren[2(✉)], Aarnout Brombacher[1], and Steven Vos[1,3]

[1] Eindhoven University of Technology, Eindhoven, The Netherlands
[2] Beijing Institute of Technology, Beijing, China
x.ren@bit.edu.cn
[3] Fontys University of Applied Science, Eindhoven, The Netherlands

Abstractcx. Eating healthier at work can substantially promote health for office workers. However, little has been investigated on designing pervasive health interventions specialized in improving workday eating patterns. This paper presents a design study of an mHealth app called EAT@WORK, which was designed to support office workers in the Netherlands in developing healthy eating behaviors in work routines. Based on semi-structured interviews with 12 office workers from a variety of occupations, we synthesized four key features for EAT@WORK, including supporting easy access to relevant knowledge, assisting goal setting, integrating with health programs, and facilitating peer supports. The user acceptance of EAT@WORK was examined through a within-subject study with 14 office workers, followed by a qualitative study on the applicability of app features to different working contexts. Quantitative results showed that EAT@WORK was experienced more useful than a benchmark app ($p < 0.01$) and EAT@WORK was also perceived easier to use than the benchmark app ($p < 0.01$). The qualitative analysis suggested that the goal assistant feature could be valuable for different working contexts, while the integrated health program was considered more suitable for office work than telework. The social and knowledge support were expected to be on-demand features that should loosely be bonded with the working contexts. Based on these findings, we discuss design implications for the future development of such mHealth technologies to promote healthy eating routines among office workers.

Keywords: Healthy eating · Office vitality · Digital health · Dutch work context

1 Introduction

The prevalent health problems related to eating habits, such as cardiovascular diseases, cancer, type 2 diabetes, and suboptimal conditions linked to obesity increasingly affect the adult working population [1]. Besides, eating-related issues may also result in high frequencies of absenteeism and productivity loss [2, 3]. Therefore, to prevent eating-related diseases and to promote healthy eating behaviors at work may not only have

© ICST Institute for Computer Sciences, Social Informatics and Telecommunications Engineering 2022
Published by Springer Nature Switzerland AG 2022. All Rights Reserved
H. Lewy and R. Barkan (Eds.): PH 2021, LNICST 431, pp. 533–549, 2022.
https://doi.org/10.1007/978-3-030-99194-4_33

economic benefits [4] but also provide improvement of personal health and quality of life [5].

According to previous research, healthy eating habits can be influenced by personal daily work routine as well as many other different aspects, for instance, accessibility of healthy foods and self-efficacy for healthy eating [6, 7]. The work routines could offer good settings to apply healthy eating interventions [6]. For instance, Campbell and colleagues [8] tailored a health program for female workers to increase fruit and vegetable consumption during working hours. Park et al. [9] found that social norms could provide benefits to healthy eating interventions. To approve this finding, they tested cultural and social supports for food choices and eating patterns among South Korean employees. Such workplace interventions are developed to improve the performance, health, and well-being of workers [10, 11], but some research states that these health-related interventions for workplaces could only produce limited effects [12–14].

The notion of mHealth (mobile health) is defined by The Global Observatory as "medical and public health practice supported by mobile devices, such as mobile phones, personal digital assistants (PDAs), and other wireless devices" [15]. In recent decades, the role of mobile technologies in healthy eating behaviors is becoming increasingly prominent and the use of diverse mHealth tools is also growing in personal health management [16]. In addition, mobile phones are increasingly used to support healthy eating behavior change. For instance, Eat&Tell [17] is a mobile application designed to facilitate the collection of eating-related data through automated tracking and self-report. MyFitnessPal [18] converts the barcode information on the food package into nutritional values to provide a clear view of intake in form of calorific or nutrient, and give related eating suggestions. Moreover, data collected from health tracking applications can also support self-reflection on eating behaviors and improve the self-awareness of eating decisions [19, 20]. There have been various digital applications developed to improve daily eating practices. For example, Hartwell et al. [21] designed the FoodSmart app to inform food consumption and give intake suggestions according to individual preferences. Sysoeva et al. [22] composed a mobile channel to provide healthy food choices via text and voice communication.

However, when applying those mHealth technologies to the working contexts, it appears to be challenging to generate desired health promotion outcomes. Recently, mHealth apps are being developed specifically aimed at preventing health risks in the working contexts [23, 24], but it only shows the potential rather than the effectiveness of such apps [25]. It comes as a surprise that little research has been done to investigate the end-users' needs to enhance the adaptivity of mHealth tools for promoting healthy eating in the daily work routines. Therefore, in this paper, we present a formative study of an mHealth app to promote healthy eating during office-based working hours. Through a series of semi-structured interviews, we derived a set of design requirements for relevant digital technologies, which led to the design of EAT@WORK, a mobile application to help individuals develop healthy eating behaviors during daily working routines. The prototype of EAT@WORK was evaluated through a within-subject user study with 14 office workers, which aimed to examine the user acceptance of EAT@WORK features and gain more design insights into updating future mHealth applications in the working context.

2 Design of EAT@WORK

To identify design opportunities of digital tools, we set out an interview study with 12 office workers (gender: 10 females and 2 males, age $= 39 \pm 11.52$, working experiences $= 16.21 \pm 13.00$), from a wide variety of occupations (e.g., secretary, researcher, administrator, human resource manager) in the societal context of the Netherlands.

All the interviews were semi-structured [32] with a set of open-ended questions. Each session was organized in two parts: We began by inquiring about participants' recent experiences with office eating routines. E.g., "How do you like your eating routine during workdays?" "Have you and your organization done anything to improve your office eating routine? And why?" and "What would you expect in the future to aid the eating aspect of your workdays?" We then discussed opportunities to design mHealth tools for enhancing their office eating routines with two open-ended questions: "How do you think to use digital technologies to improve eating routines at work?" and "What eating-related features do you expect in the future mHealth technology?" During the interview, we left enough space for participants to elaborate on their opinions freely. Besides, we asked them to explain some interesting statements that emerged from the discussion. The interview took around 18- to 39-min per session and was audio-recorded and transcribed later for thematic qualitative analysis.

All the detail of the interview study setup and results has been published in [33]. For the focus of this paper, we summarize the main findings from the interviews, which led to a design of the EAT@WORK app. The EAT@WORK app was developed as an interactive prototype using the Abode XD software for the Dutch working context (i.e., office, home office). The prototype was compatible with both Android and iOS systems with the following four key considerations.

2.1 Supporting Easy Access to Relevant Knowledge

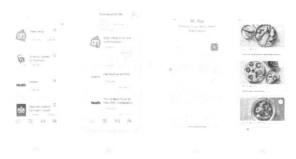

Fig. 1. The collection of relevant knowledge for improving the worker's eating routine. (a) full list of recommended knowledge providers; (b) list of subscribed knowledge providers; (c) search function; (d) specific info of one subscribed provider.

Our interviews suggested that nutrition knowledge could help office workers adhere to healthy food options and achieve eating goals. Nevertheless, the credibility and quality of health-related knowledge from the internet were critically concerned. The mixed quality of third-party resources has made it challenging for users to find the right information for the target health behaviors. One solution could be a platform that connects to reliable data resources (e.g., health authorities, food suppliers, health services, health experts) for valid knowledge of healthy eating.

The corresponding feature of EAT@WORK is an integrated tool that ensures easy access to nutrition info from the trustworthy knowledge providers, who are listed under the "*All*" view (Fig. 1(a)). In addition, the user can search for specific knowledge (Fig. 1(c)) and make their own collection by subscribing to different knowledge providers (Fig. 1(b)). Then, in the "*Subscribe*" view, it will provide the updates in real-time from those knowledge providers subscribed by the user (Fig. 1(d)).

2.2   Assisting in Setting up and Achieving Eating Goals

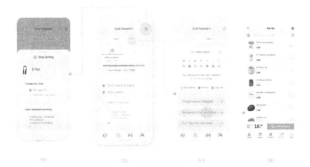

Fig. 2. The user interfaces for assisting workers in achieving eating-related health goals. (a) setting personal eating goals and keywords; (b) eating plan and intake tracking for working hours and non-working hours; (c) weekly review of goal achievement and plan for the next week; (d) direct to supermarket apps for efficient grocery shopping.

According to our interviewees' suggestions, specific and measurable eating goals could help office workers to formulate healthy eating behaviors. However, the eating conditions during working hours were always influenced by individuals' personal working routines. One solution could be a platform that connects to users' working schedules for planning proper eating time. Another challenge revealed by the interview is a long-term eating goal with limited feedback would demotivate users to adopt digital tools for healthy eating promotion. Thus, assisting users in setting short-term, achievable mini-goals and providing regular feedback could be an effective solution in establishing healthier eating routines during working hours.

For the related feature of EAT@WORK, in the "*Today*" view it facilitates the self-tracking of eating activities easily at both working hours and non-working hours through a time-dependent checklist (Fig. 2(b)). "*History*" view presents the historical data of the goal commitment as weekly summaries (Fig. 2(c)). Users can also find recipe suggestions and shopping recommendations (e.g., recipe, grocery shopping list, eating plan, etc.) based on their historical data (Fig. 2(d)).

2.3   Integrated Health Program

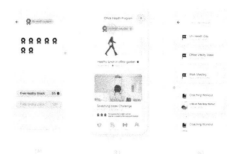

Fig. 3. The service facilitates the worker to participate in integrated health programs in the organization. (a) summary of received rewards; (b) followed health program and the completion status; (c) a list of recommended health programs.

As suggested by our interviews, a structured health program containing different interventions for promoting overall health is essential to reduce the negative influence of the daily work routine. Additionally, our interviewees believed that digital technologies (such as mHealth apps and health websites) could support their adoption of health programs in the working context over time. One suggested solution was a particular system with suggestions, challenges, and rewards for users to balance their nutrition and physical activities during working hours.

As shown in Fig. 3(b), under the "*Office Health Program*" tab of EAT@WORK, the user can follow a list of health-promoting activities organized by the company (e.g., working exercises) or suggested by the system (e.g., lunch stroll due to good weather). By completing these activities as health challenges, the user will receive some virtual rewards, such as digital coupons that can be used in the canteen and supermarkets to purchase healthy foods with a discount (Fig. 3(a)).

2.4   Facilitating Peer Support for Healthy Eating Routines

Based on our interview results, we found that interviewees preferred to eat with colleagues sharing similar eating routines. They also tended to consult others' eating patterns and food choices as guidance. Therefore, a social platform that leverages peer support between colleagues could potentially encourage healthy workaday eating patterns.

As shown in Fig. 4(a), (b), in the "*Buddy*" view the system help users with similar health goals or eating patterns to team up with each other as a health-promoting dyad at work. Once two users become buddies, they can check each other's goal completion in real-time and nudge each other via the app. The "*Community*" view facilitates a group of colleagues (e.g., coworkers from the same department, people in the same working group) to share the health-related information (e.g., external knowledge, personal experiences, questions) to encourage healthy eating via mutual interventions (Fig. 4(c), (d)).

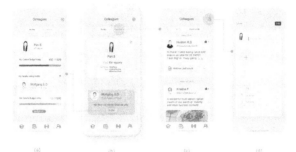

Fig. 4. The social platform leverages peer support among colleagues to encourage healthy eating. (a) health-promoting dyad with a similar eating goal; (b) a list of recommended users with similar eating goals; (c) a social platform that leverage peer support among colleagues and co-workers; (d) post personal health-related info to others.

3   Materials and Methods of User Study

This user study aimed to investigate 1) the user acceptance of EAT@WORK; and 2) design opportunities and challenges for the future application of EAT@WORK. For these purposes, Fig. 5 shows that a within-subject experiment was designed to compare the user acceptance of our interactive prototype with an existing mHealth system for healthy eating, followed by a co-creation session to qualitatively evaluate and discuss how the UX features of EAT@WORK could be improved and applied in different working contexts (i.e., telework vs. office work). The benchmark mHealth technology used in this study is called Traqq [34], which is a dietary assessment app and can be used as a recall and food record in the Dutch societal context. The study has received the Ethical Review approval at the Eindhoven University of Technology, with the reference number: ERB2020ID8.

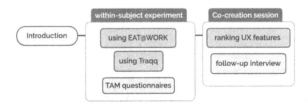

Fig. 5. A visualization of overall study procedure.

3.1   Participants

We recruited participants by spreading information via emails and public posts on social media such as Facebook and Twitter. We also invited participants from our previous semi-structured interview (as presented in Sect. 2), who contributed insights into the concept development of EAT@WORK. Due to the COVID-19 regulation, all the participants had to work from home during the period of our study (Nov–Dec 2020). Prior to the study, none of the participants had the using experiences with EAT@WORK and Traqq. They were fully informed the study's purpose and procedure and signed a consent form in advance and were given the opportunity to withdraw at any point of the study.

3.2   Study Design

In accordance with the COVID-19 regulation, we were able to conduct the study via remote meeting software (i.e., Microsoft Teams) and an online survey system (i.e., Microsoft Form). The study with each participant took around 65–80 min for the entire process, which consisted of a within-subject experiment and a co-creation session. Next, we describe the two sessions in detail.

Within-Subject Experiment.   Each experiment was divided into two conditions using EAT@WORK and Traqq respectively with the following procedure. For each condition, we firstly introduced one of the two apps by sharing our screen. We then sent a link containing the download address of the app and asked the participant to experience different features of the app for 15 min. Afterward, we asked the participant to fill in a short version Technology Acceptance Model (TAM) questionnaire, developed by Davis [35], based on their user experiences with the app. Upon the completion of the TAM questionnaire, we invited the participant to enter the next experiment with another condition following the same process as described above. The exposures to the EAT@WORK and the Traqq conditions were fully counterbalanced in our study. The comparison between these two apps was to verify whether EAT@WORK would receive reasonable high user acceptance during working hours. Thus, our first hypothesis is:

- H01: The EAT@WORK app will be deemed to be more useful and easier to use by office workers than Traqq.

Additionally, given our study involved both experienced subjects (who participated in the earlier study) and non-experienced subjects, we were also interested in knowing if such a difference would also influence their acceptance towards EAT@WORK. Therefore, the second hypothesis is:

- H02: The responses on the TAM questionnaire between the experienced and non-experienced participants will not be significantly different.

Co-creation Session.   To aid the interpretation of our quantitative comparison, at the start of this session we asked every participant: *"which app do you prefer to use during your working hours?" "Please describe the reason for your choice.",* individually. As shown in Fig. 6, We also prepared a Miro dashboard for facilitating the online co-creation. On the right side of the dashboard, we present the Four UX features of EAT@WORK (knowledge for me, goal assistant, health program, social). On the left side, we asked the participant to rank four features regarding their applicability to the office work context and the work-from-home context, respectively. The participant was then asked to explain their choices with three open-ended questions, which were developed according to Mobile App Rating Scale [36]. The Questions Were *"why do you rank features during your working hours in the office and at home in this way?" "Please describe the reason you like or dislike each feature and share your ideas for further improvement." "do you have any ideas, comments or suggestions concerning the use of digital applications during your working hours?"* Every participant was given enough space to freely express their opinions.

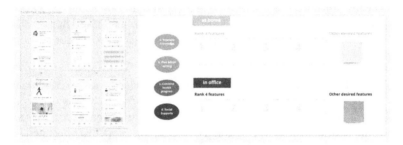

Fig. 6. The screenshot of our Miro co-creation dashboard.

3.3   Data Collection

For the quantitative data, we collected participants' responses to the TAM questionnaire and created the screenshots for the rankings of different UX features during the co-creation session. For this study, we used two subscales of TAM: Perceived Usefulness (PU) and Perceived Ease of Use (PEOU). In the questionnaire, each subscale contains six items, and each item has been designed as a seven-point Likert scale (from 1 – extremely unlikely to 7 – extremely likely). For the qualitative data, we audio-recorded each interview and transcribed interview content later for analysis.

3.4   Data Analysis

Quantitative Data. The responses to the TAM Questionnaire were analyzed using the SPSS software. Firstly, we processed the quantitative data with the descriptive statistics, in which we checked the distribution of the PU and PEOU data through Shapiro–Wilk tests, which showed that there had no significant difference with the normality ($P > 0.05$). Thus, the two-way mixed ANOVA was conducted with the user experience sessions with different prototypes (EAT@WORK vs. Traqq) as dependent variables, and the type of participants (experienced participants vs. non-experience participants) as independent factors. Where ANOVA was significant, pairwise comparisons were processed. The main objective of quantitative analyses was to examine the acceptance and usefulness of EAT@WORK.

Qualitative Data. The interview data were analyzed by thematic analysis following deductive coding [37] using the MAXQDA software. Specifically, our data analysis was proceeded as follows: to begin with, one researcher (the first author) transcribed responses and labeled statements using affinity diagrams [38] to identify clusters and themes. Next, according to the member check approach [39, 40], all the identified themes and clusters were reviewed, discussed, and revised through several iterations with all the members of the research team (all the co-authors) to validate the qualitative analysis. One main objective of qualitative data results was to indicate the importance and relevance of our quantitative data. another purpose was to gain design insights into future developments of healthy eating technologies for office workers.

4 Results

4.1 Participants' Description

Table 1. The demographics of the 14 participants (MBO: secondary vocational education, HBO: higher vocational education).

Group	ID	Sex	Age	Education level	Working years	Working hours/day	Type of occupation
Experienced Subjects (ES)	P1	F	45	HBO	21	8	Secretary
	P2	F	27	Bachelor	4	8	Secretary
	P3	F	54	HBO	36	8	Secretary
	P4	M	28	Master	3	8	Junior researcher
	P5	F	31	PhD	9	8	Researcher
	P8	M	26	Master	2	8	Junior researcher
	P10	M	30	Master	5	8	Program director
Non-Experienced Subjects (NS)	P6	F	27	MBO	1.5	8	Secretary
	P7	F	28	Master	3.5	8	Junior researcher
	P9	F	55	HBO	33	8	Office manager
	P11	M	28	Master	2	8	Office manager
	P12	F	26	Master	2.5	8	Researcher
	P13	F	38	Bachelor	15	8	Entrepreneur
	P14	F	38	Master	15	8	Program director

In total 14 participants from various working-based jobs in the Netherlands were recruited. Seven participants who took part in our early semi-structured interview study were named as experienced subjects (ES), while the rest newly recruited participants were named as non-experienced subjects (NS). These 14 participants (gender: 10 females and 4 males, age $= 34.36 \pm 10.20$, working experiences $= 12.26 \pm 13.18$) are labeled as P1 to P14. Their characteristics are summarized in Table 1.

4.2 The User Acceptance of EAT@WORK

Quantitative Findings. As shown in Fig. 7(a), the perceived usefulness (PU) of the EAT@WORK prototype was rated with a mean at 5.36 ($SE = 0.39$) by experienced subjects (ES) and 5.43 ($SE = 0.16$) by non-experienced subjects (NS). In contrast, the PU of the Traqq app was scored at 4.12 ($SE = 0.49$) by ES and 3.48 ($SE = 0.33$) by NS. The 2×2 ANOVA revealed that the PU between EAT@WORK and the Traqq app was significantly different ($F = 42.85, p < 0.01$), while the participation experiences did not affect the PU scores ($F = 2.15, p = 0.168$). The pairwise comparison showed that the usefulness of EAT@WORK ($M = 5.39, SE = 0.20$) was perceived significantly higher ($p < 0.01$) than Trapp ($M = 3.80, SE = 0.30$).

As shown in Fig. 7(b), the perceived ease of use (PEOU) of the EAT@WORK prototype was scored with a mean value of 5.71 ($SE = 0.36$) by ES and 6.10 ($SE = 0.17$) by NS. Traqq was rated at 4.86 ($SE = 0.36$) by ES and 5.14 ($SE = 0.33$) by NS in terms of PEOU. The 2x2 ANOVA revealed that the PEOU between EAT@WORK and Traqq has a significant difference ($F = 22.07, p < 0.01$), while there was no difference between the feedback from ES and NS ($F = 0.061, p = 0,809$). According to the pairwise comparison, EAT@WORK ($M = 5.90, SE = 0.20$) was perceived significantly easier to use ($p < 0.01$) than Traqq ($M = 5.00, SE = 0.24$).

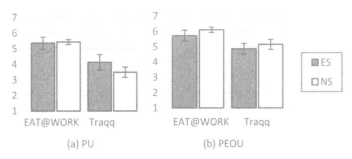

Fig. 7. Mean and SE of TAM.

Qualitative Findings. According to interview feedback, all the participants showed a positive attitude toward using digital technology for health promotion during their working hours. Compared to Traqq, all of them expressed their preference of using EAT@WORK to promote their workdays' eating routines in the future. The reasons for their choice can be summarized as the following aspects. firstly, they stated that they could see the potential benefits of this application because it included not only food tracking but also social and physical activities that are highly related to eating. for instance, some participants mentioned that *"it can also manage my physical activities, so I don't need to use another app (P1)"*, *"having an eating buddy would really help me to eat on time and share eating-related information to each other (P8)"*, *"I like reward setting in the prototype, which can motivate me to eat healthier foods."* Secondly, the responses indicated that a well-designed interface helped users adopt the system in a short term. As P12 explained, *I like the interface on this application, a clear layout helps me easily use the app during working hours.*

4.3   The Applicability of EAT@WORK UX Features in Different Contexts

The Rankings. As shown in Table 2, the 'knowledge for me' feature received similar scores in the two working contexts, with an average rank of 2.93 for office-based work (ObW) and 2.85 for work-from-home (WfH). Regarding the UX feature of 'goal assistant', it was considered mostly desirable for both contexts, as it received the first rank eight times for ObW and 12 times for WfH. The 'health program' feature received mixed feedback between those two contexts. On the one hand, for ObW nine out of 14 participants ranked this feature as the first or second, which made its average rank at 2.07. On the other hand, only four participants ranked this feature as the first half in the context of WfH, resulting its average rank at 2.86. interestingly, we found that the UX feature of 'social' in EAT@WORK was ranked the least desirable, as 50% of our participants ranked it the fourth feature in both working contexts.

Table 2. The ranking of four features in different types of working context (office-based work vs. home-based work in our case).

UX features	Office-based work					Work-from-home				
	1st	2nd	3rd	4th	Avg	1st	2nd	3rd	4th	Avg
'Knowledge for me'	1	5	2	6	2.93	0	6	4	4	2.85
'Goal assistant'	8	4	2	0	1.57	12	1	1	0	1.21
'Health program'	5	4	4	1	2.07	1	3	7	3	2.86
'Social'	0	1	6	7	3.43	1	4	2	7	3.07

Qualitative Feedback. From the follow-up interview, we learned several factors that led to the quantitative results of these UX features. First, almost all participants mentioned that a well-support goal assistant during working hours could be beneficial to their personal health. for example, some participants stated that: *"I prefer to have a scheduled eating plan no matter in the office or from home so that I can balance my working routines with it in an efficient way (P7)."* *"if the app could help me to plan my intake and achieve my eating goals step by step, it will save my time and let me pay more attention to my* *working tasks* (P11)." In addition, some participants presented that the 'health program' could be more useful to ObW than WfH. As P2 described: "*When I work in the office, I have a more overwhelming work schedule than work from home. So, I think I need the app to arrange healthy activities for me.*" Although participants thought 'social' is a contextual determinant that influences their eating patterns, it was not as essential and necessary as the first two features during working hours. P14 mentioned that "*Due to COVID-19, I have less contact with my colleagues and friends. EAT@WORK provides a remote way to have a connection with them, which is good. However, I can eat with my family and share eating-related information. I don't think I need to use an app to support my eating social activities unless I live alone.*" "*I like this function, but I prefer using other functions than this one because face-to-face eating with colleagues in the office and with family members at home is quiet enough for me* (P3)." Lastly, 'knowledge for me' was considered as an on-demand feature that would not be frequently used for the working contexts yet could be helpful on some particular occasions. For instance, some participants (P7, P8, P13, P14) stated that the feature might support them in preparing healthy work lunches, especially during the work-from-home period.

4.4 Extra Findings

From the interviews, we obtained a few qualitative suggestions for the future developments of EAT@WORK, which can be summarized into two aspects. Firstly, some participants suggested that the prototype could be embedded into the desktop software or workstations. E.g., "*I don't always use my mobile phone when I work (P3).*" "*It is better if the prototype could be a real product around me and help me to track my eating. (P6)*" "*If I can get notifications and feedbacks from my laptop, that will be easier for me to use the system in a long term* (P11)". Secondly, participants expected that the system could leverage machine learning to customize the using experiences and provide specific feedback. For example, P13 stated: "*It is better if the digital tool can learn when and how the office workers use the system and adapt its service flow according to the routine and habits of the user*". "*I really want to get some specific feedback based on my own situation, then I can decide what I should do and change accordingly to improve my eating* (P1)."

5   Discussion and Limitation

Healthy eating can contribute to the overall health and vitality of office workers [41]. The rapid advance of mHealth technologies can play a crucial role in improving the workday eating routines. In the working context, office workers can be very busy with their tasks at hand throughout the day and should keep their performance following the implicit and explicit working rules [42]. Obviously, this situation can potentially create barriers for utilizing digital health technologies as well as adhering to the health interventions during daily work. This paper reports a study that focuses on developing an mHealth application to promote healthy eating routines among office workers and examining its applicability to the context. A semi-structured interview with 12 office workers was conducted, which led to a set of design considerations, including the easy access to relevant knowledge, eating goal and planning support, the integrated workplace health programs, and social supports between coworkers. Based on these design considerations, we designed an mHealth application, called EAT@WORK, containing UX features of 'knowledge for me', 'goal assistant', 'health program', and 'social support'. To examine the usability and applicability of EAT@WORK, a formative user study was set out using a within-subject experiment and an online co-creation session. Both of our research hypotheses have been achieved. Our results revealed that EAT@WORK is more useful and easier to use by office workers than Traqq, and there has no using difference between experienced subjects as well as non-experienced subjects.

Regarding the within-subject experiment results, the two-way mixed ANOVA analysis between EAT@WORK and Traqq app revealed that EAT@WORK was an easy-to-use and useful digital tool in facilitating healthy eating for office workers. Participants showed a positive attitude toward using EAT@WORK because of its integrations among various eating-related elements (such as eating-related knowledge, health program, and social support) as well as its user-friendly and well-designed interfaces. Our results are consistent with earlier studies that embodying contextual elements (such as gaining nutrition knowledge [43], well-planned eating [44], and social influence on eating [45]) can improve the quality of individuals' diet and encourage healthy eating routines. Besides, easy-learning interfaces and natural interaction between digital tools and individuals positively influence the acceptance of digital tools [46, 47].

The results from co-creation session interviews indicated the applicability of EAT@WORK's four UX features ('knowledge for me', 'goal assistant', 'health program' and 'social'). Firstly, the 'goal assistant' feature could be helpful to plan eating routines and achieve eating goals in both office working and teleworking contexts. Secondly, 'health program' is more helpful to apply when people working in the office than working from home. Thirdly, 'social support' was a useful feature but not the main factor that affects eating routines and behaviors during working hours. Fourthly, 'knowledge for me' was considered as an on-demand feature that could be helpful on some particular occasions.

The user study also revealed several future design developments of EAT@WORK. On the one hand, our findings suggested that mHealth tools embedded into the desktop software or office necessities could be more appropriate for promoting healthy eating among office workers. This finding is in line with the research by Patrick et al. [48] that using existing infrastructures could reduce additional investments from users, thus increasing the technology adoption. On the other hand, customized user experiences and feedback were expected by most participants. This is in line with several previous pieces of research that tailored content and customized user feedback could help individuals to stick to promote their health [49, 50].

To summarize, this paper makes the following main contributions: 1) the considerations related to the design opportunities for improving the acceptance of mHealth tools for healthy eating among office workers; 2) the design of EAT@WORK prototype with four UX features.

The findings of this paper may need to be cautiously interpreted due to the following limitations. Firstly, the study was conducted with a small number of people (12 participants in the semi-structured interview and 14 participants in the user study) with an imbalanced sex ratio, which might not be adequate to quantitatively prove the acceptance of digital tools in the working context. Secondly, the findings were not representative of expected digital tool features globally. Different regions may have very varied working cultures and food cultures [51], it is valuable to evaluate digital tools in one particular cultural context.

6 Conclusion

This paper presented a formative study of an mHealth app, called EAT@WORK, for promoting healthy eating routines among office workers. Based on the societal context of the Netherlands, we set out this study to identify design considerations to appropriate mHealth technologies into the workday eating routines, as well as to develop and evaluate the related UX features. From our study, we proposed and confirmed that to support healthy eating behaviors at work, mHealth tools should be designed to enable the user to access health-relevant knowledge, planning and goal setting, involving in integrated office health programs, and creating peer support. Applying these considerations into the mHealth UX features could significantly improve user acceptance among office workers. Additionally, our qualitative study results revealed that the eating goal assistant could be generally applied in different working contexts, while the integrated health program might not very applicable to the teleworking context. Receiving social and knowledge supports for promoting healthy eating at work were considered to be on-demand experiences. These results were discussed and synthesized as design implications, including embedding the mHealth features into the existing infrastructure of the office and creating customized user experience. We look forward to consolidating and engineering our EAT@WORK prototype with nutritionists and application developers to enable the full user experiences. Eventually, we plan to conduct a longitudinal field study based on our finalized prototype to examine our design's effectiveness for promoting healthy eating during working hours.

Acknowledgment. We thank all participants who volunteered to take part in the studies. The first author is being sponsored by China Scholarship Council.

References

1. Organization, W.H.: Diet, Nutrition, and the Prevention of Chronic Diseases: Report of a Joint WHO/FAO Expert Consultation. World Health Organization, Geneva, vol. 916 (2003). ISBN 924120916X
2. Van Duijvenbode, D.C., Hoozemans, M.J.M., Van Poppel, M.N.M., Proper, K.I.: The relationship between overweight and obesity, and sick leave: a systematic review. Int. J. Obes. **33**, 807–816 (2009)
3. Berghöfer, A., Pischon, T., Reinhold, T., Apovian, C.M., Sharma, A.M., Willich, S.N.: Obesity prevalence from a European perspective: a systematic review. BMC Public Health **8**, 1–10 (2008)

4. Proper, K.I., De Bruyne, M.C., Hildebrandt, V.H., Van Der Beek, A.J., Meerding, W.J., Van Mechelen, W.: Costs, benefits and effectiveness of worksite physical activity counseling from the employer's perspective. Scand. J. Work. Environ. Health **1**, 36–46 (2004)
5. Maes, L., et al.: Effectiveness of workplace interventions in Europe promoting healthy eating: a systematic review. Eur. J. Public Health **22**, 677–683 (2012)
6. Brug, J.: Determinants of healthy eating: motivation, abilities and environmental opportunities. Fam. Pract. **25**, i50–i55 (2008)
7. Swan, E., Bouwman, L., Hiddink, G.J., Aarts, N., Koelen, M.: Profiling healthy eaters. Determining factors that predict healthy eating practices among Dutch adults. Appetite **2015**(89), 122–130 (2015)
8. Campbell, M.K., Tessaro, I., DeVellis, B., Benedict, S., Kelsey, K., Belton, L., Sanhueza, A.: Effects of a tailored health promotion program for female blue-collar workers: health works for women. Prev. Med. (Baltim) **34**, 313–323 (2002)
9. Park, S., Sung, E., Choi, Y., Ryu, S., Chang, Y., Gittelsohn, J.: Sociocultural factors influencing eating practices among office workers in urban South Korea. J. Nutr. Educ. Behav. **49**, 466–474 (2017)
10. Wierenga, D., Engbers, L.H., Van Empelen, P., Duijts, S., Hildebrandt, V.H., Van Mechelen, W.: What is actually measured in process evaluations for worksite health promotion programs: a systematic review. BMC Public Health **13**, 1–16 (2013)
11. Rongen, A., Robroek, S.J.W., van Lenthe, F.J., Burdorf, A.: Workplace health promotion: a meta-analysis of effectiveness. Am. J. Prev. Med. **44**, 406–415 (2013)
12. Drewnowski, A.: Impact of nutrition interventions and dietary nutrient density on productivity in the workplace. Nutr. Rev. **78**, 215–224 (2020)
13. Allan, J., Querstret, D., Banas, K., de Bruin, M.: Environmental interventions for altering eating behaviours of employees in the workplace: a systematic review. Obes. Rev. **18**, 214–226 (2017)
14. Jensen, J.D.: Can worksite nutritional interventions improve productivity and firm profitability? A literature review. Perspect. Public Health **131**, 184–192 (2011)
15. World Health Organization: mHealth: new horizons for health through mobile technologies (2011)
16. Šmahel, D., Macháčková, H., Šmahelová, M., Čevelíček, M., Almenara, C.A., Holubčíková, J.: Using mobile technology in eating behaviors. In: Digital Technology, Eating Behaviors, and Eating Disorders, pp. 101–118. Springer, Cham (2018). https://doi.org/10.1007/978-3-319-93221-7_6
17. Achananuparp, P., Abhishek, V., Lim, E.P., Yun, T.: Eat & tell: a randomized trial of random-Loss incentive to increase dietary self-Tracking compliance. In: ACM International Conference on Proceeding Series, April 2018, pp. 45–54 (2018)
18. Evans, D.: My fitness pal. Br J Sport. Med **51**, 1101–1102 (2017)
19. Wing, R.R., Hill, J.: Successful weight loss maintenance. Ann. Rev. Nutr. **21**, 323–341 (2001)
20. Parker, A.G., Grinter, R.E.: Collectivistic health promotion tools: accounting for the relationship between culture, food and nutrition. Int. J. Hum. Comput. Stud. **72**, 185–206 (2014)
21. Hartwell, H., et al.: Shaping smarter consumer food choices: the FoodSMART project. Nutr. Bull. **44**, 138–144 (2019)
22. Sysoeva, E., Zusik, I., Symonenko, O.: Food-to-person interaction: how to get information about what we eat? In: DIS 2017 Companion – Proceedings of 2017 ACM Conference on Designing Interactive Systems, pp. 106–110 (2017)
23. In corporate wellness programs, wearables take a step forward|Fortune. https://fortune.com/2014/04/15/in-corporate-wellness-programs-wearables-take-a-step-forward/. Accessed 24 Nov 2021

24. HR Magazine - Wearable technology for health and wellbeing Available online: https://www.hrmagazine.co.uk/content/features/wearable-technology-for-health-and-wellbeing. Accessed 25 Nov 2021

25. de Korte, E.M., Wiezer, N., Janssen, J.H., Vink, P., Kraaij, W.: Evaluating an mHealth app for health and well-being at work: mixed-method qualitative study. JMIR mHealth uHealth **6**, e6335 (2018)

26. Zhu, F., et al.: Technology-assisted dietary assessment. Comput. Imaging VI **6814**, 681411 (2008)

27. Lazar, A., Koehler, C., Tanenbaum, J., Nguyen, D.H.: Why we use and abandon smart devices. In: UbiComp 2015 – Proceedings of 2015 ACM International Joint Conference on Pervasive Ubiquitous Computing, pp. 635–646 (2015)

28. Hofstede, G.: Dimensionalizing cultures: the hofstede model in context. Online Readings Psychol. Cult. **2**, 1–26 (2011)

29. De Castro, J.M., Bellisle, F., Feunekes, G.I.J., Dalix, A.M., De Graaf, C.: Culture and meal patterns: A comparison of the food intake of free- living American, Dutch, and French students. Nutr. Res. **17**, 807–829 (1997)

30. Stajcic, N.: Understanding culture: food as a means of communication. Hemispheres. Stud. Cult. Soc. **28**, 77–87 (2013)

31. World Health Organization: WHO Guideline Recommendations on Digital Interventions for Health System Strengthening. World Health Organization, Geneva (2019). [cited 15 July 2020]

32. Kallio, H., Pietilä, A., Johnson, M., Kangasniemi, M.: Systematic methodological review: developing a framework for a qualitative semi-structured interview guide. J. Adv. Nurs. **72**, 2954–2965 (2016)

33. Pan, S., Ren, X., Vos, S., Brombacher, A.: Design opportunities of digital tools for promoting healthy eating routines among Dutch office workers. In: Stephanidis, C., et al. (eds.) HCII 2021. LNCS, vol. 13097, pp. 94–110. Springer, Cham (2021). https://doi.org/10.1007/978-3-030-90966-6_8

34. Brouwer-Brolsma, E.M., et al.: Dietary intake assessment: from traditional paper-pencil questionnaires to technology-based tools. In: Athanasiadis, I.N., Frysinger, S.P., Schimak, G., Knibbe, W.J. (eds.) ISESS 2020. IAICT, vol. 554, pp. 7–23. Springer, Cham (2020). https://doi.org/10.1007/978-3-030-39815-6_2

35. Davis, F.D.: Perceived usefulness, perceived ease of use, and user acceptance of information technology. MIS Q. Manag. Inf. Syst. **13**, 319–339 (1989)

36. Stoyanov, S.R., Hides, L., Kavanagh, D.J., Zelenko, O., Tjondronegoro, D., Mani, M.: Mobile app rating scale: a new tool for assessing the quality of health mobile apps. JMIR mHealth uHealth **3**, e27 (2015)

37. Braun, V., Clarke, V.: Using thematic analysis in psychology. Qual. Res. Psychol. **3**, 77–101 (2006)

38. Kawakita, J.: The original KJ method. Tokyo. Kawakita. Res. Inst. **5**, 1–7 (1991)

39. Birt, L., Scott, S., Cavers, D., Campbell, C., Walter, F.: Member checking: a tool to enhance trustworthiness or merely a nod to validation? Qual. Health Res. **26**, 1802–1811 (2016)

40. Koelsch, L.E.: Reconceptualizing the member check interview. Int. J. Qual. Methods **12**, 168–179 (2013)

41. Canada, H.: Eating Well with Canada's Food Guide: A Resource for Educators and Communicators. Publications Health Canada, Ottawa (2011). ISBN 0662444698

42. Reinhardt, W., Schmidt, B., Sloep, P., Drachsler, H.: Knowledge worker roles and actions—results of two empirical studies. Knowl. Process Manag. **18**, 150–174 (2011)

43. Nestle, M., et al.: Behavioral and social influences on food choice. Nutr. Rev. **56**, 50–64 (2009)

44. Hargreaves, M.K., Schlundt, D.G., Buchowski, M.S.: Contextual factors influencing the eating behaviours of African American women: a focus group investigation. Ethn. Heal. **7**, 133–147 (2002)
45. Higgs, S., Thomas, J.: Social influences on eating. Curr. Opin. Behav. Sci. **9**, 1–6 (2016)
46. Lu, J., Chen, Q., Chen, X.: App interface study on how to improve user experience. In: Proceedings of the 2012 7th International Conference on Computer Science and Education (ICCSE), pp. 726–729. IEEE (2012)
47. Zheng, Y., Gao, X., Li, L.: Information resonance in intelligent product interface design. In: Proceedings of the 2009 IEEE 10th International Conference on Computer-Aided Industrial Design and Conceptual Design, pp. 1353–1356. IEEE (2009)
48. Patrick, K., et al.: The pace of technologic change: implications for digital health behavior intervention research. Am. J. Prev. Med. **51**, 816–824 (2016)
49. Coulter, A., Entwistle, V.A., Eccles, A., Ryan, S., Shepperd, S., Perera, R.: Personalised care planning for adults with chronic or long-term health conditions. Cochrane Database Syst. Rev. **2015**, 1–120 (2015)
50. Ordovas, J.M., Ferguson, L.R., Tai, E.S., Mathers, J.C.: Personalised nutrition and health. Bmj. **361**, 1–6 (2018)
51. Silva, T.H., Vaz De Melo, P.O.S., Almeida, J., Musolesi, M., Loureiro, A.: You are what you eat (and drink): identifying cultural boundaries by analyzing food and drink habits in foursquare. In: Proceedings of 8th International Conference on Weblogs Social Media, ICWSM 2014, pp. 466–475 (2014)

Design Contributions to Pervasive Health and Care Services

Designing for and with Neurodiverse Users: Wearable Applications for Self-regulation

Vivian Genaro Motti$^{(\boxtimes)}$ ⓘ, Niloofar Kalantari, Anika Islam,
and Leela Yaddanapudi

George Mason University, Fairfax, VA 22030, USA
vmotti@gmu.edu

Abstract. Wearable Technologies have a large potential to provide assistance to neurodiverse users – thanks to their close proximity to the user, continuous usage, and discreteness. However traditional user-centric design techniques are not always suitable to attend the needs of this user population. In this paper, we discuss practical considerations for methodological approaches involving neurodiverse users front and center in the design of assistive wearables. The discussion is grounded on a longitudinal field study conducted with a cohort of eight young adults with Down Syndrome and Autism. We designed, developed, and evaluated an assistive wearable application that provides emotion regulation support on demand. Study participants provided feedback through questionnaires, weekly meetings, and interviews. This paper presents and discusses design considerations, as well as the challenges and recommendations for recruitment, design, and evaluation of the application.

Keywords: Assistive wearables · Neurodiversity · Emotion regulation · Design

1 Introduction

Wearable technologies have evolved in the past decades to include miniaturized hardware, energy-efficient batteries, and protocols for data transmission [5,6]. Wearable technologies are well-suited to serve as assistive devices [3], first, due to their conventional look they can reduce potential stigmas; second, their on-body interfaces are beneficial for on demand interventions and timely assistance; third, the availability of development frameworks allow for customized solutions for hardware and applications as well [10].

Assistive technologies aim to provide support for users with diverse needs. Assistive technologies are able to augment human abilities and/or to replace those, helping users to achieve high quality of life and to live more independently. Although assistive technologies have been extensively researched and

H. Lewy and R. Barkan (Eds.): PH 2021, LNICST 431, pp. 553–560, 2022.
https://doi.org/10.1007/978-3-030-99194-4_34

developed for many types of disabilities, including visual impairments, hearing impairments, and motor impairments [3], fewer technologies have been dedicated to meet the specific needs of neurodiverse users–a population that has been increasing in number and whose conditions largely vary.

Neurodiverse conditions include attention deficit and hyperactivity disorder (ADHD), Autism, Down Syndrome, and cerebral palsy. They are characterized by variations in cognitive abilities, information processing, and executive functions. They are lifelong and chronic, manifesting themselves in a spectrum, i.e. each individual has unique traits, abilities, assets, strengths, and limitations as well.

The field of accessibility has involved users with disabilities in the design of technology since its inception. Still, there are tendencies to focus on specific disabilities and to closely involve end users' peers (e.g., parents, caregivers, professionals) rather than users with diverse needs. Oftentimes users with diverse needs are not sufficiently involved in the design process to actively inform and iteratively shape the design of technology [4]. Moreover, several techniques employed conventionally in a user-centered design process are not suitable for neurodiverse users [2], specifically, think aloud requires participants to be verbal (which is not always the case for autistic individuals) and to concentrate on multiple tasks at a time (inspecting the user interface and describing their thought processes) [7]. Diaries for example require participants with cognitive abilities, literacy skills, and memory which may be impaired for users with Down Syndrome and dysgraphia.

To involve neurodiverse users front and center in the research and design agenda, we need to take into account their specific abilities [9], i.e. motor skills (for sketching tasks), visual thinking (for diagramming), communication skills (verbal expression), literacy levels (reading and writing), among others. Because no validated methods or best practices specific to neurodiverse populations exist in the field, we rely on recommendations from the research community [1]. Still, it is crucial to report and discuss the experiences of investigators conducting such studies in order to identify methodological approaches that have been proven to be successful to engage neurodiverse users in the design process [2]. Additionally, we must reflect on the potential sources of bias and address those [8].

This paper reflects on the authors' experience, conducting user studies for and with neurodiverse participants for the past five years. The discussion focuses on the design, development, and evaluation of assistive wearables and a gender-balanced participant population of young adults. Application domains for the technology involved contexts that range from inclusive employment, independent living facilities, and postsecondary programs. Specifically, we focus on a case study involving the design and development of assistive smartwatch applications for emotion regulation. We present the challenges faced in recruitment, data collection, analysis, and deployment of the tool. We conclude with design implications for stakeholders investigating wearables as assistive technologies for neurodiverse users.

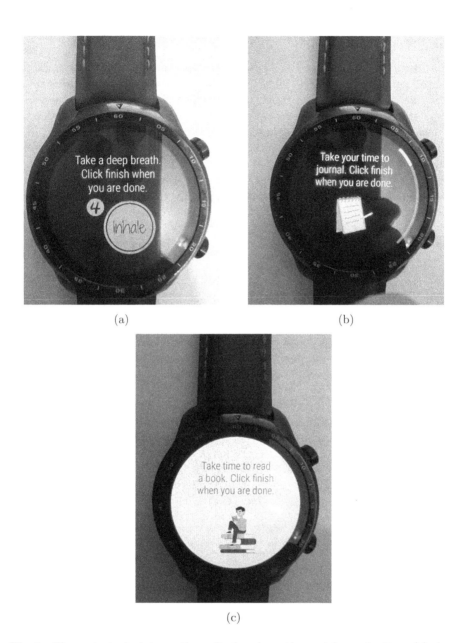

(a)

(b)

(c)

Fig. 1. Three strategic interventions displayed on the watch application: (a) deep breathing; (b) journalling; and (c) reading. Participants could suggest interventions in the beginning of the study, to customize the app. The interventions were triggered per time.

2   Methods

2.1   Recruitment

Upon Institutional Review Board approval of the study protocol by the university, we recruited neurodiverse participants. We advertised the study using flyers, emails, and word-of-mouth. Specifically, we relied on a network of contacts of alumni from a postsecondary inclusive program (email list), we also contacted the coach of the Special Olympics where the study has been conducted, and distributed the call for participation in social media channels (dedicated parent groups on Facebook). We reached out to the coordinators of independent living facilities in our region (Northeastern US) and other educational programs. More than 100 people were contacted–including neurodiverse adults, parents, and professionals, such as: coaches, analysts, therapists, and caregivers. The recruitment took place in the Spring 2021.

2.2   Experimental Design

The study consisted of three parts: onboarding, weekly meetings, and closure interviews. Initially, in the onboarding phase, we applied a demographic form, collecting profile information such as age, gender, condition, and preferred interventions. Secondly, participants joined a video conference call to watch a demo video about the watch app, and received the watch with a phone. The delivery of the devices was done via porch pick up or mail, to avoid issues related to COVID-19. A pre-paid data package was used to ensure all participants had a stable Internet connection to synchronize data. In the second phase, the participants started using the watch. The duration of their participation ranged from 4 to 8 weeks. Each participant received notifications and prompts on their watches at their preferred times (morning, afternoon, or evening) and frequency (5 to 10 times per day) as they indicated in the responses to the demographic form. Lastly, to give closure to the study, we invited participants to join a one-on-one interview and to recall the memorable events when they needed the watch.

2.3   Data Collection

We collected data using a brief questionnaire (demographic form) to characterize profile information, and gather their individual preferences regarding the types of strategic interventions (preferred regulation techniques). Also, the watch collected data about their responses (mood at the time of the notification, intervention chosen, heart rate and timestamp). We collected heart rate data in order to identify the potential success of the intervention in decreasing high heart rates. Also, we revised the transcripts from the audio recorded in weekly meetings. Lastly, for the individual interviews we asked participants to draw their ideas, describing their experiences. In case they were not comfortable with sketching or drawing they had the option to explain out loud their experiences using the watch application.

2.4 Data Analysis

We adopted a mixed-method approach for data analysis according to the nature of the data collected, amount, and research questions of interest. Specifically, to analyze the watch data (log files) we assessed the times in which the application was accessed, the choice of strategic intervention, the changes in heart rate. To analyze the video transcripts, we highlighted the comments related to their experience, suggestions for modification, challenges faced, among others. The analysis of the closure interviews was also based on review and annotation of the audio transcripts. The analysis was conducted in a collaborative effort by the research team, specifically, we meet weekly to discuss the study protocol, procedure for analysis, and key research findings.

2.5 Incentives

Each participant was compensated with a US$25 gift card, delivered by email, after participation in the final interview and return of the equipment.

3 Results

3.1 WELLI

As Fig. 1 shows, the application was implemented for Android watches (using Wear OS). In the database we stored data about the user interaction as log files. All participants received the same version of the watch and phones. A brief training was provided to explain how to use the app, and weekly calls were held online to discuss the user experience. The next sections summarize major design considerations based on the analysis of field notes.

3.2 Design Considerations

Regarding the acceptance of the watch, participants who were already familiar with a smartwatch from another brand and model (e.g., an Apple watch), hesitated to switch to another device. As they became more familiar with the watch and learned how to use it, such a concern faded. A few participants would like to continue using the device after the study ended, stating for example "Should we return the watch in one month? Can I have it longer?" [P4]. This indicates a potential for long term adoption and acceptance of the app.

Regarding the strategic interventions, initially, participants could not easily identify and suggest their preferred interventions. However, as they became more familiarized with the app during the study, they recommended interventions and asked us to update the list of pre-defined interventions. As P3 asked: "Is it possible to put watching TV on my watch as one of my things? I don't like storms, and it is storming and when the weather is like this, watching TV helps me be calm" [P3]. We observe that having their favorite interventions implemented proved to be successful for participants, whereas not having those available led to the rejection of the app.

Regarding the participatory design and inclusion (designing for and with neurodiverse users), some participants were invested in the study, even offering to assist other participants with training. Also, they offered to further advertise the study and invited their friends to join it as well. As P3 mentioned: "Is it ok if I let P2 know how she should use the watch? I can help her to learn it. I know all the things about the watch, and I can help if you want" [P3]. Such recommendation suggests that participants were engaged with the study and took ownership to exert their agency, influencing recruitment and leading to a community-based approach for onboarding.

Regarding the utility of the watch, when participants were not using the app they felt the need to have it readily available. This was remarkable in situations of extreme stress, for instance when P3 experienced a shooting event during an football match and informed that she wished she had the watch with her to calm her down. She felt upset that she could not use the watch at that moment. Also, when they could not use the watch due to technical issues they felt frustrated. P4 for instance had problems connecting her watch to the Bluetooth. Because she felt upset she asked the researchers to assist her promptly, so that she could start using the app the next day.

Regarding the effectiveness of the app and interventions, we noticed participants were overall satisfied. In weekly calls, participants shared their experience using the watch and how it impacted their routines. For P4, a delay in her work schedule caused frustration, but she stated that the breathing techniques in the watch helped her to feel better: "Getting a notification that asks me if I am feeling all right and checking on me makes me happy. I expect to see some kind of rewarding quote in the notifications, like 'you are doing great!' I like some notifications that say you have had more than 500 steps so far. Excellent job. It always feels good to receive something like this" [P4]. Positive reinforcement has been identified as a key design decision for technology implemented for neurodiverse users, such a remark confirms findings from prior work.

As noted in previous studies, positive reinforcement is highly appreciated among neurodiverse participants. Hence, in the watch app WELLI, participants accumulate stars when the strategic interventions are completed. In the weekly meetings, participants expressed excitement about the stars they had received. The rewards system also encourages them to use the app. As P1 mentioned: "...it's kind of sad because I got really excited with seeing the stars, but I haven't seen my stars in a while...". The watch app proved to be useful even during their holidays, as P1 stated "... me and my parents were on vacation at the home for a couple of days and I had to make sure to wear my watch every day and whenever we took some walk... For make star, I always click finish" [P1]. Such comments indicate that overall participants had a positive experience and enjoyed using the app.

3.3 Discussion of the Methodological Approach

Recruitment of participants during the pandemic proved to be more challenging. Specifically, it required more time and effort of investigators to find participants who were willing to join the study. Some participants already had a watch but of another brand/model (Apple Watch) and were not willing to switch devices. Also, some participants had vacation plans, and the lack of routine summed with travel prevented them from attending weekly meetings. Although more than 80 participants were contacted, the initial cohort consisted of 8 people. While no conclusive results can be obtained from a small sample size, we approach the analysis in depth investigating individual experiences longitudinally.

We observe in the findings that the technology interest of each participant influenced their device usage. In other words, participants who were more inclined to technology took the lead on training their peers, explaining how the device works, and inviting their friends to join the study. Such an appropriation is beneficial since participants took ownership of the study and engaged in a kind of community-based approach to engage others as well.

To address connectivity issues, we provided participants with a pre-paid data card since it proved to be easier than managing problems related to WiFi connections at various locations. Because we aimed at ecological validity in multiple sites, reducing the burden related to setting up devices became an essential requirement in the study.

Regarding social connections, the weekly meetings proved to be a great opportunity for participants to meet and talk to one another, even those who did not use the watch application regularly still enjoyed joining the weekly meetings as an opportunity to meet their peers, and talk to them. Still, reminders were needed to encourage participation in online meetings.

3.4 Participants' Experience

We observed in the study that the acceptance, adoption, and attachment to the watch app was tied to participants' levels of self-awareness about their emotions, or executive function, but not necessarily linked to a disability type or IQ level. Further studies with a large sample size are needed though to identify potential causation effects.

Regardless of the level of participant engagement in the study, we observed their enjoyment in interacting with other people in the call, in addition to technology use. Hence, the weekly meetings lasted longer than initially planned. Also, participants who were not using the watch app regularly, kept joining the call. This observation must consider the COVID-19 pandemic context, in which participants had their regular routines disrupted and remained in isolation, instead of going to classes, work, or practicing group activities.

Regarding need for training, the onboarding process was extended, with participants requiring reminders, prompts, and regular contact to troubleshoot watch app issues or to notify them to use the app.

4   Concluding Remarks

This paper reports on the design and evaluation of an assistive wearable application that provides support for emotion regulation for neurodiverse adults. The field study discussed involved 8 participants who used the app during 8 weeks. The analysis of the field notes yield design recommendations that can guide future research with neurodiverse users. Specifically, we discuss how we addressed challenges in recruitment, connectivity, user engagement, and adoption.

Acknowledgments. We thank all the study participants who joined the study, Dr. Evmenova and Dr. Heidi Graff from SourceAmerica for their collaborations. This research received financial support from the National Institute on Disability, Independent Living, and Rehabilitation Research (NIDILRR) under Grant No. 90DPGE0009.

References

1. Cibrian, F.L., Lakes, K.D., Schuck, S.E., Hayes, G.R.: The potential for emerging technologies to support self-regulation in children with ADHD: a literature review. Int. J. Child-Comput. Interact. **31**, 100421 (2022)
2. Frauenberger, C., Makhaeva, J., Spiel, K.: Blending methods: developing participatory design sessions for autistic children. In: Proceedings of the 2017 Conference on Interaction Design and Children, pp. 39–49 (2017)
3. Motti, V.G.: Assistive wearables: opportunities and challenges. In: Adjunct Proceedings of the 2019 ACM International Joint Conference on Pervasive and Ubiquitous Computing and Proceedings of the 2019 ACM International Symposium on Wearable Computers, pp. 1040–1043 (2019)
4. Motti, V.G.: Designing emerging technologies for and with neurodiverse users. In: Proceedings of the 37th ACM International Conference on the Design of Communication, pp. 1–10 (2019)
5. Motti, V.G.: Introduction to wearable computers. In: Motti, V.G. (ed.) Wearable Interaction, pp. 1–39. Springer, Cham (2020). https://doi.org/10.1007/978-3-030-27111-4_1
6. Motti, V.G.: Wearable Interaction. Springer, Heidelberg (2020). https://doi.org/10.1007/978-3-030-27111-4
7. Motti, V.G., Evmenova, A.: Designing technologies for neurodiverse users: considerations from research practice. In: Ahram, T., Taiar, R., Colson, S., Choplin, A. (eds.) IHIET 2019. AISC, vol. 1018, pp. 268–274. Springer, Cham (2020). https://doi.org/10.1007/978-3-030-25629-6_42
8. Spiel, K., et al.: Nothing about us without us: investigating the role of critical disability studies in HCI. In: Extended Abstracts of the 2020 CHI Conference on Human Factors in Computing Systems, pp. 1–8 (2020)
9. Wobbrock, J.O., Kane, S.K., Gajos, K.Z., Harada, S., Froehlich, J.: Ability-based design: concept, principles and examples. ACM Trans. Accessible Comput. (TACCESS) **3**(3), 1–27 (2011)
10. Zheng, H., Genaro Motti, V.: Assisting students with intellectual and developmental disabilities in inclusive education with smartwatches. In: Proceedings of the 2018 CHI Conference on Human Factors in Computing Systems, pp. 1–12 (2018)

Augmented Reality Games for Children with Cerebral Palsy

Charlotte Magnusson$^{(\boxtimes)}$, Kirsten Rassmus-Gröhn, and Cecilia Lindskog

Department of Design Sciences, Lund University, PO Box 118, 221 00 Lund, Sweden
charlotte.magnusson@certec.lth.se

Abstract. This paper describes and discusses the development of mobile exergames for children with cerebral palsy. The design process was built on co-design, and resulted in three activity games, two augmented reality (AR) games and one GPS based game. The resulting activity games were evaluated by 8 persons with cerebral palsy (CP). To complement this evaluation, the games have been evaluated against existing guidelines for accessible games. The developed games provide a proof of concept of how mobile games can be designed to encourage physical activity for children with mobility impairments.

Keywords: Physical activity · Cerebral Palsy · Exergame

1 Introduction

1.1 Background

Children and adults with cerebral palsy (CP) often participate less in physical activities, and have reduced health related fitness (muscle strength and cardiorespiratory endurance) [1], having a higher risk for negative health outcomes; eg cardiovascular disease. CP is also often associated with pain, making physical activity less attractive. At the same time, exercise can both improve fitness/function and reduce pain [2]. It is thus important to find ways to make physical activity motivating, in order to encourage children, as well as adults, with these kinds of problems to become more physically active. Video exergames have been successfully developed for children with CP [3], however video games require special equipment which is both costly and which is also tied to a specific location.

With the success of Pokémon Go, it has become clear that mobile games can promote physical activity, and that they may reach populations who are otherwise typically difficult to reach (those with established sedentary behaviors) [4]. Unfortunately, many mainstream games may be difficult to interact with for a person disabilities [5], and there is a need for more games developed for this user group.

© ICST Institute for Computer Sciences, Social Informatics and Telecommunications Engineering 2022
Published by Springer Nature Switzerland AG 2022. All Rights Reserved
H. Lewy and R. Barkan (Eds.): PH 2021, LNICST 431, pp. 561–567, 2022.
https://doi.org/10.1007/978-3-030-99194-4_35

1.2   Project GameA

The aim of the project GameA was to develop activity games specially designed for children with mobility impairments such as Cerebral Palsy (CP) or Spina bifida (MMC). The goal of these activity games should be to encourage movement and counteract a sedentary lifestyle. They should also be adapted to the abilities of our user group, while being inclusive. Within the framework of this project different technologies and designs were investigated. The project was based on co-design, and started with workshops together with users, to gather ideas and evaluate different types of technology. Covid-19 then prevented physical meetings, which meant that we had to collect opinions digitally, as well as through informal contacts with children with and without mobility impairments. The design process resulted in three activity games, two AR games and one GPS based game. We also have an overall game app "PlantAliens" incorporating the two AR games, where you develop characters by collecting points in the activity games. The app is available for iPhone[1] and Android[2]. The activity games in PlantAliens were evaluated by 8 persons with CP who rated the AR games as easy to understand and play, and on average judged the speed/difficulty as "appropriate". To complement this evaluation, the games have been evaluated against existing guidelines for accessible games.

The project team consisted of researchers from the Department of Design Sciences, Lund University, Do-Fi - a game company, RBU Skåne and Funkibator – end user organizations, Musik i Syd – an organization working with music for children, who had an existing app for children called MusikA, and a physiotherapist and health science researcher from Lund University, Annika Lundkvist Josenby, specialized in pediatrics/neurological disorders and with clinical experience of working the target user group. The project had ethical approval (2019-04069).

2   Design Process

After the initial brainstorms in the project team, it was decided together with our clinical expert not to focus on specific movements where the challenge is to perform the movement correctly, but rather to focus on encouraging movements involving the whole body such as standing or walking. In order to get initial input from our user group, we organized a technology exploration workshop. For this workshop we collected a set of existing games and demos, which all relied on physical movement for the interaction, didn't require strength/endurance and worked in a smaller area/indoors. We had a NFC-tag treasure hunt, an audio game where the phone would produce different sounds depending on how it was moved, an augmented reality (AR) game where you killed bugs and a step counting game where you could collect keys and chests (the keys would unlock the chests). Two young persons with CP attended this workshop and explored and discussed the different games. This workshop was followed by a study visit/workshop at the end user organization Funkibator, which (among other things) organizes game sessions for persons with disabilities, where we tested VR games, dance mats and also discussed the mobile games from our earlier workshop with end users. Based on the

---

[1] https://apps.apple.com/se/app/plantaliens/id1547433659.

[2] https://play.google.com/store/apps/details?id=com.DoFi.PlantAliens.

results from these two activities, we decided to focus the development primarily around AR games. The bug-shooter AR game was very clearly the most popular game at the user workshop, but AR games also have several advantages from a more technical perspective; given that AR uses the video stream from the camera, they are less heavy from a development point of view (no need to create virtual environments, it is enough to create virtual characters), AR works anywhere and doesn't necessarily require strength or endurance. In a parallel design process within a master thesis project, an additional GPS based game was developed.

At this stage in the project, the Covid pandemic hit, and all project activities had to be move on-line. While the development could continue fairly unhindered, user activities became more problematic. We were able to get some users to test game prototypes informally, but user workshops were harder. Normally, we in the research team would install and do all setup for the users (while finished apps should be easy to install and set up, prototypes are less finished and often require more tech support), but when testing is done remotely, the user or someone close to the user has to take care of the setup procedure. This turned out to be a significant hurdle, and we had to rely mainly on informal testing by persons that participants in the project were able to meet during the development process. Since the project involved both end user organizations as well as a clinician this still provided useful input, but it was a restriction. Once we had more finished prototypes, we were able to distribute our games for testing digitally, and our final game designs were tested by 8 persons with cerebral palsy (one teenager, 5 young adults, and two adults). In this final evaluation, the AR games were rated as easy to understand and play and the speed/difficulty was on average judged as "appropriate". The GPS game was built on MapBox, and unfortunately suffered from technical problems (not loading, freezing) which impacted on the user experience (about half of the testers found it easy while the rest rated the difficulty as neutral or hard). Given these technical problems, the GPS based app was not included in the released version of PlantAliens.

To complement the user evaluation, we also did a heuristic evaluation based on the Game Accessibility Guidelines[3]. In general the games follow these guidelines well, the user can select distances/difficulty, interactive elements are not too many, and are fairly big/easy to see, the game do not require great fine motor precision (eg the gun for shooting bugs fires automatically), sounds complement the visual feedback, and the games work both in landscape and portrait orientation. Still, we can also see room for improvement; more settings might make the games even more adaptable, more instructions could potentially be included in the games and of course, the games could involve even more levels/more development over time.

3 Game Design

Two AR games were designed. In one, the user can catch objects (clouds) by moving the whole phone close to the object, in the other the user can point towards a target (bugs) to shoot it. The shooting triggers automatically once the phone is pointing towards a potential target. You have to keep pointing in the same direction in order to hit the target with a couple of shots before it explodes.

---

[3] http://gameaccessibilityguidelines.com.

The two games are set within an overall framework where you collect some kind of alien plants ("PlantAliens"), in the AR games you collect resources in order to nurture your plants and unlock new ones (Fig. 1). The AR games increase in difficulty – initially targets keep still, but as you progress in the game they fade away faster (clouds) or start moving (bugs). The game area is selected every time you start the game, for the clouds you have four choices (close in front, middle in front, middle all around and far all around), while for the bugs there are two choices, in front or all around. Graphical elements that reflect different abilities, eg figures with wheels/wheelchair are included.

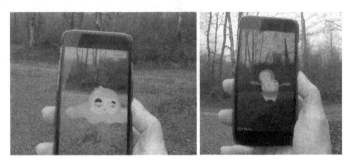

Fig. 1. Screen shots from the cloud game (left) and bug game (right). (Color figure online)

In the GPS game, the goal was to collect stars, and it allowed the user to select short, medium or long distances (Fig. 2). The game was initially intended to be used together with the AR games to unlock game features, but due to the technical problems experienced, the GPS game was not included in the final PlantAliens app. If included, the game would have allowed users to choose freely which game to play, in order to cater to differences in abilities and preferences.

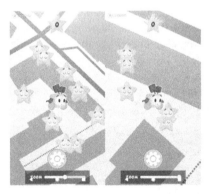

Fig. 2. Screen shots from the GPS game at two different map zoom levels. The user avatar is the yellow/red figure in the middle. When you get close to a star it wakes up, and you can catch it. (Color figure online)

3.1 Game Area

A general challenge in the game development has been how to adapt it to different abilities. It should be possible to play the game from sitting, as well as from standing (with different abilities to move around). Our initial design was based on an enclosed area where one could move the corners of the area in order to get the correct shape (Fig. 3). In order to change the shape, the user could point the cross hair to a corner-ball, put a finger anywhere on the screen, and then move the ball/corner by moving the whole phone in space until it was in the right place.

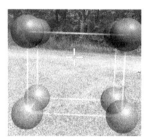

Fig. 3. Enclosed game area. The corners could be moved into any position separately, and it was also possible to move the whole shape to a new position.

Putting the finger on the screen with the cursor not on a ball, would select all the balls, and you could then move the whole shape by moving the phone. In the final version of the games, this was changed to pre-determined game areas (Fig. 4).

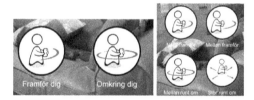

Fig. 4. Pre-determined game areas. In front of you or around you (bugs) or in front close, in front medium, all around medium and all around far (clouds).

4   Discussion and Conclusion

The developed games provide a proof of concept of how mobile AR games can be designed to encourage physical activity for children with mobility impairments (CP). In earlier projects eg [6], we had done both graphic and sound design ourselves (relying on bought material from shutterstock.com and freesound.org), while in this project we had the privilege to work with both graphic game designers and a musician, something which, as expected, made a huge difference.

By relying on AR, it is possible to design games which require quite limited movements, which are fun/engaging and which can be played anywhere there is a suitable environment.

A difficulty we struggled with during the development was the adaptation of the game area. For a person with limited mobility, it is crucial that the game can be restricted to a suitable space – it is no fun if you get stuck in a game simply because you cannot reach/hit a target. Our initial version of the games included a game area setting, where you could drag the corners of the game area into any configuration you wanted. Once you had the desired configuration it was saved and could be re-used. However, the exact location of the center of the game area would usually need to be adjusted every time, since the origin location in the AR coordinate system was where the game was started. While tests showed the initial design was in principle a working solution (the persons who tested it were able to use it), it turned out to be cumbersome. Thus, we decided to scrap this very flexible design for one with pre-set game areas. More research on how to make this type of games more flexible and adaptable, while keeping them simple and usable is needed. Still, the interaction by physically dragging virtual object, moving them by moving the whole phone worked well in itself, and could potentially be used in other contexts, eg. in puzzle games where you should move objects into the correct position.

In this kind of development, one typically relies on existing packages/environments. In the project we used Unity and existing AR packages, which generally worked well, and which allowed us to create apps both for iOS and Android. Games like these also need to work when connectivity is poor or non-existing. The GPS game relied on MapBox, and it turned out the prototype required both a working network connection as well as GPS. Unfortunately, we were unable to make it independent of connection quality within the limited time frame available. It is always a trade off between building from scratch (providing full control), and relying on code written by others (you get a lot for free, but can run into difficulties when problems occur).

Long term use remains a challenge. It is well known that players tend to lose interest in games after some time [7]. Design features recommended for engagement in AR games in general, such as outdoor and physical activities, teaming up, exploring formerly unknown environments, collection of in-game items, such as capturing Pokémon and competition and fights [8], may still be useful but need special consideration. In the presented games we relied mostly on the collection of in-game items, in combination with physical and potentially outdoor activities. Given the scarcity of exergames for our user group, further research and development on this point is important.

Acknowledgements. We wish to thank VINNOVA, Sweden's innovation agency, for funding the GameA project. We also want to thank all our testers, and we want to thank Braulio Gutiérrez and Victoria Sarria for graphic game design and Andreya Ek Frisk for music and sound design.

References

1. Verschuren, O., Peterson, M.D., Balemans, A.C.J., Hurvitz, E.A.: Exercise and physical activity recommendations for people with cerebral palsy. Dev. Med. Child Neurol. **58**, 798–808 (2016)

2. Vogtle, L.K., Malone, L.A., Azuero, A.: Outcomes of an exercise program for pain and fatigue management in adults with cerebral palsy. Disabil. Rehabil. **36**, 818–825 (2014)
3. Hernandez, H.A., Ye, Z., Graham, T.C.N., Fehlings, D., Switzer, L.: Designing action-based exergames for children with cerebral palsy. In: Proceedings of the SIGCHI Conference on Human Factors in Computing Systems, pp. 1261–1270. Association for Computing Machinery, New York (2013)
4. Wong, F.Y.: Influence of Pokémon go on physical activity levels of university players: a cross-sectional study. Int. J. Health Geogr. **16**, 8 (2017). https://doi.org/10.1186/s12942-017-0080-1
5. Yuan, B., Folmer, E., Harris, F.C.: Game accessibility: a survey. Univers. Access Inf. Soc. **10**, 81–100 (2011). https://doi.org/10.1007/s10209-010-0189-5
6. Magnusson, C., et al.: Designing motivating interactive balance and walking training for stroke survivors. ACM International Conference Proceeding Series, pp. 327–333 (2019)
7. Macvean, A., Robertson, J.: Understanding exergame users' physical activity, motivation and behavior over time. In: Proceedings of the SIGCHI Conference on Human Factors in Computing Systems, pp. 1251–1260. Association for Computing Machinery, New York (2013)
8. Söbke, H., Baalsrud Hauge, J., Stefan, I.: Long-term engagement in mobile location-based augmented reality games. In: Geroimenko, Vladimir (ed.) Augmented Reality Games I, pp. 129–147. Springer, Cham (2019). https://doi.org/10.1007/978-3-030-15616-9_9

Author Index

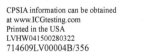